Advances in Liver Transplantation

Advances in Liver Transplantation

Editor: Dylan Long

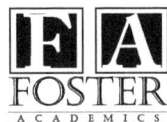

FA
FOSTER
ACADEMICS

www.fosteracademics.com

www.fosteracademics.com

FA Foster ACADEMICS

Cataloging-in-Publication Data

Advances in liver transplantation / edited by Dylan Long.
    p. cm.
Includes bibliographical references and index.
ISBN 978-1-63242-473-0
1. Liver--Transplantation. 2. Transplantation of organs, tissues, etc. I. Long, Dylan.
RD546 .A38 2017
617.556--dc23

© Foster Academics, 2017

Foster Academics,
118-35 Queens Blvd., Suite 400,
Forest Hills, NY 11375, USA

ISBN 978-1-63242-473-0 (Hardback)

Printed and bound in the United States of America.

Contents

Preface

This book traces the progress of the field of liver transplantation and highlights some of its key concepts and applications. The topics included in this book on the subject are of utmost significance and bound to provide incredible insights to readers. Liver transplantation refers to the surgical method of removing a disease infected liver and implanting a healthy liver in its place. The most common techniques used are liver-support therapy, liver dialysis, etc. The various advancements in liver transplantation are glanced at and their applications as well as ramifications are looked at in detail. It includes topics of utmost importance, which are bound to provide incredible insights to the readers. This book is a vital tool for all researching and studying this field.

Various studies have approached the subject by analyzing it with a single perspective, but the present book provides diverse methodologies and techniques to address this field. This book contains theories and applications needed for understanding the subject from different perspectives. The aim is to keep the readers informed about the progress in the field; therefore, the contributions were carefully examined to compile novel researches by specialists from across the globe.

Indeed, the job of the editor is the most crucial and challenging in compiling all chapters into a single book. In the end, I would extend my sincere thanks to the chapter authors for their profound work. I am also thankful for the support provided by my family and colleagues during the compilation of this book.

Editor

N-Acetylcysteine Attenuates Ischemia-Reperfusion-Induced Apoptosis and Autophagy in Mouse Liver via Regulation of the ROS/JNK/Bcl-2 Pathway

Chengfen Wang[9], Kan Chen[9], Yujing Xia, Weiqi Dai, Fan Wang, Miao Shen, Ping Cheng, Junshan Wang, Jie Lu, Yan Zhang, Jing Yang, Rong Zhu, Huawei Zhang, Jingjing Li, Yuanyuan Zheng, Yingqun Zhou*, Chuanyong Guo*

Department of Gastroenterology, Shanghai Tenth People's Hospital, Tongji University School of Medicine, Shanghai, China

Abstract

Background: Hepatic ischemia–reperfusion injury (HIRI) remains a pivotal clinical problem after hemorrhagic shock, transplantation, and some types of toxic hepatic injury. Apoptosis and autophagy play important roles in cell death during HIRI. It is also known that N-acetylcysteine (NAC) has significant pharmacologic effects on HIRI including elimination of reactive oxygen species (ROS) and attenuation of hepatic apoptosis. However, the effects of NAC on HIRI-induced autophagy have not been reported. In this study, we evaluated the effects of NAC on autophagy and apoptosis in HIRI, and explored the possible mechanism involved.

Methods: A mouse model of segmental (70%) hepatic warm ischemia was adopted to determine hepatic injury. NAC (150 mg/kg), a hepatoprotection agent, was administered before surgery. We hypothesized that the mechanism of NAC may involve the ROS/JNK/Bcl-2 pathway. We evaluated the expression of JNK, P-JNK, Bcl-2, Beclin 1 and LC3 by western blotting and immunohistochemical staining. Autophagosomes were evaluated by transmission electron microscopy (TEM).

Results: We found that ALT, AST and pathological changes were significantly improved in the NAC group. Western blotting analysis showed that the expression levels of Beclin 1 and LC3 were significantly decreased in NAC-treated mice. In addition, JNK, p-JNK, Bax, TNF-α, NF-κB, IL2, IL6 and levels were also decreased in NAC-treated mice.

Conclusion: NAC can prevent HIRI-induced autophagy and apoptosis by influencing the JNK signal pathway. The mechanism is likely to involve attenuation of JNK and p-JNK via scavenged ROS, an indirect increase in Bcl-2 level, and finally an alteration in the balance of Beclin 1 and Bcl-2.

Editor: Edward J. Lesnefsky, Virginia Commonwealth University, United States of America

Funding: This work was supported by the National Natural Science Foundation of China (Nos. +81101579 and 81270515), the Shanghai Science and Technology Innovation Plan of Action for international cooperation projects (No. 11430702400), the China Foundation for Hepatitis Prevention and Control WBN Liver Disease Research Fund (Nos. 20100021 and 20120005), and the Shanghai Health Bureau issues (Nos. 2011287 and 2012107). The funders had no role in study design, data collection and analysis, decision to publish, or preparation of the manuscript.

Competing Interests: The authors have declared that no competing interests exist.

* Email: yqzh02@163.com (YZ); guochuanyong@hotmail.com (CG)

9 These authors contributed equally to this work.

Introduction

Hepatic ischemia reperfusion injury (HIRI) was recognized as a main cause of pathological damage by Toledo-Pereyra et al. in 1975 during research on liver transplantation [1]. HIRI can be divided into warm ischemia reperfusion injury and cold-storage reperfusion injury [2,3]. The former is clinically relevant in liver surgery, hypovolemic shock, liver transplantation, some forms of toxic liver injury and Budd-Chiari syndrome [4]. The latter occurs during organ preservation before transplantation [5,6]. It is recognized that an excessive inflammatory response is an important mechanism of ischemia reperfusion injury [7]. The activation of Kupffer cells and neutrophils contribute to the formation of reactive oxygen [8,9,10]. There is still no explicit mechanism of HIRI, Therefore, the possible mechanism of HIRI and how to reduce ischemia reperfusion damage are important research issues. Thus, identification of an effective novel therapeutic is urgently required.

Ischemia-reperfusion injury is a complex pathophysiological process which involves Kupffer cell activation, the production of reactive oxygen species (ROS), the release of chemokines and cytokines, mitochondrial permeability transition, neutrophil recruitment and the pH paradox [11,12]. The main pathophysiological changes in HIRI are inflammatory cells infiltration, proinflammatory factors release and eventually hepatocyte death [13]. Two mechanisms are involved in the process of hepatocyte

Table 1.

Gene		Primer Sequence(5'→3')
Bax	Forward	AGACAGGGGCCTTTTTGCTAC
	Reverse	AATTCGCCGGAGACACTCG
Bcl-2	Forward	GCTACCGTCGTCGTGACTTCGC
	Reverse	CCCCACCGAACTCAAAGAAGG
Beclin 1	Forward	ATGGAGGGGTCTAAGGCGTC
	Reverse	TGGGCTGTGGTAAGTAATGGA
LC3	Forward	GACCGCTGTAAGGAGGTGC
	Reverse	AGAAGCCGAAGGTTTCTTGGG
NF-κB	Forward	ATGGCAGACGATGATCCCTAC
	Reverse	CGGATCGAAATCCCCTCTGTT
IL-6	Forward	CTGCAAGAGACTTCCATCCAG
	Reverse	AGTGGTATAGACAGGTCTGTTGG
TNF-α	Forward	CAGGCGGTGCCTATGTCTC
	Reverse	CGATCACCCCGAAGTTCAGTAG

death. One is necrosis, a type of non-programmed cell death, which is characterized by swelling of cells and organelles, membrane breakdown causing release of cell contents and activation of inflammatory factors. The other mechanism is apoptosis, named type I programmed cell death, which is characterized by cell shrinkage, DNA programmed degradation and chromatin condensation [14,15]. The mechanism of apoptosis initiation involves many stimuli including TNFα, Fas ligand and DNA damage. These stimuli lead to activation of the caspase family (cysteine-aspartate proteases) which can break cells into many small vesicles called apoptotic bodies [16,17]. The mitochondrial pathway is also involved in another mechanism of apoptosis, which is closely related to the Bcl-2 family. The Bcl-2 family includes both anti-apoptotic proteins such as Bcl-2 and Bcl-xL and pro-apoptotic proteins such as Bax, Bad and Bak [18,19]. In addition, apoptosis and necrosis are not completely independent, as they may share downstream pathways and signals. Thus, the phenomenon of necrapoptosis occurs in many pathophysiological conditions.

Autophagy is another important form of cell death, and is an intracellular degradation process where lysosomes degrade proteins, cellular organelles and invading microbes [20]. There are three different types of autophagy: macroautophagy, chaperone-mediated autophagy (CMA), and microautophagy [21]. At basal levels, autophagy contributes to cellular homeostasis. When nutrients are depleted and stresses occur in cells, autophagy can be further induced. Regulators of autophagy include the target of rapamycin (TOR), TOR kinase, 5'-AMP-activated protein kinase (AMPK), eukaryotic initiation factor 2α (eIF2α), inositol-trisphosphate (IP3) and c-Jun-N-terminal kinase [22,23]. Beclin 1, UVRAG, Vps34, Vps15 and Bif-1 play an important role in vesicle nucleation [24]. In addition, the anti-apoptotic proteins Bcl-2 and Bcl-xL bind to the pro-autophagy protein, leading to an inversely proportional relationship [25,26]. Light chain 3 (LC3) is a marker of autophagy, which contributes to the formation of autophagy vesicles during vesicle nucleation. LC3 and phosphatidylethanolamine (PE) conjugate and result in the formation of non-soluble LC3 (LC3 II). The presence of LC3 II allows autophagy to be detected by biochemical or microscopy techniques [27,28]. In brief, autophagy can promote cell survival

by digesting free fatty acids and misfolded proteins. However, auto-lysosomes may degrade cellular membrane lipids, which can activate enzymes and proinflammatory cytokines. Thus, autophagy is a double-edged sword in terms of cell survival. Autophagy plays a significant role in the liver which is a dynamic organ.

HIRI is a complex process involving necrosis, apoptosis, and autophagy. Preconditioning and pharmacologic interventions can increase the resistance of liver cells to HIRI. Therefore, an investigation of the possible mechanisms and novel treatment of HIRI is meaningful. In this study, the therapeutic effects and possible mechanisms of N-acetylcysteine (NAC) in an ischemia–reperfusion model were determined. NAC has been used as an antioxidant for the treatment of many clinical diseases such as doxorubicin-induced cardiotoxicity, acetaminophen (paracetamol) intoxication, bronchitis, heavy metal toxicity, and hepatic encephalopathy [29]. NAC is a source of glutathione (GSH) and sulfhydryl groups, and a scavenger of free radicals due to its interaction with ROS. NAC is known as an "antioxidant" in experimental models. It has been reported to prevent apoptosis and increase cell survival by activating the extracellular signal regulated kinase pathway [30]. Treatment of HIRI with NAC impedes NF-kappa B activity and ROS expression. How NAC affects the JNK signal pathway has not yet been fully elucidated.

Materials and Methods

2.1 Reagents

N-acetylcysteine (NAC) was purchased from Sigma-Aldrich (St. Louis, MO, USA). The following antibodies were used in this research: anti-TNF-α (0.1 ug/ml; Santa Cruz, CA, USA), anti-IL-6 and anti-IL-2 (both from Proteintech, CA, and USA), anti-Bax, anti-Bcl-2, anti-Beclin 1, anti-LC3, anti-JNK, anti-p-JNK, anti-NF-κB (all from Cell Signal Technology, USA). ROS Fluorescent Probe-DHE was purchased from Vigorous. (Beijing, China).

2.2 Animals

Male Balb/c mice (6-8 weeks old, 22 ± 2 g) were purchased from Shanghai SLAC Laboratory Animal Co. Ltd (Shanghai, China). They were fasted in plastic cages which were maintained at 26°Cand 55% humidity. The mice had free access to food and water. The study and the experimental design were approved by the Ethics Committee of Shanghai Tongji University.

2.3 Experimental design

The mice were randomly divided into three groups: group I (saline only) included 18 mice which were injected with saline via the tail vein before laparotomy without I/R, group II (IR model) included 18 mice which were injected with saline via the tail vein 1 h before they underwent segmental (70%) hepatic warm ischemia for 40 min, and group III (NAC + IR) which included 18 mice which were injected with NAC (dissolved in saline) via the tail vein 1 h before they underwent IR for 40 min. Six mice from each of the three groups were selected and were sacrificed 6 h, 12 h and 24 h after IR. At the end of the experiment, serum and liver tissue samples were obtained from each mouse and stored for further analysis.

2.4 Analysis of liver enzymes

Alanine aminotransferase (ALT) and aspartate aminotransferase (AST) levels in the collected serum were analyzed using an automated clinical analyzer (OLYMPUS AU1000; Olympus, Tokyo, Japan).

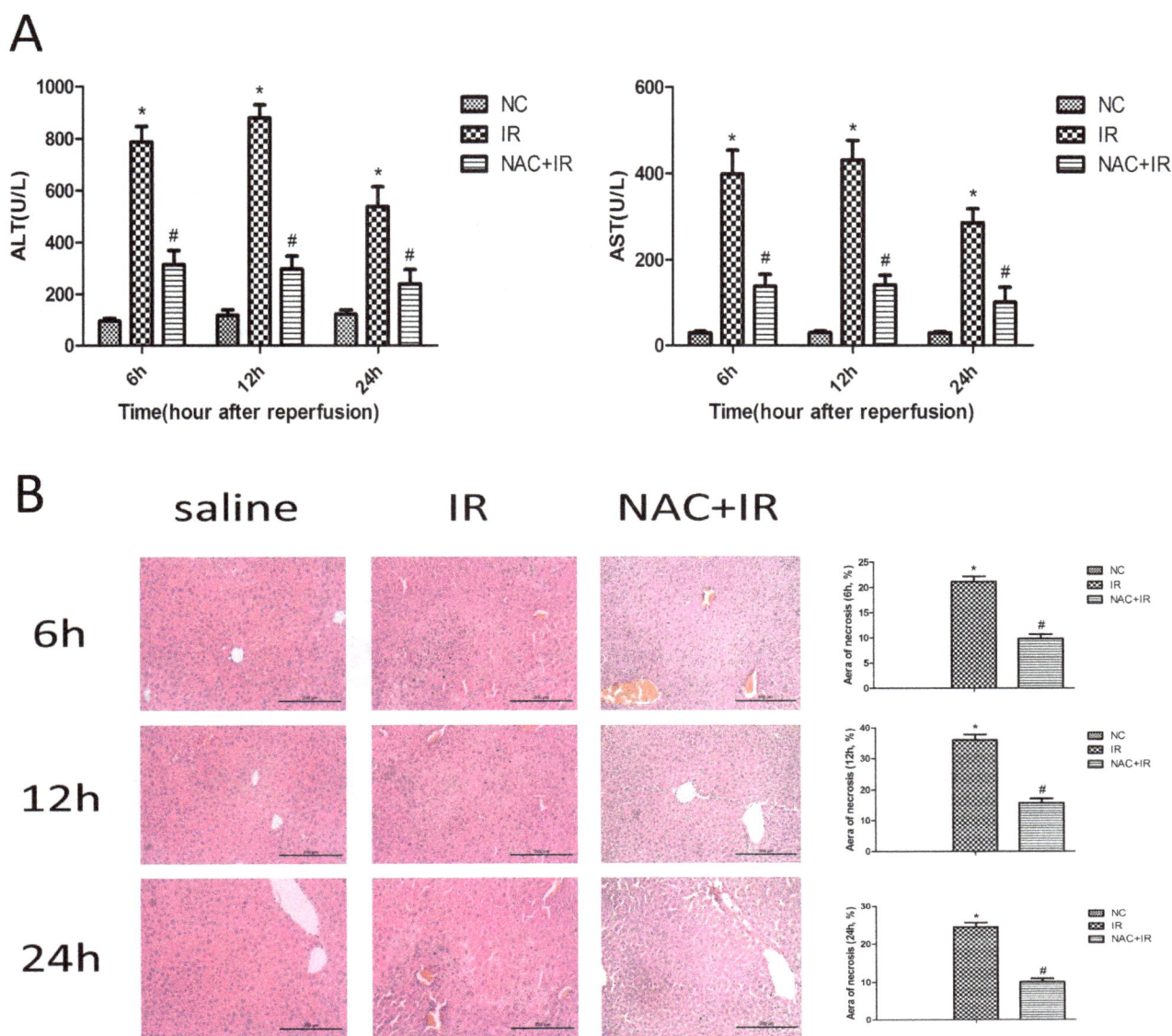

Figure 1. Effect of NAC on hepatic ischemia-reperfusion injury. The ischemia-reperfusion and sham-operated mice were pretreated with NAC (150 mg/kg) or saline. (A) Serum AST and ALT levels were measured at 6, 12 and 24 h after reperfusion of the three groups. Data represent means (SD) (n = 6 mice per time point per group). *p<0.05 for saline VS saline + IR, # p<0.05 for saline +IR VS IR + NAC (150 mg/kg). (B) Photomicrographs of representative livers collected 6, 12 and 24 h after reperfusion, stained with hematoxylin and eosin (H&E), ×200 magnification. The necrotic areas were analyzed with Image-pro Plus 6.0, indicating there existed statistical significant among different groups [n = 6, *p<0.05 for saline VS saline + IR, # p<0.05 for saline +IR VS IR + NAC (150 mg/kg)].

2.5 Histopathology

Mouse liver tissues (left lobe) were collected, stored in 4% paraformaldehyde and embedded in paraffin. Sections (5 μm thick) were stained with hematoxylin-eosin (H&E) and observed by light microscopy.

2.6 Immunohistochemical staining

The sections were heated at 67°C for 30 min and then dewaxed in dimethylbenzene. The sections were then dehydrated in a concentration gradient of alcohol and pretreated with microwave heat-induced epitope retrieval. These sections were incubated with antibodies against Bcl-2, Bax, Beclin 1, LC3, JNK and p-JNK at 1:100 dilution for 24 h at 4°C and then with a secondary antibody at 1:50 dilution for 1 h at 28°C. All the antibodies were diluted

with Tris-buffered saline (TBS), and 2% bovine serum albumin (BSA). Finally, the sections were stained by diaminobenzidine (DAB) and then observed using a digital camera (Olympus) combined with a light microscope at ×200 magnification.

2.7 Western blotting analysis

Proteins were extracted from the liver tissues by grinding with protease inhibitors and stored at -80°C. The proteins were incubated in boiling water for 10 min before the experiment. The protein samples were separated by 12.5% sodium dodecyl sulfate polyacrylamide gel electrophoresis (SDS-PAGE) and transferred onto a Polyvinylidene Fluoride (PVDF) membrane. The membranes were incubated with 5% nonfat milk for 1 h, and then incubated with antibodies against TNF-α, IL-6, IL-2, Bax, Bcl-2,

A

B

C

D

(×200 magnification). (D) Morphology of autophagosomes in hepatocytes at 12 h detected by electron microscopy (×20000 magnification). Initial autophagic vacuole (AVi) containing a mitochondrion, endoplasmic reticulum membranes, and ribosomes (arrowheads). Degradative autophagic vacuole (AVd) is found to have degradation of contents (arrowheads).

cytoplasm, and the structure of the mitochondria still had integrity (Figure 3D).

3.4 NAC inhibited the JNK signal pathway in hepatic ischemia-reperfusion injury

Previous studies proved that JNK is an important regulator of cell death including apoptosis and autophagy. To determine whether JNK signaling pathway is involved in hepatic ischemia-reperfusion induced cell death, we detected the phosphorylation of JNK in protein level in three groups respectively by western blotting (F 4A). As shown in Fig 4A, HIRI increased the activation of JNK phosphorylation. In the IR group, there was obvious up-regulation of p-JNK compared with the control group and NAC + IR group ($P<0.005$) in protein levels. And this result is concordant with the changes measured by immunohistochemistry (Fig 4A). These results suggest that NAC protects the liver from HIRI through inhibition of the p-JNK signaling pathway.

3.5 NAC attenuated cytokines and intracellular ROS generation induced by ischemia–reperfusion

Ischemia–reperfusion injury primarily occurs in hypoxic organs. The imbalance between pro- and antioxidants in the hypoxic organ leads to oxidative stress. Oxidative stress can increase the release of cytokines by activating inflammatory cells. Further activated neutrophils can generate ROS. To explore the effect of NAC attenuation on cytokines and ROS, we detected cytokines (TNF-a, IL-2, IL-6, and NF-κB) both at the cDNA and protein levels. As shown in Figure 4B, there was significantly increased expression of cytokines in the IR group compared with the NAC pretreatment group. There was also a decrease in cytokine expression in the control group. We also measured ROS generation by a ROS Fluorescent Probe-DHE in mice hepatic tissues. The proportion of ROS and normal areas were measured. Statistical analysis in three random visual fields was performed using Image-Pro plus version 6.0 software. As shown in Figure 4C, significantly increased ROS generation was observed in the IR group, compared with the control group. The level of ROS was significantly decreased in the NAC + IR group (p<0.005). Thus, pretreatment with NAC attenuated ischemia–reperfusion-induced ROS generation, cytokines release, and ROS generation.

Discussion

Hepatic ischemia–reperfusion injury remains a significant clinical problem following transplantation. HIRI is a phenomenon which depends on cellular damage in a hypoxic organ, and destroys the restoration of oxygen exchange [2]. Hypoxia increases reactive oxygen species (ROS) in injured cells. ROS then causes apoptosis and autophagy [31,32]. However, the exact mechanism involved in hepatic ischemia–reperfusion injury has not yet been fully described. We demonstrated that HIRI involves histopathologic changes, an increase of cytokines, as well as apoptotic cells, autophagosomes, and activation of the pro-apoptotic Bcl-2 family and the JNK pathway. Moreover, ischemia–reperfusion triggers cellular ROS [33]. The protective effect of NAC may involve the JNK pathway, as we observed significant changes in phosphorylation levels of JNK between the IR and NAC + IR groups.

NAC is a thiol and major precursor of L-cysteine [30]. NAC has been used in clinical practice for several years to treat clinical disorders such as stable angina pectoris, ischemia-reperfusion cardiac injury, doxorubicin-induced cardiotoxicity, acute respiratory distress syndrome and radio-contrast-induced nephropathy [34]. NAC has significant pharmacological effects on oxidative injury and is known as a source of sulfhydryl groups and a scavenger of free radicals [27]. It was demonstrated that NAC may protect cells through other mechanisms besides scavenging radicals. Our research showed that NAC protected against HIRI by attenuating hepatic apoptosis and autophagy. NAC decreased the levels of liver enzymes and attenuated histopathologic changes such as cellular swelling and cellular necrosis. Compared with the IR group, TUNEL-positive cells in the NAC + IR group were obviously reduced. This indicated that NAC can attenuate apoptosis caused by ischemia-reperfusion injury. It is thought that the Bcl-2 family plays a key role in the process of apoptosis. This family includes anti-apoptotic proteins such as Bcl-2 and Bcl-xL and pro-apoptotic proteins such as Bax and Bak [18,19]. In this study, we observed a clear decrease in Bcl-2 and an increase in Bax in the IR group compared with the NAC + IR and control groups. We suggest that NAC decreases apoptosis by stabilizing the balance between Bcl-2 and Bax. In addition, IR activated the JNK pathway, as shown by a significant increase in the levels of phosphor-JNK. The results of our study indicate that the possible mechanism of apoptosis and autophagy inhibition by NAC may involve the JNK pathway.

Apoptotic and autophagic cell death are the two main forms of hepatic ischemia-reperfusion-induced cell death [35]. Autophagy also plays a key role in the hepatic pathophysiological disorders caused by liver ischemia-reperfusion injury. NAC may be a potential treatment option for HIRI. During our evaluation of the effects of NAC on autophagy in HIRI, we detected the expression of Beclin 1 and LC3II. The levels of Beclin 1 and LC3II in group III (NAC + IR) were significantly decreased. Compared to group III (NAC+ IR) and group I (model control), the levels of Beclin1 and LC3II in group II (IR) were significantly increased. These results indicate that NAC can improve HIRI-induced autophagy and liver injury, which suggests that inhibition of autophagy may be a new pathway in NAC therapy for improving liver injury. It has been reported that ROS through the JNK pathway regulates cell death [36,37]. This pathway may be involved in many cellular events related to cell death including apoptosis and autophagy. In the present study, NAC partly attenuated apoptosis by Bcl-xL and Bcl-2, which act as important downstream factors of the JNK pathway [25]. In addition, ROS activate the JNK pathway, as shown by the increased levels of phosphorylated JNK. The findings in this study suggest that NAC may first reduce the levels of JNK and phosphorylated JNK through ROS scavenging, then causing Bcl-2 to increase. The effects of the latter interfere with Beclin 1 during the process of autophagy. The conclusion of our present research that inhibiting autophagy alleviated hepatic damage in ischemia-reperfusion induced liver injury models is in consistent with our previous studies [38,39]. Therefore, we suggest that suppression of autophagy may be a potential therapeutic method in ischemia-reperfusion liver injury.

These findings demonstrated that NAC ameliorated apoptosis and autophagy which occurred during hepatic ischemia-reperfusion. These results indicate that the ROS/JNK/Bcl-2/Beclin 1 pathway may act as an intersection between apoptosis and autophagy. Recently, many studies have indicated that JNK is a

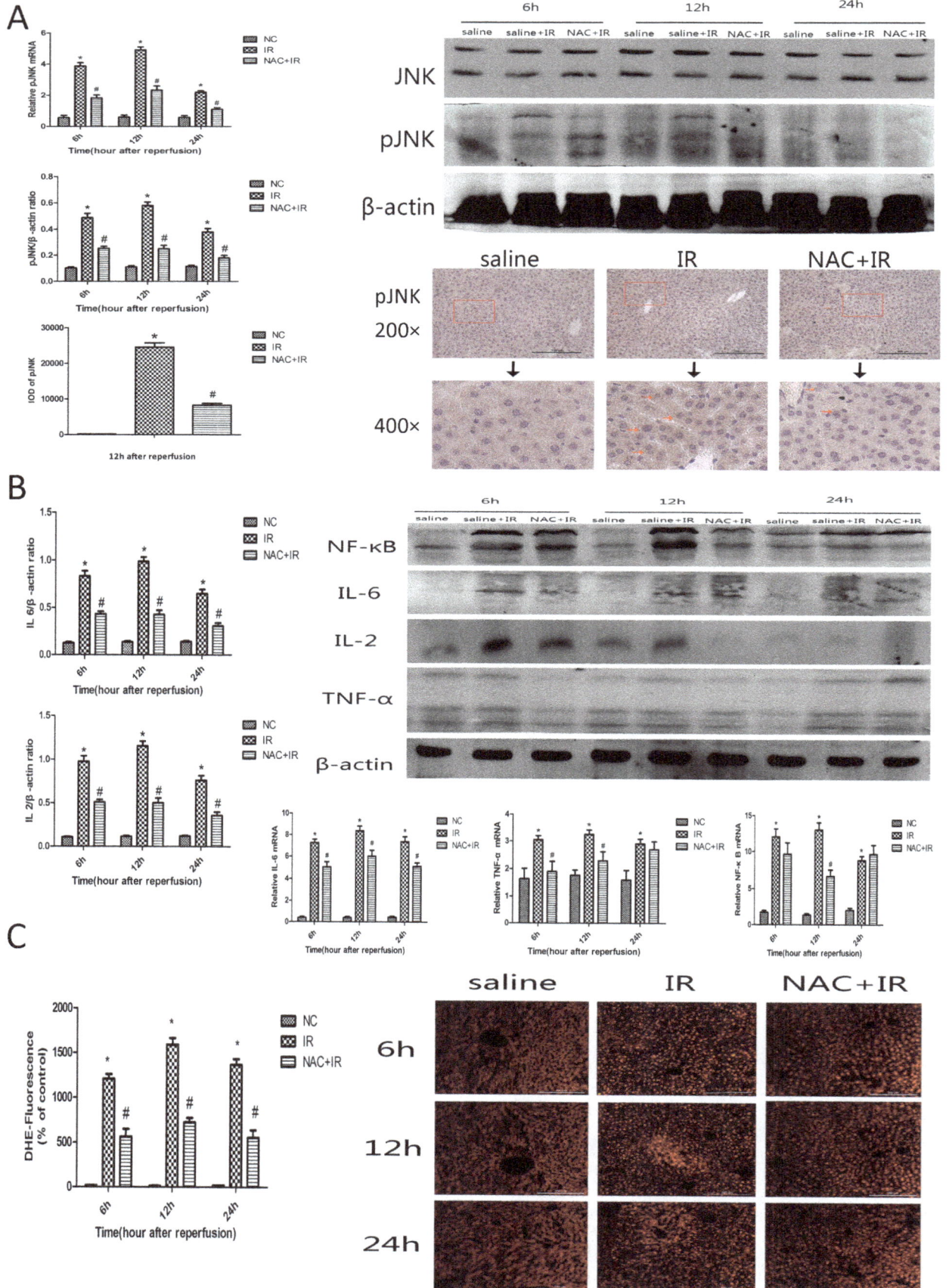

Figure 4. Effect of NAC on regulation of JNK pathway, cytokines release and ROS generation. (A) The expression of p-JNK and JNK on protein level was detected by western blot. The result of western blot were analyzed with quantity one [n = 3, *p<0.05 for saline VS saline + IR, # p< 0.05 for saline +IR VS IR + NAC (150 mg/kg)]. The expression of p-JNK in hepatic tissue of different groups were shown by immunohistochemistry at 12 h (×200 magnification). The IOD of p-JNK in cytoplasm was analyzed by Image-Pro Plus 6.0. Date are showed as mean± SD [n = 3, *p<0.05 for saline VS saline + IR, # p<0.05 for saline +IR VS IR + NAC (150 mg/kg)]. The representative positive cells were indicated with red arrows. (B) The expression of NF-κB, IL-6, TNF-αon cDNA level were detected by real time PCR. *p<0.05 for saline VS saline + IR, # p<0.05 for saline +IR VS IR + NAC (150 mg/kg). And the expression of NF-κB, IL-6, TNF-α on protein level was detected by western blot. The result of the western blot were analyzed with quantity one [n = 3, *p<0.05 for saline VS saline + IR, # p<0.05 for saline +IR VS IR + NAC (150 mg/kg)]. (C) The generation of ROS was detected with ROS Fluorescent Probe-DHE. And ROS were measured and statistical analysis in three random vision fields by Image-Pro plus 6.0.

mediator of autophagy, and demonstrated that JNK contributes to autophagic cell death via phosphorylation of Bcl-2 [40,41]. Phosphorylation of Bcl-2 can lead to Bcl-2 separating from Beclin 1, thereby alleviating the inhibitory effect on Beclin 1 [42,43]. Hence, activation of JNK can alter the balance between Bcl-2 and Beclin 1. This may be the mechanism of action of JNK in the regulation of autophagy.

In conclusion, we demonstrated that ischemia–reperfusion-induced apoptosis and autophagy occurs through activation of the JNK/Bcl-2 pathway. Hepatic protection by NAC is mediated by ROS scavenging and targeting of the JNK pathway via the JNK/Bcl-2 pathway. Numerous studies have suggested that there may be a common signal pathway between autophagy and apoptosis,

and together with our findings, this indicates that the ROS/JNK/Bcl-2 pathway may play a key role in the cross-talk between autophagy and apoptosis. Finally, these results provide insight into the mechanism of HIRI and propose a potential clinical treatment for NAC in HIRI.

Author Contributions

Conceived and designed the experiments: CG Y. Zhou. Performed the experiments: CW KC YX WD FW MS PC. Analyzed the data: CW KC JW J. Lu Y. Zhang JY RZ HZ. Contributed reagents/materials/analysis tools: PC JW J. Lu Y. Zhang JY RZ HZ J. Li Y. Zheng. Wrote the paper: CW.

References

1. Toledo-Pereyra LH, Simmons RL, Najarian JS (1975) Protection of the ischemic liver by donor pretreatment before transplantation. Am J Surg 129: 513–517.
2. Teoh NC, Farrell GC (2003) Hepatic ischemia reperfusion injury: pathogenic mechanisms and basis for hepatoprotection. J Gastroenterol Hepatol 18: 891–902.
3. Teoh NC (2011) Hepatic ischemia reperfusion injury: Contemporary perspectives on pathogenic mechanisms and basis for hepatoprotection-the good, bad and deadly. J Gastroenterol Hepatol 26 Suppl 1: 180–187.
4. Jaeschke H, Lemasters JJ (2003) Apoptosis versus oncotic necrosis in hepatic ischemia/reperfusion injury. Gastroenterology 125: 1246–1257.
5. Theodoraki K, Tympa A, Karmaniolou I, Tsaroucha A, Arkadopoulos N, et al. (2011) Ischemia/reperfusion injury in liver resection: a review of preconditioning methods. Surg Today 41: 620–629.
6. Abu-Amara M, Yang SY, Tapuria N, Fuller B, Davidson B, et al. (2010) Liver ischemia/reperfusion injury: processes in inflammatory networks–a review. Liver Transpl 16: 1016–1032.
7. Zhang S, He XS (2003) [The molecular mechanism of warm ischemia-reperfusion injury in liver graft]. Zhonghua Gan Zang Bing Za Zhi 11: 767–768.
8. Shiratori Y, Ohmura K, Hikiba Y, Matsumura M, Nagura T, et al. (1998) Hepatocyte nitric oxide production is induced by Kupffer cells. Dig Dis Sci 43: 1737–1745.
9. Rizzardini M, Zappone M, Villa P, Gnocchi P, Sironi M, et al. (1998) Kupffer cell depletion partially prevents hepatic heme oxygenase 1 messenger RNA accumulation in systemic inflammation in mice: role of interleukin 1beta. Hepatology 27: 703–710.
10. Jaeschke H, Farhood A (1991) Neutrophil and Kupffer cell-induced oxidant stress and ischemia-reperfusion injury in rat liver. Am J Physiol 260: G355–G362.
11. Currin RT, Gores GJ, Thurman RG, Lemasters JJ (1991) Protection by acidotic pH against anoxic cell killing in perfused rat liver: evidence for a pH paradox. FASEB J 5: 207–210.
12. Gores GJ, Nieminen AL, Wray BE, Herman B, Lemasters JJ (1989) Intracellular pH during "chemical hypoxia" in cultured rat hepatocytes. Protection by intracellular acidosis against the onset of cell death. J Clin Invest 83: 386–396.
13. Wanner GA, Ertel W, Muller P, Hofer Y, Leiderer R, et al. (1996) Liver ischemia and reperfusion induces a systemic inflammatory response through Kupffer cell activation. Shock 5: 34–40.
14. Georgiev P, Dahm F, Graf R, Clavien PA (2006) Blocking the path to death: anti-apoptotic molecules in ischemia/reperfusion injury of the liver. Curr Pharm Des 12: 2911–2921.
15. Weigand K, Brost S, Steinebrunner N, Buchler M, Schemmer P, et al. (2012) Ischemia/Reperfusion injury in liver surgery and transplantation: pathophysiology. HPB Surg 2012: 176723.
16. Ozaki M, Haga S, Ozawa T (2012) In vivo monitoring of liver damage using caspase-3 probe. Theranostics 2: 207–214.
17. Kim SJ, Eum HA, Billiar TR, Lee SM (2013) Role of heme oxygenase 1 in TNF/TNF receptor-mediated apoptosis after hepatic ischemia/reperfusion in rats. Shock 39: 380–388.
18. Lin HC, Lai IR (2013) Isolated mitochondria infusion mitigates ischemia-reperfusion injury of the liver in rats: reply. Shock 39: 543.

19. Neuman MG (2001) Apoptosis in diseases of the liver. Crit Rev Clin Lab Sci 38: 109–166.
20. Tsujimoto Y, Shimizu S (2005) Another way to die: autophagic programmed cell death. Cell Death Differ 12 Suppl 2: 1528–1534.
21. Choi AM, Ryter SW, Levine B (2013) Autophagy in human health and disease. N Engl J Med 368: 1845–1846.
22. Sakoda H, Ogihara T, Anai M, Fujishiro M, Ono H, et al. (2002) Activation of AMPK is essential for AICAR-induced glucose uptake by skeletal muscle but not adipocytes. Am J Physiol Endocrinol Metab 282: E1239–E1244.
23. Matsui Y, Takagi H, Qu X, Abdellatif M, Sakoda H, et al. (2007) Distinct roles of autophagy in the heart during ischemia and reperfusion: roles of AMP-activated protein kinase and Beclin 1 in mediating autophagy. Circ Res 100: 914–922.
24. Kihara A, Kabeya Y, Ohsumi Y, Yoshimori T (2001) Beclin-phosphatidylinositol 3-kinase complex functions at the trans-Golgi network. EMBO Rep 2: 330–335.
25. Maundrell K, Antonsson B, Magnenat E, Camps M, Muda M, et al. (1997) Bcl-2 undergoes phosphorylation by c-Jun N-terminal kinase/stress-activated protein kinases in the presence of the constitutively active GTP-binding protein Rac1. J Biol Chem 272: 25238–25242.
26. Shen M, Chen K, Lu J, Cheng P, Xu L, et al. (2014) Protective effect of astaxanthin on liver fibrosis through modulation of TGF-beta1 expression and autophagy. Mediators Inflamm 2014: 954502.
27. Eskelinen EL, Deretic V, Neufeld T, Levine B, Cuervo AM (2007) 4th International Symposium on Autophagy: exploiting the frontiers of autophagy research. Autophagy 3: 166–173.
28. Zhou Y, Dai W, Lin C, Wang F, He L, et al. (2013) Protective effects of necrostatin-1 against concanavalin A-induced acute hepatic injury in mice. Mediators Inflamm 2013: 706156.
29. Gillissen A, Nowak D (1998) Characterization of N-acetylcysteine and ambroxol in anti-oxidant therapy. Respir Med 92: 609–623.
30. Zafarullah M, Li WQ, Sylvester J, Ahmad M (2003) Molecular mechanisms of N-acetylcysteine actions. Cell Mol Life Sci 60: 6–20.
31. Samarasinghe DA, Tapner M, Farrell GC (2000) Role of oxidative stress in hypoxia-reoxygenation injury to cultured rat hepatic sinusoidal endothelial cells. Hepatology 31: 160–165.
32. Ohshima H, Pignatelli B, Li CQ, B5aflast S, Gilibert I, et al. (2002) Analysis of oxidized and nitrated proteins in plasma and tissues as biomarkers for exposure to reactive oxygen and nitrogen species. IARC Sci Publ 156: 393–394.
33. McCord JM (1985) Oxygen-derived free radicals in postischemic tissue injury. N Engl J Med 312: 159–163.
34. Kelly GS (1998) Clinical applications of N-acetylcysteine. Altern Med Rev 3: 114–127.
35. Thorburn A (2008) Apoptosis and autophagy: regulatory connections between two supposedly different processes. Apoptosis 13: 1–9.
36. Dhanasekaran DN, Reddy EP (2008) JNK signaling in apoptosis. Oncogene 27: 6245–6251.
37. Verma G, Datta M (2012) The critical role of JNK in the ER-mitochondrial crosstalk during apoptotic cell death. J Cell Physiol 227: 1791–1795.

38. Shen M, Lu J, Dai W, Wang F, Xu L, et al. (2013) Ethyl pyruvate ameliorates hepatic ischemia-reperfusion injury by inhibiting intrinsic pathway of apoptosis and autophagy. Mediators Inflamm 2013: 461536.

39. Cheng P, Wang F, Chen K, Shen M, Dai W, et al. (2014) Hydrogen sulfide ameliorates ischemia/reperfusion-induced hepatitis by inhibiting apoptosis and autophagy pathways. Mediators Inflamm 2014: 935251.

40. Li C, Xing G, Dong M, Zhou L, Li J, et al. (2010) Beta-asarone protection against beta-amyloid-induced neurotoxicity in PC12 cells via JNK signaling and modulation of Bcl-2 family proteins. Eur J Pharmacol 635: 96–102.

41. Liu L, Fang YQ, Xue ZF, He YP, Fang RM, et al. (2012) Beta-asarone attenuates ischemia-reperfusion-induced autophagy in rat brains via modulating JNK, p-JNK, Bcl-2 and Beclin 1. Eur J Pharmacol 680: 34–40.

42. Pattingre S, Tassa A, Qu X, Garuti R, Liang XH, et al. (2005) Bcl-2 antiapoptotic proteins inhibit Beclin 1-dependent autophagy. Cell 122: 927–939.

43. Mizushima N (2004) Methods for monitoring autophagy. Int J Biochem Cell Biol 36: 2491–2502.

2

Transplantation of ATP7B–Transduced Bone Marrow Mesenchymal Stem Cells Decreases Copper Overload in Rats

Shenglin Chen[1]◖, Cunhua Shao[2]◖, Tianfu Dong[3,4], Hao Chai[3,4], Xinkui Xiong[3,4], Daoyi Sun[3,4], Long Zhang[3,4], Yue Yu[3,4], Ping Wang[3,4]∗, Feng Cheng[3,4]∗

1 Department of Hepatobiliary Surgery Ward of General Surgery, The Affiliated Wuhu No. 2 People's Hospital of Wannan Medical College, Wuhu, Anhui Province, China, 2 Department of Hepatobiliary Surgery, Dongying People's Hospital, Dongying, Shandong Province, China, 3 Liver Transplantation Center, First Affiliated Hospital of Nanjing Medical University, Nanjing, Jiangsu Province, China, 4 Key Laboratory of Living Donor Liver Transplantation, Ministry of Public Health, Nanjing, Jiangsu Province, China

Abstract

Background: Recent studies have demonstrated that transplantation of ATP7B-transduced hepatocytes ameliorates disease progression in LEC (Long-Evans Cinnamon) rats, a model of Wilson's disease (WD). However, the inability of transplanted cells to proliferate in a normal liver hampers long-term treatment. In the current study, we investigated whether transplantation of ATP7B-transduced bone marrow mesenchymal stem cells (BM-MSCs) could decrease copper overload in LEC rats.

Materials and Methods: The livers of LEC rats were preconditioned with radiation (RT) and/or ischemia-reperfusion (IRP) before portal vein infusion of ATP7B-transduced MSCs (MSCs^{ATP7B}). The volumes of MSCs^{ATP7B} or saline injected as controls were identical. The expression of ATP7B was analyzed by real-time quantitative polymerase chain reaction (RT-PCR) at 4, 12 and 24 weeks post-transplantation. MSC^{ATP7B} repopulation, liver copper concentrations, serum ceruloplasmin levels, and alanine transaminase (ALT) and aspartate transaminase (AST) levels were also analyzed at each time-point post-transplantation.

Results: IRP-plus-RT preconditioning was the most effective strategy for enhancing the engraftment and repopulation of transplanted MSCs^{ATP7B}. This strategy resulted in higher ATP7B expression and serum ceruloplasmin, and lower copper concentration in this doubly preconditioned group compared with the saline control group, the IRP group, and the RT group at all three time-points post-transplantation ($p<0.05$ for all). Moreover, 24 weeks post-transplantation, the levels of ALT and AST in the IRP group, the RT group, and the IRP-plus-RT group were all significantly decreased compared to those of the saline group ($p<0.05$ compared with the IRP group and RT group, $p<0.01$ compared with IRP-plus-RT group); ALT and AST levels were significantly lower in the IRP-plus-RT group compared to either the IRP group or the RT group ($p<0.01$ and $p<0.05$. respectively).

Conclusions: These results demonstrate that transplantation of MSCs^{ATP7B} into IRP-plus-RT preconditioned LEC rats decreased copper overload and was associated with an increase in MSC engraftment and repopulation.

Editor: Yiru Guo, University of Louisville, United States of America

Funding: This study was financially supported, in part, by the National Natural Science Foundation of China (Grant No. 81070324), the Research Foundation of the Department of Health of Jiangsu Province (Grant No. 200906, H201102) and "Summit of the Six Top Talents" Program of Jiangsu Province (Grant No. 2009). All fundings mentioned above were received by Feng Cheng. The funders had no role in study design, data collection and analysis, decision to publish, or preparation of the manuscript.

Competing Interests: The authors have declared that no competing interests exist.

* Email: wuwpzhy@163.com (PW); docchengfeng@njmu.edu.cn (FC)

◖ These authors contributed equally to this work.

Introduction

Wilson's disease (WD), also known as hepatolenticular degeneration, is an autosomal recessive inherited disease that is caused by a mutation in the ATP7B gene and is characterized by impaired biliary copper excretion and lack of ceruloplasmin synthesis [1]. This leads to copper accumulation in the liver, brain, kidney, and other organs [2]. Because WD is a monogenic hereditary disease, gene therapy could potentially reverse the defect. Many genetic diseases could theoretically be cured by transplantation of normal cells. However, in order to have a beneficial clinical impact, transplanted cells must effectively engraft in the host, and maintain their proliferative capacity. To this point in time, the most effective treatment to correct copper metabolism and prevent the progression of WD has been orthotopic liver transplantation [3,4]. However, shortage of quality donor organs, low hepatocyte viability (only 30% of hepatocytes survive transplantation) and post-transplantation complications have hampered more widespread use of this clinical therapy [4–6]. Therefore, cell-based therapy is emerging as a potential tool in regenerative medicine [7]. This is the case because of the ease of retroviral vector–mediated integration of exogenous genes into chromosomes of target cells, with the outcome of long-term gene expression. However, retroviral vectors cannot efficiently transfect non-dividing cells. In contrast, lentiviral vectors can transfect both dividing cells as well as non-dividing cells such as hepatocytes. In addition, they can accommodate large inserts—up to 10 kb—and the inserted fragments integrate into target-cell chromosomes. The lentiviral vectors are composed of 3 basic genetic structures: gag, pol, and env genes, four auxiliary genes—vif, vpr, nef, and vpu and two regulatory genes—tat and rev [8]. Because of the presence of a transcription promoter, more efficient, long-term gene expression, and lower level of induced immune response, lentiviral vectors are superior to both retroviral and adenoviral vectors [9–11].

Bone marrow mesenchymal stem cells (BM-MSCs) are a type of adult stem cell. They have attracted much attention due to their high capacity for self-renewal, multipotent differentiation potential, ready availability, and low occurrence of adverse reactions post-transplantation. They are being studied for a variety of clinical applications [12]. Studies have found that BM-MSCs can differentiation into osteoblasts [13], chondrocytes [14], adipocytes [15], neurons [16], cardiomyocytes [17], and hepatocytes [18]. When co-cultured with hepatocytes, they promoted growth of the hepatocytes. When transplanted into liver, they likewise promoted the growth of hepatocytes in vivo, and accelerated restoration of function in damaged livers [19]. Studies have also shown that BM-MSCs migrate to a damaged liver and promote liver regeneration [20]. More importantly, because of the ease of transfection of BM-MSCs with exogenous genes, they can be used as vectors of these exogenous genes [21]. A number of studies have shown the therapeutic effects of BM-MSCs in animal models of acute liver failure and liver fibrosis. However, there have been few such studies in congenital hepatic metabolic diseases [22].

LEC (Long-Evans Cinnamon) rats have a deletion mutation of 900 bp in the 3′-terminal region of Atp7b, the rat homologue of the human WD gene, ATP7B [23,24]. This deletion leads to hepatic copper accumulation in the LEC rat [25]. Therefore, the LEC rat provides an excellent animal model for human copper overload [26]. The aim of the present study was to transfect the ATP7B gene into BM-MSCs, and determine the effects of transplantation of those cells on copper overload in LEC rats preconditioned by ischemia-reperfusion (IRP) and/or radiation (RT).

Materials and Methods

Animal Care

LEC rats were kindly provided by S. Gupta (Albert Einstein University College of Medicine, NY, USA). All animals used in this study were bred and maintained in individually ventilated cages in the animal facilities at Nanjing Medical University under controlled temperature ($23 \pm 2°C$) and humidity ($55 \pm 10\%$) under 12 hour light/12 hour dark cycle, with tap water and food available ad libitum. The experimental protocol was approved by Nanjing Medical University/Institutional Animal Care and Use Committee (NJMU/IACUC). Ninety healthy two month old LEC rats were used in this research, they were randomly divided into 5

groups:, group a were injected with saline, group b were injected with MSCs^{ATP7B}, groups c, d and e had livers preconditioned with ischemia-reperfusion (IRP), radiation (RT) and ischemia-reperfusion plus radiation (IRP-plus-RT), respectively before injection with MSCs^{ATP7B}.

Isolation of BM-MSCs

BM-MSCs were isolated from healthy 3–4 week old LEC rats using a previously described protocol [27]. The rats were sacrificed, soaked in 75% ethanol for 5 min, with subsequent isolation of femurs and tibias under sterile conditions. Samples were placed in phosphate buffered saline (PBS) containing 100 U/mL penicillin, and 100 µg/mL streptomycin (GIBCO, Grand Island, NY, USA). The ends of the diaphyses were removed, and the bone marrow cavity flushed with PBS. The cell suspension was filtered through nylon mesh and centrifuged at 300×g for 5 min at room temperature. The obtained cells were resuspended in SD rat mesenchymal stem cell growth medium (Cyagen Biosciences, Guangzhou, China) and cultured in 25 cm^2 plastic culture flasks (Corning Incorporated, Corning, NY, USA) at 37°C under 5% CO_2. Fourth-to-eighth passage BM-MSCs were used in this study.

Immunophenotyping of BM-MSCs

Flow cytometric analysis of the surface markers of BM-MSCs were performed on a BD FACS Calibur flow cytometer (BD Biosciences, San Jose, CA, USA) by a method described in our previous work [27]. The fifth passage of BM-MSCs were harvested and re-suspended in 0.1 mL PBS. The cell suspensions were incubated with the following antibodies for 15 min at 4°C: anti-rat CD29 conjugated with phycoerthrin (PE), anti-rat CD90 conjugated with PE, anti-rat CD45 conjugated with fluorescein isothiocyanate (FITC), anti-rat CD11b/c conjugated with PerCP-eFluor710 (eBioscience, San Diego, CA, USA). PE-conjugated mouse IgG2a, PE-conjugated Armenian Hamster IgG, FITC-conjugated mouse IgG1, and PerCP-e710 mouse IgG2a were used as an isotype-matched control.

Lentiviral vectors

All plasmids used in this study were kindly provided by Professor Duanqing Pei, Drug Discovery Pipeline Group, Guangzhou Institutes of Biomedicine and Health, Chinese Academy of Sciences. In order to produce ATP7B lentiviral particles, HEK293T cells were co-transfected with pRRL.PPT.SF.ATP7B.i2GFPBsd.pre and two packaging plasmids, psPAX2 and pMD2.G through calcium phosphate-mediated transient transfection, as previously described [28]. HEK293T cells were also co-transfected with pRRL.PPT.SF.i2GFPpre and the two packaging plasmids mentioned above as negative controls. Viral supernatants were harvested 48 hours post-transfection.

Transduction of BM-MSCs in Cell Culture

Fourth-or-fifth passage BM-MSCs were used for transduction. BM-MSCs 70–80% confluent, were digested with trypsin, and then seeded into six-well plates at a density of $2–3 \times 10^5$ cells/well. Twenty-four hours after subculture, the medium was discarded, cells were gently rinsed with PBS and treated with 1 mL viral supernatants and 8 µg/mL polybrene per well for 4 h. Subsequently, 1 mL conventional BM-MSC culture medium (SD rat mesenchymal stem cell growth medium) was added per well. Twenty-four hours after transduction, the medium was changed to conventional medium. Forty-eight hours after transduction, subcultured MSCs^{ATP7B} were passaged at a split ratio of 1:3. Second-or-third passage MSCs^{ATP7B} were harvested for transplantation. For additional cell culture studies, total protein was extracted from MSCs^{ATP7B} five days after transduction for analysis of ATP7B levels by Western Blot. Protein extracted from BM-MSCs transduced with pRRL.PPT.SF.i2GFPpre was used as negative control.

Preconditioning

To determine which preconditioning was optimal for stimulating proliferation of transplanted cells, LEC rat livers underwent ischemia-reperfusion (IRP) and/or radiation (RT) prior to cell transplantation. For the RT procedure, LEC rats were anesthetized with 10% chloral hydrate (3 mL/kg body weight) by intraperitoneal injection. Four days before transplantation, the whole liver received a single dose of 50 Gy at a dose rate of 320 cGy/min using a RS-2000 x-ray Biological Irradiator (Rad Source Technologies, Inc., Suwanee, GA, USA) as described previously [29]. For IRP, the left portal vein branch was isolated and occluded with a hemostatic clip for 45 min as described previously [30]. Immediately after release of the clip, MSCs^{ATP7B} were injected into the liver via the portal vein.

Cell Transplantation

Ninety-two-month old LEC rats were divided into 5 groups of 18 animals each: a) saline; b) MSCs^{ATP7B}; c) IRP + MSCs^{ATP7B} (IRP group); d) RT + MSCs^{ATP7B} (RT group); e) IRP + RT + MSCs^{ATP7B} (IRP-plus-RT group). Before transplantation, 2×10^7 MSCs^{ATP7B} were resuspended in 0.5 mL PBS (cell viability was assessed by trypan blue dye exclusion assay), then transfused into the portal vein with a 30-gauge needle for over 2 min. Rats were sacrificed 4, 12 and 24 weeks later. At each time point, fresh liver, brain, and kidney tissues, and blood were obtained for analysis.

Biochemical Analysis and Histopathology

Blood samples at each time point were collected in heparin-containing tubes and centrifuged at 5000×g for 10 min. Levels of alanine aminotransferase (ALT) and aspartate aminotransferase (AST) were measured with a biochemical analyzer (Hitachi Co. Ltd., Tokyo, Japan). Formalin-fixed liver sections (5 μm) were stained with hematoxylin and eosin (HE) and Masson's trichrome (MT). The fibrotic area by MT staining was quantified by image analysis (Image-Pro Plus 6.0; Media Cybernetics, Bethesda, MD) and the histological features were independently assessed by two pathologists who were blinded to other details of the experiments.

Immunofluorescence

To confirm that injected MSCs^{ATP7B} had differentiated into normal hepatocytes, GFP/CK-18 double fluorescence intensity was assessed using a previously described protocol [31]. Briefly, liver tissues were embedded in tissue freezing medium (Tissue-Tek OCT Compound, Sakura Finetek, Torrance, CA, USA) and frozen at −80°C. Frozen sections were cut at 4 μm, fixed in cold acetone and then blocked in bovine serum albumin (BSA). Anti-CK-18 rabbit monoclonal antibody (Abcam, Cambridge, MA, USA) and anti-GFP mouse monoclonal antibody (Abmart, Shanghai, China) diluted, respectively, to 1:100 and 1:500 in

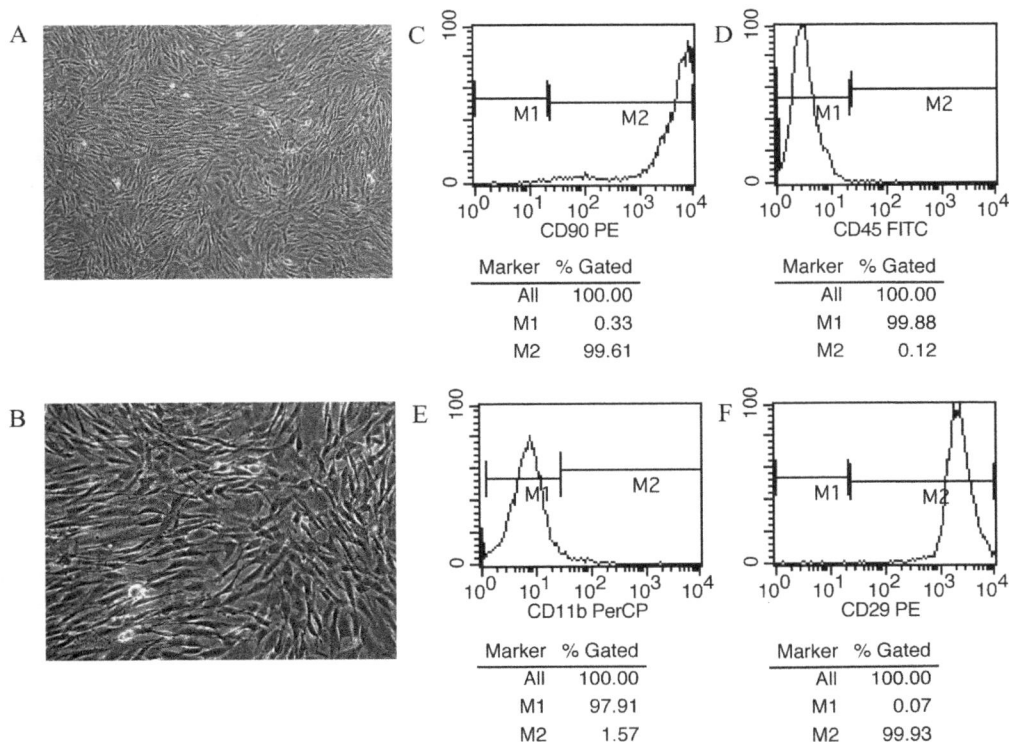

Figure 1. Morphology and characterization of BM-MSCs. (A, B): The morphology of BM-MSCs of passage 5 (×100 magnification [A] and ×200 magnification [B]). The BM-MSCs have a fibroblast-like, spindle-shaped morphology. (C–F): Immunophenotype of BM-MSCs. BM-MSCs of passage 5 were marked with antibodies specific for positive antigen (CD 90 [C] or CD 29 [F]) or negative controls (CD45 [D] and CD11b/c [E]), and analyzed by flow cytometry.

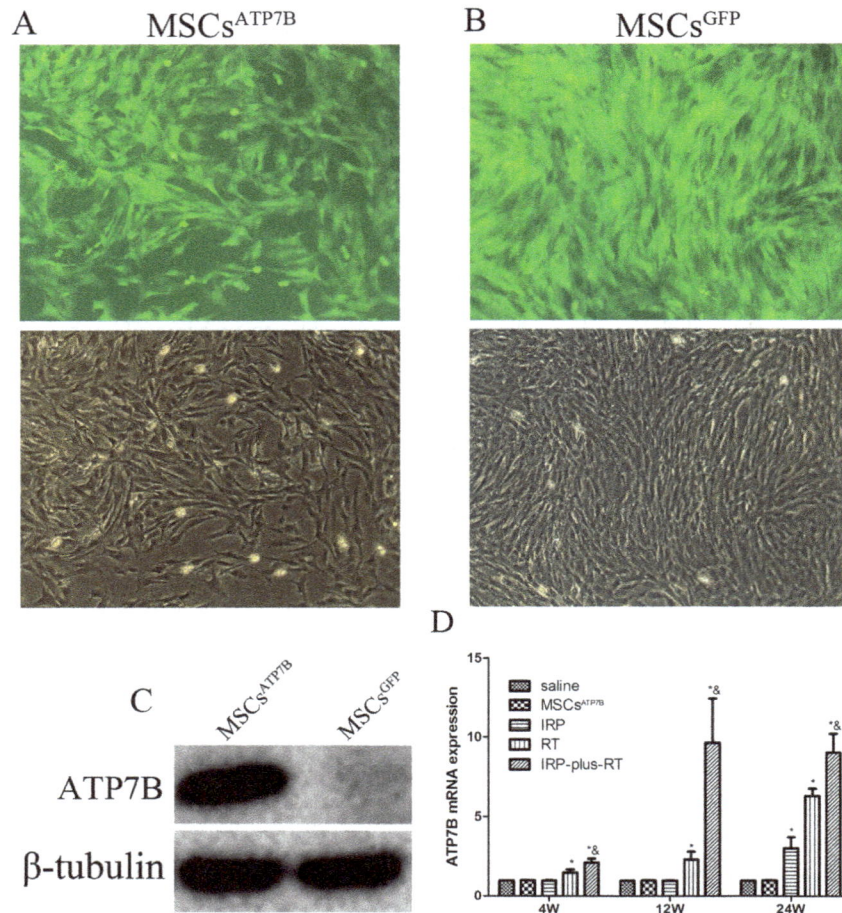

Figure 2. Transfection efficacy, expression of ATP7B post-transfection and post-transplantation. (A) Transfection efficacy of pRRL.PPT.SF.ATP7B.i2GFPBsd.pre in BM-MSCs. (B) Transfection efficacy of pRRL.PPT.SF.i2GFPpre in BM-MSCs. Transfected cells were observed under both a fluorescence microscope and a regular microscope (×100); (C) Expression of ATP7B in BM-MSCs post-transfection assessed by Western Blot. (D) Expression of ATP7B in each group at each time-point following transplantation *in vivo*. $^*p < 0.05$ compared with the saline group, $^&p < 0.05$ compared with IRP and RT group, respectively.

PBS containing 1% BSA were applied to the blocked sections for 16 hours at 4°C. Negative controls were incubated with PBS containing 1% BSA instead of primary antibody. After washing in PBS, FITC-conjugated donkey anti-rabbit IgG (1:1000, Abcam, Cambridge, MA, USA) and PE-conjugated goat anti-mouse IgG (1:400, Santa Cruz, CA, USA) were applied for 1 hour at room temperature.

Real-time Quantitative Polymerase Chain Reaction (RT-PCR)

Total RNA was extracted from frozen liver tissues using Trizol solution (Invitrogen Life Technologies, Carlsbad, CA, USA) and then treated with RNase-free DNase. mRNA was reverse transcribed using a commercially available kit (Perfect Real Time, SYBR PrimeScriP TaKaRa, Shiga, Japan). The RT-PCR analysis was carried out with the following primers: ATP7B (F: 5′-GCCAGCATTGCAGAAGGAAAG-3′ and R: 5′ -TGA-TAAGTGATGACGGCCTCT-3′) and cDNAs for 40 cycles of 95°C for 5 min, 95°C for 30 s, 60°C for 30 s and 72°C for 30 s according to the manufacturer's protocol using the ABI Prism 7000 Sequence Detection system (Applied Biosystems, Tokyo,

Japan). Ct values produced by ATP7B primers were normalized to the expression of the ß-actin housekeeping gene ($2^{-\Delta\Delta Ct}$ method).

Western Blot Analysis

Western Blots were performed with slight modifications to a previous protocol [32]. Cell lysates were prepared by incubation in cold lysis buffer containing 25 mmol/L Tris-Cl (pH 7.5), and 5 mmol/L EDTA 1% SDS; the samples were then mixed with loading buffer and boiled at 100°C for 5 min. The concentration of protein was determined using the bicinchoninic acid (BCA) protein assay kit (Beyotime Institute of Biotechnology, Shanghai, China). Samples were subjected to electrophoresis in SDS-PAGE and transferred to polyvinylidene fluoride membranes. Membranes were blocked in 5% blocking buffer for 2 hours at room temperature, and incubated with the primary antibodies, overnight at 4°C. After washing in TBS with 0.1% Tween-20, membranes were incubated with secondary antibodies for 1 hour at room temperature. The primary antibodies used in this study were rabbit monoclonal anti-ATP7B antibody (1:3000 dilution, Abcam, Cambridge, MA, USA) and rabbit polyclonal anti-β-

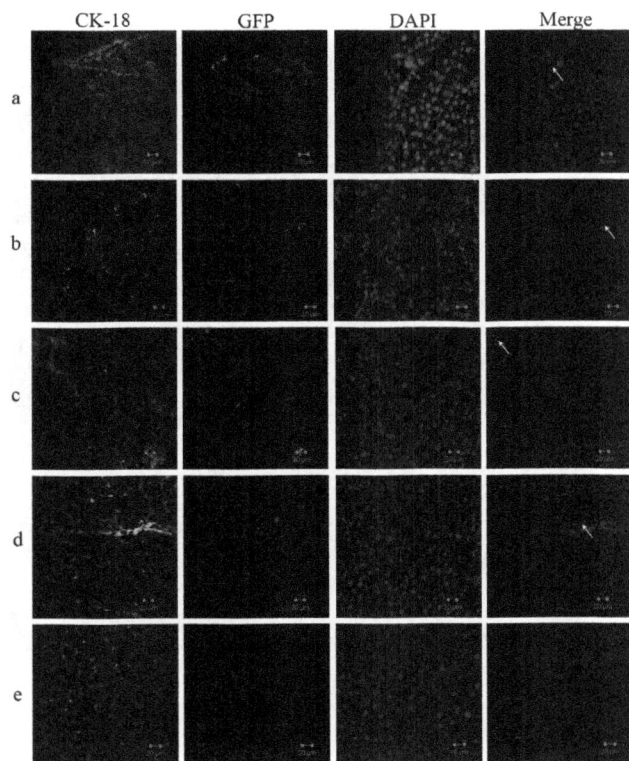

Figure 3. Migration and population of transplanted BM-MSCs in vivo. Expression of CK-18 in GFP labeled BM-MSCs engrafted in liver tissues 4 weeks after transplantation; detection by immunofluorescence histochemistry. (DAPI, 4′,6-diamidino-2-phenylindole). The collected figure illustrates hepatocytes differentiated from transplanted MSCs^{ATP7B}: (a) IRP-plus-RT group, (b) RT group, (c) IRP group, (d) MSCs^{ATP7B} group, (e) saline group.

tubulin antibody (1:1000 dilution, Cell Signaling Technology, Danvers, MA, USA).

Copper Measurement

Fresh liver samples at each time-point were desiccated under vacuum at 65°C for 16 hours, then solubilized in nitric acid. Levels of copper were determined by atomic absorption spectroscopy (AAS) at the Center of Modern Analysis, Nanjing University, according to a protocol described previously [33]. Results were expressed as μg/g dry weight of tissue.

Serum ceruloplasmin analysis

Serum ceruloplasmin at each time-point was determined using the method of Malhi et al. [33]. Results were expressed as mg/dL.

Statistical analysis

All data were expressed as mean ± standard deviation, and were compared by ANOVA followed by Student-Newman-Keuls (SNK) post-hoc analysis using GraphPad Prism 5 software. Differences were considered significant at p values <0.05.

Results

Ninety healthy two month old LEC rats were used in this research. They were randomly divided into 5 groups: group a were injected with saline, group b were injected with MSCs^{ATP7B}, groups c, d and e had livers preconditioned with ischemia-reperfusion (IRP), radiation (RT) and ischemia-reperfusion plus radiation (IRP-plus-RT), respectively before injection with MSCs^{ATP7B}.

Characterization of BM-MSCs derived from LEC rat bone marrow

BM-MSCs were isolated from rat bone-marrow mononuclear cell fractions by the direct plastic adherence method. BM-MSCs were observed to be spindle-shaped, fibroblast-like (figures 1A–B), and maintained their undifferentiated status.

The surface markers of BM-MSCs were identified by flow cytometry. Over 99% of the isolated BM-MSCs expressed CD29 and CD90, but not CD11b/c and CD45 (figures 1C–F).

Transduction of BM-MSCs in cell culture

At 48-hours post-transduction, nearly 100% of cells were transduced (figures 2A and 2B). To analyze the functional activity of BM-MSCs, 5 days after transduction, total proteins extracted from MSCs^{ATP7B} and MSCs^{GFP} were analyzed by Western Blots. The protein levels of ATP7B were markedly enhanced in MSCs^{ATP7B} (figure 2C).

Expression of ATP7B, post-transplantation, as a function of time

Liver ATP7B expression was measured by RT-PCR at 4, 12, and 24 weeks post-transplantation. As shown in Figure 2D, at all three time points, the ATP7B expression of both the RT group and the IRP-plus-RT group were significantly higher than the saline group (for all, $p<0.05$). The same comparison between the IRP group and the saline group showed a significant difference only at 24 weeks post-transplantation. It was also found that ATP7B expression in the IRP-plus-RT group was markedly higher than that in either the IRP or the RT group at each time point post-transplantation ($p<0.05$, for all).

Engraftment and repopulation of MSCs^{ATP7B} after transplantation

To track hepatocytes that had differentiated from MSCs^{ATP7B}, a red-fluorescent second antibody was used to detect GFP transduced into MSCs as a marker of mature hepatocytes. A green-fluorescent second antibody was used to mark CK-18 of the hepatocytes. GFP/CK-18 positive cells (figure 3) were detected around both hepatic sinusoids and within the parenchyma of recipient livers of the IRP-plus-RT group and the RT group at 4 weeks post-transplantation. These cells remained present in recipient livers through 24 weeks following transplantation. However, there were few GFP/CK-18 positive cells in the livers of either the IRP group or the MSCs^{ATP7B} group and no GFP-positive cells in the liver of the saline group were observed at any time point post-transplantation. No GFP fluorescence intensity was detected in other organs such as brain and kidney (data not shown).

Protective effect of transplantation of MSCs^{ATP7B} on liver histopathology

HE staining showed that cholangiocarcinomas were present in the livers of both the saline (4/6) and MSCs^{ATP7B} (5/6) groups 24 weeks post-transplantation, while only chronic hepatitis was observed in the IRP, RT and IRP-plus-RT groups (figure 4A). Moreover, as shown in Figure 4B–C, compared with saline group, a significant decrease in liver fibrosis were observed in the IRP,

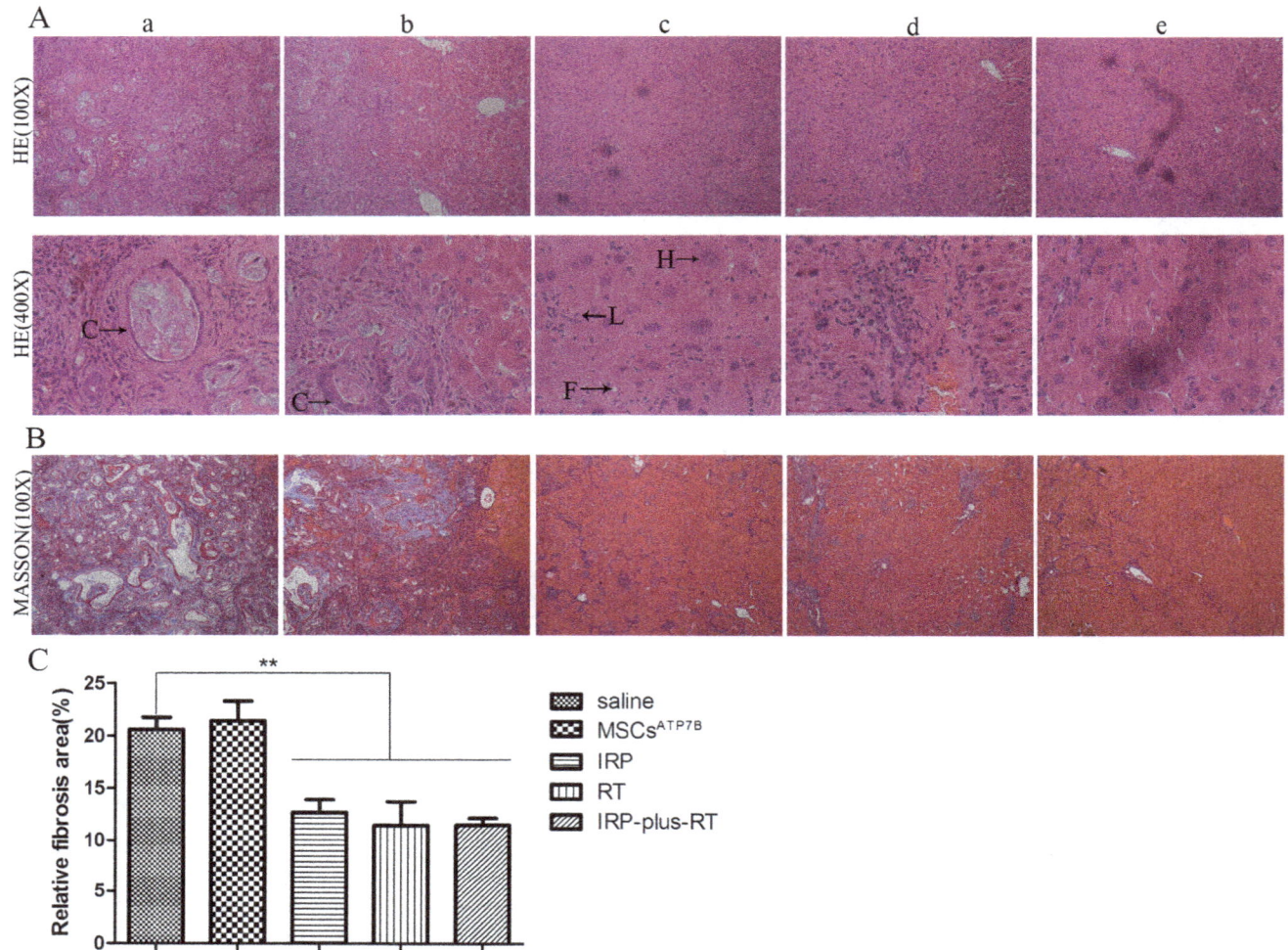

Figure 4. Hematoxylin and eosin and Masson's trichrome staining of liver sections 24 weeks post-transplantation. A. H&E staining, (a, b): Typical histological finding of cholangiocarcinoma seen in the liver of saline and MSCs^{ATP7B} groups. (c–e): Livers of IRP, RT, and IRP-plus-RT rats, respectively. The typical histological finding of cholangiocarcinoma is absent, but the histological finding of chronic hepatitis is present. Enlarged nuclei and fatty changes are visible in some of the hepatocytes; lymphocytes are irregularly distributed among hepatocytes. (C: cholangiocarcinoma; H: regenerated hepatocytes; L: lymphocytes; F: fine fatty droplets); B. MT staining. C. Quantitation of MT staining. The liver fibrosis of IRP, RT, and IRP-plus-RT groups are compared with the saline group, respectively; IRP and RT groups are also compared with IRP-plus-RT group, respectively. $^{**}p < 0.01$.

Table 1. Changes in Hepatic Copper Content of LEC Rats as a Function of Time after MSC^{ATP7B} Transplantation (μg/g dry weight tissue).

Preconditioning	n	4W	12W	24W
Saline	6	466±39	907±20	1240±106
MSCs^{ATP7B}	6	454±42	890±30	1246±100
IRP	6	453±36	893±14	758±92*
RT	6	308±23*	646±17*	450±33*
IRP-plus-RT	6	229±20$^{*&}$	509±24$^{*&}$	341±28$^{*&}$

IRP: Ischemia Reperfusion, RT: radiation.
$^{*}p < 0.05$, compared with the saline group.
$^{&}p < 0.05$, compared with IRP and RT groups, respectively.

Table 2. Serum Ceruloplasmin Levels in LEC Rats 4, 12, and 24 weeks after MSCs^{ATP7B} Transplantation (mg/dL).

Preconditioning	n	4W	12W	24W
Saline	6	7.1±1.6	6.8±3.0	6.1±1.5
MSCs^{ATP7B}	6	8.5±1.9	7.6±1.9	7.0±3.4
IRP	6	7.7±2.6	9.3±3.0	16.2±2.0*
RT	6	15.2±2.4*	11.5±2.2*	21.5±2.0*
IRP-plus-RT	6	19.3±3.2$^{*&}$	17.0±2.8$^{*&}$	25.0±2.2$^{*&}$

IRP: Ischemia Reperfusion, RT: radiation.
*$p<0.05$, compared with the saline group.
&$p<0.05$, compared with IRP group and RT group, respectively.

RT and IRP-plus-RT groups (12.66±1.26% for IRP group, 11.42±2.30% for RT group and 11.46±0.68% for IRP-plus-RT group versus 20.60±1.19% for saline group, $p<0.01$, for all). However, there were no significant differences in liver fibrosis between the IRP-plus-RT group and IRP or RT groups, both $p>0.05$.

Liver copper concentration

Liver copper concentration (μg/g dry weight tissue) was determined 4, 12, and 24 weeks following MSCs^{ATP7B} transplantation. As shown in Table 1, liver copper concentration increased from 466±39 μg/g to 1240±106 μg/g in the saline group, and 454±42 μg/g to 1246±100 μg/g in the MSCs^{ATP7B} group. Liver copper concentrations increased from 453±36 μg/g to 758±92 μg/g in the IRP group, 308±23 μg/g to 450±33 μg/g in the RT group and 229±20 μg/g to 341±28 μg/g in the IRP-plus-RT group. There were no significant differences in liver copper concentrations between the saline group and MSCs^{ATP7B} group ($p>0.05$) at any time-point. Twenty-four weeks after transplantation, liver copper concentrations in the IRP group were significantly lower than in the saline group ($p<0.05$). Moreover, liver copper concentration of the RT group and the IRP-plus-RT group was significantly lower than that of the saline group at all time-points ($p<0.05$, for all). Additionally, rats preconditioned with IRP-plus-RT demonstrated decreased liver copper concentration compared with rats preconditioned with IRP alone or RT alone at each time-point post-transplantation ($p<0.05$, respectively). No significant differences in the copper concentration of brain and kidney were found between treatment groups and the saline group at all time points (data not shown).

Serum ceruloplasmin analysis

Serum ceruloplasmin levels (mg/dL) were compared between treatment and the saline groups as well as between rats preconditioned with IRP-plus-RT and rats preconditioned with either IRP alone or RT alone at each time-point following MSCs^{ATP7B} transplantation. The results are shown in table 2. Briefly, serum ceruloplasmin was decreased from 7.1±1.6 mg/dL to 6.1±1.5 mg/dL in the saline group, and from 8.5±1.9 mg/dL to 7.0±3.4 mg/dL in MSCs^{ATP7B} group. Serum ceruloplasmin increased from 7.7±2.6 mg/dL to 16.2±2.0 mg/dL in the IRP group. Serum ceruloplasmin increased from 15.2±2.4 mg/dL to 21.5±2.0 mg/dL in the RT group, and from 19.3±3.2 mg/dL to 25.0±2.2 mg/dL in the IRP-plus-RT group. Rats treated with IRP-plus-RT and RT alone showed a higher serum ceruloplasmin level than rats in the saline group at all time points ($p<0.05$, for all). In the IRP group, serum ceruloplasmin levels were only higher than the saline group at 24 weeks following MSCs^{ATP7B} transplantation ($p<0.05$). In the treated groups, serum ceruloplasmin levels in rats treated with IRP-plus-RT were higher than those in rats treated with IRP alone or RT alone at each time-point ($p<0.05$, for all).

Effect of MSCs^{ATP7B} transplantation on ALT and AST levels

Serum ALT and AST levels were analyzed at each time-point following MSCs^{ATP7B} transplantation, in order to compare the

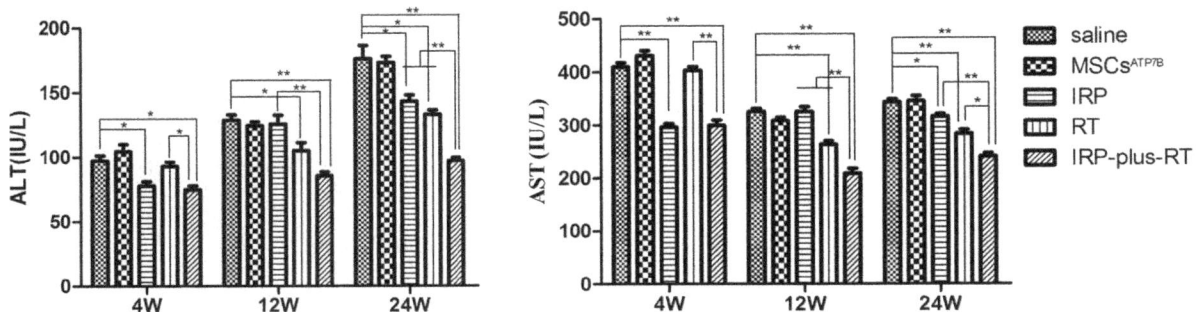

Figure 5. Effect of BM-MSCs on serum biomarkers. Values are expressed as mean ± SD. For ALT and AST levels at each time point, IRP, RT, and IRP-plus-RT groups are compared with the saline group, respectively; IRP and RT groups are also compared with IRP-plus-RT group, respectively. *$p<0.05$, **$p<0.01$.

recovery of liver damage in the rats of different groups. As shown in figure 5, 4 weeks after transplantation, a significant reduction in ALT and AST levels was found in the IRP group and the IRP-plus-RT group compared to the saline group (for ALT, 19.8% and 22.9%, both $p<0.05$; for AST, 27.6% and 27%, both $p<0.01$). The levels of ALT and AST in the IRP-plus-RT group were significantly lower than those in the RT group (for ALT, 75 ± 5.29 U/L versus 93 ± 6 U/L, $p<0.05$; for AST, 299.3 ± 18.45 U/L versus 403.3 ± 12.66 U/L, $p<0.01$). At 12 weeks post-transplantation, the ALT and AST levels of the RT group and the IRP-plus-RT group were significantly decreased compared to the saline group (for ALT, 18.4% and 33.4%, $p<0.05$ or 0.01; for AST, 19.2% and 35.9%, both $p<0.01$); and compared with the IRP group, both ALT and AST levels were significant decreased in the IRP-plus-RT group (for ALT, 31.8%, for AST, 35.9%, both $p<0.01$). There was no significant difference in ALT levels between the RT group and the IRP-plus-RT group ($p>0.05$). There was a significant decrease in the AST levels of the IRP-plus-RT group (20.7%, $p<0.01$) compared with those of the RT group. In contrast, 24 weeks post-transplantation, the levels of ALT and AST in the IRP group, the RT group, and the IRP-plus-RT group were all significantly decreased compared to those of the saline group (for ALT, 18.6%, 24.4%, and 44.9%; for AST, 7.9%, 17.4%, and 29.8%, compared with IRP and RT group, $p<0.05$; compared with IRP-plus-RT group, $p<0.01$). Furthermore, ALT levels were significantly lower in the IRP-plus-RT group compared to both IRP and RT groups (32.3% and 27%, $p<0.01$, respectively). The same comparison for results for AST level showed 23.8% and 15% differences, ($p<0.01$ and $p<0.05$, respectively).

Discussion

In recent years, LEC rats and Atp7b$^{-/-}$ mice have been shown to be suitable models for gene therapy of WD [34]. Terada *et al.* [35] administered recombinant adenovirus containing WND (ATP7B) cDNA into LEC rats by tail vein injection, and showed that the holoceruloplasmin levels were partially restored within two weeks. However, the expression of the WND gene tended to disappear after two weeks. Moreover, adenovirus vectors have a relatively strong toxicity and can induce an immune response. To overcome this shortcoming, Merle *et al.* rescued LEC rats with modified lentiviral vectors. However, quantitative immunofluorescence analysis of liver tissue sections showed a lower percentage of ATP7B-positive hepatocytes 24 weeks after treatment when compared to 2 weeks after treatment [36]. Two problems remained unresolved in this research. First, implanted hepatocytes could not correct the liver injury caused by the disorder of copper metabolism. Second, although several studies have confirmed that hepatocyte transplantation is effective for correcting the copper metabolism of LEC rats [37–40], the inability of transplanted cells to proliferate in normal liver prevents cell therapy from being clinically useful. In the current experiments, we obtained prolonged expression of ATP7B which is consistent with our previous results using BM-MSCs and lentiviral vectors in gene therapy [41,42].

Oxidative hepatic DNA damage induced by IRP or RT is known to impair the survival of native cells, and promote proliferation of transplanted cells. Malhi *et al.* [29] preconditioned F344 rats with whole liver radiation and warm ischemia-reperfusion followed by intrasplenic transplantation of syngeneic F344 rat hepatocytes, and found that the proliferation of transplanted cells in the animals treated with IRP-plus-RT was far more successful than that in control animals as well as in animals preconditioned with either IRP or RT alone. A similar study was also conducted in LEC rats, and showed that the resulting long-term reversal of copper toxicity in the animals preconditioned with IRP-plus-RT occurred because of superior engraftment and proliferation [33]. Consistent with these two results, we found that ATP7B expression lasted up to 24 weeks post-transplantation, and that the copper concentration, serum ceruloplasmin, and liver functions of the IRP-plus-RT group were obviously improved compared to those of the saline, IRP, or RT groups. The possible mechanisms by which IRP and RT promote engraftment and proliferation may lie in the selective pressure of liver damage. Selective pressure in the form of liver injury has been proven to be required for donor cell engraftment of the liver [43]. However, the limitations of IRP and/or RT preconditioning such as acute hepatitis cannot be ignored, although such preconditioning was well-tolerated by all animals. Malhi *et al.* [29] have confirmed that acute liver injury could be produced by such strategies.

Recently, Sauer *et al.* [44] mimicked high hepatic copper conditions in cell culture and found that ATP7B overexpression confers an important viability and selective advantage to cells in toxic copper microenvironments. Furthermore, previous researchers have shown that human MSCs can integrate into the livers of rats and mice and differentiate into functional hepatocytes [18,45], suggesting that ATP7B-transduced MSCs might be suitable for therapy of WD. Also, *in vivo* application of ATP7B encoding viral vectors to the liver was found to restore copper metabolism and holoceruloplasmin synthesis in LEC rats [35,46]. This is the best evidence that the expression of ATP7B is necessary for therapy of WD. However, such experimental conditions are not directly applicable to WD patients in the clinic, our present study included. Reasons for this may be the following: (1) the safety of the viral vectors in humans is still unknown; (2) infusion of cells into the portal vein is known to cause sinusoidal occlusion and portal hypertension; and (3) in our present study, we rescued the LEC rats with MSCs^{ATP7B} when the rats were 8 weeks old. LEC rats have no signs of WD at this time point. In other words, the treatment was preemptive, but not proof of disease improvement. However, in clinical situations, the livers of WD patients are often cirrhotic when WD symptoms appear. Treatment of such patients by stem cell transplantation may not be very effective due to the damaged hepatic architecture. Therefore, further studies are needed to determine the timing and the best infusion approach for stem cell transplantation of WD patients.

In summary, transplantation of ATP7B-transduced bone marrow mesenchymal stem cells decreases copper overload in rats.

Acknowledgments

We thank Professor S. Gupta for kindly providing us LEC rats and Professor Duanqing Pei for kindly providing all plasmids used in our research. We thank *Medjaden* Bioscience Limited for assisting in the preparation of this manuscript.

Author Contributions

Conceived and designed the experiments: FC PW. Performed the experiments: SC CS TD HC XX DS LZ. Analyzed the data: SC YY. Contributed reagents/materials/analysis tools: TD HC XX DS LZ. Wrote the paper: SC CS.

References

1. Gollan JL, Gollan TJ (1998) Wilson disease in 1998: genetic, diagnostic and therapeutic aspects. J Hepatol 28 Suppl 1: 28–36.
2. Scheinberg IH (1981) Wilson's disease. J Rheumatol Suppl 7: 90–93.
3. Medici V, Mirante VG, Fassati LR, Pompili M, Forti D, et al. (2005) Liver transplantation for Wilson's disease: The burden of neurological and psychiatric disorders. Liver Transpl 11: 1056–1063.
4. Polson RJ, Rolles K, Calne RY, Williams R, Marsden D (1987) Reversal of severe neurological manifestations of Wilson's disease following orthotopic liver transplantation. Q J Med 64: 685–691.
5. Wertheim JA, Petrowsky H, Saab S, Kupiec-Weglinski JW, Busuttil RW (2011) Major challenges limiting liver transplantation in the United States. Am J Transplant 11: 1773–1784.
6. Bataller R, Brenner DA (2005) Liver fibrosis. J Clin Invest 115: 209–218.
7. Nussler A, Konig S, Ott M, Sokal E, Christ B, et al. (2006) Present status and perspectives of cell-based therapies for liver diseases. J Hepatol 45: 144–159.
8. Solaiman F, Zink MA, Xu G, Grunkemeyer J, Cosgrove D, et al. (2000) Modular retro-vectors for transgenic and therapeutic use. Mol Reprod Dev 56: 309–315.
9. Buchschacher GL, Jr., Wong-Staal F (2000) Development of lentiviral vectors for gene therapy for human diseases. Blood 95: 2499–2504.
10. Naldini L, Blomer U, Gallay P, Ory D, Mulligan R, et al. (1996) In vivo gene delivery and stable transduction of nondividing cells by a lentiviral vector. Science 272: 263–267.
11. Yu X, Zhan X, D'Costa J, Tanavde VM, Ye Z, et al. (2003) Lentiviral vectors with two independent internal promoters transfer high-level expression of multiple transgenes to human hematopoietic stem-progenitor cells. Mol Ther 7: 827–838.
12. Abdallah BM, Kassem M (2008) Human mesenchymal stem cells: from basic biology to clinical applications. Gene ther 15: 109–116.
13. Bruder SP, Jaiswal N, Ricalton NS, Mosca JD, Kraus KH, et al. (1998) Mesenchymal stem cells in osteobiology and applied bone regeneration. Clin Orthop Relat Res: S247–256.
14. Kobayashi T, Ochi M, Yanada S, Ishikawa M, Adachi N, et al. (2008) A novel cell delivery system using magnetically labeled mesenchymal stem cells and an external magnetic device for clinical cartilage repair. Arthroscopy 24: 69–76.
15. Murphy JM, Dixon K, Beck S, Fabian D, Feldman A, et al. (2002) Reduced chondrogenic and adipogenic activity of mesenchymal stem cells from patients with advanced osteoarthritis. Arthritis Rheum 46: 704–713.
16. Wang N, Sun C, Huo S, Zhang Y, Zhao J, et al. (2008) Cooperation of phosphatidylcholine-specific phospholipase C and basic fibroblast growth factor in the neural differentiation of mesenchymal stem cells in vitro. Int J Biochem Cell Biol 40: 294–306.
17. Pasha Z, Wang Y, Sheikh R, Zhang D, Zhao T, et al. (2008) Preconditioning enhances cell survival and differentiation of stem cells during transplantation in infarcted myocardium. Cardiovasc Res 77: 134–142.
18. Sato Y, Araki H, Kato J, Nakamura K, Kawano Y, et al. (2005) Human mesenchymal stem cells xenografted directly to rat liver are differentiated into human hepatocytes without fusion. Blood 106: 756–763.
19. Yagi K, Kojima M, Oyagi S, Ikeda E, Hirose M, et al. (2008) [Application of mesenchymal stem cells to liver regenerative medicine]. Yakugaku zasshi 128: 3–9.
20. Lemoli RM, Catani L, Talarico S, Loggi E, Gramenzi A, et al. (2006) Mobilization of bone marrow-derived hematopoietic and endothelial stem cells after orthotopic liver transplantation and liver resection. Stem Cells 24: 2817–2825.
21. Baccarani U, De Stasio G, Adani GL, Donini A, Sainz-Barriga M, et al. (2006) Implication of stem cell factor in human liver regeneration after transplantation and resection. Growth Factors 24: 107–110.
22. Enns GM, Millan MT (2008) Cell-based therapies for metabolic liver disease. Mol Genet Metab 95: 3–10.
23. Muramatsu Y, Yamada T, Moralejo DH, Cai Y, Xin X, et al. (1995) The rat homologue of the Wilson's disease gene was partially deleted at the 3' end of its protein-coding region in Long-Evans Cinnamon mutant rats. Res Commun Mol Pathol Pharmacol 89: 421–424.
24. Yamamoto F, Kasai H, Togashi Y, Takeichi N, Hori T, et al. (1993) Elevated level of 8-hydroxydeoxyguanosine in DNA of liver, kidneys, and brain of Long-Evans Cinnamon rats. Jpn J Cancer Res 84: 508–511.
25. Sakai H, Horiguchi N, Endoh D, Nakayama K, Hayashi M (2011) Radiofrequency radiation at 40 kHz induces hepatic injury in Long-Evans

Cinnamon (LEC) rats, an animal model for human Wilson disease. J Vet Med Sci 73: 299–304.
26. Wu J, Forbes JR, Chen HS, Cox DW (1994) The LEC rat has a deletion in the copper transporting ATPase gene homologous to the Wilson disease gene. Nat Genet 7: 541–545.
27. Shao CH, Chen SL, Dong TF, Chai H, Yu Y, et al. (2014) Transplantation of bone marrow-derived mesenchymal stem cells after regional hepatic irradiation ameliorates thioacetamide-induced liver fibrosis in rats. J Surg Res 186: 408–416.
28. Follenzi A, Ailles LE, Bakovic S, Geuna M, Naldini L (2000) Gene transfer by lentiviral vectors is limited by nuclear translocation and rescued by HIV-1 pol sequences. Nat Genet 25: 217–222.
29. Malhi H, Gorla GR, Irani AN, Annamaneni P, Gupta S (2002) Cell transplantation after oxidative hepatic preconditioning with radiation and ischemia-reperfusion leads to extensive liver repopulation. Proc Natl Acad Sci U S A 99: 13114–13119.
30. Frederiks WM, James J, Bosch KS, Schroder MJ, Schuyt HC (1982) A model for provoking ischemic necrosis in rat liver parenchyma and its quantitative analysis. Exp Pathol 22: 245–252.
31. Chen X, Xing S, Feng Y, Chen S, Pei Z, et al. (2011) Early stage transplantation of bone marrow cells markedly ameliorates copper metabolism and restores liver function in a mouse model of Wilson disease. BMC Gastroenterol 11: 75.
32. Zhang H, Huang CJ, Tian Y, Wang YP, Han ZG, et al. (2012) Ectopic overexpression of COTE1 promotes cellular invasion of hepatocellular carcinoma. Asian Pac J Cancer Prev 13: 5799–5804.
33. Malhi H, Joseph B, Schilsky ML, Gupta S (2008) Development of cell therapy strategies to overcome copper toxicity in the LEC rat model of Wilson disease. Regen Med 3: 165–173.
34. Bartee MY, Lutsenko S (2007) Hepatic copper-transporting ATPase ATP7B: function and inactivation at the molecular and cellular level. Biometals 20: 627–637.
35. Terada K, Nakako T, Yang XL, Iida M, Aiba N, et al. (1998) Restoration of holoceruloplasmin synthesis in LEC rat after infusion of recombinant adenovirus bearing WND cDNA. J Biol Chem 273: 1815–1820.
36. Merle U, Encke J, Tuma S, Volkmann M, Naldini L, et al. (2006) Lentiviral gene transfer ameliorates disease progression in Long-Evans cinnamon rats: an animal model for Wilson disease. Scand J Gastroenterol 41: 974–982.
37. Park SM, Vo K, Lallier M, Cloutier AS, Brochu P, et al. (2006) Hepatocyte transplantation in the Long Evans Cinnamon rat model of Wilson's disease. Cell Transplant 15: 13–22.
38. Sauer V, Siaj R, Stoppeler S, Bahde R, Spiegel HU, et al. (2012) Repeated transplantation of hepatocytes prevents fulminant hepatitis in a rat model of Wilson's disease. Liver Transpl 18: 248–259.
39. Yoshida Y, Tokusashi Y, Lee GH, Ogawa K (1996) Intrahepatic transplantation of normal hepatocytes prevents Wilson's disease in Long-Evans cinnamon rats. Gastroenterology 111: 1654–1660.
40. Irani AN, Malhi H, Slehria S, Gorla GR, Volenberg I, et al. (2001) Correction of liver disease following transplantation of normal rat hepatocytes into Long-Evans Cinnamon rats modeling Wilson's disease. Mol Ther 3: 302–309.
41. Gao Y, Yao A, Zhang W, Lu S, Yu Y, et al. (2010) Human mesenchymal stem cells overexpressing pigment epithelium-derived factor inhibit hepatocellular carcinoma in nude mice. Oncogene 29: 2784–2794.
42. Yu Y, Lu L, Qian X, Chen N, Yao A, et al. (2010) Antifibrotic effect of hepatocyte growth factor-expressing mesenchymal stem cells in small-for-size liver transplant rats. Stem Cells Dev 19: 903–914.
43. Wang X, Montini E, Al-Dhalimy M, Lagasse E, Finegold M, et al. (2002) Kinetics of liver repopulation after bone marrow transplantation. Am J Pathol 161: 565–574.
44. Sauer V, Siaj R, Todorov T, Zibert A, Schmidt HH (2010) Overexpressed ATP7B protects mesenchymal stem cells from toxic copper. Biochem Biophys Res Commun 395: 307–311.
45. Aurich I, Mueller LP, Aurich H, Luetzkendorf J, Tisljar K, et al. (2007) Functional integration of hepatocytes derived from human mesenchymal stem cells into mouse livers. Gut 56: 405–415.
46. Meng Y, Miyoshi I, Hirabayashi M, Su M, Mototani Y, et al. (2004) Restoration of copper metabolism and rescue of hepatic abnormalities in LEC rats, an animal model of Wilson disease, by expression of human ATP7B gene. Biochim Biophys Acta 1690: 208–219.

3

Accuracy of Estimation of Graft Size for Living-Related Liver Transplantation: First Results of a Semi-Automated Interactive Software for CT-Volumetry

Theresa Mokry[1], Nadine Bellemann[1], Dirk Müller[2], Justo Lorenzo Bermejo[3], Miriam Klauß[1], Ulrike Stampfl[1], Boris Radeleff[1], Peter Schemmer[4], Hans-Ulrich Kauczor[1], Christof-Matthias Sommer[1]*

1 Department of Diagnostic and Interventional Radiology, University Hospital Heidelberg, Heidelberg, Germany, 2 Philips Healthcare Germany, Hamburg, Germany, 3 Department of Medical Biometry and Informatics, University Hospital Heidelberg, Heidelberg, Germany, 4 Department of General and Transplant Surgery, University Hospital Heidelberg, Heidelberg, Germany

Abstract

Objectives: To evaluate accuracy of estimated graft size for living-related liver transplantation using a semi-automated interactive software for CT-volumetry.

Materials and Methods: Sixteen donors for living-related liver transplantation (11 male; mean age: 38.2 ± 9.6 years) underwent contrast-enhanced CT prior to graft removal. CT-volumetry was performed using a semi-automated interactive software (P), and compared with a manual commercial software (TR). For P, liver volumes were provided either with or without vessels. For TR, liver volumes were provided always with vessels. Intraoperative weight served as reference standard. Major study goals included analyses of volumes using absolute numbers, linear regression analyses and inter-observer agreements. Minor study goals included the description of the software workflow: degree of manual correction, speed for completion, and overall intuitiveness using five-point Likert scales: 1–markedly lower/faster/higher for P compared with TR, 2–slightly lower/faster/higher for P compared with TR, 3–identical for P and TR, 4–slightly lower/faster/higher for TR compared with P, and 5–markedly lower/faster/higher for TR compared with P.

Results: Liver segments II/III, II–IV and V–VIII served in 6, 3, and 7 donors as transplanted liver segments. Volumes were 642.9 ± 368.8 ml for TR with vessels, 623.8 ± 349.1 ml for P with vessels, and 605.2 ± 345.8 ml for P without vessels ($P < 0.01$). Regression equations between intraoperative weights and volumes were $y = 0.94x + 30.1$ ($R^2 = 0.92$; $P < 0.001$) for TR with vessels, $y = 1.00x + 12.0$ ($R^2 = 0.92$; $P < 0.001$) for P with vessels, and $y = 1.01x + 28.0$ ($R^2 = 0.92$; $P < 0.001$) for P without vessels. Inter-observer agreement showed a bias of 1.8 ml for TR with vessels, 5.4 ml for P with vessels, and 4.6 ml for P without vessels. For the degree of manual correction, speed for completion and overall intuitiveness, scale values were 2.6 ± 0.8, 2.4 ± 0.5 and 2.

Conclusions: CT-volumetry performed with P can predict accurately graft size for living-related liver transplantation while improving workflow compared with TR.

Editor: Nupur Gangopadhyay, University of Pittsburgh, United States of America

Funding: This work was technically supported by Philips Healthcare Germany, Hamburg, Germany. There was no financial funding. The funder taught us how to use the software prototype, and helped in data interpretation, statistics and manuscript editing. The funder had no influence on data acquisition and manuscript writing (but language proof).

Competing Interests: This work was technically supported by Philips Healthcare Germany, Hamburg, Germany. There are no other conflicts of interest regarding this study.

* Email: christof.sommer@med.uni-heidelberg.de

Introduction

Computer-assisted image analysis is an emerging technology for diagnosis, therapy and follow-up in making observer-independent and reproducible readings, and can improve the workflow compared with conventional image analysis. Time-efficient image post-processing with correct interpretation is of great importance, considering the increasing speed of data acquisition on the one hand and the extremely large amount of data available for interpretation on the other. Computer-assisted image analysis is a special challenge for the liver because of motion and deformation during respiration, multi-phase image acquisition and segmental anatomy with four different tubular systems. Although multiple approaches for computer-assisted image analysis have been introduced for oncologic liver resection, living-related liver transplantation and interventional oncology there seems to be still a lack of satisfactory solutions for the clinical routine [1]. For patients with end-stage liver disease, liver transplantation is the most effective treatment [2]. The great increase in the number of patients awaiting liver transplantation during the past years has led to a significant shortage of cadaveric organs [3]. Living-related liver transplantation has emerged as a valuable alternative, and allows healthy adults to donate a part of their own liver to a compatible recipient [4,5]. Since the convincing results associated with low risk for the healthy donor and improved outcome for the diseased recipient compared with cadaveric liver transplantation, living-related liver transplantation becomes more and more common [6,7]. For the clinical success after living-related liver transplantation, the liver volume plays a key role [8,9]. For donor and recipient, the post-operative liver volume must be large enough to fulfill metabolic demands [10]. Additionally, the liver graft should not be oversized since compression can lead to liver necrosis and impaired wound healing with potentially fatal outcome for the recipient (large-for-size) [11]. Currently, non-automated CT-volumetry can be regarded as the preoperative standard to assess liver anatomy and the future graft size [12]. After clinical estimation of the adequate graft size for the recipient (e.g. using the "graft weight to body weight ratio"), the most suitable segments for liver donation can be defined on the basis of CT-volumetry [13–15]. With this background, we defined the objective of our study: to evaluate accuracy of estimation of graft size for living-related liver transplantation using a semi-automated interactive software for CT liver volumetry (P). We hypothesized that CT-volumetry performed with P can predict accurately graft size while improving workflow compared with a manual commercial software (TR).

Materials and Methods

Ethics Statement

The Institutional Review Board (Ethikkommission der Medizinischen Fakultät Heidelberg, Heidelberg, Germany) approved the study. Every donor underwent an individual standardized evaluation process for living-related liver donation in regards of ethical as well as medical issues. Written informed consent was obtained for all donors. The data was analyzed retrospectively from a prospective digital database.

Donors for Living-Related Liver Transplantation

From January 2008 until December 2011, donors for living-related liver transplantation were enrolled. Inclusion criteria were (I) typical liver resection for living-related liver donation as well as (II) CT examination according to our standard protocol "living-related liver donor evaluation". Sixteen donors (11 male) with a mean age of 38.2±9.6 years were identified. All donors were healthy adults. Suitability for living-related liver donation was approved according to standard operating procedures including history, clinical examination, blood analysis, echocardiography, lung function, chest x-ray, and psychosocial evaluation [16]. Detailed patient demographics are presented in Table 1.

CT Examination

A 64-row multi-detector CT scanner (Somatom Definition DS, Siemens Medical Solutions, Forchheim, Germany) was used. The CT scan protocol consisted of multiple different phases of the liver: non-enhanced, biliary, arterial, and portal-venous. A late phase was acquired in the case of focal lesions. Prior to acquisition of the non-enhanced phase, all donors received an intravenous premedication consisting of 4 mg clemastine fumarate (Tavegil; Novartis, Basel, Switzerland) and 20 mg ranitidine hydrochloride (Ranitic; Hexal, Holzkirchen, Germany) to prevent potential adverse effects to the intravenous contrast materials. After continuous intravenous infusion of 100 ml biliary contrast material at a flow rate of 150 ml/h (iotroxate dimeglumine, Biliscopin; Bayer Schering Pharma, Berlin, Germany), the biliary phase was obtained. After intravenous injection of 100 ml of iodinated contrast material at a flow rate of 5 ml/s (iomeprol, Imeron 350; Bracco, Konstanz, Germany), arterial and portal-venous phases were acquired. Automated bolus tracking in the aorta at the level of the celiac trunc ensured accurate timing of the arterial phase (trigger threshold of 100 HU). The portal-venous phase was obtained with a delay of 50 s. The optional late phase was acquired with an additional delay of 180 s. Major scanning parameters included a tube voltage of 120 kVp, a reference current-time product of 240 mAs (CARE Dose 4D), a pitch of 0.55 and a collimation of 64×0.6 mm. Raw-data of all phases were reconstructed to obtain transverse and coronal images with a slice thickness of 3 mm and an increment of 1 mm, as well as transverse and coronal images with a slice thickness of 1 mm and an overlap of 0.7 mm. All reconstructions were performed in a medium soft tissue kernel (B30f, Siemens Medical Solutions, Siemens, Forchheim). All phases were used to study the liver, and no relevant anatomical variants or pathological conditions (e.g. focal liver lesions) were detected.

CT-Volumetry

Transverse images of the portal-venous phase (slice thickness of 3 mm and increment of 1 mm) were used for CT-volumetry. Two different software tools were used and compared: a semi-automated interactive commercial software called "IntelliSpace Portal Liver Analysis application" (Philips Medical Systems, Best, The Netherland) (P) and a manual commercial software (TR; Aquarius iNtuition; TeraRecon, Foster City, USA). For P, the images were uploaded, and then the outline of the entire liver was determined between liver tissue and surrounding fatty tissue. The algorithm responsible for the segmentation of the liver in contrast-emhanced CT images belongs to the family of variational approaches. It is based on a deformable mesh guided by Hounsfield units as well as surrounding anatomical structures.

Table 1. Patient Demographics.

Parameter	Study group
Age (years)	38.2±9.6 (19–63)*
Gender (male/female)	11/5
Height (cm)	173.4±10.5 (148–189)*
Weight (kg)	74.3±13.4 (53–105)*
BMI (kg/m^2)	24.6±2.9 (20–32)*
BSA (m^2)	1.9±0.2 (1.48–2.29)*

Note: given numbers are mean±SD (range).

The algorithm is composed of four different steps. (1) Surrounding anatomical structures are coarsely segmented to provide spatial context. (2) A region inside the liver is localized. (3) Liver tissue likelihood is estimated and refined as the mesh evolves. (4) The mesh is evolved based on likelihood and proximity to surrounding structures. False-positive and false-negative extractions could be corrected using manual correction tools. After manual positioning of 9 anatomical landmarks proposed by the software using the "work-me-through" tool in the "landmark selection mode", the segments of Couinaud were then calculated automatically, and volumes of transplanted liver segments were obtained subsequently (Fig. 1). Since the opportunity to segment automatically liver veins and portal veins between liver tissue and vasculature, P provided liver volumes with and without vessels. For TR, the images were uploaded in the 'CTA Abdomen' workflow. Using the free region-of-interest (ROI) tool, the outline of the entire liver and transplanted liver segments were set manually on every image slice, and respective liver volumes were provided always with vessels. A forth study group with TR without vessels was not performed since the proceeding would have been extremely time consuming.

Weight of Transplanted Liver Segments

The intraoperative weight of transplanted liver segments was defined as reference standard for the graft size. After resection of the respective liver segments, the grafts were flushed with normal saline to remove the blood. Grafts were prepared and weighed on the back table with a precision balance with an accuracy of 0.5 g.

Study Goals, Data Acquisition, and Statistical Analysis

The primary study goal was the definition of volumes of transplanted liver segments. Two observers (Observer 1 (T.M.) and Observer 2 (N.B.) with 1 and 3 years experience with preoperative CT-volumetry, respectively) independently performed CT-volumetry twice (interval between both reads>30 days). Consequently, 4 reads (Read 1 and Read 2 for Observer 1 as well as Read 1 and Read 2 for Observer 2) were available for P with vessels, P without vessels, and TR with vessels. To describe statistically significant differences of volume of transplanted liver segments between the 3 different techniques, ANOVA for repeated measures was applied. Linear regression analysis between intraoperative weights and volumes was performed with volume on the x-axis and intraoperative weight on the y-axis. Disagreement between intraoperative weights and volumes was calculated

as published previously [3]:

$$\text{error ratio} = (\text{volume - intraoperative weight}) / \text{intraoperative weight x 100}$$

.

To describe statistically significant differences for the error ratio between the 3 different techniques, ANOVA for repeated measures was applied. Intra-observer and inter-observer agreements of volumes were calculated applying the Blant-Altman analysis with bias and 95% limits of agreement. The secondary study goal was to describe the software workflow. The degree of manual correction during CT-volumetry was rated for each read applying a five-point Likert scale: 1–markedly lower for P compared with TR, 2–slightly lower for P compared with TR, 3–identical for P and TR, 4–slightly lower for TR compared with P, and 5–markedly lower for TR compared with P. The speed for completion of CT-volumetry (from the start of the uploading of the images to the final report) was rated for each read applying a five-point Likert scale: 1–markedly faster for P compared with TR, 2–slightly faster for P compared with TR, 3–identical for P and TR, 4–slightly faster for TR compared with P, and 5–markedly faster for TR compared with P. The overall software intuitiveness for both software types was rated by each observer applying a five-point Likert scale: 1 – markedly higher for P compared with TR, 2 – slightly higher for P compared with TR, 3 – identical for P and TR, 4 – slightly higher for TR compared with P, and markedly higher for TR compared with P. The issues impacting the workflow were described qualitatively. All procedures were performed with a commercial software (Prism 4.00, GraphPad Software, LaJolla, USA). Quantitative data were also expressed as mean and standard deviation with range. P<0.05 was considered as the level of statistical significance.

Results

Liver segments II/III, II–IV and V–VIII served in 6, 3 and 7 donors as transplanted liver segments, respectively.

Primary Study Goal

Intraoperative Weight and Volume of Transplanted Liver Segments. Full data are presented in Table 2. Volumes of transplanted liver segments were 642.9±368.8 ml for TR with

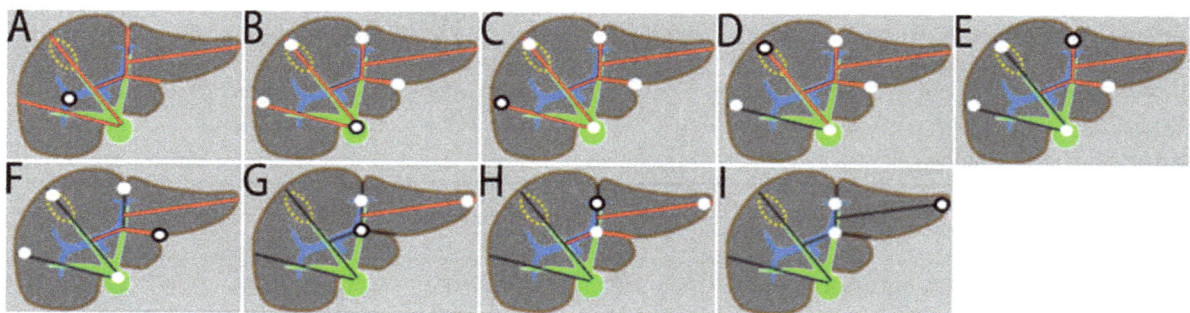

Figure 1. Semi-automated Interactive Software for CT-volumetry (P) – Manual Positioning of 9 Anatomical Landmarks to Define the Segments of Couinaud (Schematic Illustration; Courtesy of Philips Healthcare Germany, Hamburg, Germany). A first bifurcation of the right portal vein (black circle). B inferior caval vein (black circle). C right hepatic vein (black circle). D middle hepatic vein (black circle). E left hepatic vein (black circle). F superficial ligamentum venosum (black circle). G deep ligamentum venosum (black circle). H end of left portal vein (black circle). I left liver tip (black circle) Note: after automated outline of the entire liver with correction of false-positive and false-negative extractions, and then after manual positioning of the 9 anatomical landmarks, volumes of transplanted liver segments are obtained.

Table 2. Intraoperative Weights and Volumes of Transplanted Liver Segments.

Intraoperative weight (g)	TR volume with vessels (ml)	P volume with vessels (ml)	P volume without vessels (ml)	P-value*
636.1±363.1 (225.0–1310.0)*	642.9±368.8 (210.8–1345.0)*	623.8±349.1 (211.5–1281.0)*	605.2±345.8 (200.8–1291.0)*	<0.01

Note: *statistically significant differences between the 3 different techniques were evaluated applying ANOVA for repeated measures; mean of 4 reads (Read 1 and Read 2 for Observer 1 as well as Read 1 and Read 2 for Observer 2); given numbers are mean±SD (range).

vessels, 623.8±349.1 ml for P with vessels, and 605.2±345.8 ml for P without vessels. Statistically significant differences were detected between the 3 different techniques (P<0.01).

Linear Regression Analysis between Intraoperative Weight and Volume of Transplanted Liver Segments. Regression equations between intraoperative weights and volumes were y = 0.94x+30.1 (R^2 = 0.92; P<0.001) for TR with vessels, y = 1.00x+12.0 (R^2 = 0.92; P<0.001) for P with vessels, and y = 1.01x+28.0 (R^2 = 0.92; P<0.001) for P without vessels (Fig. 2).

Disagreement between Intraoperative Weight and Volume of Transplanted Liver Segments. Error ratios were −1.5±14.2% (−21.7–20.2) for TR with vessels, −2.7±13.0% (−20.4–20.6) for P with vessels, and −6.5±14.1% (−27.3–17.2) for P without vessels. Statistically significant differences were detected between the 3 different techniques (P<0.01).

Intra-observer and Inter-observer Agreement of Volume of Transplanted Liver Segments. Full data are presented in Table 3. Intra-observer agreement regarding volume for Observer 1/2 showed a bias of 25.9/−17.5 ml for TR with vessels, 2.4/−37.4 ml for P with vessels, and 5.1/−26.5 ml for P without vessels (Fig. 3). Inter-observer agreement regarding volume showed a bias of 1.8 ml for TR with vessels, 5.4 ml for P with vessels, and 4.6 ml for P without vessels. For inter-observer agreement regarding volume, the 95% limits of agreements were −20.6–24.4 ml for TR with vessels, −16.6–27.4 ml for P with vessels, and −12.8–22.1 ml for P without vessels.

Secondary Study Goal

For the degree of manual interaction, the mean scale value was 2.6±0.8 (1–5) (Fig. 4, 5). Accordingly, the degree of manual interaction was slightly lower for P compared with TR. For TR, the process of manual outline of the liver applying the free ROI tool was perceived as the major reason for the higher degree of interaction for TR. For P, manual correction tools were used on average in 8 reads (6–10 reads) per series (each series consisting of 16 reads) for correction of too large or too small Couinaud segments. For the time for completion of CT-volumetry, a scale value of 2.4±0.5 (1–5) resulted. Accordingly, the speed for completion of CT-volumetry was faster for P compared with TR. For TR, uploading of images and manual outline of the liver applying the free ROI tool were perceived as the most time consuming steps. Subsequent calculation of volume of transplanted liver segments was very fast. For P, uploading of images was perceived as a time consuming step, whereas automatic outline of the entire liver was fast. The time required for the correction of false-positive and false-negative extractions was on average 3 min (1–8) for the reads with the use of manual correction tools. The latter was also perceived as the overall most time consuming step for P. The time necessary to position the landmarks in the "work-me-through" tool was on average 2 min (1–4). Subsequent calculation of the volume of transplanted liver segments was very fast, irrespective of whether the vessels were considered or not. For the overall software intuitiveness, both observers rated a scale value of 2. Accordingly, the software intuitiveness was rated slightly lower for TR compared with P. For TR, software intuitiveness was perceived "good", and both observers reported multiple years experience with this software. For P, the "work-me-through" tool was perceived "very helpful", and the clinical implementation of this new software was perceived "auspicious".

Discussion

In this study, accuracy of estimation of graft size for living-related liver transplantation was evaluated using a semi-automated interactive software (P), and compared with a manual commercial software (TR). Prediction of graft size was good with strong linear relationships and low error ratios between intraoperative weights

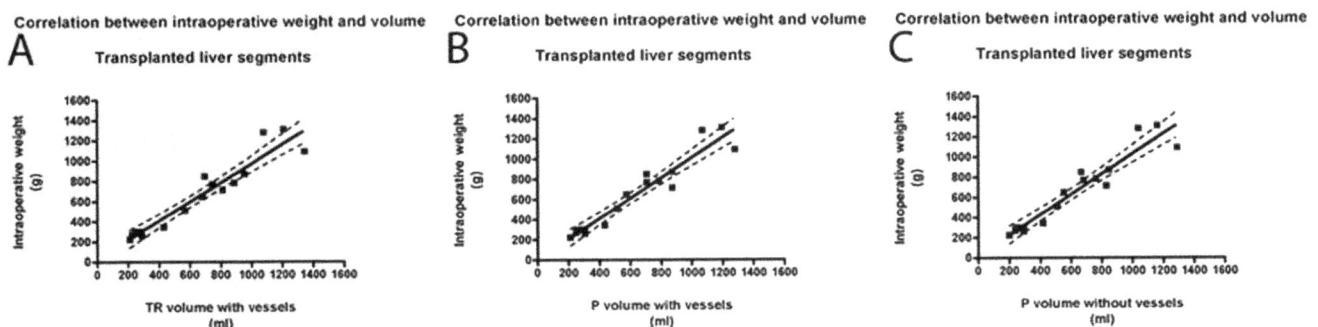

Figure 2. Linear Regression Analysis between Intraoperative Weights and Volumes of Transplanted Liver Segments. A For the manual commercial software (TR) with vessels, the regression equation was y = 0.94x+30.1 (R^2 = 0.92; P<0.001). B For the semi-automated interactive software (P) with vessels, the regression equation was y = 1.00x+12.0 (R^2 = 0.92; P<0.001). C For semi-automated interactive software (P) without vessels, the regression equation was y = 1.01x+28.0 (R^2 = 0.92; P<0.001). Note: dotted curves mark the 95% confidence bands; linear regression analysis demonstrated a strong linear relationship between intraoperative weights and volumes with comparable results between the 3 different techniques.

Table 3. Intra-observer and Inter-observer Agreement of Volume of Transplanted Liver Segments.

Volume type	Intra-observer agreement		Inter-observer agreement
	O 1	O 2	O1* versus O2*
TR volume with vessels (ml)	25.9 (−37.8–89.5)	−17.5 (−72.0–37.0)	1.8 (−20.6–24.4)
P volume with vessels (ml)	2.4 (−99.9–104.8)	−37.4 (−163.3–88.6)	5.4 (−16.6–27.4)
P volume without vessels (ml)	5.1 (−85.4–95.7)	−26.5 (−115.5–62.4)	4.6 (−12.8–22.1)

Note: O for Observer; intra-observer and inter-observer agreement was evaluated applying the Blant-Altman analysis: bias (95% limits of agreement); *mean of Read 1 and Read 2 of Observer 1 and Observer 2, respectively; given numbers are mean±SD (range).

and volumes for the different transplanted liver segments. Inter-observer and intra-observer agreements were good. Compared with TR, the workflow was better for P. The results confirmed our hypothesis that CT-volumetry performed with P can accurately predict graft size while improving workflow compared with TR.

Yoneyama et al. estimated the liver graft weight from preoperative CT [17]. The coefficient factor between estimated graft volume and actual graft weight was 0.84 for right lobes and 0.85 for left lobes. Their data indicate that CT-volumetry overestimated the actual graft weight. In our study, there was a slight trend of underestimation of the intraoperative weight of transplanted liver segments. In this context, the different approaches for CT-volumetry should be mentioned. In the study of Yoneyama et al., the volume was calculated automatically by summation of the products of section thickness and area in each section of the segmented liver. In our study, CT-volumetry was performed as voxel analysis within the outlined liver. Li et al. published results for CT-volumetry in left lobe liver donation [3]. The outline of the future liver graft was traced and marked section by section by means of a cursor with manual exclusion of non-parenchymal structures (e.g. portal vein). They found an error ratio of $13.8 \pm 8.1\%$, and as in the study by Yoneyama et al., the graft weight was overestimated although vascular structures were not segmented. From our 3 different techniques, P without vessels showed the largest differences between intraoperative weight and volume. It is likely that the significant differences of Table 2 result from this observation (since the results for TR and P with vessels were comparable). We recommend therefore to use P with vessels for the preoperative evaluation of the graft volume for potential liver donors.

Kim et al. performed a study with 88 living-related liver donors applying automated blood-free CT-volumetry [2]. The five main steps of this automated software consisted of "pre-processing", "initial shape detection", "liver segmentation", "vessel segmentation" and "liver resection". The authors found a CT volume of 789.0 ± 126.4 ml for blood-filled right lobe and 713.9 ± 114.4 ml for blood-free right lobe, whereas the intraoperative weight was 717.8 ± 110.4 g. The slight underestimation of the graft weight according to blood-free CT-volumetry is in line with our results. Kim et al., however, found the best prediction of graft weight for blood-free CT-volumetry. The corresponding linear regression equation was $y = 0.88x + 88.5$ ($R2 = 0.83$; $P < 0.001$). Our results for linear regression analysis demonstrated also a strong linear relationship between intraoperative weights and volumes, with comparable results between the 3 different techniques.

For intra-observer and inter-observer agreement regarding CT-volumetry, there is a lack of data in living-related liver donation. Our results for inter-observer agreement regarding volume were excellent, with a maximum bias of 5.4 ml. For intra-observer agreement of volume, a maximum bias of −37.5 ml was found. In view of the absolute values, this agreement could be rated as "clinically acceptable". The latter is also encouraged by the study of Dello et al., who discussed that mean liver resection volume differences of 62.3 ml (987.7 ± 64.0 ml for Surgeon 1 and 1050.0 ± 78.6 ml for Surgeon 2 applying the same software) should have no clinical consequences [18]. This statement is particularly remarkable as the weight of the resected specimen (788.8 ± 53.7g) was lower by approximately one fourth.

The different software algorithms available for CT-volumetry could also impact significantly the accuracy of estimation of future graft size. A word of caution, however, should be given to the reference standard "intraoperative weight". According to the publication of Satou et al., back-table procedures can affect the weight of transplanted liver segments [9]. During surgical

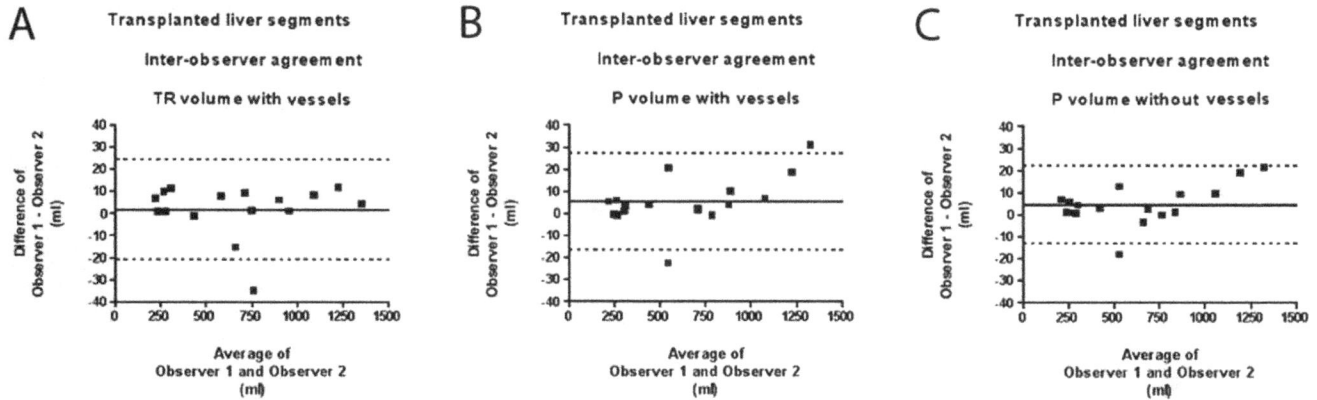

Figure 3. Blant-Altman Analysis for Inter-observer Agreement Regarding Volume of Transplanted Liver Segments. A Manual commercial software (TR) with vessels. B Semi-automated interactive software (P) with vessels. C Semi-automated interactive software (P) without vessels. Note: straight lines define bias; dotted lines define 95% limits of agreement; the inter-observer agreement can be regarded as "good" for the 3 different techniques.

preparation, the graft weight decreased significantly from "blood-filled" over "blood-free" over "after perfusion" to "after venoplasty". The authors discussed dehydration effects (e.g. induced by high osmotic preservative solution) and preparation (e.g. trimming for venous reconstruction) as relevant. Another interesting point to discuss is the perfusion pressure. Müller et al. analyzed liver volumes in an experimental setting [19]. Ten pig livers were studied in-vivo, and additionally in an ex-vivo perfusion simulator. The deviation for perfused and non-perfused livers applying ex-vivo CT-volumetry was 22.9% (15.5–37.8). The paired in-vivo results applying the water displacement technique were comparable, with a deviation for perfused and non-perfused liver volumes of 22.9% (19.0–25.6). Those observations should be kept in mind when in-vivo (perfused) CT-volumetry is compared with ex-vivo (non-perfused) gravimetry.

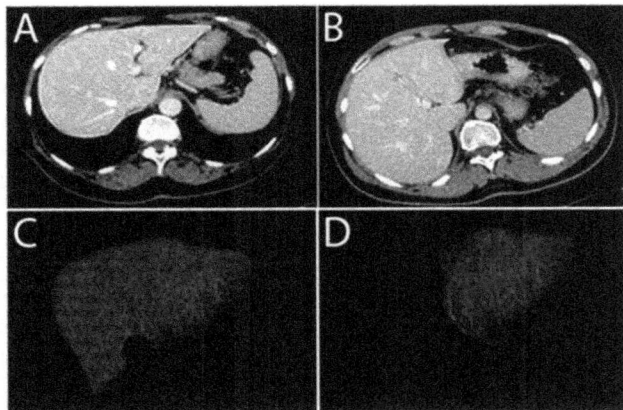

Figure 4. Manual Commercial Software (TR) – Image Example. A Transverse image of the portal-venous phase – manual outline of the entire liver (yellow). B Transverse image of the portal-venous phase – manual outline of liver segments II/III (yellow). C Volume rendering (coronal view) resulting after manual outline of the entire liver. D Volume rendering (coronal view) resulting after manual outline of liver segments II/III. Note: in each live liver donor, CT-volumetry of the entire liver as well as of the future liver graft (transplanted liver segments) were performed to ensure that the postoperative liver volume is adequate.

The workflow with a special focus on CT slice thickness was analyzed by Hori et al. [20]. The mean time required for completion of the volumetric analyses was 98 min. Although four segmentations were included (four different slice thicknessess), the time necessary per segmentation seems to be markedly longer compared with our study. Dello et al. concluded that a slice thickness of 10 mm provides an optimal balance between accuracy and time efficiency [18]. On the contrary, Puesken et al. published that a CT slice thickness of no more than 3mm should be used because of the significant deviations in measurements for thicker slices [21]. The dependency between user interaction and the different software algorithm was published by Zhou et al. [22]. As one result, the more tasks are shifted to the software, the more degrees of freedom are introduced and the larger the variations that occur. In our study, the degree of manual correction/interaction was lower for P compared with TR. Both observers reported some degree of freedom for the positioning of the anatomical landmarks (e.g. multiple slices fulfilled the landmark criteria of Fig. 1). It can be speculated that further specification in the "work-me-through" tool could lead to better volumetric results. Finally, the learning curve was better for P which is not surprising since both observers were accustomed to use TR for years. While for TR, the procedural steps regarding time and accuracy were "almost identical" between Read 1 and Read 2, for P both observers were more efficient in Read 2.

This study has limitations, most important is the small number of living-related liver donors. Although the potentially low statistical power, our concept showed feasibility in this first-in-man analysis, and opened the way to analyze more clinical data. Secondly, the absolute time to perform CT-volumetry was not recorded systematically, and therefore the description of representative quantitative data is impossible. In order to still indicate results for the duration of CT-volumetry, we used semi-quantitative methods in the form of a Lickert scale.

In conclusion, CT-volumetry performed with P can accurately predict graft size for living-related liver transplantation while improving the workflow compared with TR. The clinical use of the presented semi-automated interactive software might facilitate the radiological routine without reducing reporting quality.

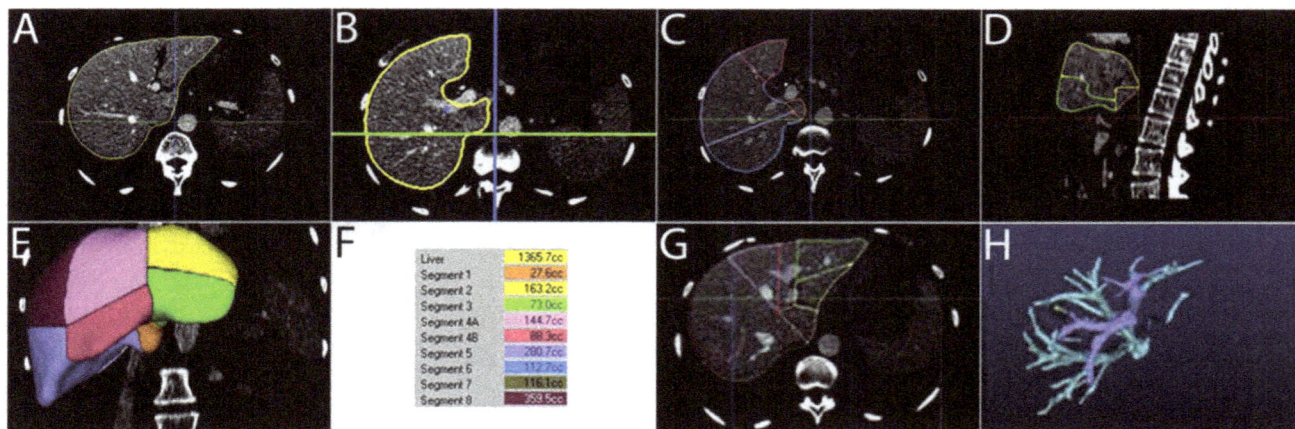

Figure 5. Semi-automated Interactive Software (P) – Image Example. A Transverse image of the portal-venous phase – automated outline of the entire liver after manual correction of false-positive and false-negative extractions. B Manual positioning of the anatomical landmark "first bifurcation of the right portal vein" (blue circle) according to Fig. 1A. C Automated definition of segments of Couinaud for right liver - transverse image. D Automated definition of segments of Couinaud for left liver - sagittal image. E Volume rendering (coronal view) with automated definition of segments of Couinaud of the entire liver. F List of volumes for the different segments of Couinaud. G Transverse image of the portal-venous phase – automated outline of the entire liver after manual correction of false-positive and false-negative extractions. H Volume rendering (coronal view) with automated definition of vessels (liver veins in light blue and portal veins in dark blue). Note: in each live liver donor, CT-volumetry of the entire liver was performed to ensure that the postoperative liver volume, calculated on the basis of Fig. 5F, is adequate.

Acknowledgments

The authors would like to thank the technicians of the Department of Diagnostic and Interventional Radiology, University Hospital Heidelberg, Heidelberg, Germany, for the performance of the time-consuming CT examinations "living-related liver donor evaluation". We thank the staff of the institutional living-donation liver transplantation program for the excellent cooperation.

Author Contributions

Conceived and designed the experiments: DM MK HUK CMS. Performed the experiments: TM NB BR PS CMS. Analyzed the data: TM NB DM JLB MK US BR PS HUK CMS. Contributed reagents/materials/analysis tools: DM. Wrote the paper: TM NB DM MK US BR PS HUK CMS. Statistics: JLB CMS. Literature research: TM NB DM US PS CMS.

References

1. Ringe KI, Ringe BP, von Flack C, Shin HO, Becker T, et al. (2012) Evaluation of living liver donors using contrast enhanced CT – The radiologists impact on donor selection. BMC Imaging 12: 21

2. Kim KW, Lee J, Lee H, Jeong WK, Won HJ, et al. (2010) Right Lobe Estimated Blood-free Weight for Living Donor Liver Transplantation: Accuracy of Automated Blood-free CT Volumetry – Preliminary Results. Radiology 256(2):433–40

3. Li YC, Hu Y, Zhang MM, Jin XQ, Fan X, et al. (2011) Usage of 64-detector-row spiral computed tomography volumetry in preoperative volume prediction in living donor liver transplantation in children. Pediatr Surg Int 27(5):445–9

4. Tango A, Pomfret EA, Pomposelli JJ (2012) Accurate Estimation of Living Donor Right Hemi-Liver Volume from Portal Vein Diameter Measurement and Standard Liver Volume Calculation. Am J Transplant 12(5):1229–39

5. Kamel IR, Raptopoulos V, Pomfret EA, Kruskal JB, Kane RA, et al. (2000) Living adult right lobe liver transplantation: imaging before surgery with multidetector multiphase CT. AJR Am J Roentgenol 175(4):1141–3.

6. Schemmer P, Mehrabi A, Friess H, Sauer P, Schmidt J, et al. (2005) Living related liver transplantation: the ultimate technique to expand the donor pool? Transplantation 80(1):S138–41.

7. Grant RC, Sandhu L, Dixon PR, Greig PD, Grant DR, et al. (2013) Living vs. deceased donor liver transplantation for hepatocellular carcinoma: a systematic review and meta-analysis. Clin Transplant 27(1):140–7

8. Müller SA, Mehrabi A, Schmied BM, Welsch T, Fonouni H, et al. (2007) Partial liver transplantation – living donor liver transplantation and split liver transplantation. Nephrol Dial Transplant 22(8):12–22

9. Satou S, Sugawara Y, Tamura S, Yamashiki N, Kaneko J, et al. (2011) Discrepancy between estimated and actual weight of partial liver graft from living donors. J Hepatobiliary Pancreas Sci 18(4):586–91

10. Lemke A-J, Brinkmann MJ, Schott T, Niehues SM, Settmacher U, et al. (2006) Living Donor Right Liver Lobes: Preoperative CT Volumetric Measurement for Calculation of Intraoperative Weight and Volume. Radiology 240: 736–42

11. Fukazawa K, Yamada Y, Nishida S, Hibi T, Arheart KL, et al. (2013) Determination of the safe range of graft size mismatch using body surface area index in deceased liver transplantation. Transpl Int. 26(7):724–33

12. Nakayama Y, Li Q, Katsuragawa S, Ikeda R, Hiai Y, et al. (2006) Automated Hepatic Volumetry for Living Related Liver Transplantation At Multisection CT. Radiology 240(3):743–8

13. Fischer L, Tetzlaff R, Schöbinger M, Radeleff B, Bruckner T, et al. (2010) How many CT detector rows are necessary to perform adequate three dimensional visualization? Eur J Radiol 74(3):114–8

14. Krawczyk M, Paluszkiewicz R, Pacho R, Hevelke P, Zieniewicz, et al. (2003) Liver regeneration in living-related donors after harvesting of liver segments II and III or II, III and IV. HPB (Oxford) 5(3):146–51

15. Neumann JO, Thorn M, Fischer L, Schöbinger M, Heimann T, et al. (2006) Branching patterns and drainage territories of the middle hepatic vein in computer-simulated right living-donor hepatectomies. Am J Transplant 6(6):1407–15

16. Sauer P, Schemmer P, Uhl W, Encke J (2004) Living-donor liver transplantation: evaluation of donor and recipient. Nephrol Dial Transplant 19(4):11–5

17. Yoneyama T, Asonuma K, Okajima H, Lee KJ, Yamamoto H, et al. (2011) Coefficient factor for graft weight estimation from preoperative computed tomography volumetry in living donor liver transplantation. Liver Transpl 17(4):369–72

18. Dello SA, Stoot JH, van Stiphout RS, Bloemen JG, Wigmore SJ, et al. (2011) Prospective volumetric assessment of the liver on a personal computer by nonradiologists prior to partial hepatectomy. World J Surg 35(2):386–92

19. Müller SA, Pianka F, Schöbinger M, Mehrabi A, Fonouni H, et al. (2011) Computer-based liver volumetry in the liver perfusion simulator. J Surg Res 171(1):87–93

20. Hori M, Suzuki K, Epstein ML, Baron RL (2011) Computed tomography liver volumetry using 3-dimensional image data in living donor liver transplantation: effects of the slice thickness on the volume calculation. Liver Transpl 17(12):1427–36

21. Puesken M, Buerke B, Fortkamp R, Koch R, Seifarth H, et al. (2011) Liver lesion segmentation in MSCT: effect of slice thickness on segmentation quality, measurement precision and interobserver variability. Rofo 183(4):372–80

22. Zhou J-Y, Wong DWK, Ding F, Venkatesh SK, Tian Q, et al. (2010) Liver tumour segmentation using contrast-enhanced multi-detector CT data: performance benchmarking of three semiautomated methods. Eur Radiol 20: 1738–48.

4

Proton Pump Inhibitor Intake neither Predisposes to Spontaneous Bacterial Peritonitis or Other Infections nor Increases Mortality in Patients with Cirrhosis and Ascites

Mattias Mandorfer[1,4], Simona Bota[1,4], Philipp Schwabl[1,4], Theresa Bucsics[1,4], Nikolaus Pfisterer[1,4], Christian Summereder[1,4], Michael Hagmann[2], Alexander Blacky[3], Arnulf Ferlitsch[1,4], Wolfgang Sieghart[1,4], Michael Trauner[1,4], Markus Peck-Radosavljevic[1,4], Thomas Reiberger[1,4]*

1 Division of Gastroenterology and Hepatology, Department of Internal Medicine III, Medical University of Vienna, Vienna, Austria, 2 Section for Medical Statistics, Center for Medical Statistics, Informatics, and Intelligent Systems, Medical University of Vienna, Vienna, Austria, 3 Clinical Institute of Hospital Hygiene, Vienna General Hospital, Vienna, Austria, 4 Vienna Hepatic Hemodynamic Lab, Division of Gastroenterology and Hepatology, Department of Internal Medicine III, Medical University of Vienna, Vienna, Austria

Abstract

Background and Aim: The aim of this study was to assess the impact of proton pump inhibitor (PPI) intake on the development of spontaneous bacterial peritonitis (SBP) or other infections, as well as on mortality, in a thoroughly documented cohort of patients with cirrhosis and ascites.

Patients and Methods: We performed a retrospective analysis of follow-up data from 607 consecutive patients with cirrhosis undergoing their first paracentesis at a tertiary center. A binary logistic regression model investigating the association between PPI intake and SBP at the first paracentesis was calculated. Competing risk analyses and Cox models were used to investigate the effect of PPIs on the cumulative incidence of SBP or other infections and transplant-free survival, respectively. Adjustments were made for age, hepatocellular carcinoma, history of variceal bleeding, varices and model of end-stage liver disease score.

Results: Eighty-six percent of patients were receiving PPIs. After adjusting for potential confounding factors, PPI intake was neither associated with increased SBP prevalence at the first paracentesis (odds ratio (OR):1.11,95% confidence interval (95%CI):0.6–2.06; $P = 0.731$) nor cumulative incidence of SBP (subdistribution hazard ratio (SHR): 1.38; 95%CI:0.63–3.01; $P = 0.42$) and SBP or other infections (SHR:1.71; 95%CI:0.85–3.44; $P = 0.13$) during follow-up. Moreover, PPI intake had no impact on transplant-free survival in both the overall cohort (hazard ratio (HR):0.973,95%CI:0.719–1.317; $P = 0.859$) as well as in the subgroups of patients without SBP (HR:1.01,95%CI:0.72–1.42; $P = 0.971$) and without SBP or other infections at the first paracentesis (HR:0.944,95%CI:0.668–1.334; $P = 0.742$).

Conclusions: The proportion of cirrhotic patients with PPI intake was higher than in previous reports, suggesting that PPI indications were interpreted liberally. In our cohort with a particularly high prevalence of PPI intake, we observed no association between PPIs and SBP or other infections, as well as mortality. Thus, the severity of liver disease and other factors, rather than PPI treatment *per se* may predispose for infectious complications.

Editor: Erica Villa, University of Modena & Reggio Emilia, Italy

Funding: The authors have no support or funding to report.

Competing Interests: The authors have declared that no competing interests exist.

* Email: thomas.reiberger@meduniwien.ac.at

Introduction

Cirrhosis, which accounts for 1.8% of all deaths in Europe [1], is the 12th leading cause of death in the United States, though a recent report suggests even this rank to be an underestimation [2].

According to a prognostic model proposed by D'Amico and co-workers [3], the occurrence of varices initiates the second stage of cirrhosis, the third stage is defined by the development of ascites and variceal hemorrhage initiates the fourth stage. The occurrence

of bacterial infections, which delineates an additional fifth stage of cirrhosis termed the "critically ill" patient with cirrhosis [4], as it increases mortality of patients with decompensated cirrhosis up to four-fold. Thirty percent of patients die within 1 month and another 30% die during the first year after onset of infection [4]. These bacterial infections predominately occur in decompensated patients with advanced cirrhosis who typically have ascites. Spontaneous bacterial peritonitis (SBP) is the most common infection among patients with cirrhosis [5] and a consequence of quantitative and qualitative changes in gut microbiota, increased intestinal permeability and bacterial translocation [6]. In addition immunologic impairments observed in patients with advanced cirrhosis may play a role [5]. Small intestinal bacterial overgrowth (SIBO), a quantitative change of the gut microbiota, has been found to be associated with SBP development [7] and Chang and co-workers observed higher rates of SIBO among patients with a history of SBP [8]. Moreover, an association between SIBO and the presence of bacterial DNA in the peripheral blood of cirrhotic patients has been observed [9]. Impaired small intestinal motility [8], portal hypertension [10] and acid-suppressive therapy, such as proton pump inhibitors (PPIs) [11], have been reported as factors contributing to SIBO in patients with cirrhosis.

Several studies have observed an association between PPI intake and SBP development [12–18] and this relationship has recently been confirmed by a meta-analysis [19]. However, this association was not observed in all cohorts [16,20], as demonstrated by one of the few prospective studies on the association between PPI intake and SBP development [20]. In fact, Kwon and co-workers [12] reported increased mortality after SBP development among patients with PPI intake, while other studies have observed a lack of effect on mortality [13,20]. Moreover, several major limitations related to the study design as well as the consideration of potential confounding factors substantially limit the conclusions drawn from previous studies and the meta-analysis based on their results.

The aim of this study was to assess the impact of PPI intake on (i) the development of SBP or other infections, as well as (ii) on mortality, in a large, thoroughly documented cohort of patients with cirrhosis and ascites.

Patients and Methods

Study design

A total of 607 previously investigated [21] consecutive patients with cirrhosis who underwent their first paracentesis at the Medical University of Vienna between 2006 and 2011 were included in this retrospective study. Patients were followed up until 2011. Patients with other causes of ascites, such as severe cardiovascular disease, renal insufficiency, extra-hepatic malignancies and non-cirrhotic portal hypertension were excluded from the study.

Assessed parameters

Epidemiological characteristics, etiology of cirrhosis, presence of hepatocellular carcinoma (HCC), liver transplantation, varices as well as information on history of variceal bleeding were assessed from patients' medical records. Thus, information on varices was not only based on endoscopic examinations exactly at the time of the first paracententesis. Moreover, information on PPI, non-selective beta blocker (NSBB) and rifaximin intake was obtained from patients' medical records. Laboratory parameters were assessed at the first paracentesis and at the first diagnosis of SBP including platelet count, albumin, bilirubin, international normalized ratio (INR), creatinine and ascitic fluid polymorphnuclear neutrophil (PMN) count. Hepatic venous pressure gradient (HVPG) measurements were performed as described previously [22]. The model for end-stage liver disease (MELD) [23] and Child-Pugh score (CPS) [24] were calculated based on laboratory parameters and patients' medical history.

Paracenteses, diagnosis of SBP and other infections and definition of resolution of infection

Patients were grouped according to the presence of signs or symptoms or laboratory abnormalities suggestive of or associated with infection (e.g., abdominal pain or tenderness, fever, unexplained encephalopathy, AKI, leukocytosis and variceal bleeding) and paracentesis volume: diagnostic paracentesis (paracentesis volume <5 L), diagnostic large-volume paracentesis (LVP; paracentesis volume $\geq$5 L), and therapeutic LVP (no clinical or laboratory evidence for infection and paracentesis volume $\geq$5 L).

In accordance with national guidelines [25,26], albumin was administered in LVPs and patients received long-term prophylaxis with quinolones after SBP development. SBP was diagnosed if the ascitic PMN count was >250 cells x mL^{-1} in absence of an intra-abdominal source of infection or any other explanation for an elevated PMN count [26–28].

In addition, patients' medical records were reviewed for hospitalizations resulting from infections other than SBP or development of systemic infections during hospitalizations due to other reasons. The standardized work up at hospital admission included laboratory blood and urine tests, as well as a chest X-ray. Systemic infections were diagnosed based on the American College of Chest Physicians (ACCP)/Society of Critical Care Medicine (SCCM) definitions for systemic inflammatory response syndrome (SIRS) and sepsis [29].

Resolution of SBP or other infections was defined by the regression of clinical or laboratory evidence for infection within 7 days after the diagnosis, as well as the absence or regression of infection-related complications such as grade 3/4 hepatic encephalopathy according to West Haven criteria [30] and acute kidney injury (AKI) within 7 days after the diagnosis of infection. AKI was defined as group C of the modified acute kidney injury classification proposed by Fagundes and co-workers [31].

Statistics

Statistical analyses were conducted using IBM SPSS Statistics 21 (SPSS Inc., Armok, USA) and R.3.0.2 (R Core Team, R Foundation for Statistical Computing, Vienna, Austria). Continuous variables were reported as mean $\pm$standard deviation or median (interquartile range), while categorical variables were reported as numbers (proportions) of patients with the certain characteristic. Student's t-test was used for group comparisons of continuous variables when applicable. Otherwise, Mann-Whitney U test was applied. Group comparisons of categorical variables were performed using either Pearson's chi-squared or Fisher's exact test.

A binary logistic regression model investigating the association between PPI intake and SBP at the first paracentesis adjusted for all variables (age, HCC, history of variceal bleeding, varices and MELD score) that were not comparable between PPI and no-PPI patients (Table 1) was calculated.

The impact of PPI intake on the cumulative incidence of SBP or other infections was analyzed by a competing risk analyses [32] treating death as a competing risk. Cumulative incidence functions are shown for the models investigating the incidence of SBP or other infections (Figure 1). Transplant-free survival was analyzed using Cox proportional hazards models. Patients who underwent a liver transplantation were censored on the day of surgery. Transplant-free survival time was defined as the time to liver transplantation, death or end of follow-up. Kaplan-Meier curves are presented for transplant-free survival models (Figure 2). In addition to PPI intake, age, HCC, history of variceal bleeding, varices and MELD score were considered as covariates in all of the above-mentioned models, as they were not comparable between PPI and no-PPI patients (Table 1).

All patients without SBP entered the SBP cumulative incidence model (Model 1) with their first paracentesis, while the SBP or

Table 1. Patient Characteristics.

Patient characteristics	All patients, n = 607	no-PPI, n = 87	PPI, n = 520	P value
Age, years	57.5±11.8	60.2±12.1	57.1±11.7	0.02
Sex				
Male	426 (70%)	59 (68%)	367 (71%)	0.602
Female	181 (30%)	28 (32%)	153 (29%)	
Etiology				
ALD	336 (55%)	41 (47%)	295 (57%)	0.38
Viral	113 (19%)	20 (23%)	93 (18%)	
ALD and viral	49 (8%)	9 (10%)	40 (8%)	
Other	109 (18%)	17 (20%)	92 (18%)	
HCC	129 (21%)	28 (32%)	101 (19%)	0.007
History of variceal bleeding	111 (18%)	9 (10%)	102 (20%)	0.038
Varices	443 (73%)	52 (60%)	391 (75%)	0.003
Upper-gastrointestinal bleeding	46 (8%)	6 (7%)	40 (8%)	0.795
At Hospital admission	32 (5%)	4 (5%)	28 (5%)	0.808
During hospitalization	14 (2%)	2 (2%)	12 (2%)	1
Portal hypertensive bleeding	35 (6%)	4 (5%)	31 (6%)	0.642
HVPG*, mmHg	18.7±6.5	17.3±5.8	18.8±6.6	0.273
MELD	17.5 (10.6)	15.2 (7.7)	18 (10.3)	0.037
CPS				
A	22 (4%)	5 (6%)	17 (3%)	0.361
B	281 (46%)	43 (49%)	238 (46%)	
C	304 (50%)	39 (45%)	265 (51%)	
Platelet count, G x L^{-1}	117 (107)	138 (104)	117 (110)	0.17
Albumin, g x L^{-1}	27.2±5.7	27.8±5.9	27.1±5.6	0.337
Bilirubin, mg x dL^{-1}	3.2 (6.02)	2.43 (4.07)	3.34 (6.34)	0.046
INR	1.38 (0.58)	1.33 (0.47)	1.39 (0.59)	0.135
Creatinine, mg x dL^{-1}	1.14 (0.78)	1.14 (0.64)	1.14 (0.78)	0.949
Rifaximin treatment	63 (10%)	6 (7%)	57 (11%)	0.25
NSBB treatment	245 (40%)	32 (37%)	213 (41%)	0.462
Hospitalization prior to paracentesis, days	1 (4)	1 (6)	1 (4)	0.343
Paracentesis indication				
Diagnostic paracentesis	258 (43%)	45 (52%)	213 (41%)	0.133
Diagnostic LVP	270 (44%)	30 (34%)	240 (46%)	
Therapeutic LVP	79 (13%)	12 (14%)	67 (13%)	
SBP at first paracentesis	114 (19%)	15 (17%)	99 (19%)	0.691
Systemic infection at first paracentesis	34 (6%)	1 (1%)	33 (6%)	0.072

*Information on HVPG was available in 220 patients.
Patient characteristics at the first paracentesis and comparison of patients with (PPI) and without (no-PPI) proton pump inhibitor therapy.
Abbreviations: PPI proton pump inhibitor; ALD alcoholic liver disease; HCC hepatocellular carcinoma; HVPG hepatic venous pressure gradient; MELD model for end-stage liver disease; CPS Child-Pugh score; INR international normalized ratio; NSBB non-selective beta blocker; LVP large-volume paracentesis.

other infections cumulative incidence model (Model 2) was restricted to patients without SBP or another infection at the first paracentesis.

Moreover, we assessed the effect of PPI intake on transplant-free survival in the overall cohort (Model 3), among patients without SBP (Model 4) and among patients without SBP or other infections at the first paracentesis (Model 5).

P values <0.05 were considered as statistically significant.

Ethics

This study was conducted in accordance with the Declaration of Helsinki and approved by the local ethics committee of the Medical University of Vienna (EK Nr. 1008/2011). Due to the retrospective design of the study, the local ethics committee did not require a written informed consent from the study participants. Patient data was pseudonymized prior to statistical analysis.

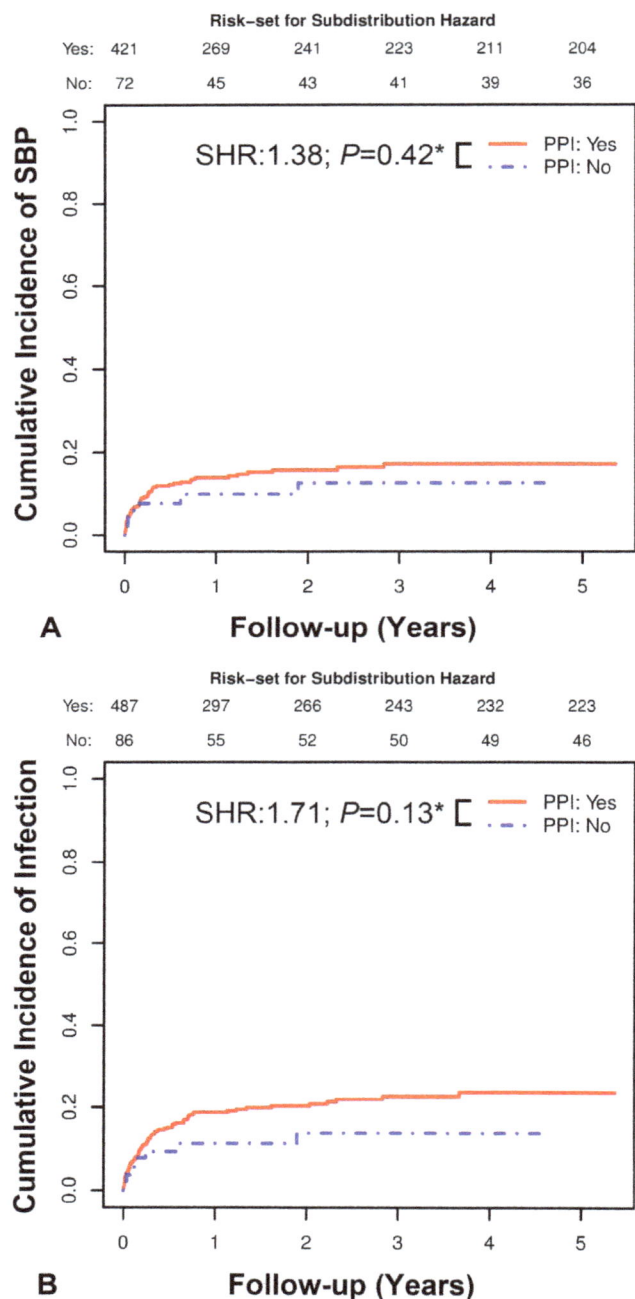

Figure 1. PPI Intake and Cumulative Incidence of SBP or other Infections. Impact of PPI intake on **A** cumulative incidence of SBP among patients without SBP at the first paracentesis and **B** cumulative incidence of SBP or other infections among patients without SBP or another infection at the first paracentesis. Statistics: The impact of PPI intake on the cumulative incidence of SBP or other infections was analyzed by a competing risk analysis [32] treating death as a competing risk. *In addition to PPI intake, age, HCC, history of variceal bleeding, varices and MELD score were considered covariates. Cumulative incidence functions are shown for the models investigating the incidence of SBP or other infections. Abbreviations: PPI proton pump inhibitor; SBP spontaneous bacterial peritonitis; SHR subdistribution hazard ratio; HCC hepatocellular carcinoma; MELD model for end-stage liver disease.

Results

Patient characteristics at the first paracentesis (Table 1)

The majority of patients (70%) were male, with a mean age of 57.5 ± 11.8 years. The predominant etiology of cirrhosis was alcoholic liver disease (ALD) (55%), followed by chronic viral hepatitis (19%) and the combination of ALD and chronic viral hepatitis (8%). In 18% percent of patients, other etiologies of cirrhosis were reported. Twenty-one percent of patients were diagnosed with HCC and 18% had a history of variceal bleeding, though varices were present in 73% of patients. Five percent of patients presented with upper-gastrointestinal bleeding at hospital admission, while 2% developed upper-gastrointestinal bleeding during hospitalization. Portal hypertensive bleeding at admission or during hospitalization was observed in 6% of patients. Information on HVPG was available in a subgroup of 220 patients, with a mean HVPG of 18.7 ± 6.5 mmHg. The median MELD score was 17.5 (10.6) and the distribution of CPS stage was as follows: A: 4%, B: 46% and C: 50%. Ten percent of patients received rifaximin, while 40% of patients were administered NSBB treatment. The median duration of hospitalization prior to the paracentesis was 1 (4) day. Forty-three percent of paracenteses were diagnostic, 44% were diagnostic LVPs and 13% were therapeutic LVPs.

Among 607 cirrhotic patients with ascites, PPI intake was present in 520 (86%) of patients. At the first paracentesis, mean age was lower (PPI: 57.1 ± 11.7 vs. no-PPI: 60.2 ± 12.1 years; $P = 0.02$), while median MELD score was higher (PPI: 18 (10.3) vs. no-PPI: 15.2 (7.7); $P = 0.037$) among patients with PPI intake. While the proportion of patients with HCC was higher among patients without PPI intake (PPI: 19% vs. no-PPI: 32%; $P = 0.007$), history of variceal bleeding (PPI: 20% vs. no-PPI: 10%; $P = 0.038$) and varices (PPI: 75% vs. no-PPI: 60%; $P = 0.003$) were more frequently observed in the PPI group. No other statistically significant differences in patient characteristics between patients with PPI intake, and without, were observed.

Patient characteristics of the subgroups of patients without SBP and patients without SBP or other infections at the first paracentesis are shown in Table S1 and Table S2, respectively.

Follow-up of patients

A total of 607 patients were followed for 486 person-years after their first paracentesis. Of these, 59% underwent a liver transplantation or died and 7% were lost to follow-up. The proportion of patients who were lost to follow-up was similar in the subgroups of patients with PPI intake (7%) and without (6%; $P = 0.642$).

Impact of PPI intake on SBP prevalence at the first paracentesis and SBP incidence during follow-up

The proportion of patients with SBP at the first paracentesis was comparable between the PPI (19%) and no-PPI (17%; $P = 0.691$) group. In multivariate logistic regression analysis, neither PPI treatment (odds ratio (OR): 1.11, 95% confidence interval (95%CI): 0.602–2.061; $P = 0.731$), nor any of the other covariates including age (per 10 years, OR: 1, 95%CI: 0.99–1; $P = 0.704$), HCC (OR: 1.48, 95%CI: 0.91–2.41; $P = 0.116$), history of variceal bleeding (OR: 0.673, 95%CI: 0.376–1.205; $P = 0.183$), varices (OR: 1.54; 95%CI: 0.93–2.55; $P = 0.093$) and MELD score (per point, OR: 1.02, 95%CI: 1–1.05; $P = 0.077$) were associated with SBP prevalence.

Among patients without SBP at the first paracentesis, PPI intake was not associated with the cumulative incidence of SBP (subdistribution hazard ratio (SHR): 1.38; 95%CI: 0.63–3.01;

A

B

C

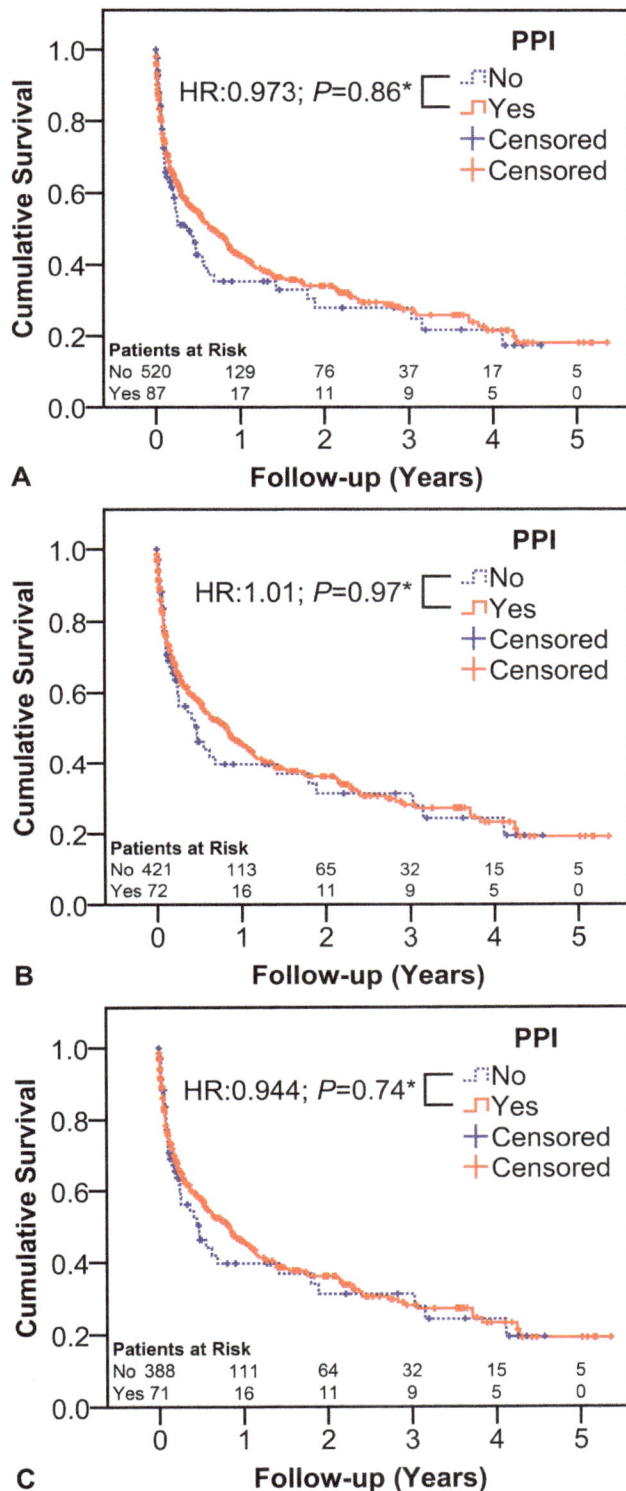

Figure 2. PPI Intake and Transplant-free Survival. Influence of PPI intake on transplant-free survival in **A** the overall cohort, **B** among patients without SBP and **C** among patients without SBP or others infections at the first paracentesis. Statistics: Transplant-free survival was analyzed using Cox proportional hazards models. *In addition to PPI intake, age, HCC, history of variceal bleeding, varices and MELD score are considered covariates in all of the above-mentioned models. Kaplan-Meier curves are presented for transplant-free survival models. Abbreviations: PPI proton pump inhibitor; SBP spontaneous bacterial peritonitis; HR hazard ratio; HCC hepatocellular carcinoma; MELD model for end-stage liver disease.

$P = 0.42$) during follow-up when adjusting for age, HCC, history of variceal bleeding, varices and MELD score (Figure 1; Table 2). We observed a trend toward an increased cumulative incidence of SBP among patients with a history of variceal bleeding (SHR: 1.71, 95%CI: 0.96–3.05; $P = 0.07$).

Influence of PPI intake on the prevalence of systemic infections at the first paracentesis and incidence of SBP or other infections during follow-up

Systemic non-SBP infections were classified as sepsis (31%), pneumonia (22%), urinary tract infections (11%), cellulitis (5%), C. difficile infection (4%) and other specific infections (11%). In 16% of patients, no specific type of infection could be identified, although they presented with clinical or laboratory evidence for systemic infection.

There was a trend toward a higher proportion of patients with systemic infections other than SBP at the first paracentesis in the PPI group (PPI: 6% vs. no-PPI: 1%; $P = 0.072$). When considering both SBP and other systemic infections as a combined event, prevalence rates at the first paracentesis were comparable between treatment groups (PPI: 25% vs. no-PPI: 18%; $P = 0.16$).

Among patients without SBP or another infection at the first paracentesis, the association between PPI intake and the cumulative incidence of the combined event (SHR: 1.71; 95%CI: 0.85–3.44; $P = 0.13$) during follow-up did not attain statistical significance, when adjusting for age, HCC, history of variceal bleeding, varices and MELD score (Figure 1; Table 2).

Impact of PPI intake on resolution of SBP or other infections

Resolution was assessed for all SBPs and other systemic infections at the first paracentesis, as well as all incident SBPs and other systemic infections during follow-up (n = 233). The proportion of patients in which the infection was resolved was similar among patients with PPI intake (56%), and without (52%; $P = 0.686$). Moreover, we observed similar rates of infection resolution in the subgroup of patients with SBP (PPI: 60% vs. no-PPI: 50%; $P = 0.36$).

Impact of PPI intake on transplant-free survival

The influence of PPI intake on transplant-free survival was studied in the overall cohort, among patients without SBP and among patients without SBP or other infections at the first paracentesis (Figure 2; Table 3). While higher age (per 10 years, HR: 1.38, 95%CI: 1.25–1.53, $P<0.001$), the presence of HCC (HR: 2.41, 95%CI: 1.88–3.08; $P<0.001$) and higher MELD score (per point, HR: 1.56, 95%CI: 1.45–1.68; $P<0.001$) were associated with decreased transplant-free survival in the overall cohort, no association with PPI intake (HR: 0.97, 95%CI: 0.72–1.32; $P = 0.859$) was observed.

Discussion

The emergence of alarming results from recent studies [12–18] has initiated an intense debate on whether PPI intake has an adverse effect on the occurrence of infectious complications among patients with cirrhosis and ascites. However, in addition to their retrospective design, most previous studies display limitations, which must be considered. The majority of studies either

Table 2. PPI Intake and Cumulative Incidence of SBP or other Infections.

Patient characteristics	A Cumulative incidence of SBP n=493, Model 1				B Cumulative incidence of SBP or systemic infection n=459, Model 2			
	SHR	95%CI lower	upper	P value	SHR	95%CI lower	upper	P value
Age, per 10 years	1	0.98	1.02	0.71	1	0.98	1.02	0.96
HCC, yes	1.35	0.74	2.46	0.33	1.01	0.61	1.68	0.97
History of variceal Bleeding, yes	1.71	0.96	3.05	0.07	1.46	0.91	2.35	0.12
Varices, yes	0.82	0.48	1.64	0.69	0.9	0.55	1.48	0.68
MELD, per point	0.99	0.96	1.02	0.4	0.98	0.96	1.01	0.18
PPI, yes	1.38	0.63	3.01	0.42	1.71	0.85	3.44	0.13

Impact of PPI intake on **A** cumulative incidence of SBP among patients without SBP at the first paracentesis and **B** cumulative incidence of SBP or other infections among patients without SBP or another infection at the first paracentesis.

Statistics: The impact of PPI intake on the cumulative incidence of SBP or other infections was analyzed by a competing risk analysis [32] treating death as a competing risk. In addition to PPI intake, age, HCC, history of variceal bleeding, varices and MELD score were considered covariates.

Abbreviations: PPI proton pump inhibitor; SBP spontaneous bacterial peritonitis; SHR subdistribution hazard ratio; HCC hepatocellular carcinoma; MELD model for end-stage liver disease.

Table 3. PPI Intake and Transplant-free Survival.

Patient characteristics	A Transplant-free mortality All patients n=607, Model 3				B Transplant-free mortality No SBP at first paracentesis, n=493, Model 4				C Transplant-free mortality No SBP or systemic infection at first paracentesis n=459, Model 5			
	HR	95%CI lower	upper	P value	HR	95%CI lower	upper	P value	HR	95%CI lower	upper	P value
Age, per 10 years	1.38	1.25	1.53	<0.001	1.32	1.17	1.48	<0.001	1.33	1.18	1.51	<0.001
HCC, yes	2.41	1.88	3.08	<0.001	2.59	1.96	3.43	<0.001	2.79	2.09	3.74	<0.001
History of variceal bleeding, yes	1.01	0.77	1.34	0.923	1.17	0.86	1.59	0.322	1.14	0.82	1.57	0.433
Varices, yes	1.13	0.88	1.44	0.35	1.07	0.81	1.42	0.617	1.15	0.86	1.56	0.35
MELD, per point	1.56	1.45	1.68	<0.001	1.54	1.41	1.69	<0.001	1.51	1.37	1.66	<0.001
PPI, yes	0.97	0.72	1.32	0.859	1.01	0.72	1.42	0.971	0.94	0.67	1.33	0.742

Influence of PPI intake on transplant-free survival in **A** the overall cohort, **B** among patients without SBP and **C** among patients without SBP or others infections at the first paracentesis.

Statistics: Transplant-free survival was analyzed using Cox proportional hazards models. In addition to PPI intake, age, HCC, history of variceal bleeding, varices and MELD score were considered covariates in all of the above-mentioned models.

Abbreviations: PPI proton pump inhibitor; SBP spontaneous bacterial peritonitis; HR hazard ratio; HCC hepatocellular carcinoma; MELD model for end-stage liver disease.

investigated a relatively small sample size [13–17,20], or had a case-control, rather than a longitudinal cohort design [13–17]. Moreover, some studies insufficiently controlled for potential confounding factors or did not consider death as a competing risk when investigating the impact of PPI treatment on the incidence of SBP or other infections.

Our study, although retrospective, is a longitudinal study based on a large, thoroughly documented cohort of patients with cirrhosis and ascites and applied competing risk analyses [32] treating death as a competing risk. Previous studies reporting an association between PPI intake and SBP incidence were based on cohorts with a lower proportion of patients on PPI treatment [12,13], suggesting indications for PPI administration were followed more rigorously. In contrast, in our cohort, the particularly high prevalence of PPI intake (86%) suggests that the indications for PPI treatment were interpreted liberally in daily clinical practice. However, in the context of rather high PPI intake, we observed no association between PPI intake and SBP, as well as mortality. Although the prevalence of peptic ulcers is increased among cirrhotic patients and correlates with the severity of liver disease [33], PPI intake might have been initiated based on indications which are not sufficiently supported by evidence, such as portal hypertensive gastropathy, varices or history of variceal bleeding, abdominal pain or discomfort induced by distension of the abdomen, as well as polypharmacy [34].

In our study, the proportion of patients with HCC was higher in the no-PPI group, while the proportions of patients with varices and a history of variceal bleeding were higher in the PPI group. PPI intake was associated with higher age and MELD score, factors that were associated with lower transplant-free survival in our study. In addition, patients with a history of variceal bleeding had a numerically higher risk of SBP development during follow-up. Other potential confounding factors, such as the portal hypertensive bleeding at admission or during hospitalization, duration of hospitalization prior to paracentesis and indication for paracentesis were assessed and found to be comparable between patients with PPI intake, and without. However, the retrospective assessment of the indication for paracentesis has limitations and since the American Association for the Study of the Liver (AASLD) practice guideline for the management of adult patients with ascites due to cirrhosis [28] recommends paracentesis at the first development of ascites and at hospital admission, none of the paracenteses might have been solely therapeutic. Importantly, most previous studies did not provide sufficient information on these potential confounding factors. Thus, it cannot be excluded that the severity of the underlying liver disease and other factors, rather than PPI treatment *per se,* may predispose for infectious complications in patients with cirrhosis and ascites.

Moreover, hospitalization due to infections other than SBP or development of systemic infections during hospitalization for other reasons was assessed. Systemic infections during follow-up were not very common in our cohort of cirrhotic patients with ascites. The retrospective assessment of systemic inflammatory response syndrome (SIRS) and sepsis according to the American College of Chest Physicians (ACCP)/Society of Critical Care Medicine (SCCM) definitions [29] has inherent weaknesses, especially in patients with liver cirrhosis, in which the diagnostic capacity of SIRS criteria might already be limited [35,36]. The retrospective assessment could have had an impact on the prevalence and

incidence of systemic infections observed in our study, although there was a standardized work up at hospital admission including laboratory blood and urine tests, as well as a chest X-ray. Moreover, infections treated in an outpatient setting were not assessed. Since hospitalization is generally recommended for cirrhotic patients with ascites presenting with signs and symptoms of systemic infection, this might not have significantly affected our results. Moreover, as patients have not been prospectively followed, we cannot entirely rule out that some events were missed, especially if patients were treated outside of Vienna or in private hospitals. We observed a trend toward a higher prevalence of systemic infections other than SBP at the first paracentesis in the PPI group. However, this was an unadjusted analysis not considering the previously mentioned unfavorable baseline characteristics of the PPI group, as multivariate analysis was not feasible due to the low number of events. When considering both SBP and other systemic infections as a combined event, prevalence rates at the first paracentesis were comparable between the treatment groups. Importantly, there was no association between PPI intake and the combined event during follow-up, when adjusting for potential confounding factors.

In conclusion, we observed no association between PPIs and SBP or other infections, as well as mortality, in our large, thoroughly documented cohort of patients with cirrhosis and ascites with a particularly high prevalence of PPI intake. The severity of the underlying liver disease and other factors, rather than PPI treatment *per se* may predispose for complications in patients with cirrhosis and ascites. Nevertheless, the restriction of PPI treatment to evidence-based indications should be emphasized.

Supporting Information

Table S1 Patient characteristics of patients without SBP at the first paracentesis and comparison of patients with (PPI) and without (no-PPI) proton pump inhibitor therapy. Abbreviations: PPI proton pump inhibitor; ALD alcoholic liver disease; HCC hepatocellular carcinoma; HVPG hepatic venous pressure gradient; MELD model for end-stage liver disease; CPS Child-Pugh score; INR international normalized ratio; NSBB non-selective beta blocker; LVP large-volume paracentesis.

Table S2 Patient characteristics of patients without SBP or other infection at the first paracentesis and comparison of patients with (PPI) and without (no-PPI) proton pump inhibitor therapy. Abbreviations: PPI proton pump inhibitor; ALD alcoholic liver disease; HCC hepatocellular carcinoma; HVPG hepatic venous pressure gradient; MELD model for end-stage liver disease; CPS Child-Pugh score; INR international normalized ratio; NSBB non-selective beta blocker; LVP large-volume paracentesis.

Author Contributions

Study concept and design: MM PS MH AF WS MT MP TR. Acquisition of data: SB PS TB NP CS AB TR. Statistical analysis: MM MH. Interpretation of data: MM MH AF WS MT MP TR. Drafting of the manuscript: MM MH TR. Critical revision for important intellectual content and approval of the final version of the manuscript: MM SB PS TB NP CS MH AB AF WS MT MP TR.

References

1. Blachier M, Leleu H, Peck-Radosavljevic M, Valla DC, Roudot-Thoraval F (2013) The burden of liver disease in Europe: a review of available epidemiological data. J Hepatol 58: 593–608.

2. Asrani SK, Larson JJ, Yawn B, Therneau TM, Kim WR (2013) Underestimation of liver-related mortality in the United States. Gastroenterology 145: 375–382.

3. D'Amico G, Garcia-Tsao G, Pagliaro L (2006) Natural history and prognostic indicators of survival in cirrhosis: a systematic review of 118 studies. J Hepatol 44: 217–231.

4. Arvaniti V, D'Amico G, Fede G, Manousou P, Tsochatzis E, et al. (2010) Infections in patients with cirrhosis increase mortality four-fold and should be used in determining prognosis. Gastroenterology 139: 1246–1256.

5. Jalan R, Fernandez J, Wiest R, Schnabl B, Moreau R, et al. (2014) Bacterial infections in cirrhosis: A position statement based on the EASL Special Conference 2013. J Hepatol 60: 1310–24.

6. Reiberger T, Ferlitsch A, Payer BA, Mandorfer M, Heinisch BB, et al. (2013) Non-selective betablocker therapy decreases intestinal permeability and serum levels of LBP and IL-6 in patients with cirrhosis. J Hepatol 58: 911–921.

7. Morencos FC, de las Heras Castano G, Martin Ramos L, Lopez Arias MJ, Ledesma F, et al. (1995) Small bowel bacterial overgrowth in patients with alcoholic cirrhosis. Digestive Diseases and Sciences 40: 1252–1256.

8. Chang CS, Chen GH, Lien HC, Yeh HZ (1998) Small intestine dysmotility and bacterial overgrowth in cirrhotic patients with spontaneous bacterial peritonitis. Hepatology 28: 1187–1190.

9. Jun DW, Kim KT, Lee OY, Chae JD, Son BK, et al. (2010) Association between small intestinal bacterial overgrowth and peripheral bacterial DNA in cirrhotic patients. Digestive Diseases and Sciences 55: 1465–1471.

10. Gunnarsdottir SA, Sadik R, Shev S, Simren M, Sjovall H, et al. (2003) Small intestinal motility disturbances and bacterial overgrowth in patients with liver cirrhosis and portal hypertension. Am J Gastroenterol 98: 1362–1370.

11. Bauer TM, Steinbruckner B, Brinkmann FE, Ditzen AK, Schwacha H, et al. (2001) Small intestinal bacterial overgrowth in patients with cirrhosis: prevalence and relation with spontaneous bacterial peritonitis. Am J Gastroenterol 96: 2962–2967.

12. Kwon JH, Koh SJ, Kim W, Jung YJ, Kim JW, et al. (2014) Mortality associated with proton pump inhibitors in cirrhotic patients with spontaneous bacterial peritonitis. Journal of Gastroenterology and Hepatology 29: 775–781.

13. de Vos M, De Vroey B, Garcia BG, Roy C, Kidd F, et al. (2013) Role of proton pump inhibitors in the occurrence and the prognosis of spontaneous bacterial peritonitis in cirrhotic patients with ascites. Liver Int 33: 1316–1323.

14. Choi EJ, Lee HJ, Kim KO, Lee SH, Eun JR, et al. (2011) Association between acid suppressive therapy and spontaneous bacterial peritonitis in cirrhotic patients with ascites. Scandinavian Journal of Gastroenterology 46: 616–620.

15. Goel GA, Deshpande A, Lopez R, Hall GS, van Duin D, et al. (2012) Increased rate of spontaneous bacterial peritonitis among cirrhotic patients receiving pharmacologic acid suppression. Clin Gastroenterol Hepatol 10: 422–427.

16. Campbell MS, Obstein K, Reddy KR, Yang YX (2008) Association between proton pump inhibitor use and spontaneous bacterial peritonitis. Digestive Diseases and Sciences 53: 394–398.

17. Bajaj JS, Zadvornova Y, Heuman DM, Hafeezullah M, Hoffmann RG, et al. (2009) Association of proton pump inhibitor therapy with spontaneous bacterial peritonitis in cirrhotic patients with ascites. Am J Gastroenterol 104: 1130–1134.

18. Bajaj JS, Ratliff SM, Heuman DM, Lapane KL (2012) Proton pump inhibitors are associated with a high rate of serious infections in veterans with decompensated cirrhosis. Alimentary Pharmacology and Therapeutics 36: 866–874.

19. Deshpande A, Pasupuleti V, Thota P, Pant C, Mapara S, et al. (2013) Acid-suppressive therapy is associated with spontaneous bacterial peritonitis in cirrhotic patients: a meta-analysis. Journal of Gastroenterology and Hepatology 28: 235–242.

20. van Vlerken LG, Huisman EJ, van Hoek B, Renooij W, de Rooij FW, et al. (2012) Bacterial infections in cirrhosis: role of proton pump inhibitors and intestinal permeability. European Journal of Clinical Investigation 42: 760–767.

21. Mandorfer M, Bota S, Schwabl P, Bucsics T, Pfisterer N, et al. (2014) Nonselective beta Blockers Increase Risk for Hepatorenal Syndrome and Death in Patients with Cirrhosis and Spontaneous Bacterial Peritonitis. Gastroenterology 146: 1680–1690.

22. Reiberger T, Ulbrich G, Ferlitsch A, Payer BA, Schwabl P, et al. (2013) Carvedilol for primary prophylaxis of variceal bleeding in cirrhotic patients with haemodynamic non-response to propranolol. Gut 62: 1634–1641.

23. Kamath PS, Kim WR (2007) The model for end-stage liver disease (MELD). Hepatology 45: 797–805.

24. Child C, Turcotte J, editors (1964) Surgery and portal hypertension. Philadelphia: Saunders. 50–64.

25. Peck-Radosavljevic M, Trauner M, Schreiber F (2005) Austrian consensus on the definition and treatment of portal hypertension and its complications. Endoscopy 37: 667–673.

26. Peck-Radosavljevic M, Angermayr B, Datz C, Ferlitsch A, Ferlitsch M, et al. (2013) Austrian consensus on the definition and treatment of portal hypertension and its complications (Billroth II). Wien Klin Wochenschr 125: 200–219.

27. (2010) EASL clinical practice guidelines on the management of ascites, spontaneous bacterial peritonitis, and hepatorenal syndrome in cirrhosis. J Hepatol 53: 397–417.

28. Runyon BA (2013) Introduction to the revised American Association for the Study of Liver Diseases Practice Guideline management of adult patients with ascites due to cirrhosis 2012. Hepatology 57: 1651–1653.

29. (1992) American College of Chest Physicians/Society of Critical Care Medicine Consensus Conference: definitions for sepsis and organ failure and guidelines for the use of innovative therapies in sepsis. Critical Care Medicine 20: 864–874.

30. Ferenci P, Lockwood A, Mullen K, Tarter R, Weissenborn K, et al. (2002) Hepatic encephalopathy—definition, nomenclature, diagnosis, and quantification: final report of the working party at the 11th World Congresses of Gastroenterology, Vienna, 1998. Hepatology 35: 716–721.

31. Fagundes C, Barreto R, Guevara M, Garcia E, Sola E, et al. (2013) A modified acute kidney injury classification for diagnosis and risk stratification of impairment of kidney function in cirrhosis. J Hepatol 59: 474–481.

32. Fine JP, Gray RJ (1999) A Proportional Hazards Model for the Subdistribution of a Competing Risk. Journal of the American Statistical Association 94: 496–509.

33. Siringo S, Burroughs AK, Bolondi L, Muia A, Di Febo G, et al. (1995) Peptic ulcer and its course in cirrhosis: an endoscopic and clinical prospective study. J Hepatol 22: 633–641.

34. Lodato F, Azzaroli F, Di Girolamo M, Feletti V, Cecinato P, et al. (2008) Proton pump inhibitors in cirrhosis: tradition or evidence based practice? World Journal of Gastroenterology 14: 2980–2985.

35. Jalan R, Fernandez J, Wiest R, Schnabl B, Moreau R, et al. (2014) Bacterial infections in cirrhosis: a position statement based on the EASL Special Conference 2013. J Hepatol 60: 1310–1324.

36. Fernandez J, Gustot T (2012) Management of bacterial infections in cirrhosis. J Hepatol 56 Suppl 1: S1–12.

5

The Corepressor *Tle4* Is a Novel Regulator of Murine Hematopoiesis and Bone Development

Justin C. Wheat[1,☸,¤], Daniela S. Krause[2,3,☸], Thomas H. Shin[1,4,☸], Xi Chen[1], Jianfeng Wang[1], Dacheng Ding[1], Rae'e Yamin[1], David A. Sweetser[1]*

1 Department of Pediatrics, Divisions of Pediatric Hematology/Oncology and Medical Genetics, Massachusetts General Hospital, Boston, Massachusetts, United States of America, 2 Center for Regenerative Medicine and Cancer Center, Massachusetts General Hospital, Boston, Massachusetts, United States of America, 3 Department of Pathology, Massachusetts General Hospital, Boston, Massachusetts, United States of America, 4 Department of Molecular and Translational Medicine, Boston University School of Medicine, Boston, Massachusetts, United States of America

Abstract

Hematopoiesis is a complex process that relies on various cell types, signaling pathways, transcription factors and a specific niche. The integration of these various components is of critical importance to normal blood development, as deregulation of these may lead to bone marrow failure or malignancy. *Tle4*, a transcriptional corepressor, acts as a tumor suppressor gene in a subset of acute myeloid leukemia, yet little is known about its function in normal and malignant hematopoiesis or in mammalian development. We report here that *Tle4* knockout mice are runted and die at around four weeks with defects in bone development and BM aplasia. By two weeks of age, *Tle4* knockout mice exhibit leukocytopenia, B cell lymphopenia, and significant reductions in hematopoietic stem and progenitor cells. *Tle4* deficient hematopoietic stem cells are intrinsically defective in B lymphopoiesis and exhaust upon stress, such as serial transplantation. In the absence of *Tle4* there is a profound decrease in bone mineralization. In addition, *Tle4* knockout stromal cells are defective at maintaining wild-type hematopoietic stem cell function *in vitro*. In summary, we illustrate a novel and essential role for *Tle4* in the extrinsic and intrinsic regulation of hematopoiesis and in bone development.

Editor: Pranela Rameshwar, Rutgers - New Jersey Medical School, United States of America

Funding: This work was supported by National Institutes of Health grants K08 CA138916-02 (DSK), R01 CA115772 (DAS, JCW, XC, JW), and T32 CA071345 (JW) as well as funding by Hyundai Hope on Wheels (DAS; http://www.hyundaihopeonwheels.org) and the Mattina Proctor Foundation (DAS; 75 Federal St, Boston, Massachusetts 02110). The funders had no role in study design, data collection and analysis, decision to publish, or preparation of the manuscript.

Competing Interests: The authors have declared that no competing interests exist.

* Email: dsweetser@partners.org

¤ Current address: Department of Cell Biology, Albert Einstein College of Medicine, Bronx, New York, United States of America

☸ These authors contributed equally to this work.

Introduction

The bone marrow (BM) is a heterotypic organ that dynamically integrates a variety of signals to modulate both quantitative and qualitative output of hematopoiesis to meet specific needs such as oxygen transport, immunity, and clotting. It is increasingly recognized that the differentiation of blood cells is affected not only by factors intrinsic to hematopoietic stem and progenitor cells (HSPC) but also a variety of cell types in the HSPC niche, including endothelial cells, osteolineage cells, sympathetic neurons, Cxcl12-activated reticular (CAR) cells, and nestin expressing stromal cells [1]. Together, these external and internal regulators work in concert to dynamically respond to physiological demand.

Genetic aberrations in these HSPC can lead to clonal expansions of progenitor cells as in leukemia. One such recurrent genetic mutation occurring in approximately 2% of acute myeloid leukemia (AML) patients is del(9q), which is enriched in patients with the t(8:21) fusion protein *AML1-ETO* [2]. Previously, we showed that loss of two genes, *Tle1* and *Tle4*, within the commonly deleted region of 9q can cooperate specifically with

the *AML1-ETO* fusion product in a zebrafish model of myeloblastic expansion. Moreover, modulation of these genes in cell lines harboring t(8; 21) can influence the proliferative and apoptotic rate of these cells [3]. Additionally, *Tle1* has been shown to be silenced by methylation in a broader set of AML samples, as well as in non-Hodgkin's lymphoma and diffuse large B-cell lymphomas [4].

The TLE family of genes is a group of highly conserved transcriptional corepressors. The TLE homologue in Drosophila, *Groucho* (Gro), plays a crucial role in multiple developmental processes including neurogenesis, segmentation, and sex determination [5]. Gro also has instructive roles in many signaling pathways including receptor tyrosine kinase/Ras/MAPK, Notch, Wingless (Wg)/Wnt, and Decapentaplegic (Dpp) [6]. Proteins in the *TLE* family can influence transcription by either direct binding to a variety of transcription factors essential to both hematopoiesis and leukemogenesis, including members of the Hes, Runx, LEF1/ Tcf, Pax, and Myc families, as well as recruitment of histone deacetylases and methylases, leading to chromatin silencing via condensation over large domains [7]. A combination of these effects likely underlies the ability of this protein family to influence cell fate and malignant transformation. Depending on context, these proteins may behave as either tumor suppressor genes or as facilitators of oncogenesis as in invasive breast cancer and synovial cell sarcoma, respectively [8,9].

To better understand the role of *Tle4* in development and oncogenesis, we developed a *Tle4* knockout (KO) mouse. *Tle4* KO mice have significant postnatal growth abnormalities, including skeletal and hematological defects. By three weeks of age, KO mice are leukopenic and display specific deficiencies of B cells and HSPC. We show that these defects arise from a combination of both intrinsic and extrinsic defects.

Materials and Methods

Generation of *Tle4* null Mice

A conditional *Tle4* null mouse was constructed by targeting LoxP sites to flank exon 2 via homologous recombination using the 129S6/SvEvTac ES cell line (Figure 1a). Resultant mice were crossed with *β-actin: Cre* mice (gift of Susan Dymecki) to delete exon 2 in all tissues. Heterozygote mice were backcrossed to C57BL/6 background for over 6 generations and interbred to generate *Tle4* null mice.

Whole Mount Staining Of Skeletons to Visualize Cartilage and Calcified Bone

Embryos at embryonic age day 19.5 (E19.5) and one day old newborn pups were euthanized and skeletons subsequently cleared of skin and viscera. Specimens were fixed in 95% ETOH for at least five days, followed by at least two days in 100% acetone to remove adipose tissue. Specimens were then stained in 0.3% Alcian blue, 0.1% Alizarin red in 70% ETOH, and 5% acetic acid for three days. After rinsing in water, specimens were cleared in 2% KOH for 24 hours, 1% KOH/20% glycerol for 5–7 days, 1% KOH/50% glycerol 5–7 days, 1% KOH/80% glycerol 5–7 days, and finally stored in 100% glycerol.

Terminal Deoxynucleotidyl transferase dUTP nick end labeling Stain (TUNEL)

Paraffin-embedded humeri harvested from two week old *Tle4* WT and KO mice were sectioned for TUNEL staining using the Apoptag kit per manufacturer's protocol (EMD Millipore, Billerica, MA). Briefly, sections were bathed in Tris buffer with Tween X, followed by proteinase K, peroxidase block, and TdT enzyme treatments. All antibodies used for TUNEL staining were included in the kit and sections were counterstained using Methyl Green.

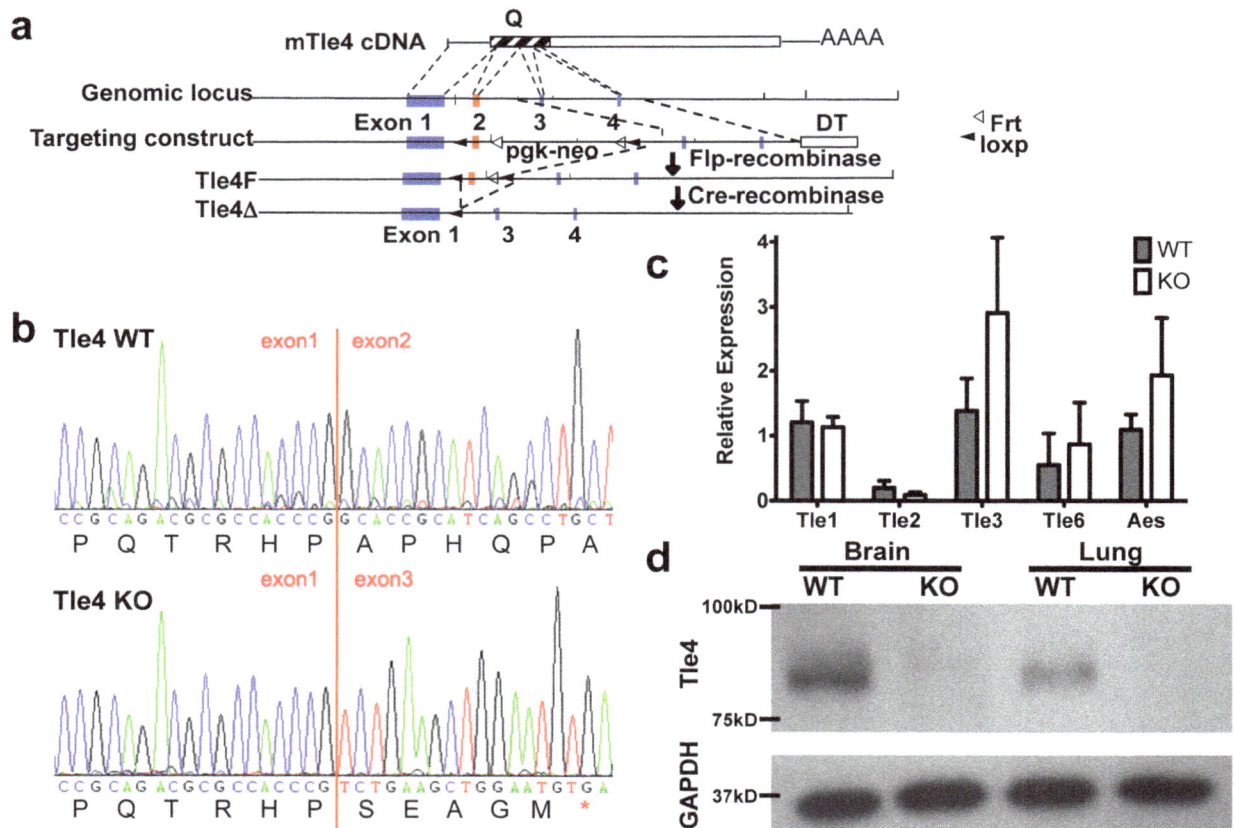

Figure 1. The development of a novel *Tle4* null mouse model. (a) Targeting schema for generation of *Tle4* null animals. Conditional *Tle4* null mice were created by homologous recombination with an original construct containing a pgk-neo positive selection cassette and a Diptheria toxin (Dt) negative selection sequence, The pgk-neo selection cassette was excised between flanking Frt sites (white arrow head) by breeding mice to beta actin-Flp mice, leaving loxp sites flanking exon 2. These conditionally *Tle4* null mice were bred to beta-actin cre mice to generate *Tle4* null mice with a deleted exon 2 between flanking Loxp sites (black arrowheads). (b) RT-PCR showed exon 2 was cleanly excised. Loss of exon 2 creates a frameshift in the cDNA and a truncated non-functional Tle4 peptide. (c) Loss of Tle4 does not significantly affect the expression of other Tle family members as shown by RT-PCR of cDNA from the bone marrow of 2 week old mice. (d) Loss of Tle4 expression in *Tle4* null mice was demonstrated by Western blot with protein from brain and lung.

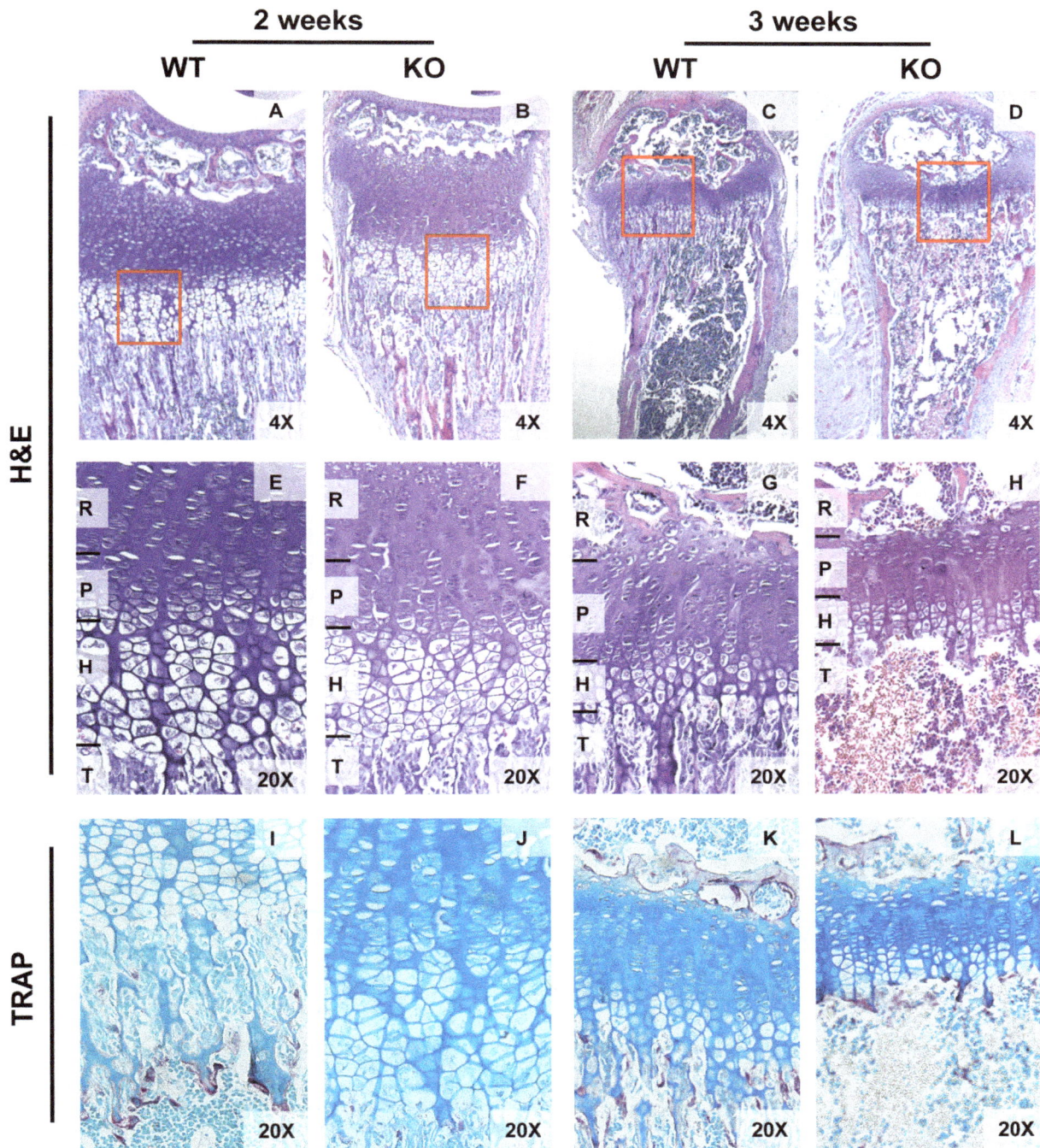

Figure 3. Progressive bone marrow hypoplasia with defective ossification, loss of trabecular bone and thinning of cortical bone is seen by 3 and 4 weeks in *Tle4* null mice. A–D. Hematoxylin and Eosin (H&E) staining of tibiae of 3 and 4 week old WT and *Tle4* null (KO) mice demonstrate multiple abnormalities in *Tle4* null mice including progressive pancytopenia of the bone marrow (BM), loss of trabecular bone (T), and thinning of the cortical bone layer (C). A higher power view shows a thinner proximal tibial growth plate in *Tle4* null mice with a decrease in thickness of the resting (R), proliferative (P), and hypertrophic (H) zones and near complete loss of the trabeculae. E–H. Tartrate-resistant acid phosphatase (TRAP) staining (pink) demonstrates osteoclasts clustering under the hypertrophic zone at the boundary of the bone marrow cavity in *Tle4* null mice at 3 and 4 weeks of age.

fold reduction in CD34$^+$ LKS cells (Figure 7a). Interestingly, the total number of long-term HSC, defined by surface expression of SLAM markers CD150$^+$ and CD48$^-$, were not reduced in KO mice despite the five-fold reduction in total BM leukocytes at this age (Figure 7a). However, total numbers of common myeloid (CMP) and more so common lymphoid progenitors (CLP) were significantly reduced in *Tle4* null mice (Figure 7b). Finally, *Tle4* null mice also have significant reductions in Pre/ProB fractions A through C (Figure 7c). *Pax5*, which derives its repressive activity via interaction with *Tle4*, is necessary for progression through the

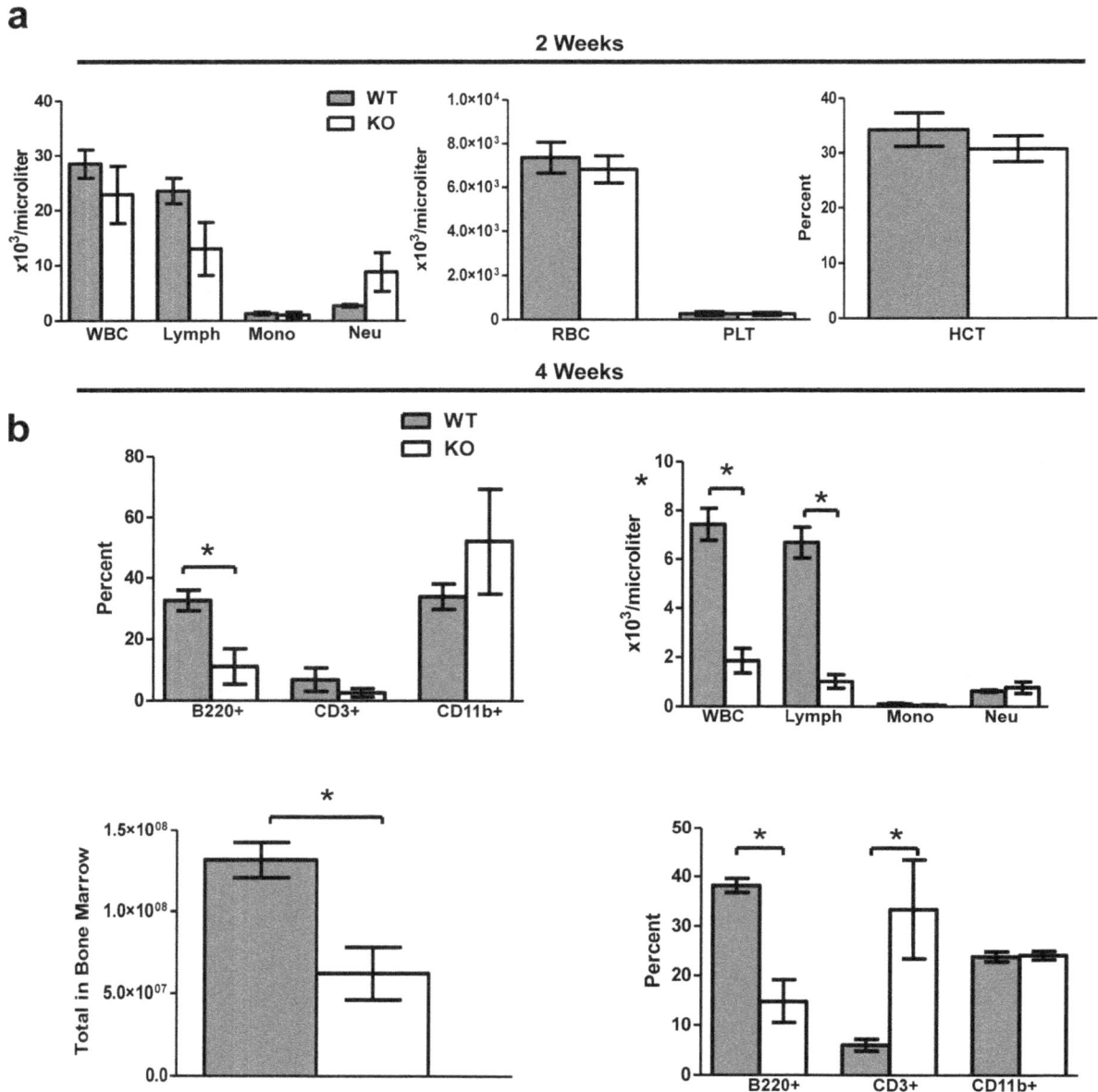

Figure 4. Peripheral blood counts are normal in *Tle4* null mice at 2 weeks of age, but significant abnormalities are seen in peripheral blood and bone marrow at 4 weeks of age. (a) At 2 weeks of age there was no significant difference in any of the cell compartments in the peripheral blood of *Tle4* null mice (KO) as compared with normal control littermates (WT). However, by 4 weeks of age *Tle4* null mice exhibit a marked leukopenia (decreased WBC) and lymphopenia in the peripheral blood, that primarily affects the B-cells (B220+ cells), and not T-cell (CD3+) or myeloid cells (CD11b+). (b) *Tle4* null mice exhibit severe bone marrow aplasia with a 2-fold decrease in bone marrow cellularity. Within the remaining population of lymphoid cells, B-cell development appears particularly affected with a significant decrease in the percentage of B-cells (B220+) and relative increase in the percentage of T-cells (CD3+).

Pre/ProB checkpoints. Deletion of *Pax5* results specifically in a block in B cell development between Fractions B (early pro-B) and C (late pro-B) [15,16]. Therefore, while some component of the *Tle4* null ProB phenotype may be derived from deregulated Pax5 signaling, it also appears that loss of *Tle4* led to more deleterious effects on B cell development than mere phenocopy of *Pax5* deficiency. Taken together, loss of *Tle4* appears to decrease the frequency of LKS cells and especially B lymphoid progenitors, but not of LKS SLAM cells.

To further typify the above-described difference in LKS frequency between WT and KO mice, additional studies were done to examine cell proliferation and apoptosis within LKS populations. There is no difference in cell proliferation and cell cycling between two-week old WT and KO LKS, as indicated by flow cytometry analysis of Ki-67 (Figure 8a). Interestingly, however, Annexin V analysis showed LKS cells from two-week old KO mice exhibiting significantly reduced viability and increased apoptotic and dead cells (Figure 8b). This suggests the decrease in LKS frequency in KO mice may be due to Tle4-dependent increased apoptosis rather than changes in cell proliferation or cycling.

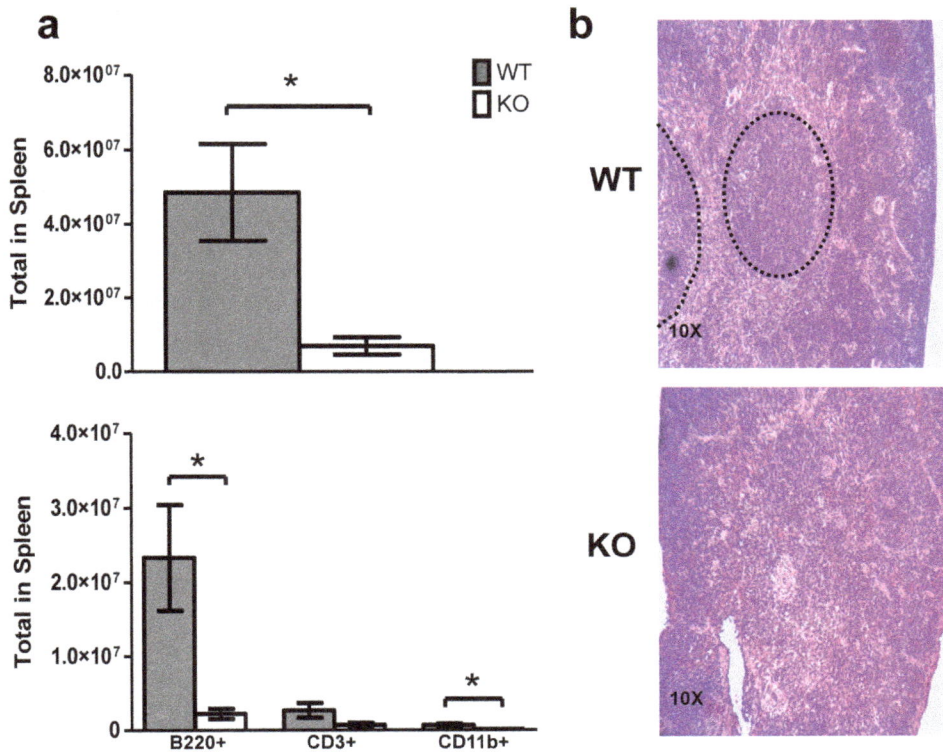

Figure 5. *Tle4* null mice develop splenic atrophy with abnormal splenic architecture. (a) At three weeks of age there is marked splenic atrophy and decreased cellularity especially of the major B-cell (B220+) compartment. (b) H&E staining of the spleen reveals an absence of splenic follicles (dashed oval) in two week old *Tle4* null mice (KO). (n = 3–4 per genotype; mean +/−SEM; *: $P < .05$).

Co-culture of wild-type HSC on *Tle4* null stromal cells impairs long term colony forming ability

Given the critical importance of the BM niche on hematopoiesis, we hypothesized that the abnormalities in the skeletal or stromal compartments of the BM were contributing to defective hematopoiesis [17,18]. This was confirmed by TUNEL staining of paraffin-embedded humeri harvested from two-week old WT and KO mice (Figure 8c). Compared to WT, various compartments of KO bone exhibited increased TUNEL staining, including the periosteal cells lining lacunae in the epiphysis (Figure 8c, panel C vs H) and periosteal cells under the cortex of the diaphyseal portion of the humerus (Figure 8c, panel D vs I). Moreover, TUNEL staining was more extensively pervasive throughout trabeculae and bone marrow in KO compared to WT mice (Figure 8c, panel B vs G, E vs J). This further suggested the possibility that the hematopoietic abnormalities seen in KO mice might be at least in part due to the absence of support from the osteoblastic niche.

To further elucidate whether impaired HSC maintenance by KO BM was dependent on stromal cell irregularities, western blots using whole bone lysates from two week old WT and KO mouse were performed using antibodies against *Scf*, a known factor involved in the maintenance of HSC [1] [27]. Though some KO mice displayed a complete lack of Scf expression, others showed modest protein levels (results not shown). The considerable animal to animal variation suggests that down-regulation of *Scf* expression is not a direct effect of Tle4 loss, but might reflect a loss of an *Scf* producing cell type in *Tle4* null mice. Other factors may account for the impairment of HSC maintenance.

Since *Tle4* null animals do not survive long enough to serve as bone marrow recipients of wild-type HSPC, we adapted a co-culturing assay to determine whether HSC-extrinsic factors may have influenced the observed hematological phenotype [11]. Wild-type LKS cells from two week old mice were co-cultured on WT or KO stroma cells derived from 3 day old mice for two weeks (Figure 9a). Non-adherent cells were harvested and analyzed for expression of c-Kit and Sca-1. In WT co-cultures, 6–15% of recovered cells were positive for both markers. In stark contrast, less than 1% of cells recovered from WT LKS cells plated on KO stromal co-cultures were C-kit$^+$ Sca-1$^+$ (Figure 9b). Long-term co-culture experiments plated in methylcellulose revealed an even more pronounced effect. Cells recovered from WT co-cultures exhibited an average of 10-fold more colonies than their KO counterparts (Figure 9c). Some KO co-cultures failed to exhibit any colony forming ability. Thus, *Tle4* null stromal cells cannot maintain and support HSPC growth as efficiently as WT stromal cells.

Tle4 null HSPC are intrinsically impaired in B cell differentiation and exhaust after serial transplantation

Due to the progressive leukopenia in primary *Tle4* null mice and the extrinsic effects noted above, we tested the colony-forming ability of sorted LKS cells from 2 week old WT or *TLE4* null mice. After seven days in methylcellulose, *TLE4* null LKS were significantly less efficient at forming colonies than WT LKS cells, suggesting intrinsic defects in HSC and HSPC and impaired HSC-self renewal in *Tle4* null mice (Figure 10a). These observations were further reinforced by a continued decrease in the ability of KO LKS cells to produce colonies when serially replated in

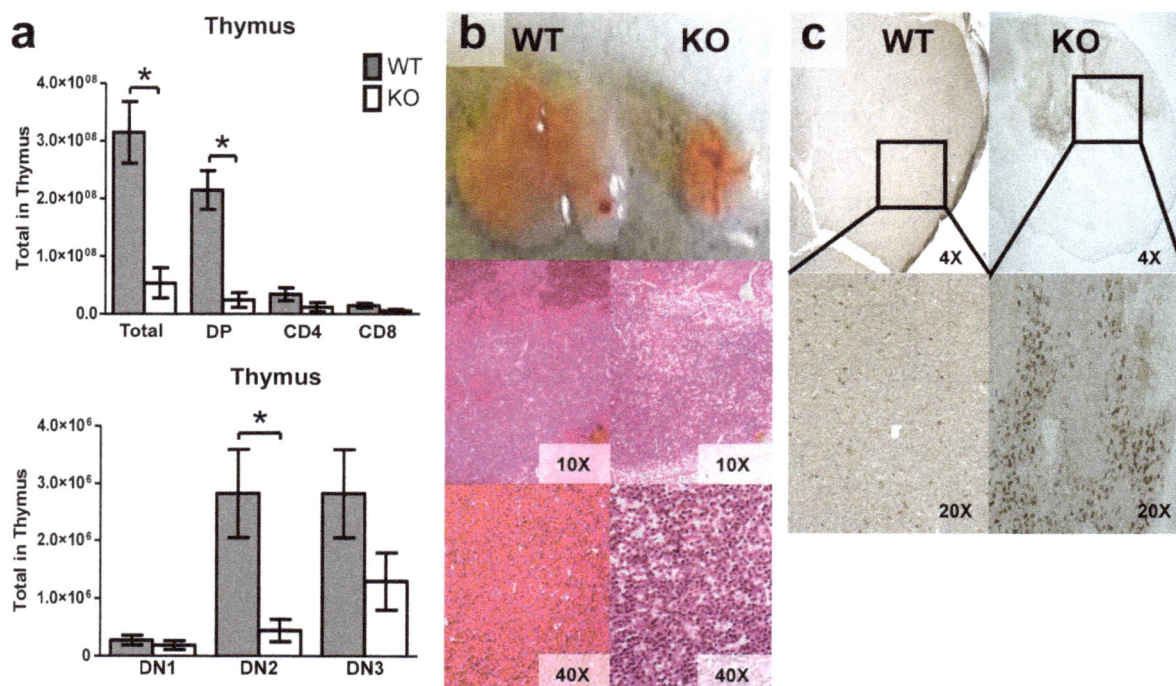

Figure 6. *Tle4* **null mice develop thymic atrophy with a block in T-cell differentiation.** (a) There is a dramatic decrease in total thymocytes in 3 week old Tle4 null mice as compared to wild-type littermates. The majority of this decrease is due to loss of double positive CD4+CD8+ cells. Within the double negative (DN) T progenitor populations there appears to be a block between DN1 (CD44+CD25−) and DN2 (CD44+CD25+) with a significant decrement in DN2 cells and an insignificant decrease in DN3 (CD44−, CD25+) cells. (n = 3–4 per genotype; mean +/−SEM; *: P<.05). (b) The thymus of 3 week old Tle4 null mice is atrophied with a loss in the demarcation between cortex and medulla as seen by H&E. (c) TUNEL staining demonstrates thymic apoptosis in Tle4 mice.

methylcellulose at 14 days (Figure 10a). Additionally, these colonies were also typified as granulocyte/macrophage-forming (CFU-GM), erythroid-forming (BFU-E), or granulocyte/erythrocyte/monocyte/megakaryocyte-forming (CFU-GEMM) colony forming units to identify any *Tle4*-dependent HSC-intrinsic effects on progenitor differentiation. After 13 days in methylcellulose culture, sorted LKS cells from KO were less efficient in forming CFU-GM and CFU-GEMM compared to their WT counterparts (Figure 10b).

To further test this effect, we performed *in vivo* transplantation assays using BM from 2 week old animal or fetal liver hematopoietic cells to determine whether loss of *Tle4* intrinsically affected HSC self-renewal and repopulation efficiency. Whole BM from two-week-old CD45.2+ KO and WT animals was isolated and transplanted into lethally irradiated allogeneic WT mice expressing CD45.1 (Figure 11a). Given our observation of non-significant differences in LKS SLAM populations, representing long-term HSC, between WT and KO BM, equal numbers of cells from donor KO and WT BM were transplanted into recipient mice. Sixteen weeks after BM transplant (BMT), recipients of KO and WT BM showed non-significant differences in donor chimerism in blood (Figure 11b). However, FACS analysis of peripheral blood showed that recipient mice of KO BM had significant reductions in the frequency of B cells, with concomitant increases in both T and myeloid cell frequencies (Figure 11b). At 32 weeks after transplant, CBC analysis of KO BM recipients demonstrated the development of significant leukopenia, especially a decrease in myeloid and lymphoid lineages (Figure 11c, left panel). Immunophenotypic analysis showed that the leukopenia was mostly due to a decreased frequency of B cells (Figure 11c,

right panel). Fractionation of B cell precursors in recipients 32 weeks post-transplant showed a reduction in the absolute number of Fraction D and E cells and an increase in Fraction C before progression to fraction D (Figure 11d). This suggests that transplanted *Tle4* null BM cells have a block in B cell development at the late pro-B to pre-B-cell stage, more restricted than seen in situ with Tle4 null mice, but still distinct from the early pro-B to late pro-B block reported with *Pax5* deficiency [15,16,19].

Analysis of HSPC in recipients 32 weeks after transplant, which has been shown to reflect long term repopulating activity of HSC [32], revealed no significant differences between KO and WT recipients in the absolute number of LKS, CLP, CMP, or GMP compartments. However, MEPs were significantly reduced in KO recipient mice (Figure 11e). A competitive homing experiment revealed that at 18 hours after transplant, KO HSC were able to home to the recipient niche as efficiently as WT cells (Figure 11f), indicating the observed abnormalities were not due to homing defects of these cells. These findings suggest that BMT with *Tle4* null HSC results in leukopenia, specifically B lymphopenia arising from partial blocks in ProB development. However, KO donor BM retained normal frequencies of most HSPC fractions after transplantation into a normal BM niche.

To test self-renewal capacity of KO versus WT HSC while excluding confounding effects possibly due to prior exposure to a defective *Tle4* null BM niche, we performed serial transplantations of fetal liver hematopoietic cells (FL) of E13.5 WT and KO CD45.2+ fetuses (Figure 12a). Recipients of KO and WT FL primary transplants exhibited peripheral leukopenia and specific B cell lymphopenia (Figure 7b, left and middle panels), recapitulating the phenotype observed in recipients of KO BM in prior BMT

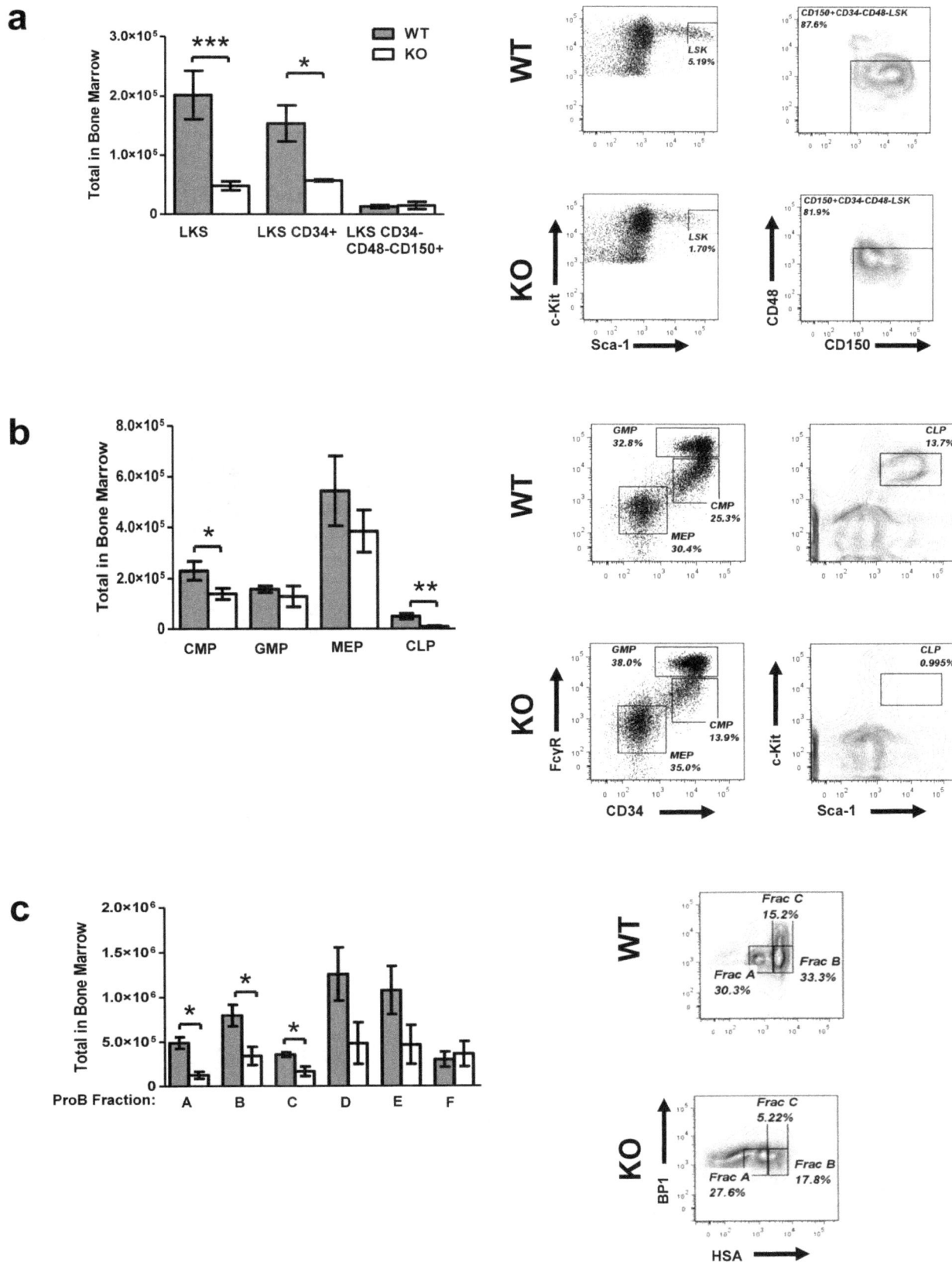

Figure 7. *Tle4* null mice have significant aberrations in hematopoietic stem and progenitor cells (HSPC). Bar graphs with representative flow cytometry plots in two week old littermates (a) show significant loss of LSK and LKS CD34+ cells, though the most immature long-term HSC population (LKS CD34+CD48−CD150+ HSC) is relatively preserved. (b) Examination of CMP, GMP, MEP, and CLP progenitor fractions demonstrated

significant decreases in CMP and CLP populations. (c) Amongst the Pre/Pro B cell progenitors the decrement is most prominent in the early Fractions A through C. (n = 3–8 per genotype; mean +/− SEM; *: $P<.05$, **: $P<.001$, ***: $P<.0001$). See methods for gating strategy of stem and progenitor cell compartments.

experiments (Figure 11c and 11d). Additionally, there were no differences in the frequency of HSC between primary recipients of KO or WT FL (Figure 12b, right). Upon serial transplantation of FL into secondary transplant recipients, we again saw highly significant leukopenia and lymphopenia 16 weeks after transplant in KO recipient mice (Figure 12c, left). Interestingly, secondary KO FL recipients also exhibited a significant reduction in *Tle4* null-derived LKS (Figure 12c, right). Moreover, these LKS cells

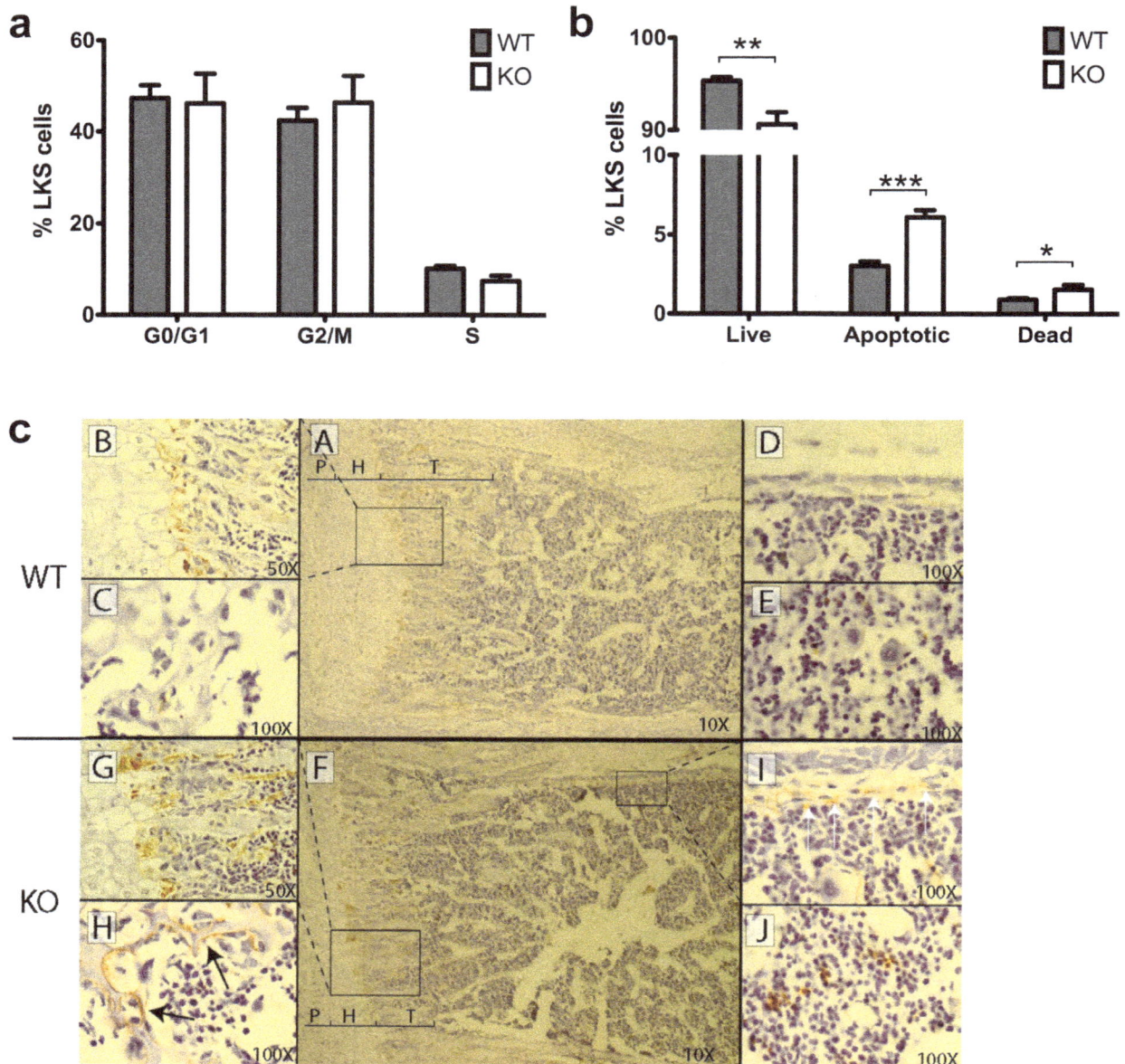

Figure 8. The decrease in LKS cells in Tle4 null mice is due to an increase in apoptosis and cell death rather than a decrease in proliferation and is accompanied by abnormalities of the bone marrow stroma. (a) LKS cells isolated from the bone marrow of two week old mice show no difference in cell cycle distribution. (b) There is however an increase in apoptotic and dead LKS cells in the Tle4 null mice. (c) TUNEL staining of the growth plate of the femur in two week old mice marks the normal zone of cell death between the hypertrophic (H) layer and forming trabecular (T) bone (A, B) with an increase in staining in Tle4 null mice (F, G). Lacunae in the epiphysis are lined with periosteal cells undergoing apoptosis in Tle4 null mice (H), but was not seen in wild type (WT) littermates. Similar periosteal cells undergoing apoptosis and stained by TUNEL are seen under the cortex of diaphyseal bone in Tle4 null mice (I) but absent in wild-type mice (D). An increase in TUNEL staining is also observed in cells of the bone marrow in Tle4 null mice (J) as compared to wild-type bone marrow (E).

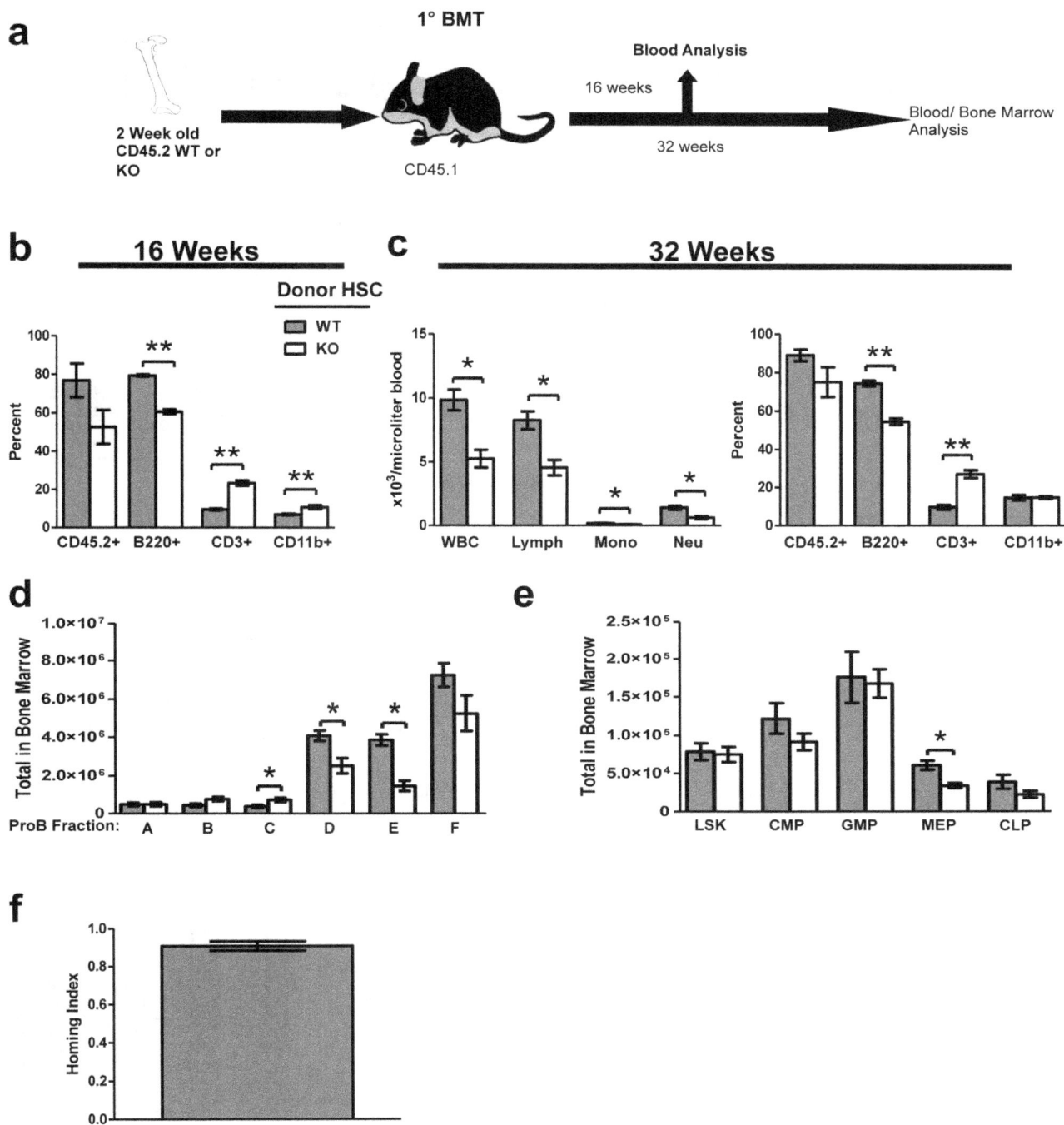

Figure 11. *Tle4* null mice have cell-intrinsic defects in HSPC self-renewal and B-cell development. Bone marrow transplants of wild-type (WT) or Tle4 null (KO) bone marrow from 2 week old mice into normal recipients were performed to evaluate cell intrinsic defects. (a) Schematic of BMT experimental design. (b) Analysis of peripheral blood at 16 after transplant by flow cytometry and CBC demonstrated insignificant differences in engraftment as measured by the percent CD45.2+ cells, but impaired B-cell numbers (B220+) with relatively increased T-cells (CD3+) and myeloid cells (CD11b+). (c) 32 weeks after transplant mice receiving Tle4 null bone marrow developed leukopenia (decreased WBC) primarily accounted for by a decrease in lymphocytes (c, left panel), which by immunophenotyping represented a decrease in B-cells (B220+). (n = 9–10 per transplant group, *: $P < .005$ **: $P < .0001$). (d) Analysis of B-cell differentiation in the BM of recipient mice 32 weeks after transplant by quantitation of ProB Fractions shows an increase in Fraction C, but decreased Fractions D and E indicating a relative block in differentiation between Fractions C and D (n = 5 per genotype, *: $P < .05$). (e) Analysis of bone marrow 32 weeks after transplant showed no significant differences between KO and WT recipients in the absolute number of LKS, CLP, CMP, or GMP compartments, but did show a decrease in MEPs in KO recipient mice. (f) Competitive homing 18 hours after transplantation using whole BM from two week old WT and KO littermates showed no defect in homing ability (n = 3). The homing index is represented as: Input/Output or $(KOi/WTi)/(KOo/WTo)$.

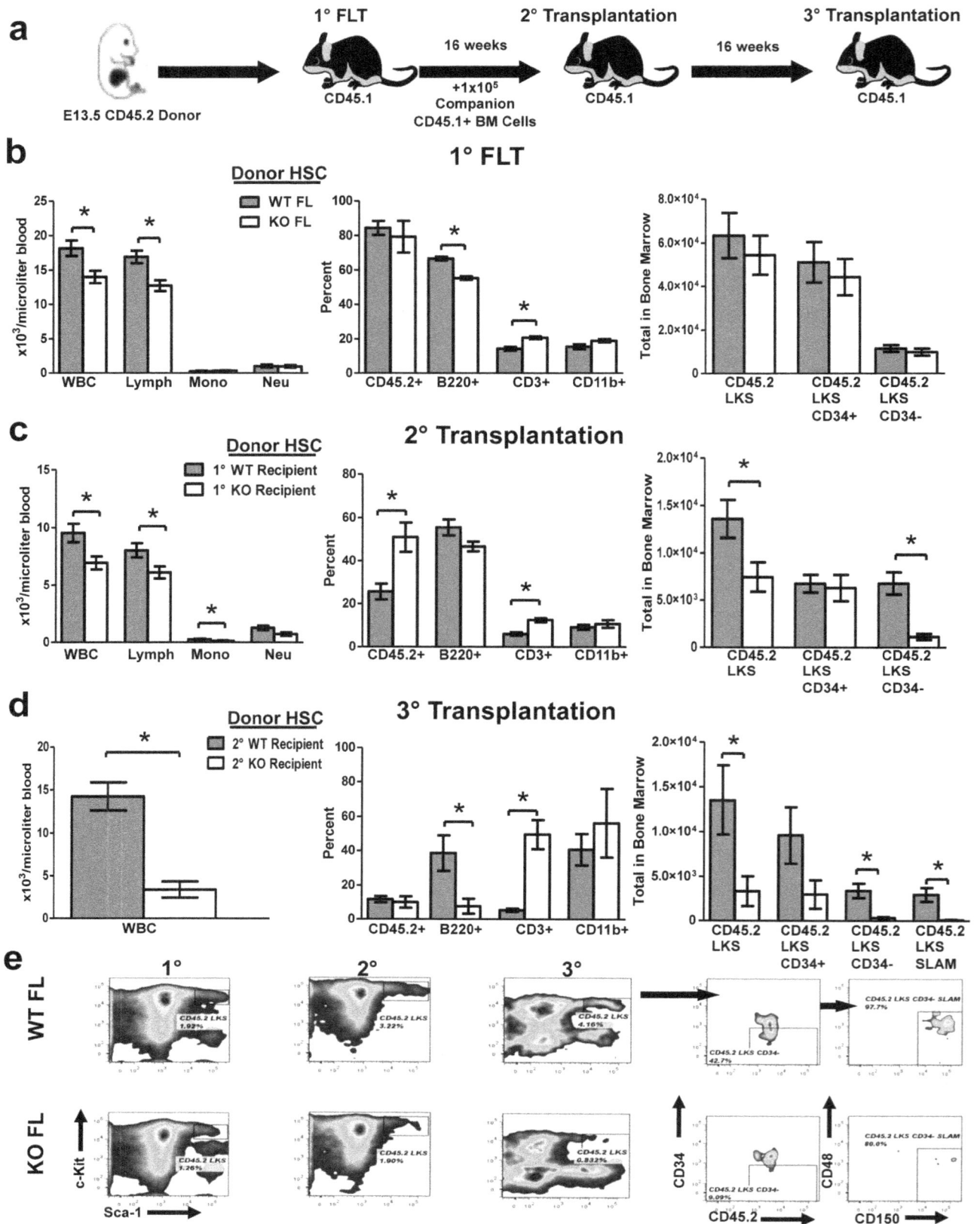

Figure 12. *Tle4* null fetal liver HSCs have impaired B cell development and exhaust with serial transplantation. (a) Schematic of serial FL transplantation experimental design. (b) Peripheral blood and LKS analysis of FL transplant recipients 16 weeks after transplant revealed peripheral leukopenia (WBC) and specifically B cell (B220+) lymphopenia in the absence of Tle4 with no difference in LKS, LKS, CD34+, LKS CD34− populations

(n = 10 per genotype for blood analysis, n = 6–7 per genotype for LKS analysis, ***: P<.0001). (c) Peripheral blood and LKS analysis 16 weeks after secondary transplantation also indicates leukopenia and lymphopenia in Tle4 null cells, but at this time also a significant decrease in LKS and LKS, CD34– populations (n = 5 KO recipients, n = 10 WT recipients for blood analysis, n = 5 mice per group for LKS analysis, *: P<.05 **: P<.001). (d) Peripheral blood analysis and LKS analysis 16 weeks after tertiary transplantation again showed leukopenia, B-cell lymphopenia, and a profound decrease in all HSC containing populations (n = 4 per genotype for blood and LKS analysis, *: P<.05, **: P<.01, ***: P<.001). (e) Representative flow cytometry plots showing progressive loss of Tle4 null HSCs over successive transplantation.

Several reports have described the role of the BM microenvironment on hematopoiesis [23,24]. Osteoblasts have a well-defined role in supporting B lymphopoiesis via expression of the heterotrimeric G protein alpha subunit G(s)alpha [25,26]. While we have not yet determined whether osteoblasts are specifically affected in our model *per se*, it is reasonable to assume that the compromise of trabecular bone is at least contributory to the observed B cell and HSPC defects. The inability of *Tle4* null stromal cells cultured *in vitro* to maintain WT HSC suggests that the hematopoietic phenotype seen in KO mice may derive in part from niche-induced deregulation. Furthermore, as evidenced by TUNEL staining of bones harvested from WT and KO mice, it is clear that the absence of *Tle4* has an effect on the viability and integrity of the BM niche and stroma, Further experiments are needed to better characterize the nature of this defective stromal support of HSPC.

Loss of *Tle4* appears to significantly impair LSK differentiation into granulocyte, monocyte, macrophage progenitors and LSK self-renewal, at least in part due to increased cellular apoptosis. The finding of preserved numbers of long term stem cells as marked by CD34+ LSK CD48– CD150+ in two week old *Tle4* knockout mice, despite decreases in more mature lineages, further studies are need to understand the mechanisms of this preservation.

Concurrently, BM and fetal liver serial transplantation experiments demonstrate a robust HSPC-intrinsic effect of *Tle4* deletion. In both transplant models, mice receiving KO HSPC develop peripheral leukopenia. Moreover, this finding in FL serial transplantation illustrates the potential HSPC-intrinsic defects of Tle4 loss leading to decreased capacity of HSPC self-renewal. Additionally, our study provides the first direct *in vivo* evidence of a role of Tle4 on B-cell development, an effect previously inferred based on interactions of Tle4 and Pax5 [28,29]. The somewhat distinct block in B-cell differentiation seen with Tle4 loss compared to that reported with Pax5 loss suggests Tle4 may exert some B-cell effects independent from Pax5, although we can't exclude potential animal models differences as accounting for this effect. Taken together, our data demonstrates the critical importance of *Tle4* in regulating various developmental processes central to bone maturation, medullary hematopoiesis, and HSPC

maintenance. These findings may have significant implications for understanding hematopoiesis in both normal and disease states. Moreover, our observations provide further insight and affirmation to previous findings that implicate *Tle4* as a critical regulator of leukemia and other states of hematological dysregulation.

Conclusion

In summary, by the development of the first model for *Tle4* deletion in mammals, our data provide evidence for an essential role for *Tle4* in mammalian bone and blood development. *Tle4* deficient B cells exhibit intrinsic developmental defects and HSC exhibit stem cell depletion after serial transplantation. *Tle4* null bone marrow stromal cells fail to support hematopoiesis *in vitro*, suggesting a potentially novel extrinsic role of *Tle4* in the regulation of hematopoiesis. *Tle4* null mice have profound defects in bone mineralization and growth plate organization, which apparently affects skeletal growth.

Our work has shed light on a novel regulatory function for this corepressor in normal hematopoiesis and bone development. As such, elucidating the regulatory mechanisms controlled by *Tle4* offers a significant challenge and opportunity for expanding our understanding of bone development and the multicellular orchestration of hematopoiesis. This work further potentially offers novel insight into the transcriptional processes underlying malignant transformation.

Acknowledgments

The authors thank Laura Prickett-Rice, Katherine Folz-Donohue, Meredith Weglarz, and David Dombkowski for assistance with flow cytometry and sorting. We thank Dr. Yiyun Zhang and Dr. Joanna Yeh for their helpful comments and discourse.

Author Contributions

Conceived and designed the experiments: JCW DSK THS. Performed the experiments: JCW DSK THS XC JW DD RY DAS. Analyzed the data: JCW DSK THS DAS. Contributed reagents/materials/analysis tools: DAS. Contributed to the writing of the manuscript: JCW DSK THS DAS.

References

1. Nwajei F, Konopleva M (2013) The bone marrow microenvironment as niche retreats for hematopoietic and leukemic stem cells. Adv Hematol 2013: 953982.
2. Grimwade D, Walker H, Oliver F, Wheatley K, Harrison C, et al. (1998) The importance of diagnostic cytogenetics on outcome in AML: analysis of 1,612 patients entered into the MRC AML 10 trial. The Medical Research Council Adult and Children's Leukaemia Working Parties. Blood 92: 2322–2333.
3. Dayyani F, Wang J, Yeh JR, Ahn EY, Tobey E, et al. (2008) Loss of TLE1 and TLE4 from the del(9q) commonly deleted region in AML cooperates with AML1-ETO to affect myeloid cell proliferation and survival. Blood 111: 4338–4347.
4. Fraga MF, Berdasco M, Ballestar E, Ropero S, Lopez-Nieva P, et al. (2008) Epigenetic inactivation of the Groucho homologue gene TLE1 in hematologic malignancies. Cancer Res 68: 4116–4122.
5. Paroush Z, Finley RL Jr, Kidd T, Wainwright SM, Ingham PW, et al. (1994) Groucho is required for Drosophila neurogenesis, segmentation, and sex determination and interacts directly with hairy-related bHLH proteins. Cell 79: 805–815.
6. Turki-Judeh W, Courey AJ (2012) Groucho: a corepressor with instructive roles in development. Curr Top Dev Biol 98: 65–96.
7. Jennings BH, Ish-Horowicz D (2008) The Groucho/TLE/Grg family of transcriptional co-repressors. Genome Biol 9: 205.
8. Brunquell C, Biliran H, Jennings S, Ireland SK, Chen R, et al. (2012) TLE1 is an anoikis regulator and is downregulated by Bit1 in breast cancer cells. Mol Cancer Res 10: 1482–1495.
9. Seo SW, Lee H, Lee HI, Kim HS (2011) The role of TLE1 in synovial sarcoma. J Orthop Res 29: 1131–1136.
10. Krause DS, Lazarides K, von Andrian UH, Van Etten RA (2006) Requirement for CD44 in homing and engraftment of BCR-ABL-expressing leukemic stem cells. Nat Med 12: 1175–1180.
11. Mukherjee S, Raje N, Schoonmaker JA, Liu JC, Hideshima T, et al. (2008) Pharmacologic targeting of a stem/progenitor population in vivo is associated with enhanced bone regeneration in mice. J Clin Invest 118: 491–504.
12. Krause DS, Fulzele K, Catic A, Sun CC, Dombkowski D, et al. (2013) Differential regulation of myeloid leukemias by the bone marrow microenvironment. Nat Med in press.

13. Chen G, Nguyen PH, Courey AJ (1998) A role for Groucho tetramerization in transcriptional repression. Mol Cell Biol 18: 7259–7268.

14. McLarren KW, Lo R, Grbavec D, Thirunavukkarasu K, Karsenty G, et al. (2000) The mammalian basic helix loop helix protein HES-1 binds to and modulates the transactivating function of the runt-related factor Cbfa1. J Biol Chem 275: 530–538.

15. Hardy RR, Hayakawa K (2001) B cell development pathways. Annu Rev Immunol 19: 595–621.

16. Nutt SL, Urbanek P, Rolink A, Busslinger M (1997) Essential functions of Pax5 (BSAP) in pro-B cell development: difference between fetal and adult B lymphopoiesis and reduced V-to-DJ recombination at the IgH locus. Genes Dev 11: 476–491.

17. Walkley CR, Olsen GH, Dworkin S, Fabb SA, Swann J, et al. (2007) A microenvironment-induced myeloproliferative syndrome caused by retinoic acid receptor gamma deficiency. Cell 129: 1097–1110.

18. Fulzele K, Krause DS, Panaroni C, Saini V, Barry KJ, et al. (2013) Myelopoiesis is regulated by osteocytes through Gsalpha-dependent signaling. Blood 121: 930–939.

19. Milili M, Gauthier L, Veran J, Mattei MG, Schiff C (2002) A new Groucho TLE4 protein may regulate the repressive activity of Pax5 in human B lymphocytes. Immunology 106: 447–455.

20. Wang WF, Wang YG, Reginato AM, Plotkina S, Gridley T, et al. (2002) Growth defect in Grg5 null mice is associated with reduced Ihh signaling in growth plates. Dev Dyn 224: 79–89.

21. Beagle B, Johnson GV (2010) AES/GRG5: more than just a dominant-negative TLE/GRG family member. Dev Dyn 239: 2795–2805.

22. Choi JY, Pratap J, Javed A, Zaidi SK, Xing L, et al. (2001) Subnuclear targeting of Runx/Cbfa/AML factors is essential for tissue-specific differentiation during embryonic development. Proc Natl Acad Sci U S A 98: 8650–8655.

23. Calvi LM, Adams GB, Weibrecht KW, Weber JM, Olson DP, et al. (2003) Osteoblastic cells regulate the haematopoietic stem cell niche. Nature 425: 841–846.

24. Asada N, Katayama Y, Sato M, Minagawa K, Wakahashi K, et al. (2013) Matrix-embedded osteocytes regulate mobilization of hematopoietic stem/progenitor cells. Cell Stem Cell 12: 737–747.

25. Zhu J, Garrett R, Jung Y, Zhang Y, Kim N, et al. (2007) Osteoblasts support B-lymphocyte commitment and differentiation from hematopoietic stem cells. Blood 109: 3706–3712.

26. Wu JY, Purton LE, Rodda SJ, Chen M, Weinstein LS, et al. (2008) Osteoblastic regulation of B lymphopoiesis is mediated by Gs{alpha}-dependent signaling pathways. Proc Natl Acad Sci U S A 105: 16976–16981.

27. Ding L, Saunders TL, Enikolopov G, Morrison SJ (2012) Endothelial and perivascular cells maintain haematopoietic stem cells. Nature 481: 457–462.

28. Eberhard D, Jimenez G, Heavey B, Busslinger M (2000) Transcriptional repression by Pax5 (BSAP) through interaction with corepressors of the Groucho family. EMBO J 19: 2292–2303.

29. Linderson Y, Eberhard D, Malin S, Johansson A, Busslinger M, et al. (2004) Corecruitment of the Grg4 repressor by PU.1 is critical for Pax5-mediated repression of B-cell-specific genes. EMBO Rep 5: 291–296.

6

Personalized Tacrolimus Dose Requirement by CYP3A5 but Not ABCB1 or ACE Genotyping in Both Recipient and Donor after Pediatric Liver Transplantation

Yi-kuan Chen[⑨], Long-zhi Han[⑨], Feng Xue*, Cong-huan Shen, Jun Lu, Tai-hua Yang, Jian-jun Zhang, Qiang Xia*

Department of Liver Surgery and Liver Transplantation, Ren Ji Hospital, School of Medicine, Shanghai Jiao Tong University, Shanghai, P.R. China

Abstract

Tacrolimus (TAC) is the backbone of an immunosuppressive drug used in most solid organ transplant recipients. A single nucleotide polymorphism (SNP) at position 6986G>A in *CYP3A5* has been notably involved in the pharmacokinetic variability of TAC. It is hypothesized that *CYP3A5* genotyping in patients may provide a guideline for TAC therapeutic regimen. To further evaluate the impact of *CYP3A5* variants in donors and recipients, *ABCB1* and *ACE* SNPs in recipients on TAC disposition, clinical and laboratory data were retrospectively reviewed from 90 pediatric patients with liver transplantation and their corresponding donors after 1 year of transplantation. The recipients with *CYP3A5* *1/*1 or *1/*3 required more time to achieve TAC therapeutic range during the induction phase, and needed more upward dose during the late induction and the maintained phases, with lower C/D ratio, compared with those with *CYP3A5* *3/*3. And donor *CYP3A5* genotypes were found to impact on TAC trough concentrations after liver transplantation. No association between *ABCB1* or *ACE* genotypes and TAC disposition post-transplantation was found. These results strongly suggest that *CYP3A5* genotyping both in recipient and donor, not *ABCB1* or *ACE* is necessary for establishing a personalized TAC dosage regimen in pediatric liver transplant patients.

Editor: Lorna Marson, Centre for Inflammation Research, United Kingdom

Funding: This project was supported by National Ministry of Public Health grant (IHECCO8-201213) (http://www.nhfpc.gov.cn/gjhzs/index.shtml) and Shanghai Science and Technology Committee grant (12ZR1418300) (http://www.stcsm.gov.cn/). The funders had roles in study design, data collection and analysis.

Competing Interests: The authors have declared that no competing interests exist.

* Email: fengxue6879@163.com (FX); xiaqiang@medmail.com.cn (QX)

[⑨] These authors contributed equally to this work.

Introduction

Tacrolimus (TAC) is the backbone of immunosuppressive drug used worldwide in organ transplantation and characterized by a narrow therapeutic range and high inter-individual variability in its pharmacokinetics [1,2]. To achieve the desired target blood concentrations is of critical importance to avoid rejection and dose-related adverse effects after transplantation [3]. The variability makes it difficult to establish an empirical dose regimen for this drug, especially in pediatric patients, in whom 100-fold variability in pharmacokinetic parameters and blood concentration after a fixed dose is routinely observed [4,5]. Underexposure to TAC may result in immunosuppression failure and acute rejection in recipients. On the other hand, overexposure to it may put patients at risk for its considerable toxicity. Therefore, maintaining the drug exposure within this narrow safe therapeutic window becomes a critical aspect in patient management. Concerning the concept that young children need a higher TAC dose than adult patients [4,6], the blood TAC concentration should be monitored regularly to maintain a therapeutic range, especially during the induction phase post-transplantation therapy, when the risk of rejection is the highest. Although various factors, such as age, sex, body weight, drug interactions and other factors lead to the wide range of interpatient variability ineffective dosage of TAC [7], among them genetic factors play a critical role in the pharmacokinetic properties and therapeutic levels of TAC.

Cytochrome P450 (CYP) 3A5 is the major enzyme responsible for the metabolism of TAC and is found in small intestine as well as in the liver [8]. A single nucleotide polymorphism (SNP) in the *CYP3A5* gene involving an A to G transition at position 6986 within intron 3 was found strongly associated with CYP3A5 protein expression. At least one *CYP3A5*1* allele were found to express large amounts of CYP3A5 protein, whereas homozygous for the *CYP3A5*3* allele did not express significant quantities of CYP3A5 protein, which causes alternative splicing and results in a truncated protein and a severe decrease of functional *CYP3A5* [9]. It has become clear that *CYP3A5*1/*1* or *1/*3 (hereinafter defined 'expressor') are significantly associated with lower dose-adjusted TAC exposure and increased TAC dose requirements in order to achieve target blood concentrations compared with variant *CYP3A5*3/*3* (hereinafter defined 'nonexpressor') [7,9–12]. However, it is controversial that, for liver transplantation, the impact of the *CYP3A5* genotype of both the recipients (intestine) and the donors (graft liver) should be taken into account when evaluating TAC pharmacokinetics.

TAC is also substrate of P-glycoprotein, a member drug efflux transporter encoded by the multidrug resistance *ABCB1* gene [13,14]. It has been suggested that some SNPs of the *ABCB1* gene in exons 12 (1236C>T), 21 (2677G>A/T) and 26 (3435C>T) maybe affect synthesis and function of P-glycoprotein. In addition, angiotensin converting enzyme (ACE), which is a key enzyme in the renin-angiotensin system, catalyzes the conversion of angiotensin I to II in the liver and kidney. A line of evidence suggests that variation in intron 16 of the ACE gene (14091–14378) may impact on pharmacokinetics and pharmacodynamics of TAC [15]. However, the impact of SNPs of *ABCB1* and *ACE* on pediatric liver transplants remains unclear.

Although much effort has been devoted to the better understanding of inter-individual differences in response to TAC, little data are available about these relationships in Chinese liver transplanted recipients [16,17], particularly in the pediatric population. Moreover, the effects of *CYP3A5*, *ABCB1* and *ACE* variants on clinical outcomes are not well established in China. The aim of this study was, therefore to retrospectively determine the impact of *CYP3A5* genotype of recipients (intestine) and donors (graft liver), age, sex, body weight, primary diseases and other factors on TAC dosing requirements and disposition in a cohort of pediatric liver recipients during the 12 months following transplantation. We evaluated the effect of *CYP3A5*, *ABCB1* and *ACE* variants on the clinical outcomes in our pediatric liver recipients, and attempted understanding the relationship between *CYP3A5*, *ABCB1* or *ACE* genotype and TAC pharmacokinetics may improve our knowledge of how to most effectively administer this drug, leading to considerable benefit to pediatric liver transplant patients.

Materials and Methods

1. Patients

The patients in this retrospective study were 90 consecutive de novo liver graft recipients who underwent living-donor liver transplantation at Shanghai Ren Ji Hospital between October 2008 and December 2012. Median age of the pediatric patients at liver transplantation was 10 months (range, 5–72 months). This study was reviewed and approved by Shanghai Jiao Tong University School of Medicine Ren Ji Hospital Ethical Board (Approval No.: 2013010), and written informed consent was obtained from all their parents during enrollment.

All pediatric patients were administered the immunosuppressive therapy on day 2 to 3 after liver transplantation. TAC (Astella Pharma Co., Limited) was administered orally (dissolved in water for young children) twice daily with an initial dose of 0.15 mg/kg/day, and subsequently adjusted to archiving target blood trough concentration (termed C_0) through routine monitoring. The target C_0 was between 10 and 15 ng/ml during the first month, between 8 and 12 ng/ml during 2–6 months, and between 5 and 8 ng/ml thereafter. In general, repeat or multiple post-operative infections were considered as over-immunosupressive, which needs to reduce the dose of TAC, whereas when an acute cellular rejection happens, it was considered as under-immunosupressive, which needs to increase the dose of TAC. For acute cellular rejection cases, additional immunosuppressive therapy consisted of a maintenance dose of mycophenolate mofitil and steroid.

2. Tacrolimus C_0 monitoring and C/D ratio assessment

Analysis of all patients' clinical and laboratory assessments on day 3, 7, 14, and in month 1, 3, 6, and 12 post-transplantation

were performed. EDTA-treated blood (1 ml) was collected every 12 h after the previous dose and then blood TAC C_0 was measured by a microparticulate enzyme immunoassay (Abbott Co., Ltd, Tokyo, Japan). The daily dose of TAC was recorded and weight-adjusted dosage (mg/kg/day) was calculated. The blood concentration was measured and normalized using the corresponding dose. A dose ratio was obtained by the concentration/dose (C/D) ratio, which was used for estimating TAC concentration. When the blood TAC C_0 was not measured at a given time point, the data were excluded.

3. Genotyping of *CYP3A5*, *ABCB1* and *ACE*

The 90 pediatric recipients and 90 adult donors were genotyped for the single nucleotide polymorphism of *CYP3A5* at position 6986A>G (the *3 or *1 allele, rs776746), *ABCB1* at exons 12 (1236C>T, rs1128503), 21 (2677G>A/T, rs2032582) and 26 (3435C>T, rs1045642) and *ACE* at intron 16 (14091–14378). The genotyping was detected using the PCR-based sequencing. In brief, whole blood samples (1.0 ml) were collected in EDTA-treated tubes. The genomic DNAs were extracted from leukocytes with a QIAamp Blood kit (Qiagen, Hilden, Germany). A fragment containing the 6986A>G polymorphism was amplified in ABI 7900 system (Applied biosystems, Foster City, CA, USA), using Taq polymerase qPCR kit (TaKaRa Bio. Inc., Dalian, China). The primers 5′-ACTGCCCTTGCAGCATTTA-3′ (forward) and 5′-CCAGGAAGCCAGACTTTGA-3′ (reverse) for *CYP3A5*, primers 5′-ACTTCAGTTACCCATCTCG-3′ (forward) and 5′-TTTCCCGTAGAAACCTTAC-3′ (reverse) (1236C>T), primers 5′-ATAGCAAATCTTGGGACAG-3′ (forward) and 5′-GCATAGTAAGCAGTAGGGA-3′ (reverse) (2677G>A/T), primers 5′-TGGCAGTTTCAGTGTAAGA-3′ (forward) and 5′-CTCCCAGGCTGTTTATTTG-3′ (reverse) (3435C>T) for *ACBC1* and primers 5′-GCCCTGCAGGTGTCTGCAG-CATGT-3′ (forward) and 5′-GGATGGCTCTCCCCGCCTTGTCTC-3′ (reverse) (1st), primers 5′-TGGGACCACAGCGCCCGCCACTAC-3′ (forward) and 5′-TCGCCAGCCCTCCCATGCCCATAA-3′ (reverse) (2nd) for *ACE* were employed. The qPCR process was carried out as following: 95°C for 10 min, then 94°C for 30 s, 55°C for 30 s, 72°C for 60 s for total 40 cycles and finally 72°C for 7 min. The products were then purified with a QIAquick PCRPurification kit (Qiagen, Hilden, Germany) and run on an ABI 3730XL Genetic Analyzer (Applied biosystems, Foster City, CA, USA) according to the manufacturer's recommendations.

4. Outcome measures

The primary outcomes were TAC dosing requirement (normalized for body weight) and C/D ratio (the latter as surrogate marker) at indicated time points of day (d) 3, d 7, d 14, month (m) 1, m 3, m 6 and m12 for TAC clearance. Secondary outcome measures were acute rejection, acute and chronic infection, as well as liver function.

A one-year follow up after liver transplantation was performed to investigate the possible correlation of various infections with the *CYP3A5*1 status of donors and recipients, and with the SNPs of *ABCB1* and *ACE* of recipients. Incidence of post-operative infections and acute cellular rejection were determined by double-blind physicians. Viral infections were classified by viral pathogens, including CMV, EBV, rotavirus, herpes virus, and HBV. The overlap and relative severity of these infections were also recorded. Viral infections differed according to the intensity of immunosuppression and the serologic status of the recipient. Diagnosis of acute cellular rejection or immunosuppressant-induced hepatic toxicity was based on pathological criteria.

Table 1. Demographic characteristics of recipients and donors.

Age (Median, Range)	Recipient 10 (4–120 month)	Donor 30 (21–56 year)
Sex		
Male (%)	52 (57.8)	37 (41.1)
Female (%)	38 (42.2)	53 (58.9)
Body weight (Mean ± Sd; kg)	8.88±3.28	59.35±9.47
Height (Mean ± Sd; cm)	72.97±13.69	162±8.48
Surface area (m²)	0.41±0.12	
CYP3A5 genotype		
AA, *1/*1 (%)	3 (3.3)	11 (12.2)
AG, *1/*3 (%)	37 (41.1)	34 (37.8)
GG, *3/*3 (%)	50 (55.6)	45 (50.0)
ABCB1 genotype		
1236C>T CT (%)	38 (42.2)	
TT (%)	42 (46.7)	
CC (%)	10 (11.1)	
2677G>AT AT (%)	13 (14.4)	
GA (%)	11 (12.2)	
GG (%)	21 (23.4)	
GT (%)	33 (36.7)	
TT (%)	12 (13.3)	
3435C>T CC (%)	36 (40.0)	
CT (%)	40 (44.4)	
TT (%)	14 (15.6)	
ACE genotype		
I/I (%)	40 (44.4)	
D/I (%)	37 (41.1)	
D/D (%)	13 (14.5)	
Primary diseases		
Congenital biliary atresia (%)	89 (98.9)	
Postoperative chologenic infection (%)	1 (1.1)	

5. Statistical analyses

All data were collected and expressed as the mean ± standard deviation or the median with deviation range. Data among several groups or continuous variables between two groups were compared using one-way ANOVA, while continuous variables among several groups were compared using two-way ANOVA analysis and followed by Bonferroni adjustment. Categorical variables were compared using Chi-square test or Fisher's exact test. Other data between two groups was analyzed with T-test. A value $p<0.05$ was considered statistically significant in all analyses, which were performed using SPSS 19.0 soft (SPSS inc., Chicago, IL).

Results

1. Pediatric patient clinical characteristics

We summarized the demographic characteristics of the patients and showed them in Table 1. The total of 90 eligible Chinese pediatric liver transplant recipients (52 boys and 38 girls) and 90 Chinese healthy donors (37 men and 53 women) were enrolled. The median age of patient age was 10 months (between 4 months and 10 years), whereas that of donor age median was 30 years (between 21 and 56 years). The primary diseases of the pediatric recipients included 89 congenital biliary atresias (98.9%) and 1 postoperative chologenic infection (1.1%). *CYP3A5**1/*1 (AA allele), *CYP3A5**1/*3 (AG allele) and *CYP3A5**3/*3 (GG allele) were 3 (3.3%), 37 (41.1%) and 50 (55.6%) cases respectively in recipients, whereas three variants were 11 (12.2%), 34 (37.8%) and 45 (50%) cases in donors. The allele frequencies of *ABCB1* 1236CT, TT, CC, 2677AT, GA, GG, GT, TT, 3435CC, CT and TT were 42.2%, 46.7%, 11.1%, 14.4%, 12.2%, 23.4%, 36.7%, 13.3%, 40.0%, 44.4% and 15.6% in recipients respectively. While the allele frequencies of *ACE* I/I, D/I, and D/D were 44.4%, 41.1% and 14.5% in recipients respectively. The allele frequencies of *CYP3A5*, *ABCB1* at 1236C>T, 2677G>AT and 2677G>AT, and *ACE* were detailedly shown in Table 2.

2. Effect of *CYP3A5* genotype in recipient (intestine) on TAC dosing requirements and disposition

According to *CYP3A5* genotypic results, pediatric recipients were divided into tow groups: expressor (*1/*1 and *1/*3 allele),

Table 2. Frequency of Genotyping from recipients and donors.

Genotype	Recipient	Donor	Tolerance/Total
CYP3A5	AA	AA	1/2
	AA	AG	0/1
	AA	GG	0/0
	AG	AA	2/8
	AG	AG	7/18
	AG	GG	5/11
	GG	AA	0/1
	GG	AG	7/15
	GG	GG	9/34
ABCB1 (1236C>T)	CC	CC	1/2
	CC	CT	3/8
	CC	TT	0/0
	CT	CC	2/7
	CT	CT	7/20
	CT	TT	3/11
	TT	CC	0/1
	TT	CT	8/19
	TT	TT	7/22
ABCB1 (2677G>AT)	AA	AA	0/0
	AA	AT	0/0
	AA	GA	0/0
	AA	GG	0/0
	AA	GT	0/0
	AA	TT	0/0
	AT	AA	1/2
	AT	AT	1/3
	AT	GA	2/4
	AT	GG	0/0
	AT	GT	1/2
	AT	TT	1/2
	GA	AA	0/0
	GA	AT	1/2
	GA	GA	1/1
	GA	GG	0/5
	GA	GT	0/3
	GA	TT	0/0
	GG	AA	0/0
	GG	AT	1/1
	GG	GA	2/5
	GG	GG	1/4
	GG	GT	3/9
	GG	TT	0/2
	GT	AA	0/0
	GT	AT	2/2
	GT	GA	0/2
	GT	GG	3/6
	GT	GT	5/15
	GT	TT	2/8
	TT	AA	0/0
	TT	AT	1/1

Table 2. Cont.

Genotype	Recipient	Donor	Tolerance/Total
	TT	GA	0/0
	TT	GG	0/0
	TT	GT	2/5
	TT	TT	1/6
ABCB1 (3435C>T)	CC	CC	6/19
	CC	CT	3/17
	CC	TT	0/0
	CT	CC	3/11
	CT	CT	9/21
	CT	TT	3/8
	TT	CC	0/1
	TT	CT	5/7
	TT	TT	2/6
ACE	D/D	D/D	1/4
	D/D	D/I	1/9
	D/D	I/I	0/0
	D/I	D/D	2/9
	D/I	D/I	7/17
	D/I	I/I	4/11
	I/I	D/D	0/0
	I/I	D/I	3/8
	I/I	I/I	12/32

and nonexpressor (*3/*3 allele). We compared clinical character-istics between two groups and showed them in Table 3. There was no significant difference in age, sex, body weight, height, primary diseases and postoperative complications between the recipients with expressor and those with nonexpressor. And there was no significant difference in donors' age, sex, body weight and height between the recipients with expressor and those with nonexpres-sor.

However, the peak time of TAC in the recipients with expressor was significantly longer than that in the recipients with non-expressor (9.95±8.25 *vs.* 5.90±4.23, p<0.01; **Table 3**). We further investigated the difference of dose and C/D ratio between the recipients with expressor and those with nonexpressor. As shown in Figure 1, although the two groups had the same TAC initial dose (ng/kg/day) and early induction dose (from day 3 to day 14, **Fig. 1A and 1B**), the C/D ratio in the recipients with nonexpressor was significantly higher than those with expressor (**Fig. 1C and 1D**). And then a higher TAC dose was adjusted on day 14 after transplantation according to their C/D ratio in both expressor and nonexpressor groups. Importantly, the highest dose used on day 30 was almost two-fold of the initial dose in the recipients with expressor, which was significantly higher than that in the recipients with nonexpressor at the same time point (0.27±0.12 *vs.* 0.22±0.09, p=0.013; **Fig. 1A**). Then the TAC maintenance dose was progressively reduced in both groups. At the month12 time point, the TAC dose was almost reached the initial dose in the recipients with expressor (0.14±0.06), whereas the dose was lower than the initial dose in those with nonexpressor (0.10±0.06; **Fig. 1A**). While the normalized trough concentra-tions, the C/D ratios in the recipients with nonexpressor were

significantly higher than those in the recipients with expressor at every time points during a year following transplantation (**Fig. 1C**). Therefore, the correlation between *CYP3A5* genotype and TAC late induction and maintenance doses was observed: expressor group had higher doses and lower C/D ratios, whereas nonexpressor group had lower doses and higher C/D ratios (**Fig. 1B and 1D**). Those results indicate that the recipients with expressor require more time to achieve TAC therapeutic range during the induction phase, need more upward dose during the late induction and the maintained phases, and have lower C/D ratio. In contrast, the recipients with nonexpressor require less time to achieve TAC therapeutic range during the induction phase, need lower dose during the late induction and the maintained phases, and have higher C/D ratio.

3. Impact of *CYP3A5* genotype in donors (graft liver) on TAC dosing requirements and disposition

There was significant difference in donors' *CYP3A5* genotypes between the recipients with expressor and those with nonexpres-sor, when Chi-square test was used (**Table 3**). We therefore further investigated whether *CYP3A5* expressor and nonexpressor from donors affect TAC dosing requirements and C/D ratio of recipients. According to recipients' and donors' *CYP3A5* geno-typing, pediatric recipients were divided into four groups: the recipients with expressor/the donor with expressor (ReDe), the recipients with expressor/the donor with nonexpressor (ReDn), the recipients with nonexpressor/the donor with expressor (RnDe) and the recipients with nonexpressor/the donor with nonexpressor (RnDn). We found that the initial, induction and maintenance doses are very close to those in ReDe, ReDn and RnDe groups,

Table 3. Comparison of characteristics of recipients by *CYP3A5* genotyping.

	Expressor	Nonexpressor	P value
Age (Mean ± Sd; month)	19.0±23.0	16.0±14.4	0.448
Sex			0.702
Male (%)	24 (60.0)	28 (56.0)	
Female (%)	16 (40.0)	22 (44.0)	
Body weight (Mean ± Sd; kg)	9.2±3.7	8.6±2.9	0.426
Height (Mean ± Sd; cm)	73.4±14.6	72.7±13.1	0.809
Surface area (m²)	0.41±0.13	0.40±0.12	0.663
CYP3A5 genotype			
AA, *1/*1 (%)	3 (3.3)	0 (0)	
AG, *1/*3 (%)	37 (41.1)	0 (0)	
GG, *3/*3 (%)	0 (0)	50 (55.6)	
Primary diseases			0.368
Congenital biliary atresia (%)	40 (100.0)	49 (98.0)	
Postoperative chologenic infection (%)	0 (0)	1 (2.0)	
TAC peak time (day)	9.95±8.25	5.90±4.23	0.004
Donor			
Age (Mean ± Sd; year)	32.4±8.9	30.5+5.3	0.260
Male (%)	21 (52.5)	16 (32)	0.050
Female (%)	19 (47.5)	34 (68)	
Body weight (Mean ± Sd; kg)	59.2±9.9	59.5±9.2	0.891
Height (Mean ± Sd; cm)	164.4±8.0	164.2±8.9	0.929
AA, *1/*1 (%)	10 (25.0)	1 (2.0)	
AG, *1/*3 (%)	19 (47.5)	15 (30.0)	
GG, *3/*3 (%)	11 (27.5)	34 (68.0)	0.000

Note: Expressor, *CYP3A5* *1/*1 and *1/*3; Nonexpressor, *CYP3A5* *3/*3.

respectively, while the late induction and the maintenance doses in RnDn group were significantly less than those in other three groups (**Fig. 2A and 2B**). However, TAC C/D ratios were observed with a different phenotype compared with TAC dosing phenotypes. With time, C/D ratio in RnDn group significantly increasingly higher than those in other three groups, especially in the maintenance phase (**Fig. 2C**). Moreover, ReDn group had higher C/D ratio than ReDe at month1, month3 and month12 time points (**Fig. 2C**). The overall dosing in very group was analyzed and showed in Figure 2D. The RnDn group had significantly higher TAC C/D ratio than other three groups. Although ReDn and RnDe groups had higher C/D ratio than ReDe group, no statistically significant relationship was observed among them (**Fig. 2D**). More importantly, the RnDe group had significantly lower C/D ratio than RnDn group (**Fig. 2D**), suggesting that although two groups share the same intestine *CYP3A5* expressor, graft livers with *CYP3A5* expressor or with *CYP3A5* nonexpressor play important impact on TAC trough concentrations after liver transplantation.

4. Effects of *ABCB1* and *ACE* genotypes in recipient (intestine) on TAC dosing requirements and disposition

Considering the possible influence of *ABCB1* and *ACE* SNPs in recipients on TAC pharmacokinetics, we finally assessed the effects of SNPs of *ABCB1* and *ACE* in intestine on TAC. As shown in Figure 3, we didn't find any significant difference of the C/D ratios among the recipients with *ABCB1* at position 1236CT, TT

and CC (**Fig. 3A**), among those with *ABCB1* at position 2677AT, GT, GG, GT and TT (**Fig. 3B**), among those with ABCB1 at position 3435CC, CT and TT (**Fig. 3C**), and among those with *ACE* at intron 16 (14901–14378) (**Fig. 3D**). These results indicate that the variants of *ABCB1* and *ACE* have minimal impact on TAC disposition in pediatric liver transplant patients.

5. Analysis of relationship between donors and recipients

We investigated the family relationship between donors and recipients. As shown in Table 4, parental relationship between donors and recipients with *CYP3A5*1/*1, *CYP3A5*1/*3 and *CYP3A5*3/*3 were 2 (2.2%), 35 (38.9%) and 48 (53.3%) cases respectively, whereas grandparental relationship between those were 1 (1.1%), 2 (2.2%) and 2 (2.2%) cases respectively. Parental relationship between those with *ABCB1* 1236CT, TT, CC, 2677AT, GA, GG, GT, TT, 3435CC, CT and TT were 37 (41.1%), 39 (43.3%), 9 (10.0%), 12 (13.3%), 11 (12.2%), 20 (22.2%), 31 (34.4%), 11 (12.2%), 34 (37.8%), 38 (42.2%) and 13 (14.4%) respectively, whereas grandparental relationship between those were 1 (1.1%), 3 (3.3%), 1 (1.1%), 1 (1.1%), 0 (0%), 1 (1.1%), 2 (2.2%), 1 (1.1%), 2 (2.2%), 2 (2.2%) and 1 (1.1%) cases respectively. Parental relationship between those with *ACE I/I*, *D/I*, and *D/D* were 38 (42.2%), 36 (40.0%) and 11 (12.2%) cases respectively, whereas grandparental relationship between those were 2 (2.2%), 1 (1.1%) and 2 (2.2%) cases respectively.

We further analyzed frequency and rejection of pairing genotype of donors and recipients. As shown in Table 5, recipients

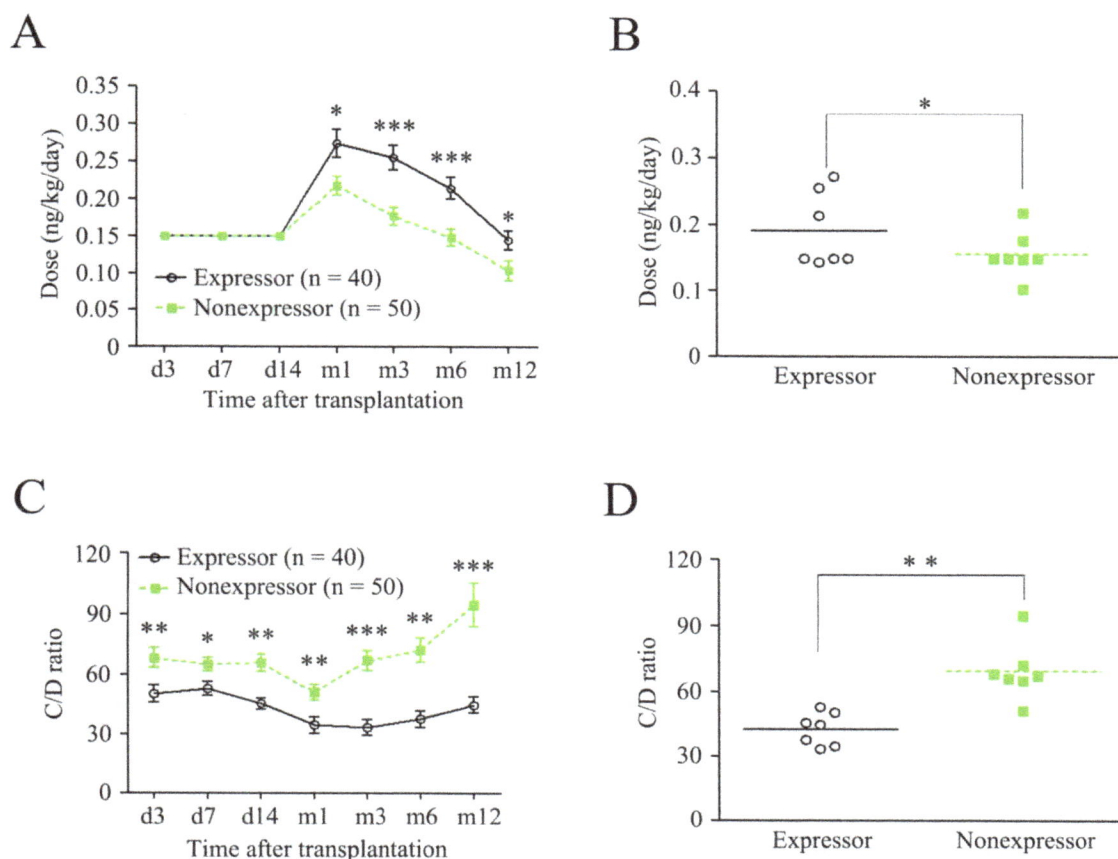

Figure 1. Doses and C/D ratios of TAC compared between recipients with *CYP3A5* expressor and those with nonexpressor. (A) Dose-time curves; (B) Doses in dots, every dot represents a dose at a time point; (C) C/D ratio-time curves; (D) C/D ratios in dots, every dot represents a C/D ratio at a time point. TAC, tacrolimus; Expressor, *CYP3A5* *1/*1 and *1/*3; Nonexpressor, *CYP3A5* *3/*3; *p<0.05; **p<0.01; ***p<0.001.

with concomitant rejection in the same and different genotyping of donors with recipients in *CYP3A5* were 15 (34.1%) and 11 (30.6%) cases respectively. Recipients with concomitant rejection in the same and different genotyping of donors and recipients in *ABCB1* at 1236, 2677 and 3435 sites were 15 (34.1%), 11 (23.9%), 6 (20.7%), 21 (34.4%), 14 (30.4%) and 12 (27.3%) respectively. While recipients with concomitant tolerance in the same and different genotyping of donors and recipients in *ACE* were 12 (22.6%) and 14 (37.8%) respectively. Interestingly, no statistical difference between those with and without concomitant rejection in the same and different genotyping, including *CYP3A5*, *ABCB1* and *ACE*, was observed.

Discussion

Therapeutic drug monitoring of TAC in blood is necessary to provide an effective immunosuppression and avoid adverse effects after organ transplantation. With regard to TAC pharmacokinetic variability, *CYP3A5* genotype has been reported to consistently associate with TAC dosing requirement [9]. In pediatric recipients, however, it is difficult to perform frequently blood samplings for measurement. Therefore, it is very important to investigate the relationship of *CYP3A5* genotyping with TAC pharmacokinetics for establishing a personalized dosage regimen including the initial, the induction and the maintenance doses. In this study, the general consistency in the concept that *CYP3A5* expressor requires higher TAC doses than nonexpressor to reach

target trough concentrations strongly suggests that *CYP3A5* genotyping not only in recipient (intestine) but also in donor (graft liver) is necessary for establishing a personalized dosage regimen in pediatric liver transplant patients. In addition, we didn't find any significant impact of *ABCB1* and *ACE* SNPs on TAC disposition. Although a recent study suggested a safer dosing and monitoring of TAC coadministered with rabeprazole early on after liver transplantation regardless of *CYP3A5* genotypes of recipients and their donors [18], our finding in this study is important as it emphasizes the combined effects of recipient's and donor's genetic variation in relation to TAC disposition. Moreover, although primary outcome time focused on the early postoperative period in most studies, we set one year of primary outcome time. It is necessary, we think, because impact on recipients, especially for pediatric liver transplant patients, will be long time period because of immunosuppressive regimen for his whole life.

TAC is characterized by narrow therapeutic index and interindividual variability in its exposure, and achieving target therapeutic level is difficult, especially during the early period of transplantation. Therefore, the TAC dosing regimens require a regular drug monitoring system based on its trough blood concentration [9]. On the other hand, TAC blood concentration is monitored to allow therapeutic levels to be maintained, to avoid toxicity and to improve efficacy. In general, post-operative infections were considered as over-immunosupressive, which needs to reduce the dose of TAC, whereas acute cellular rejection was

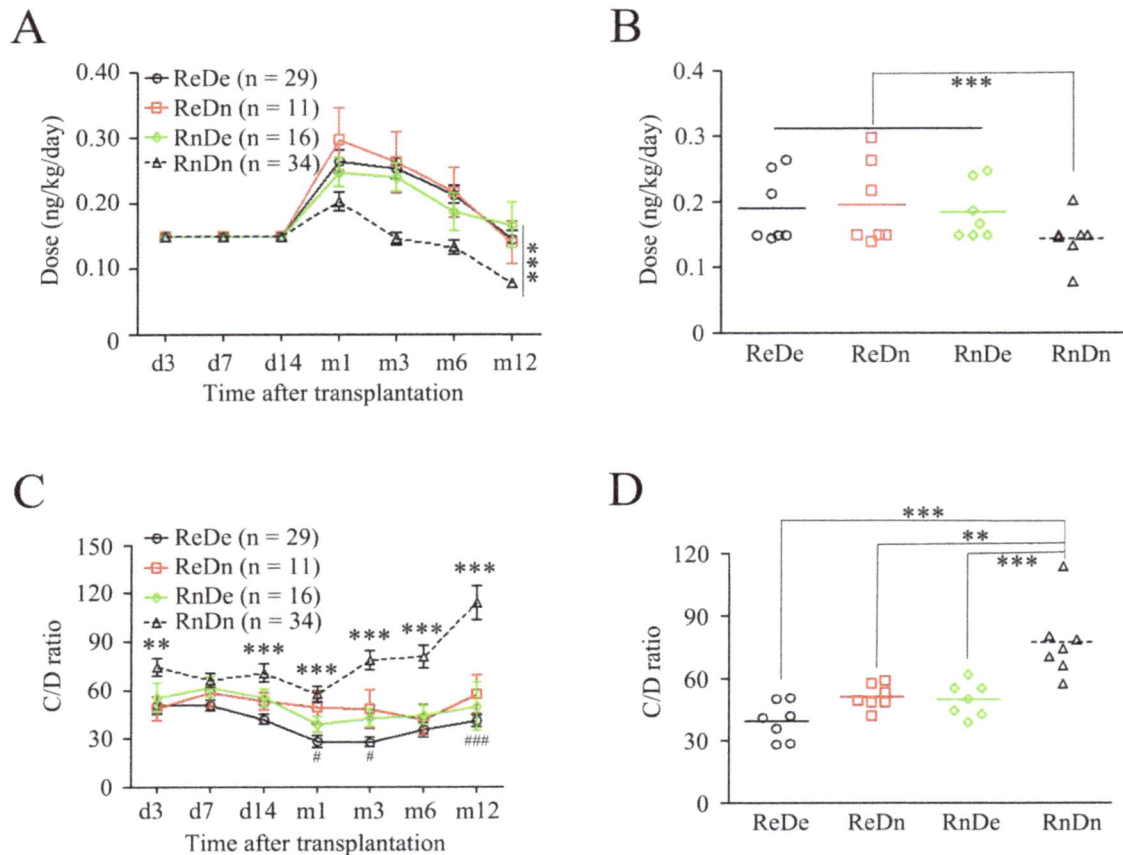

Figure 2. Doses and C/D ratios of TAC compared among four groups: ReDe, ReDn, RnDe and RnDn. (A) Dose-time curves; (B) Doses in dots, every dot represents a dose at a time point; (C) C/D ratio-time curves; * compared with ReDe; # compared with ReDn; (D) C/D ratios in dots, every dot represents a C/D ratio at a time point. TAC, tacrolimus; Expressor, *CYP3A5* *1/*1 and *1/*3; Nonexpressor, *CYP3A5* *3/*3; ReDe, recipient with expressor/donor with expressor; ReDn, recipient with expressor/donor with nonexpressor; RnDe, recipient with nonexpressor/donor with expressor; RnDn, recipient with nonexpressor/donor with nonexpressor; *p<0.05; **p<0.01; ***p<0.001; #p<0.05, ###p<0.001.

considered as under-immunosupressive, which needs to increase the dose of TAC. But the former needs to exclude the ordinary post-operative infections. Although the same initial TAC dose and the same early induction dose (~two weeks) were used, we were surprised to find a *CYP3A5* genotype effect so early after transplant, in which the C/D ratio was significantly higher in nonexpressor than expressor on day 3 (**Fig. 1**). For pediatric liver recipients, in contrast, another study claimed that they did not identify any relationship between recipient *CYP3A5* genotype and TAC dosing [19]. They supposed that the main reason for this lack of association was probably that variations in TAC deposit are largely dependent on hepatic metabolism and to a lesser extent on intestinal metabolism in the first 14 days after transplantation [19]. In addition, a similar data in pediatric renal transplant recipients have also shown that the independent impact of *CYP3A5* genotype on TAC pharmacogenetic was not evident [20]. We postulate that the main reason for this inconsistence with our results is probably that we had enrolled more cases, demonstrating a further large-scale study is necessary. Although CYP3A5 genotype has been convincingly impacted on TAC clearance in many ethic groups [1–3,5–7,9–12,16,17,19,21,22], there is limited evidence to prove that *CYP3A5* genotype-guided TAC dosing will benefit clinical outcomes.

In this study, we found that the association between TAC dosing and *CYP3A5* genotyping not only in recipients but also in

donors for liver transplantation (**Fig. 1** and **Fig. 2**). Recent a report has also shown that a more significant effect of donor genotype as early as 2 weeks after transplantation in liver transplant recipients [23]. In any case, the relative importance of recipient and donor genotyping during the early post-transplantation period is of particular significance, especially in liver transplantation, concerning the risk of graft rejection is the highest in this period. To maximize the immunosuppressive effect and minimize adverse effects, TAC dosing regimen of in the induction phase (~3 months after transplantation) and the maintenance phase (3–12 months after transplantation) should be changed [7]. Generally, TAC dosing requirement for the induction phase is higher than that requirement for the maintenance phase. In the present study, a higher TAC dose was adjusted on day 14 after transplantation basing on C/D ratio monitor. The highest dose used on day 30 was almost two-fold of the initial dose in the recipients (**Fig. 1A**), then the TAC maintenance dose was progressively reduced, and on day 365 after transplantation, the TAC dose was almost reduced to the initial dose in the recipients (**Fig. 1A**). It is very clear that pharmacogenetics-based approach to TAC dosing may prove to be more clinically relevant in terms of preventing early overexposure and toxicity. Possibly, starting with a lower TAC dose in such patients may prevent early nephrotoxicity or the development of new-onset diabetes after transplantation.

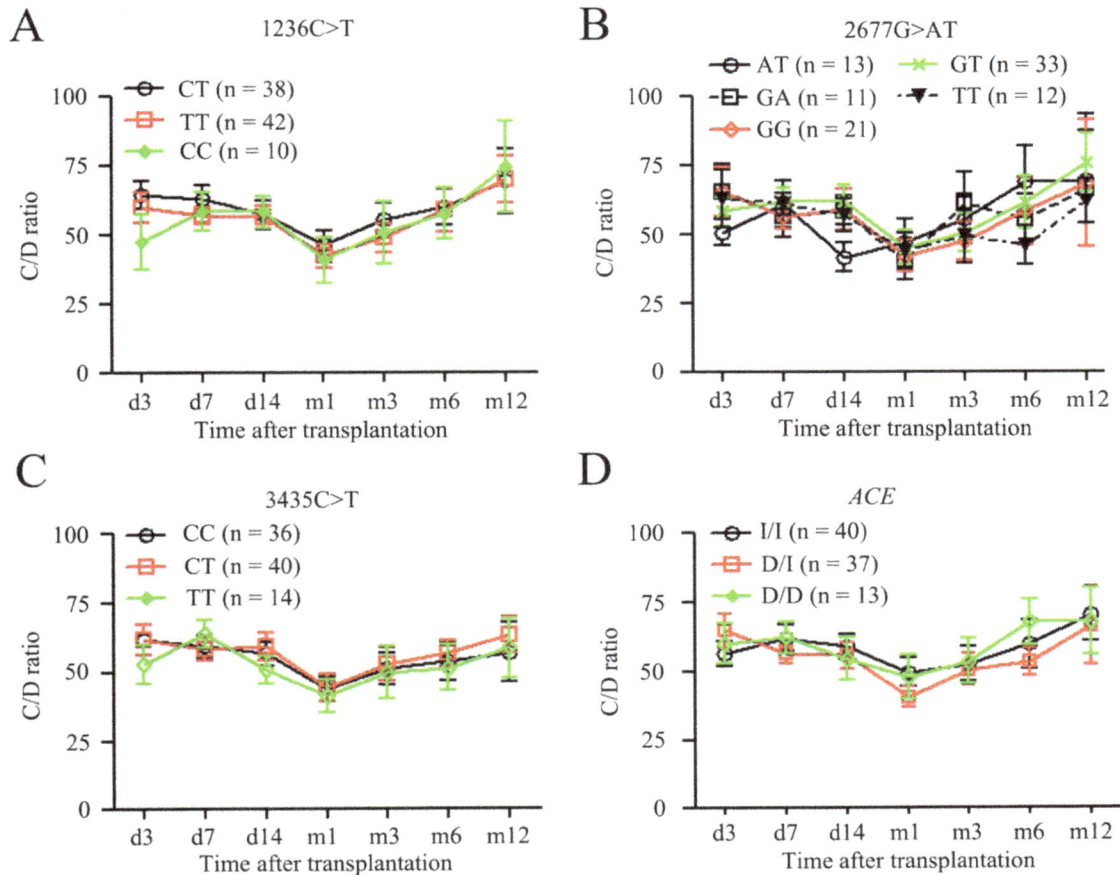

Figure 3. C/D ratios of TAC compared among *ABCB1* genotypes and among *ACE* genotypes. (A) C/D ratio-time curves of *ABCB1* variants at 1236C>T; (B) C/D ratio-time curves of *ABCB1* variants at 2677G>AT; (C) C/D ratio-time curves of *ABCB1* variants at 3435C>T; (D) C/D ratio-time curves of *ACE* variants. TAC, tacrolimus.

Patients with *CYP3A5* expressor require a higher TAC dose than *CYP3A5* nonexpressers to reach the same whole-blood exposure. Therefore, these expressor patients are prone to have subtherapeutic drug concentrations in the early phase after surgery and theoretically maybe increase acute rejection risk [9]. It is not surprising that, from a clinical point of view, TAC is prescribed to prevent acute rejection. However, an exception to this general pattern is a study of Korean kidney graft patients, which found a greater incidence of acute rejection with *CYP3A5* expressor [11]. A previous study reported that children younger than five years of age needed higher TAC doses than older children after both kidney and liver transplant and suggested that TAC starting dosing guidelines in children should reflect both age and *CYP3A5* genotype to quickly reach therapeutic concentrations after transplantation [19]. However, we didn't find an association between age and *CYP3A5* genotype (Table 3). We supposed that pediatric recipients in our study caused this inconsistence, which are almost younger children with only few cases above 5 years of age. Regarding that our results revealed the influence of CYP3A5 variant recipient or donor genotypes on TAC metabolic variables, we did not agree the idea that the impact of age and genetic variation appears to be weakened in the immediate post-transplantation period, while intraindividual variation appears larger [21].

The wide range of interpatient variability in effective dosage of TAC is caused by various factors, such as age, weight, and drug interactions. Similarly, inflammation and/or organ failure maybe reduce drug metabolism in patients [19]. In particular, genetic factors play an important role in the pharmacokinetic properties and therapeutic levels of TAC. The *CYP3A5* genotype is currently the strongest predictor of an individual's TAC dose requirement. However, it does not explain all variability. Other genetic variants may explain additional variation in TAC dose requirement. As has been illustrated in adults, the drug transporter ABCB1, the CYP3A4, the human pregnane X receptor (NR1I2), interleukin 6 and COMT SNP may be associated with early TAC exposure [9,24–26]. Although the association of *ABCB1*, *ACE* with the C/D ratios of TAC was investigated, we didn't observe any significant impact on TAC disposition in pediatric liver transplants (**Fig. 3**). Although a few reports found that high intestinal levels of P-glycoprotein were associated with TAC disposition after liver transplantation [16,27], most studies didn't find any influence of ABCB1 genotypes on TAC pharmacokinetics [28–30], especially in pediatric recipients [6,31,32]. Consistent with the majority, we couldn't find any significant association between ABCB1 genotypes and the disposition of TAC (**Fig. 3**). With regard to *ACE* SNPs, although the *ACE* study suggested an association between *ACE* and renal dysfunction in adult liver recipients who receive TAC [32], we couldn't find any significant association between its genotypes and the disposition of TAC too (**Fig. 3**). Taken together, their influence appears to be smaller than that of *CYP3A5* SNPs. If these additional genetic variants do indeed

Table 4. Relationship between recipients and donors.

Genotype of recipients	Recipients' relationship to donors	
	Parents (%)	Grandparents (%)
CYP3A5 genotype		
AA, *1/*1	2 (2.2)	1 (1.1)
AG, *1/*3	35 (38.9)	2 (2.2)
GG, *3/*3	48 (53.3)	2 (2.2)
ABCB1 genotype		
1236C>T CT	37 (41.1)	1 (1.1)
TT	39 (43.3)	3 (3.3)
CC	9 (10.0)	1 (1.1)
2677G>AT AT	12 (13.3)	1 (1.1)
GA	11 (12.2)	0 (0)
GG	20 (22.2)	1 (1.1)
GT	31 (34.4)	2 (2.2)
TT	11 (12.2)	1 (1.1)
3435C>T CC	34 (37.8)	2 (2.2)
CT	38 (42.2)	2 (2.2)
TT	13 (14.4)	1 (1.1)
ACE genotype		
I/I	38 (42.2)	2 (2.2)
D/I	36 (40.0)	1 (1.1)
D/D	11 (12.2)	2 (2.2)

explain residual variability in TAC dose requirement, it may become possible to develop personalized therapeutic strategy that helps clinicians to decide on an individual's initial dose. It is to be expected that with such an approach early TAC overexposure and toxicity may be expectantly prevented [9]. Further prospective studies of liver transplant recipients are needed to evaluate the impact of these genetic polymorphisms on TAC dosing requirement and determine whether routine genotyping would be improve in personalized TAC therapy. Since the actions of these genes appear to be cooperative. Moreover, the combination of some drugs with lower TAC dose may be safely coadministered

[33]. However, our results provided evidence that *CYP3A5* plays a more dominant role than other genetic variants in the metabolism of TAC in pediatric liver transplant recipients and their donors.

In this study, we analyzed the relationship of pairing of donors and recipients. Among pairing of donors and recipients, parental relationship cases were more than grandparental those (Table 4). In addition, there were not significantly different in occurrence of rejection between the same or different genotypes in pairing of donors and recipients (Table 5). In additional, not only donors but also recipients were genotyped with their peripheral blood samples. It seems no difference for genotyping regardless of basing

Table 5. Profiles of pairing genotypes of donors and recipients on Rejection of TAC.

Genes		Donor and recipient	Rejection (total)	Non-rejection (total)	P value
CYP3A5		Same genotype	15 (54)	39 (54)	
		Different genotypes	11 (36)	25 (36)	0.776
ABCB1					
	1236C>T	Same genotype	15 (44)	29 (44)	
		Different genotypes	11 (46)	35 (46)	0.175
	2677G>AT	Same genotype	6 (29)	23 (29)	
		Different genotypes	21 (61)	40 (61)	0.170
	3435G>AT	Same genotype	14 (46)	32 (46)	
		Different genotypes	12 (44)	32 (44)	0.110
ACE		Same genotype	12 (53)	41 (53)	
		Different genotypes	14 (37)	23 (37)	0.105

on intestinal biopsies or blood samples, but using intestinal biopsies will have high novelty, especially for recipients. More importantly, intestinal biopsies from recipients will provide us more valued information about mRNA transcription and protein expression of interesting genes and second pass of metabolism of TAC.

The main limitations of this study are the retrospective design from a single center and a limited number of patients. Also, the confounding effects of *CYP3A4* with *ABCB1* or *ACE* variants that may affect TAC pharmacokinetics were not examined. A prospective study with a large number of pediatric recipients and standard timing of ImmuKnow assay is required to establish an effective monitoring tool of immune response in children following liver transplantation. Furthermore, for recipient genotyping, periphery blood has limited novelty.

In conclusion, this study further confirmed that the *CYP3A5* polymorphism at position 6986G>A of pediatric liver transplants

and their donors, but not *ABCB1* or *ACE* SNPs in recipients, impacts on TAC dosing requirement, suggesting that early determination of the *CYP3A5* genotype in both recipients and donors would be helpful in the design of adequate immunosuppressive treatment and in lower adverse effects by predicting TAC dosing requirement for the induction and maintenance phases in individual liver transplant recipients.

Author Contributions

Conceived and designed the experiments: FX JJZ QX. Performed the experiments: YKC LZH. Analyzed the data: FX YKC. Contributed reagents/materials/analysis tools: LZH CHS JL THY. Contributed to the writing of the manuscript: YKC FX.

References

1. Penninga L, Moller CH, Gustafsson F, Steinbruchel DA, Gluud C (2010) Tacrolimus versus cyclosporine as primary immunosuppression after heart transplantation: systematic review with meta-analyses and trial sequential analyses of randomised trials. Eur J Clin Pharmacol 66: 1177–1187.
2. Kim JS, Aviles DH, Silverstein DM, Leblanc PL, Matti Vehaskari V (2005) Effect of age, ethnicity, and glucocorticoid use on tacrolimus pharmacokinetics in pediatric renal transplant patients. Pediatr Transplant 9: 162–169.
3. Provenzani A, Notarbartolo M, Labbozzetta M, Poma P, Biondi F, et al. (2009) The effect of CYP3A5 and ABCB1 single nucleotide polymorphisms on tacrolimus dose requirements in Caucasian liver transplant patients. Ann Transplant 14: 23–31.
4. Kausman JY, Patel B, Marks SD (2008) Standard dosing of tacrolimus leads to overexposure in pediatric renal transplantation recipients. Pediatr Transplant 12: 329–335.
5. Ferraris JR, Argibay PF, Costa L, Jimenez G, Coccia PA, et al. (2011) Influence of CYP3A5 polymorphism on tacrolimus maintenance doses and serum levels after renal transplantation: age dependency and pharmacological interaction with steroids. Pediatr Transplant 15: 525–532.
6. Gijsen V, Mital S, van Schaik RH, Soldin OP, Soldin SJ, et al. (2011) Age and CYP3A5 genotype affect tacrolimus dosing requirements after transplant in pediatric heart recipients. J Heart Lung Transplant 30: 1352–1359.
7. Vannaprasaht S, Reungjui S, Supanya D, Sirivongs D, Pongskul C, et al. (2013) Personalized tacrolimus doses determined by CYP3A5 genotype for induction and maintenance phases of kidney transplantation. Clin Ther 35: 1762–1769.
8. Iwasaki K (2007) Metabolism of tacrolimus (FK506) and recent topics in clinical pharmacokinetics. Drug Metab Pharmacokinet 22: 328–335.
9. Hesselink DA, Bouamar R, Elens L, van Schaik RH, van Gelder T (2014) The role of pharmacogenetics in the disposition of and response to tacrolimus in solid organ transplantation. Clin Pharmacokinet 53: 123–139.
10. Macphee IA, Fredericks S, Mohamed M, Moreton M, Carter ND, et al. (2005) Tacrolimus pharmacogenetics: the CYP3A5*1 allele predicts low dose-normalized tacrolimus blood concentrations in whites and South Asians. Transplantation 79: 499–502.
11. Min SI, Kim SY, Ahn SH, Min SK, Kim SH, et al. (2010) CYP3A5 *1 allele: impacts on early acute rejection and graft function in tacrolimus-based renal transplant recipients. Transplantation 90: 1394–1400.
12. Cho JH, Yoon YD, Park JY, Song EJ, Choi JY, et al. (2012) Impact of cytochrome P450 3A and ATP-binding cassette subfamily B member 1 polymorphisms on tacrolimus dose-adjusted trough concentrations among Korean renal transplant recipients. Transplant Proc 44: 109–114.
13. Saeki T, Ueda K, Tanigawara Y, Hori R, Komano T (1993) Human P-glycoprotein transports cyclosporin A and FK506. J Biol Chem 268: 6077–6080.
14. Glowacki F, Lionet A, Buob D, Labalette M, Allorge D, et al. (2011) CYP3A5 and ABCB1 polymorphisms in donor and recipient: impact on Tacrolimus dose requirements and clinical outcome after renal transplantation. Nephrol Dial Transplant 26: 3046–3050.
15. Gijsen VM, Madadi P, Dube MP, Hesselink DA, Koren G, et al. (2012) Tacrolimus-induced nephrotoxicity and genetic variability: a review. Ann Transplant 17: 111–121.
16. Wei-lin W, Jing J, Shu-sen Z, Li-hua W, Ting-bo L, et al. (2006) Tacrolimus dose requirement in relation to donor and recipient ABCB1 and CYP3A5 gene polymorphisms in Chinese liver transplant patients. Liver Transpl 12: 775–780.
17. Li L, Li CJ, Zheng L, Zhang YJ, Jiang HX, et al. (2011) Tacrolimus dosing in Chinese renal transplant recipients: a population-based pharmacogenetics study. Eur J Clin Pharmacol 67: 787–795.
18. Hosohata K, Masuda S, Yonezawa A, Sugimoto M, Takada Y, et al. (2009) Absence of influence of concomitant administration of rabeprazole on the pharmacokinetics of tacrolimus in adult living-donor liver transplant patients: a case-control study. Drug Metab Pharmacokinet 24: 458–463.
19. de Wildt SN, van Schaik RH, Soldin OP, Soldin SJ, Brojeni PY, et al. (2011) The interactions of age, genetics, and disease severity on tacrolimus dosing requirements after pediatric kidney and liver transplantation. Eur J Clin Pharmacol 67: 1231–1241.
20. Shilbayeh S, Zmeili R, Almardini RI (2013) The impact of CYP3A5 and MDR1 polymorphisms on tacrolimus dosage requirements and trough concentrations in pediatric renal transplant recipients. Saudi J Kidney Dis Transpl 24: 1125–1136.
21. Satoh S, Kagaya H, Saito M, Inoue T, Miura M, et al. (2008) Lack of tacrolimus circadian pharmacokinetics and CYP3A5 pharmacogenetics in the early and maintenance stages in Japanese renal transplant recipients. Br J Clin Pharmacol 66: 207–214.
22. Xue F, Zhang J, Han L, Li Q, Xu N, et al. (2010) Immune cell functional assay in monitoring of adult liver transplantation recipients with infection. Transplantation 89: 620–626.
23. Yu S, Wu L, Jin J, Yan S, Jiang G, et al. (2006) Influence of CYP3A5 gene polymorphisms of donor rather than recipient to tacrolimus individual dose requirement in liver transplantation. Transplantation 81: 46–51.
24. Jacobson PA, Oetting WS, Brearley AM, Leduc R, Guan W, et al. (2011) Novel polymorphisms associated with tacrolimus trough concentrations: results from a multicenter kidney transplant consortium. Transplantation 91: 300–308.
25. Chen D, Fan J, Guo F, Qin S, Wang Z, et al. (2013) Novel single nucleotide polymorphisms in interleukin 6 affect tacrolimus metabolism in liver transplant patients. PLoS One 8: e73405.
26. Uesugi M, Hosokawa M, Shinke H, Hashimoto E, Takahashi T, et al. (2013) Influence of cytochrome P450 (CYP) 3A4*1G polymorphism on the pharmacokinetics of tacrolimus, probability of acute cellular rejection, and mRNA expression level of CYP3A5 rather than CYP3A4 in living-donor liver transplant patients. Biol Pharm Bull 36: 1814–1821.
27. Fukudo M, Yano I, Masuda S, Goto M, Uesugi M, et al. (2006) Population pharmacokinetic and pharmacogenomic analysis of tacrolimus in pediatric living-donor liver transplant recipients. Clin Pharmacol Ther 80: 331–345.
28. Hawwa AF, McElnay JC (2011) Impact of ATP-binding cassette, subfamily B, member 1 pharmacogenetics on tacrolimus-associated nephrotoxicity and dosage requirements in paediatric patients with liver transplant. Expert Opin Drug Saf 10: 9–22.
29. Staatz CE, Goodman LK, Tett SE (2010) Effect of CYP3A and ABCB1 single nucleotide polymorphisms on the pharmacokinetics and pharmacodynamics of calcineurin inhibitors: Part II. Clin Pharmacokinet 49: 207–221.
30. Gomez-Bravo MA, Salcedo M, Fondevila C, Suarez F, Castellote J, et al. (2013) Impact of donor and recipient CYP3A5 and ABCB1 genetic polymorphisms on tacrolimus dosage requirements and rejection in Caucasian Spanish liver transplant patients. J Clin Pharmacol 53: 1146–1154.
31. Grenda R, Prokurat S, Ciechanowicz A, Piatosa B, Kalicinski P (2009) Evaluation of the genetic background of standard-immunosuppressant-related toxicity in a cohort of 200 paediatric renal allograft recipients–a retrospective study. Ann Transplant 14: 18–24.
32. Hawwa AF, McKiernan PJ, Shields M, Millership JS, Collier PS, et al. (2009) Influence of ABCB1 polymorphisms and haplotypes on tacrolimus nephrotoxicity and dosage requirements in children with liver transplant. Br J Clin Pharmacol 68: 413–421.
33. Hosohata K, Masuda S, Katsura T, Takada Y, Kaido T, et al. (2009) Impact of intestinal CYP2C19 genotypes on the interaction between tacrolimus and omeprazole, but not lansoprazole, in adult living-donor liver transplant patients. Drug Metab Dispos 37: 821–826.

7

The Suppressive Effect of Resveratrol on HIF-1α and VEGF Expression after Warm Ischemia and Reperfusion in Rat Liver

Mei Zhang[1⍭], Wujun Li[2⍭], Liang Yu[1], Shengli Wu[1]*

1 Department of Hepatobiliary Surgery, the First Affiliated Hospital of Xi'an Jiaotong University, Xi'an, P.R. China, 2 Department of General Surgery, the First Affiliated Hospital of Xi'an Medical University, Xi'an, P.R. China

Abstract

Background: Hypoxia-inducible factor-1α (HIF-1α) is overexpressed in many human tumors and their metastases, and is closely associated with a more aggressive tumor phenotype. The aim of the present study was to investigate the effect of resveratrol (RES) on the expression of ischemic-induced HIF-1α and vascular endothelial growth factor (VEGF) in rat liver.

Methods: Twenty-four rats were randomized into Sham, ischemia/reperfusion (I/R), and RES preconditioning groups. I/R was induced by portal pedicle clamping for 60 minutes followed by reperfusion for 60 minutes. The rats in RES group underwent the same surgical procedure as I/R group, and received 20 mg/kg resveratrol intravenously 30 min prior to ischemia. Blood and liver tissue samples were collected and subjected to biochemical assays, RT-PCR, and Western blot assays.

Results: I/R resulted in a significant ($P<0.05$) increase in liver HIF-1α and VEGF at both mRNA and protein levels 60 minutes after reperfusion. The mRNA and protein expressions of HIF-1α and VEGF decreased significantly in RES group when compared to I/R group ($P<0.05$).

Conclusion: The inhibiting effect of RES on the expressions of HIF-1α and VEGF induced by I/R in rat liver suggested that HIF-1α/VEGF could be a promising drug target for RES in the development of an effective anticancer therapy for the prevention of hepatic tumor growth and metastasis.

Editor: Aditya Bhushan Pant, Indian Institute of Toxicology Reserach, India

Funding: The authors have no support or funding to report.

Competing Interests: The authors have declared that no competing interests exist.

* Email: victorywu2000@163.com

⍭ These authors contributed equally to this work.

Introduction

Hepatocellular carcinoma (HCC) is one of the most common malignancies in the world [1]. Surgical resection and liver transplantation are conventional treatment modalities that can offer long-term survival for patients with HCC. However, the high incidence of tumor recurrence and metastasis after liver surgery remains a major problem [2]. Hepatic ischemia/reperfusion (I/R) injury is a phenomenon inevitable during liver surgery and promotes liver tumor growth and metastases through activation of cell adhesion, invasion, and angiogenesis pathways [3]. Hypoxia-inducible factor-1 alpha (HIF-1α) is one of the key regulators of hypoxia/ischemia [4]. Accumulating evidence indicated that the outgrowth of hepatic micrometastases is stimulated by I/R injuries during surgery and may at least in part, be stimulated by an increased HIF-1α stabilization [5,6]. HIF-1α stimulates transcription of multiple genes, including angiogenic vascular endothelial growth factor (VEGF) [7], an important growth factor involved in tumor angiogenesis [8], and HIF-1α/VEGF pathway have been implicated in the development of multiple tumors [9–11].

Resveratrol (trans-3,4′,5-trihydroxystilbene, RES) is a natural polyphenolic phytoalexin found in various plant species [12]. Numerous studies have demonstrated its diverse pharmacological activities, including antitumor and chemopreventive properties [13]. Studies in animal models have demonstrated that RES exerts potent anticarcinogenic effects via affecting diverse cellular events associated with tumor initiation, promotion, and progression [14]. Recently, RES has been found to inhibit angiogenesis and its antiangiogenic effects had been investigated in the setting of in vitro hypoxia, but the underlying mechanism of its antiangiogenic activity remains unclear [15].

In this study, we aimed to investigate whether RES inhibited I/R induced HIF-1α accumulation and VEGF expression in a rat model. The findings will provide further evidence that RES can be a potential chemopreventive and anticancer agent for reducing liver tumor recurrence and metastasis after liver surgery for HCC patients.

Materials and Methods

Animals

Male Sprague-Dawley (SD) rats 9–10 weeks old weighing 190–210 g were purchased from the Animal Center of Xi'an Jiaotong University (Xi'an, China). All rats were allowed free access to water and standard laboratory chow. Before operation the rats were fasted for 12 h and only allowed free access to water. Care was provided in accordance with the "Guide for the care and use of laboratory animals" (NIH publication No. 85–23, revised in 1996). The study was approved by the Xi'an Jiaotong University Institutional Animal Care and Use Committee.

Reagents

Resveratrol and dimethyl sulfoxide (DMSO) were purchased from Sigma Chemical Co., USA. RPMI-1640 was from Gibco-BRL, USA. The RES was dissolved and sterilized in DMSO and then diluted in RPMI-1640 to 4 mg/mL.

Experimental design

Rats were anesthetized with an intraperitoneal injection of pentobarbital sodium (50 mg/kg; Nembutal, Abbott Laboratories, North Chicago, IL). Twenty-four rats were randomly divided into three experimental groups (eight rats in each group) as follows: Sham operation group, a 6-cm midline abdominal incision was made to expose the liver and laparotomy was carried out for 60 min with no hepatic ischemia; I/R group: I/R was induced by portal pedicle clamping with an atraumatic microvascular clip for 60 minutes followed by removal of the clip for 60 minutes, and rats received an equivalent volume of placebo solution (RPMI-1640); and RES preconditioning group: rats in this group underwent the same surgical procedure as I/R group, and received one-shot injection of RES (4 mg/mL) at a dose of 20 mg/kg body weight through vena dorsalis penis 30 min prior to ischemia. All rats were euthanized with an overdose of pentobarbital (100 mg/kg IV) followed by exsanguinations at 60 min after clip removal, while Sham operation group animals were killed at the same time points after surgery. The liver was removed, and the inferior vena cava was cannulated so that blood samples could be taken from its suprahepatic segment. Blood samples were centrifuged at 4000 r/min at 4°C for 3 min and serum was taken and immediately processed. Liver tissues were snap-frozen in liquid nitrogen and stored at −80°C for further analysis.

Measurement of Serum Liver Enzymes

In all three groups serum alanine aminotransaminase (ALT), alkaline phosphates (ALP), and total bilirubin (TBIL) concentrations were measured using Hitachi AU5400 automatic biochemical analyzer (Hitachi Corp., Japan) and Roche Diagnostics kit (Roche, USA) at 60 min after reperfusion.

Real-time RT-PCR

After homogenization of liver tissue by the use of a MM301 Mixer Mill (Retsch, Haan, Germany), total cellular RNA was extracted from the liver tissue by using TriPure Reagent Isolation Reagent (Roche). RNA concentration was determined using UV spectrophotometer. Five hundred nanograms of RNA were reverse-transcribed and amplified to cDNA using real time RT-PCR with iScript One-Step RT-PCR Kit with SYBR Green (BioRad, USA). β-actin gene was used as an internal control. Primer sequences used in this study were designed using NCBI Primer-Blast (http://www.ncbi.nlm.nih.gov/tools/primer-blast) as follows: for the HIF-1α, sense 5′-ACTGCACAGGCCACATT-

CAT-3′ and antisense 5′-CGAGGCTGTGTCGACTGAGA-3′; for the VEGF, sense 5′-AGGCGAGGCAGCTTGAGTTA-3′ and antisense 5′-CTGTCGACGGTGACGATGGT-3′; for the β-actin, sense 5′-CCTAGGCACCAGGGTGTGAT-3′ and antisense 5′-TTGGTGACAATGCCGTGTTC-3′. The initial denaturation phase was 3 min at 95 °C followed by 39 cycles of denaturation at 95 °C for 10 s and annealing at 55 °C for 30 s. Relative quantification of PCR products was performed after normalization to β-actin.

Western blot analysis

After homogenization of liver tissue by the use of a MM301 Mixer Mill (Retsch, Haan, Germany), total cellular protein was extracted from the liver tissue by using tissue protein extraction buffer (Pierce, Rockford, IL, USA) containing protease inhibitors (Protease Inhibitor Cocktail 100X, Pierce). Protein concentrations were determined and the samples were subjected to sodium dodecyl sulfate/polyacrylamide gel electrophoresis and transferred to a nitrocellulose membrane (ECL, Amersham, Buckinghamshire, UK). The membranes were then blocked for 60 min and subsequently incubated with primary antibodies (1:3000) overnight at 4°C prior to incubation with anti-mouse IgG conjugated to horseradish peroxidase (1:6000) for 120 min at room temperature. Finally, the signals were detected using an enhanced chemiluminescence detection kit (Amersham, Piscataway, NJ, USA). The chemiluminescent signal was captured by a UVP BioSpectrum500 imaging system (UVP, Upland, CA, USA). Protein expression was quantified by densitometry and normalized to β-actin expression. Anti-HIF-1α, anti-VEGF, and anti-β-actin antibodies were obtained from Santa Cruz Biotechnology, Inc. (Santa Cruz, CA, United States).

Statistical analysis

All data are presented as the means ± standard deviation of the mean. Statistical analysis was performed using SPSS 16.0 software. Differences among groups were tested by one-way analysis of variance (ANOVA) with post-hoc Student-Newman-Keuls method. A P-value <0.05 was considered to indicate a statistically significant result.

Results

Liver function

Serum ALT, ALP and TBIL concentrations in different groups are shown in Table. 1. At 60 min post reperfusion, serum ALT, ALP and TBIL levels were significantly higher in I/R group than in the sham operation group (all $P<0.05$). Pretreatment with RES (20 mg/kg) showed a significant decrease in levels of serum ALT, ALP and TBIL than in I/R group (all $p<0.05$).

HIF-1α expression

The expression of HIF-1α in livers of experimental rats was examined by real-time RT-PCR and western blotting methods. Compared to sham operation group, both mRNA and protein expressions of HIF-1α were significantly increased in the livers of rats in I/R group (all $P<0.05$). Compared to I/R group, a significant reduction in HIF-1α mRNA and protein expression levels in RES preconditioning group was observed (all $P<0.05$; Fig. 1A and B).

VEGF expression

The expression of VEGF in livers of experimental rats was examined by real-time RT-PCR and western blotting methods. Compared to sham operation group, both mRNA and protein

Table 1. Serum biochemical parameters in different groups (mean ±SD).

Groups	n	ALT (U/L)	ALP(U/L)	TBIL (umol/L)
Sham	8	43.85±15.64	85.39±21.65	6.57±1.12
I/R	8	1465.50±316.37*	415.71±68.43*	35.41±5.87*
RES	8	837.65±205.53**	297.42±23.44**	21.47±3.69**

*p<0.05 vs Sham operation group;
**p<0.05 vs I/R group.

expressions of VEGF were significantly increased in the livers of rats in I/R group (all P<0.05). Compared to I/R group, a significant reduction in VEGF mRNA and protein expression levels in RES preconditioning group was observed (all P<0.05; Fig. 2A and B).

Discussion

Hepatic I/R injury may cause metabolic and structural hepatic damage [16] and has been proposed as a key clinical problem associated with liver transplantation and major liver surgery [17]. It involves a complex series of events, such as mitochondrial deenergization, adenosine-5′-triphosphate depletion, alterations of electrolyte homeostasis, as well as Kupffer cell activation, oxidative stress changes and upregulation of proinflammatory cytokine signaling [18]. At the same time, cellular response to low tissue oxygen concentrations is mediated by HIF-1 to protect liver from I/R injury.

HIF-1 is composed of HIF-1α and HIF-1β subunits [19]. HIF-1α was firstly described by Semenza in 1992 and the expression of which is tightly regulated by low oxygen tension [20], whereas

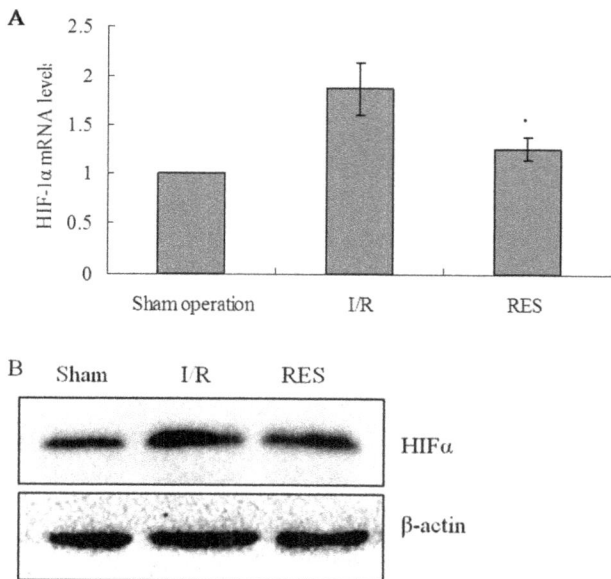

Figure 1. Expression of HIFα mRNA in rat livers. (A) HIFα mRNA levels were determined by real-time RT-PCR. Relative fold induction for HIFα mRNA (means ±SD) in I/R and RES group rat livers is presented relative to the expression in Sham operation group rat livers (*P<0.05 compared with I/R group). (B) Western blot analysis for HIFα protein expression in the indicated groups. β-actin was used as a loading control.

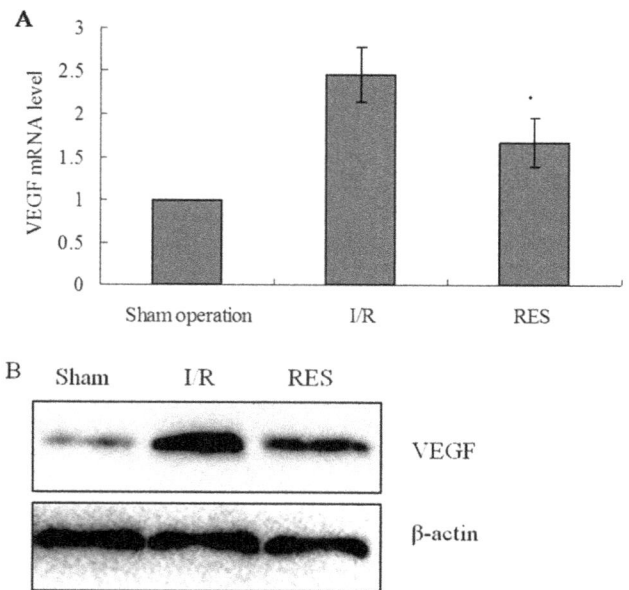

Figure 2. Expression of VEGF mRNA in rat livers. (A) VEGF mRNA levels were determined by real-time RT-PCR. Relative fold induction for VEGF mRNA (means ± SD) in I/R and RES group rat livers is presented relative to the expression in Sham operation group rat livers (*P<0.05 compared with I/R group). (B) Western blot analysis for VEGF protein expression in the indicated groups. β-actin was used as a loading control.

HIF-1β is constitutively expressed. Under normoxic conditions, HIF-1α protein is induced and continuously degraded by the ubiquitin-proteasome pathway in the cytoplasmic cellular compartment. However, under hypoxic conditions the blockade of degradation lead to the remarkable accumulation and translocation of HIF-1α protein to the nucleus, where it heterodimerizes with HIF-1β. This HIF-1 complex then initiates transcriptional activation via binding with hypoxia responsive elements in the promoter regions of target genes [21], including VEGF, erythropoietin, glycolytic enzymes, transferrin and a variety of other proteins that are important for adaptation and survival under hypoxic stress [22].

VEGF, an immediate downstream target gene of HIF-1α, plays a pivotal role in tumor angiogenesis [23], especially under conditions of intratumoral hypoxia. It promotes the proliferation of vessel endothelial cells, inhibits the apoptosis of vessel endothelial cells, and stimulates the formation of blood vessels [20]. Furthermore, it stimulates the production of hepatocyte growth factor (HGF), which is regarded as an initiator of liver regeneration [24]. Therefore, a stimulation of HIF-1α via liver ischemia, could be a double-edged sword; i.e., it protects the liver against I/R injuries, but a side effect could be the promotion of recurrence and metastasis of HCC through angiogenesis.

RES has been reported to have several biologic effects such as a potent antioxidative effect via prevention of lipid peroxidation, anti-platelet activity, an estrogenic activity, and anti-inflammatory activity attributed to cyclooxygenase inhibition [25]. Previous study had reported the hepatoprotective effects of RES in hepatic I/R and the protective effects of RES may be associated with its antioxidant activity and free radical scavenging activity which are released during the reperfusion period [26]. In recent years, RES has been found to inhibit tumor angiogenesis [27], but the mechanism of its antiangiogenic activity remains to be elucidated. Yu et al. reported that RES inhibits VEGF expression of HepG2 cells through a NF-kappa B-mediated mechanism [28]. Cao et al. reported that RES may inhibit human ovarian cancer progression and angiogenesis by inhibiting HIF-1α and VEGF expression through multiple mechanisms, including the inhibition of AKT and mitogen-activated protein kinase activation, the inhibition of several protein translational regulators, and inducing HIF-1α protein degradation through the proteasome pathway [29]. Zhang et al. showed that RES directly inhibits hypoxia-mediated HIF-1α protein accumulation by inhibiting its degradation via the proteasomal pathway in both SCC-9 and HepG2 cells [30]. In the present study, as expected, serum ALT, ALP and TBIL levels were significantly higher in I/R group than in the sham operation group at 60 min post reperfusion, while pretreatment with RES (20 mg/kg) showed a significant decrease in levels of serum ALT,

ALP and TBIL than in I/R group. Moreover, we further showed that the mRNA and protein expressions of HIF-1α and VEGF were increased significantly in rats subjected to 60 minutes of warm liver ischemia and 60 minutes of reperfusion compared to the control group, while the mRNA and protein expressions of HIF-1α and VEGF decreased significantly in RES group when compared to I/R group. These findings affirmed the results of previous studies showing the hepatoprotective effects of RES in hepatic I/R. More importantly, we provided the first evidence supporting the antiangiogenic effects of RES in the setting of in vivo hypoxia, which are consistent with previous findings, suggesting that RES inhibits angiogenesis at least partly through regulating the expressions of HIF-1α and VEGF. However, additional studies are needed to identify the detailed mechanisms by which RES regulated the expressions of HIF-1α and VEGF.

Taken together, our present study has provided evidence that RES, exerts its antiangiogenic effects through inhibiting HIF-1α and its downstream target gene, VEGF, in a rat model of hepatic I/R injury. HIF-1α/VEGF axis, as a key regulator of tumor growth and metastasis, could be a promising drug target for RES in the development of an effective anticancer therapy for the prevention of hepatic tumor growth and metastasis.

Author Contributions

Conceived and designed the experiments: SW. Performed the experiments: MZ WL. Analyzed the data: LY. Contributed reagents/materials/analysis tools: MZ. Wrote the paper: SW.

References

1. Bosch FX, Ribes J, Díaz M, Cléries R (2004) Primary liver cancer: worldwide incidence and trends. Gastroenterology 127: S5–S16.
2. Zhang Y, Shi ZL, Yang X, Yin ZF (2014) Targeting of circulating hepatocellular carcinoma cells to prevent postoperative recurrence and metastasis. World J Gastroenterol 20: 142–147.
3. Li CX, Shao Y, Ng KT, Liu XB, Ling CC, et al. (2012) FTY720 suppresses liver tumor metastasis by reducing the population of circulating endothelial progenitor cells. PLoS One 7: e32380.
4. Cursio R, Miele C, Filippa N, Van Obberghen E, Gugenheim J (2008) Liver HIF-1 alpha induction precedes apoptosis following normothermic ischemia-reperfusion in rats. Transplant Proc 40: 2042–2045.
5. van der Bilt JD, Kranenburg O, Nijkamp MW, Smakman N, Veenendaal LM, et al. (2005) Ischemia/reperfusion accelerates the outgrowth of hepatic micrometastases in a highly standardized murine model. Hepatology 42: 165–175.
6. Knudsen AR, Kannerup AS, Grønbæk H, Andersen KJ, Funch-Jensen P, et al. (2011) Effects of ischemic pre- and postconditioning on HIF-1α, VEGF and TGF-β expression after warm ischemia and reperfusion in the rat liver. Comp Hepatol 10: 3.
7. Boros P, Tarcsafalvi A, Wang L, Megyesi J, Liu J, et al. (2001) Intrahepatic expression and release of vascular endothelial growth factor following orthotopic liver transplantation in the rat. Transplantation 72: 805–811.
8. Tamagawa K, Horiuchi T, Uchinami M, Doi K, Yoshida M, et al. (2008) Hepatic ischemia-reperfusion increases vascular endothelial growth factor and cancer growth in rats. J Surg Res 148: 158–163.
9. Chai ZT, Kong J, Zhu XD, Zhang YY, Lu L, et al. (2013) MicroRNA-26a inhibits angiogenesis by down-regulating VEGFA through the PIK3C2α/Akt/HIF-1α pathway in hepatocellular carcinoma. PLoS One 8: e77957.
10. An X, Xu G, Yang L, Wang Y, Li Y, et al. (2014) Expression of hypoxia-inducible factor-1α, vascular endothelial growth factor and prolyl hydroxylase domain protein 2 in cutaneous squamous cell carcinoma and precursor lesions and their relationship with histological stages and clinical features. J Dermatol 41: 76–83.
11. Shi D, Xie F, Zhang Y, Tian Y, Chen W, et al. (2014) TFAP2A Regulates Nasopharyngeal Carcinoma Growth and Survival by Targeting HIF-1α Signaling Pathway. Cancer Prev Res (Phila) 7: 266–277.
12. Soleas GJ, Diamandis EP, Goldberg DM (1997) Wine as a biological fluid: history, production, and role in disease prevention. J Clin Lab Anal 11: 287–313.
13. Singh CK, George J, Ahmad N (2013) Resveratrol-based combinatorial strategies for cancer management. Ann N Y Acad Sci 1290: 113–121.
14. Aziz MH, Kumar R, Ahmad N (2003) Cancer chemoprevention by resveratrol: in vitro and in vivo studies and the underlying mechanisms. Int J Oncol 23: 17–28.
15. Wen D, Huang X, Zhang M, Zhang L, Chen J, et al. (2013) Resveratrol attenuates diabetic nephropathy via modulating angiogenesis. PLoS One 8: e82336.
16. Shin T, Kuboki S, Huber N, Eismann T, Galloway E, et al. (2008) Activation of peroxisome proliferator-activated receptor-gamma during hepatic ischemia is age-dependent. J Surg Res 147: 200–205.
17. Ito K, Ozasa H, Noda Y, Koike Y, Arii S, et al. (2008) Effect of non-essential amino acid glycine administration on the liver regeneration of partially hepatectomized rats with hepatic ischemia/reperfusion injury. Clin Nutr 27: 773–780.
18. Papadopoulos D, Siempis T, Theodorakou E, Tsoulfas G (2013) Hepatic ischemia and reperfusion injury and trauma: current concepts. Arch Trauma Res 2: 63–70.
19. Wang GL, Jiang BH, Rue EA, Semenza GL (1995) Hypoxia-inducible factor 1 is a basic-helix-loop-helix-PAS heterodimer regulated by cellular O2 tension. Proc Natl Acad Sci U S A 92: 5510–5514.
20. Xu LF, Ni JY, Sun HL, Chen YT, Wu YD (2013) Effects of hypoxia-inducible factor-1α silencing on the proliferation of CBRH-7919 hepatoma cells. World J Gastroenterol 19: 1749–1759.
21. Semenza GL, Jiang BH, Leung SW, Passantino R, Concordet JP, et al. (1996) Hypoxia response elements in the aldolase A, enolase 1, and lactate dehydrogenase A gene promoters contain essential binding sites for hypoxia-inducible factor-1. J Biol Chem 271: 32529–32537.
22. Vaupel P (2004) The role of hypoxia-induced factors in tumor progression. Oncologist 9: 10–17.
23. Semenza GL (2003) Targeting HIF-1 for cancer therapy. Nat Rev Cancer 3: 721–732.
24. Michalopoulos GK (2007) Liver regeneration. J Cell Physiol 213: 286–300.
25. Wu SL, Yu L, Jiao XY, Meng KW, Pan CE (2006) The suppressive effect of resveratrol on protein kinase C theta in peripheral blood T lymphocytes in a rat liver transplantation model. Transplant Proc 38: 3052–3054.
26. Gedik E, Girgin S, Ozturk H, Obay BD, Ozturk H, et al. (2008) Resveratrol attenuates oxidative stress and histological alterations induced by liver ischemia/reperfusion in rats. World J Gastroenterol 14: 7101–7106.
27. Tseng SH, Lin SM, Chen JC, Su YH, Huang HY, et al. (2004) Resveratrol suppresses the angiogenesis and tumor growth of gliomas in rats. Clin Cancer Res 10: 2190–2202.

28. Yu HB, Zhang HF, Zhang X, Li DY, Xue HZ, et al. (2010) Resveratrol inhibits VEGF expression of human hepatocellular carcinoma cells through a NF-kappa B-mediated mechanism. Hepatogastroenterology 57: 1241–1246.

29. Cao ZX, Fang J, Xia C, Shi XL, Jiang BH (2004) Trans-3,4,5'-trihydrox-ystibene inhibits hypoxia-inducible factor-1α and vascular endothelial growth factor expression in human ovarian cancer cells. Clin Cancer Res 10: 5253–5263.

30. Zhang Q, Tang X, Lu QY, Zhang ZF, Brown J, et al. (2005) Resveratrol inhibits hypoxia-induced accumulation of hypoxia-inducible factor-1alpha and VEGF expression in human tongue squamous cell carcinoma and hepatoma cells. Mol Cancer Ther 4: 1465–1474.

8

Tacrolimus-Based versus Cyclosporine-Based Immunosuppression in Hepatitis C Virus-Infected Patients after Liver Transplantation: A Meta-Analysis and Systematic Review

Zhenmin Liu[1], Yi Chen[1], Renchuan Tao[1]*, Jing Xv[2], Jianyuan Meng[2], Xiangzhi Yong[1]

1 Department of Periodontology and Oral Medicine, College of Stomatology, Guangxi Medical University, Nanning, Guangxi, China, 2 Department of Hepato-biliary Surgery, First Affiliated Hospital of Guangxi Medical University, Nanning, Guangxi, China

Abstract

Background: Most liver transplant recipients receive calcineurin inhibitors (CNIs), especially tacrolimus and cyclosporine, as immunosuppressant agents to prevent rejection. A controversy exists as to whether the outcomes of hepatitis C virus (HCV)-infected liver transplant patients differ based on the CNIs used. This meta-analysis compares the clinical outcomes of tacrolimus-based and cyclosporine-based immunosuppression, especially cases of HCV recurrence in liver transplant patients with end-stage liver disease caused by HCV infection.

Methods: Related articles were identified from the Cochrane Hepato-Biliary Group Controlled Trials Register, the Cochrane Central Register of Controlled Trials (CENTRAL) in the Cochrane Library, Medline, and Embase. Meta-analyses were performed for the results of homogeneous studies.

Results: Nine randomized or quasi-randomized controlled trials were included. The total effect size of mortality (RR = 0.98, 95% CI: 0.77–1.25, $P = 0.87$) and graft loss (RR = 1.05, 95% CI: 0.83–1.33, $P = 0.67$) showed no significant difference between the two groups irrespective of duration of immunosuppressant therapy after liver transplantation. In addition, the HCV recurrence-induced mortality (RR = 1.11, 95% CI: 0.66–1.89, $P = 0.69$), graft loss (RR = 1.62, 95% CI: 0.64–4.07, $P = 0.31$) and retransplantation (RR = 1.40, 95% CI: 0.48–4.09, $P = 0.54$), as well as available biopsies, confirmed that histological HCV recurrences (RR = 0.92, 95% CI: 0.71–1.19, $P = 0.51$) were similar.

Conclusion: These results suggested no difference in posttransplant HCV recurrence-induced mortality, graft loss and retransplantation, as well as histological HCV recurrence in patients treated with tacrolimus-based and cyclosporine-based immunosuppresion.

Editor: Rafael Aldabe, Centro de Investigación en Medicina Aplicada (CIMA), Spain

Funding: This study was supported by National Natural Science Foundation of China (NSFC81260167), funder's website: http://www.nsfc.gov.cn. The funders had no role in study design, data collection and analysis, decision to publish, or preparation of the manuscript.

Competing Interests: The authors have declared that no competing interests exist.

* Email: taorenchuan@gmail.com

Introduction

Hepatitis C virus (HCV) infection constitutes a serious challenge to global health, and accounts for the loss of approximately 12,111,000 Disability-Adjusted Life Years (DALYs) [1]. Also, end-stage liver diseases caused by HCV infection are the leading indication for orthotropic liver transplantation. Unfortunately, recurrent hepatitis C is universal, resulting in accelerated progression to cirrhosis with 5 years of transplantation for 10%–30% of patients [2] and causing graft loss as well as the need for retransplantation. Thus, good control of the virus before and after transplantation to alleviate recurrence, as well as accessing sufficient numbers of liver grafts, are both enormous challenges in liver transplantation. Attempts to prevent reinfection and

rejection via antiviral treatment with a combination of immunosuppressant regimens gave promising results [3]. However, options for antiviral therapy are limited and are associated with a significant side-effect profile mainly caused by pegylated interferon and ribavirin therapy [4]; future interferon-free antiviral therapies will be more efficacious with fewer side effects. In addition, the dosage, duration, and composition of immunosuppressant regimens vary in different liver transplant centers.

Cyclosporine has been used as an effective immunosuppressant after liver transplantation since 1983, showing significant clinical advances in graft survival and patient survival in organ transplants [5,6]. Subsequently, tacrolimus was found to have a mechanism of action in inhibition of calcineurin phosphatase (CNI) consistent with that of cyclosporine, even though they bind different intracellular immunophilins [7]. As for better efficacy with respect to reduced mortality and graft loss with immunosuppressant therapy, tacrolimus has been the primary immunosuppressant agent. However, cyclosporine has been reported to have antiviral effects by suppressing the replication of the hepatitis C virus [8,9] and increasing the chance of a sustained virological response after transplantation [10], an effect that was not detected with tacrolimus [11]. Controversy exists as to whether the clinical outcomes of HCV infection-related liver transplants differ depending on the types of CNIs used. However, immunosuppression is a major factor responsible for accelerated recurrence and faster progression of recurrent HCV infection [12]. A meta-analysis [13] reported patient and graft survivals in HCV-positive liver transplant patients were similar regardless of the CNIs selected as the basic immunosuppressant. However, few studies focused on the differences in efficacy between tacrolimus and cyclosporine which might affect HCV recurrence. Therefore, the purpose of our meta-analysis was to evaluate clinical outcomes, especially cases of HCV recurrence in liver transplantation comparing tacrolimus-based and cyclosporine-based immunosuppression.

Patients and Methods

Inclusion criteria

The inclusion criteria were: 1) Randomised and quasi-randomised controlled trials which compared tacrolimus with cyclosporine solution (Sandimmune) or cyclosporine microemulsion (Neoral) as immunosuppressive therapy in patients with end-stage liver disease caused by HCV infection who underwent a primary liver transplant; 2) Trials in which a group of HCV patients were considered as a subgroup, and results reported the variables of interest in our studies, with sufficient data for calculating the risk ratio (RR) with 95% confidence interval (CI). 3) A minimum of one year duration of follow-up. If the results of interest from patients in a clinical trial were reported more than once, data from the publication with the longest follow-up were extracted. In addition, studies on patients who underwent multi-organ transplantation or had previously received a liver transplant were excluded.

Search strategy

We performed an electronic search of the following databases: The Cochrane Hepato-Biliary Group Controlled Trials Register (up to March 2014), the Cochrane Central Register of Controlled Trials (CENTRAL) in the Cochrane Library (up to March 2014), Medline (1948 to March 2014), and Embase (1980 to March 2014). Key words used in the search were: "tacrolimus" or "FK506", and "cyclosporine" or "Neoral" or "calcineurin inhibitors" or "cyclosporine A (CyA)", as well as "liver transplantation". In addition, hepatitis C or HCV-related and HCV recurrence were included.

Data extraction

Standardized forms were designed for data extraction; two investigators entered the data on patient demographics, duration of follow-up, methodology, blood concentration of tacrolimus and cyclosporine in the first three months and in the 12th month of immunosuppressant therapy, combination regimens, and occurrence of the following outcomes: mortality, graft loss, histological HCV recurrence; and mortality, graft loss as well as retransplantation due to HCV respectively. Any inconsistencies were addressed by further discussion.

Statistical analysis

Assessment of effect sizes and heterogeneity were performed using Review Manager 5.2 software. Pooled RR and 95% CIs were calculated for categorical outcomes using fixed effects models; if no significant heterogeneity was present, random effects models were used. Heterogeneity among trials was assessed by Cochran's Q-statistic and I^2 index, when the P-value for heterogeneity was <0.1 or I^2>50%, significant heterogeneity was detected; if statistic heterogeneity was present in meta-analysis, sensitivity analysis was conducted by subsequent exclusion of the single study with the highest weight to assess the validity of outcome.

Publication bias including funnel plot and Egger's test was performed using STATA version 10.0.

Results

Study description

The search was performed in March 2014, and 82 studies were found in four public databases. Nine randomized and quasi-randomized controlled trials allocated 1180 participants of whom 570 were randomized to tacrolimus-based and 610 to cyclosporine-based. Studies were excluded if they were not originally designed to compare tacrolimus to cyclosporine. Additionally, duplicated publication or non-randomized controlled trials were also excluded (Fig 1). Across these nine studies, all participants received a primary liver transplantation with end-stage liver disease caused by HCV infection. HCV recurrence was measured and assessed using liver biopsy. The characteristics of randomized and quasi-randomized trials included in the systematic review are shown in Table 1.

Meta-Analysis of treatment efficacy

Mortality. By virtue of our selection criteria, mortality was reported in all of the included trials. There was no significant statistical difference in mortality between the two groups in the fixed-effects model (RR = 0.98, 95% CI: 0.77–1.25, P = 0.87) (Fig 2). Moreover, no heterogeneity among the included trials (P = 0.51, I^2 = 0%) was observed.

Mortality due to HCV recurrence. Mortality due to HCV recurrence was reported in five trials. The total effect size of mortality due to HCV recurrence was similar (RR = 1.11, 95% CI: 0.66–1.89, P = 0.69) (Fig 3) in fixed-effects model. Moreover, no heterogeneity among the included trials (P = 0.85, I^2 = 0.0%) was observed.

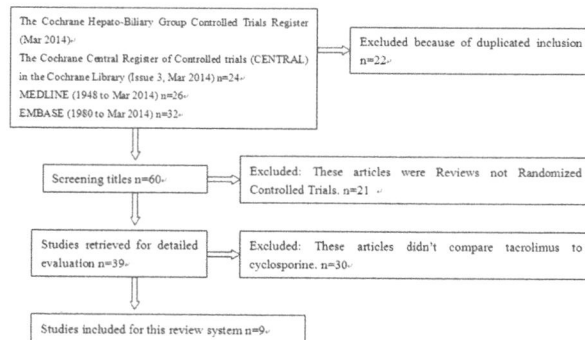

Figure 1. Flow chart of the selection process for including articles.

Table 1. Characteristics of randomized and quasi-randomized trials included in the systematic review.

Trials	Methods	N	Tacrolimus concentration (ng/ml)		Cyclosporine concentration(ng/ml)		Anti-proliferative agent	Steroids	Duration of follow-up
			0–3 month	1 year	0–3 month	1 year			
Levy 2014 [25]	Multicenter, randomized, open-label study	Tac n = 182 CsA n = 169	NS	NS	NS	NS	MMF/AZA	Not stated detail regimen of steroids OR steroids-free	12 months
Berenguer 2010 [24]	Pseudo-randomized controlled trial	Tac n = 117 CsA n = 136	5–15	3–10	150–350	100–150	MMF	Methyl-prednisolone &prednisone	7 years
Shenoy 2008 [18]	Single-center, prospective, randomized trial	Tac n = 14 CsA n = 18	8–12	5–10	800–1200	600–1000	MMF	Methyl-prednisolone &prednisone	12 months
Villamil 2006 [26]	Multicenter open-label randomized study	Tac n = 48 CsA n = 47	NS	NS	NS	NS	AZA	Not stated the detail of Steriods	34–37 months
Levy 2006 [17]	Multicenter, randomized, open-label, parallel-group, prospective study	Tac n = 85 CsA n = 88	5–15	5–10	800–1200	500–700	AZA	Methyl-prednisolone &prednisone	12 months
Martin 2004 [37]	Prospective, randomized, multicenter, open-label study	Tac n = 38 CsA n = 41	10–12	5–10	200–250	100–250	AZA	Prednisone	12 months
Zervos 1998 [31]	Randomized, prospective study	Tac n = 25 CsA n = 24	15	NS	300–400	NS	NS	Methyl-prednisolone &prednisone/ Prednisone	18 months
Wiesner 1998 [38]	Randomized comparative open-label study	Tac n = 57 CsA n = 56	10–25	10–12	250–400	200–300	AZA	Methyl-prednisolone	5 years
Mueller 1995 [39]	Single-center, prospective, randomized trial	Tac n = 17 CsA n = 18	NS	NS	NS	NS	NS	Methyl-prednisolone	12 months

NS = not stated.
MMF = mycophenolate mofetil; AZA = azathioprine.

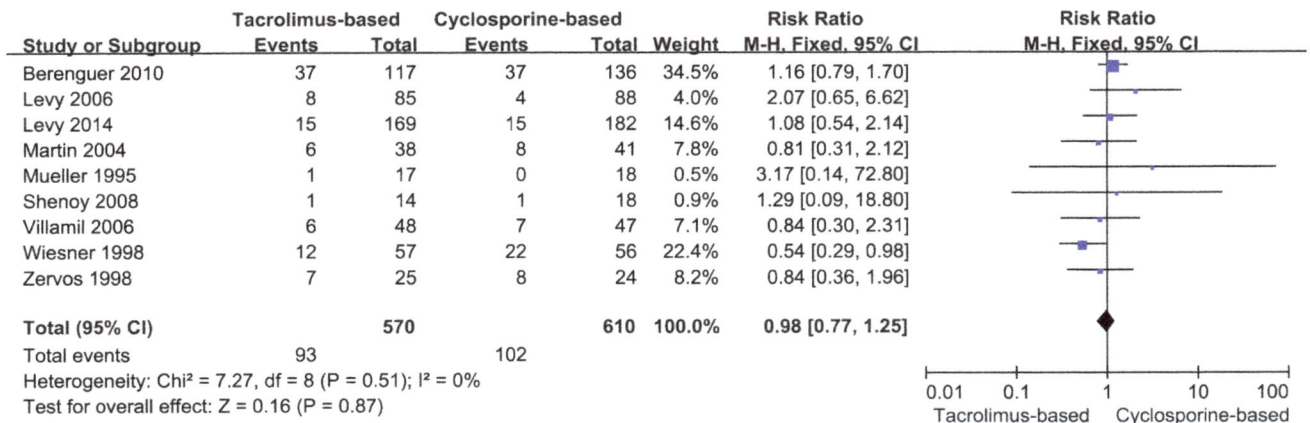

Figure 2. Forest plot of mortality comparing tacrolimus-based to cyclosporine-based immunosuppressant group.

Graft loss. Graft loss was reported in seven trials. A meta-analysis using fixed-effects model was performed with respect to graft loss, but the difference was too small to reach statistical significance (RR = 1.05, 95% CI: 0.83–1.33, $P = 0.67$) (Fig 4). Moreover, moderate inconsistencies existed among the trials ($P = 0.22$, $I^2 = 28\%$).

Graft loss due to HCV recurrence. Data on graft loss due to recurrent HCV was only available in three trials. Eleven of the 255 patients in the tacrolimus-based group compared to 7 of 270 in the cyclosporine-based group lost their grafts owing to HCV recurrence. The difference did not reach statistical significance in the fixed-effects model (RR = 1.62, 95% CI: 0.64–4.07, $P = 0.31$) (Fig 5). No heterogeneity among the included trials was detected ($I^2 = 0\%$, $P = 0.91$).

Retransplantation Due to HCV Recurrence. Retransplantation due to HCV recurrence was reported in three trials. Seven patients in the tacrolimus-based group (n = 179) and 5 in the cyclosporine-based group (n = 181) were retransplanted due to HCV recurrence after the primary transplantation during the follow-up period. When a meta-analysis using fixed-effects model was performed concerning the incidence of retransplantation due to HCV recurrence, the outcome showed no significant statistical difference between the two groups (RR = 1.40, 95% CI: 0.48–4.09, $P = 0.54$) (Fig. 6). No heterogeneity among the included trials was detected ($I^2 = 0\%$, $P = 0.47$).

Histological HCV Recurrence. Histological HCV recurrence was reported in five trials. A meta-analysis was performed using random-effects model, and the data referred to the number of the patients biopsied and the patients who were diagnosed as HCV recurrence by protocol biopsy. There was no significant statistical difference detected in the two groups (RR = 0.92, 95% CI: 0.71–1.19, $P = 0.51$), while the heterogeneity was substantially significant, ($I^2 = 72\%$, $P = 0.006$) (Fig 7). In order to conduct a sensitivity analysis to assess the validity of outcome, the trial with highest weight was excluded. The remaining four trials, which showed 107 instances of histological HCV recurrence in the tacrolimus-based group (n = 200) and 128 instances in the cyclosporine-based group (n = 207), were included. Difference in the recurrence of HCV was not statistically significant in the two groups (RR = 0.86, 95% CI: 0.73–1.01, $P = 0.06$) (Fig 8).

Publication bias

The funnel plots for publication bias for risk ratio in mortality show little asymmetry, but the Egger's test result was insignificant ($P = 0.443$). The result indicated no publication bias for the risk ratio pooled mortality in tacrolimus-based and cyclosporine-based groups.

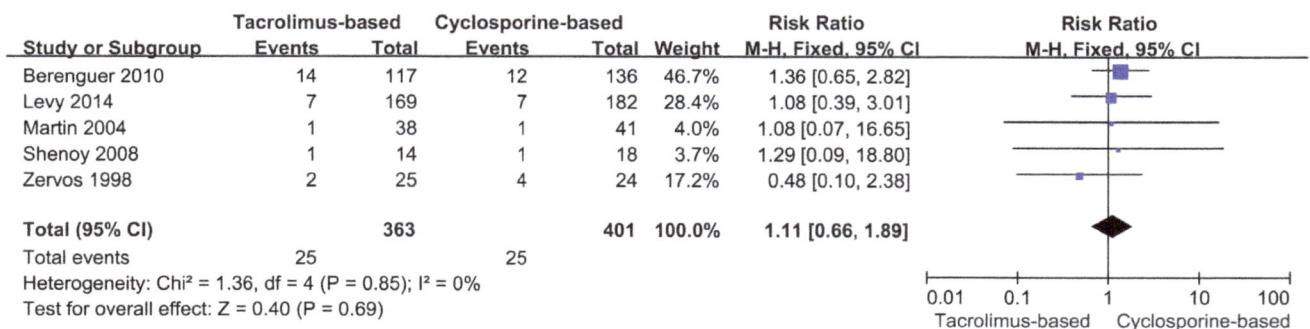

Figure 3. Forest plot of mortality due to HCV recurrence comparing tacrolimus-based to cyclosporine-based group.

| Study or Subgroup | Tacrolimus-based | | Cyclosporine-based | | | Risk Ratio | Risk Ratio |
	Events	Total	Events	Total	Weight	M-H, Fixed, 95% CI	M-H, Fixed, 95% CI
Berenguer 2010	40	117	43	136	40.8%	1.08 [0.76, 1.54]	
Levy 2006	8	85	2	88	2.0%	4.14 [0.91, 18.94]	
Levy 2014	13	169	8	182	7.9%	1.75 [0.74, 4.12]	
Martin 2004	9	38	11	41	10.9%	0.88 [0.41, 1.89]	
Villamil 2006	6	48	5	47	5.2%	1.18 [0.38, 3.59]	
Wiesner 1998	15	57	23	56	23.8%	0.64 [0.37, 1.09]	
Zervos 1998	8	25	9	24	9.4%	0.85 [0.40, 1.84]	
Total (95% CI)		539		574	100.0%	1.05 [0.83, 1.33]	
Total events	99		101				
Heterogeneity: Chi² = 8.32, df = 6 (P = 0.22); I² = 28%							
Test for overall effect: Z = 0.43 (P = 0.67)							

Tacrolimus-based   Cyclosporine-based

0.01   0.1   1   10   100

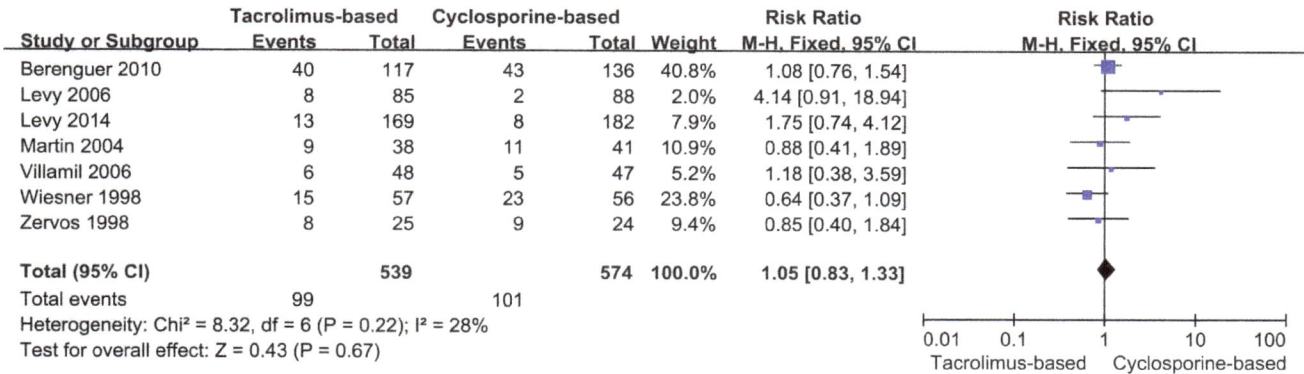

Figure 4. Forest plot of graft loss comparing tacrolimus-based to cyclosporine-based group.

Discussion

Calcineurin inhibitors (CNIs) represent the cornerstone of immunosuppression in liver transplantation, especially tacrolimus and cyclosporine. Although in recent years many clinical trials reported the distinction between these two typical calcineurin inhibitors, there is a paucity of prospective studies comparing tacrolimus with cyclosporine in terms of their ability to reduce HCV recurrence. However, the progression of HCV-related disease is accelerated in immunosuppressed liver transplant recipients compared to immunocompetent patients, with a progressive increase in patients who have recently undergone liver transplantation [2,14]. Hence, a meta-analysis was performed using prospective randomized studies to evaluate clinical outcomes, especially cases of HCV recurrence after liver transplantation in HCV-infected patients treated with tacrolimus-based and cyclosporine-based immunosuppression.

There was no significant statistical difference detected in terms of HCV recurrence-induced mortality, graft loss and retransplantation. In addition, the severity of histological HCV recurrence was similar in these two groups, which confirmed the outcome of a meta-analysis and some retrospective reviews [13,15,16]. However, two included trials [17,18] found the mean time to histological recurrence was significantly shorter in the tacrolimus-based group. Furthermore, previous reports suggested that HCV recurrence may be more aggressive with tacrolimus therapy compared to cyclosporine microemulsion [19]. A retrospective study was established in patients who underwent liver transplantation for hepatitis C virus-induced liver disease to evaluate the impact of calcineurin inhibitors, and the cyclosporine group showed improved histological hepatitis C virus recurrence-free survival compared to the tacrolimus group (55.4% vs. 30.8% at 1 year, 18.6% vs. 10.3% at 3 years, 16.7% vs. 8.1% at 5 years, p<0.001) [20]. As for the risk factors associated with survival and histological HCV recurrence, donor age and gender combined with tacrolimus use were taken into account in previous studies [20–23]. Donor age was reported in only four included trials [17,24–26]. The mean donor ages of these four studies ranged from 43 to 56 years, and there was no significant difference between patient populations in the two treatment groups in terms of donor age. As for the risk of the usage of tacrolimus, a randomized controlled pilot study in vivo showed that changing from tacrolimus to cyclosporine led to a modest HCV RNA drop and appeared to enhance the antiviral response of PEG/RBV [27]. Selzner et al. reported a retrospective study of 446 patients who received liver allograft for HCV-related cirrhosis; results suggested that the overall sustained virological response (SVR) was higher on CyA than on tacrolimus. Furthermore, cyclosporine improved the efficacy of the antiviral therapy in liver transplant patients compared to tacrolimus [28]. Because there is little established evidence of clinical benefits, further studies are needed to compare the therapeutic effect of CNIs in hepatitis C-infected patients after liver transplantation.

The trials included were enrolled from multiple centers, and the dosages, blood levels, durations and composition of the immunosuppressant regimens varied. In general, higher doses were used during the early post-transplantation weeks, and a gradual reduction was achieved during the first 12 months. Standard

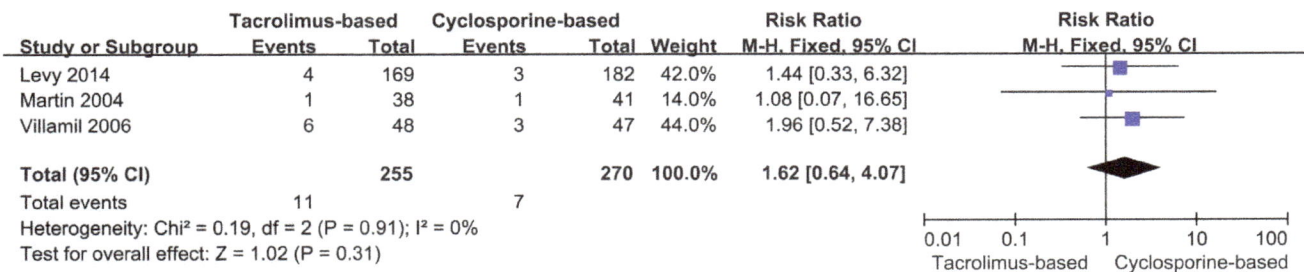

| Study or Subgroup | Tacrolimus-based | | Cyclosporine-based | | | Risk Ratio | Risk Ratio |
	Events	Total	Events	Total	Weight	M-H, Fixed, 95% CI	M-H, Fixed, 95% CI
Levy 2014	4	169	3	182	42.0%	1.44 [0.33, 6.32]	
Martin 2004	1	38	1	41	14.0%	1.08 [0.07, 16.65]	
Villamil 2006	6	48	3	47	44.0%	1.96 [0.52, 7.38]	
Total (95% CI)		255		270	100.0%	1.62 [0.64, 4.07]	
Total events	11		7				
Heterogeneity: Chi² = 0.19, df = 2 (P = 0.91); I² = 0%							
Test for overall effect: Z = 1.02 (P = 0.31)							

Tacrolimus-based   Cyclosporine-based

0.01   0.1   1   10   100

Figure 5. Forest plot of graft loss due to HCV recurrence comparing tacrolimus-based to cyclosporine-based group.

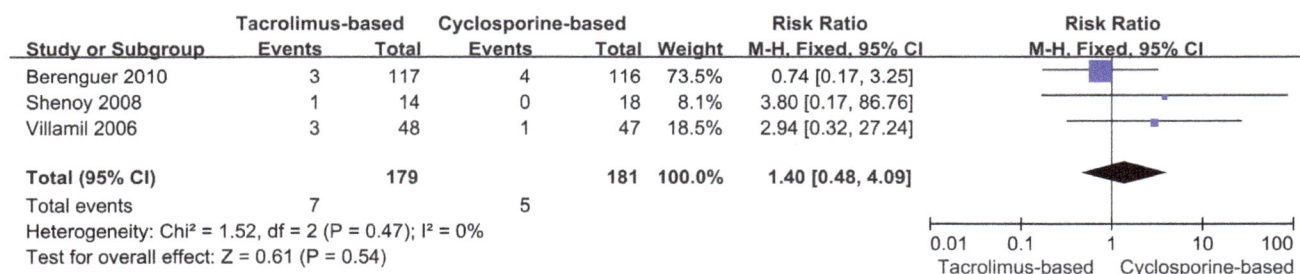

Study or Subgroup	Tacrolimus-based		Cyclosporine-based		Weight	Risk Ratio M-H, Fixed, 95% CI	Risk Ratio M-H, Fixed, 95% CI
	Events	Total	Events	Total			
Berenguer 2010	3	117	4	116	73.5%	0.74 [0.17, 3.25]	
Shenoy 2008	1	14	0	18	8.1%	3.80 [0.17, 86.76]	
Villamil 2006	3	48	1	47	18.5%	2.94 [0.32, 27.24]	
Total (95% CI)		179		181	100.0%	1.40 [0.48, 4.09]	
Total events	7		5				

Heterogeneity: Chi² = 1.52, df = 2 (P = 0.47); I² = 0%
Test for overall effect: Z = 0.61 (P = 0.54)

Figure 6. Forest plot of retransplantation due to HCV recurrence comparing tacrolimus-based to cyclosporine-based group.

dosages of CNIs and immunosuppressant regimens have not been developed, but Barbier et al. were in favor of the minimum effective dose that would achieve reduced risk of chronic rejection in the majority of liver transplant patients [29]. In addition, conversion from a tacrolimus twice-daily formulation to a once-daily formulation was considered a safe and effective strategy for the management of stable liver transplantation patients [30]. However, minimization (reduction and withdrawal) regimens of calcineurin inhibitors were scarcely reported and remain in need of study. As for the use of steroids, the details were not reported in most of the included articles, but similar dosage of steroids was administered in both arms [17,26,31]. Different usage of steroids as immunosuppressant regimen might affect the clinical outcome. A meta-analysis comprising 19 RCT was conducted to evaluate the comparison of steroid-free with steroid-based immunosuppression: HCV recurrence was lower with steroid avoidance, although no individual trial reached significant statistical difference [32]. Another meta-analysis demonstrated a significant advantage of steroid-free protocols with respect to HCV recurrence [33]. However, a retrospective analysis [34] suggested that rapid tapering off of steroid dose was associated with a significantly higher rate of HCV recurrence.

More heterogeneity was detected between the trials when analyzed for histological HCV recurrence than for other clinical outcomes. The trial with highest weight was excluded so as to conduct a sensitivity analysis, and the results showed no statistically significant difference between the two groups, which was consistent with the original results that included all five trials reporting histological HCV. This may suggest that the

meta-analysis outcomes were not affected by heterogeneity and their validity was acceptable.

Limitations

Overall, several limitations of this study should be considered. The major limitation was the small number of trials available for analysis. In addition, some of the included trials were not originally designed to compare tacrolimus versus cyclosporine in hepatitis C patients after liver transplantation; rather, HCV-infected patients were considered as one subgroup in these trials. Furthermore, because of the small sample size, tests for heterogeneity were analyzed irrespective of the dosage/blood levels of different immunosuppressant agents.

The methodological quality of some included trials had medium scores, as they were not double-blind and/or the methods of randomization were not described explicitly, which might have led to exaggerated estimates of intervention benefit or contributed to discrepancies between the results [35,36]. In other words, the heterogeneity in analyzing histological HCV recurrence might be due to the medium scores of the trials.

In addition, most authors of the included articles didn't defined graft loss in their manuscripts, and only one [26] defined graft loss as: 1) graft loss with subsequent death; 2) graft loss with retransplantation; 3) graft loss without retransplantation and loss of subsequent follow-up. In addition, the number of deaths is inferior to the number of graft loss in four manuscripts [24,31,37,38]. However, the number of deaths is superior to the number of graft loss in three manuscripts [17,25,26]. It's a hint that the definition of graft loss in their manuscripts might be different,which may lead to different result of the meta-analysis of graft loss.

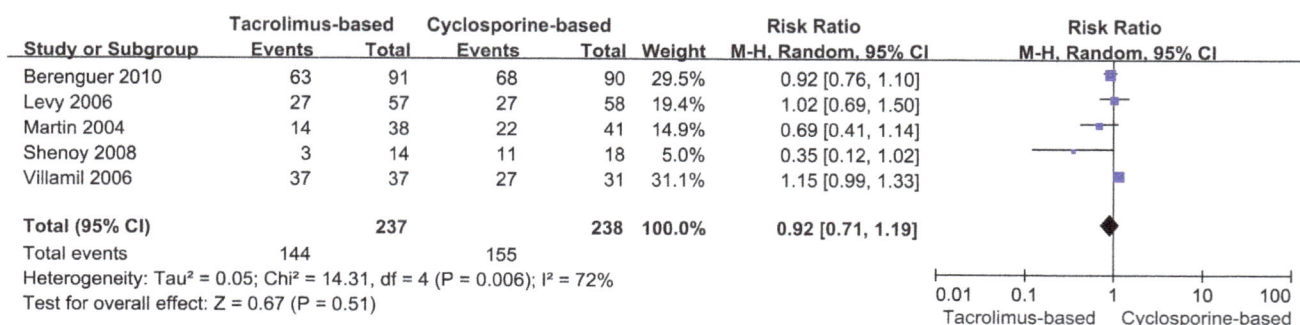

Study or Subgroup	Tacrolimus-based		Cyclosporine-based		Weight	Risk Ratio M-H, Random, 95% CI	Risk Ratio M-H, Random, 95% CI
	Events	Total	Events	Total			
Berenguer 2010	63	91	68	90	29.5%	0.92 [0.76, 1.10]	
Levy 2006	27	57	27	58	19.4%	1.02 [0.69, 1.50]	
Martin 2004	14	38	22	41	14.9%	0.69 [0.41, 1.14]	
Shenoy 2008	3	14	11	18	5.0%	0.35 [0.12, 1.02]	
Villamil 2006	37	37	27	31	31.1%	1.15 [0.99, 1.33]	
Total (95% CI)		237		238	100.0%	0.92 [0.71, 1.19]	
Total events	144		155				

Heterogeneity: Tau² = 0.05; Chi² = 14.31, df = 4 (P = 0.006); I² = 72%
Test for overall effect: Z = 0.67 (P = 0.51)

Figure 7. Forest plot of histological HCV recurrence included trials comparing tacrolimus-based to cyclosporine-based group.

Study or Subgroup	Tacrolimus-based		Cyclosporine-based		Weight	Risk Ratio M-H, Fixed, 95% CI	Risk Ratio M-H, Fixed, 95% CI
	Events	Total	Events	Total			
Berenguer 2010	63	91	68	90	54.3%	0.92 [0.76, 1.10]	
Levy 2006	27	57	27	58	21.3%	1.02 [0.69, 1.50]	
Martin 2004	14	38	22	41	16.8%	0.69 [0.41, 1.14]	
Shenoy 2008	3	14	11	18	7.6%	0.35 [0.12, 1.02]	
Total (95% CI)		200		207	100.0%	0.86 [0.73, 1.01]	
Total events	107		128				

Heterogeneity: Chi² = 4.72, df = 3 (P = 0.19); I² = 36%
Test for overall effect: Z = 1.86 (P = 0.06)

0.01   0.1   1   10   100
Tacrolimus-based   Cyclosporine-based

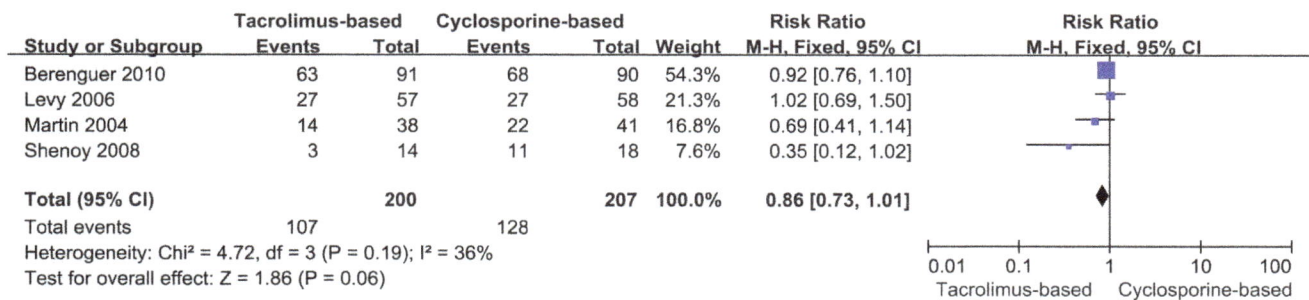

Figure 8. Sensitivity analysis of histological HCV recurrence.

Conclusions

In summary, our results demonstrated that HCV recurrence-induced mortality, graft loss and retransplantation, as well as the incidence of histological HCV recurrence, were not associated with the selection of different CNIs as the basic immunosuppressant in hepatitis C-infected patients.

Acknowledgments

We thank Ms.Collins Linda at Seattle, USA for her critical reading and language improvement of this paper.

Author Contributions

Conceived and designed the experiments: ZML YC RCT. Performed the experiments: ZML YC RCT XZY. Analyzed the data: ZML YC RCT JX JYM XZY. Contributed reagents/materials/analysis tools: RCT. Contributed to the writing of the manuscript: ZML YC RCT.

References

1. Cooke GS, Lemoine M, Thursz M, Gore C, Swan T, et al. (2013) Viral hepatitis and the Global Burden of Disease: a need to regroup. J Viral Hepat 20: 600–601.
2. Gane EJ (2008) The natural history of recurrent hepatitis C and what influences this. Liver Transpl 14 Suppl 2: S36–44.
3. Ciria R, Pleguezuelo M, Khorsandi SE, Davila D, Suddle A, et al. (2013) Strategies to reduce hepatitis C virus recurrence after liver transplantation. World J Hepatol 5: 237–250.
4. Agarwal K, Barnabas A (2013) Treatment of chronic hepatitis C virus infection after liver transplantation. Dig Liver Dis 45 Suppl 5: S349–354.
5. Gordon RD, Shaw BW, Jr., Iwatsuki S, Esquivel CO, Starzl TE (1986) Indications for liver transplantation in the cyclosporine era. Surg Clin North Am 66: 541–556.
6. Canafax DM, Ascher NL (1983) Cyclosporine immunosuppression. Clin Pharm 2: 515–524.
7. Zeevi A, Duquesnoy R, Eiras G, Rabinowich H, Todo S, et al. (1987) Immunosuppressive effect of FK-506 on in vitro lymphocyte alloactivation: synergism with cyclosporine A. Transplant Proc 19: 40–44.
8. Watashi K, Hijikata M, Hosaka M, Yamaji M, Shimotohno K (2003) Cyclosporin A suppresses replication of hepatitis C virus genome in cultured hepatocytes. Hepatology 38: 1282–1288.
9. Nakagawa M, Sakamoto N, Tanabe Y, Koyama T, Itsui Y, et al. (2005) Suppression of hepatitis C virus replication by cyclosporin a is mediated by blockade of cyclophilins. Gastroenterology 129: 1031–1041.
10. Firpi RJ, Zhu H, Morelli G, Abdelmalek MF, Soldevila-Pico C, et al. (2006) Cyclosporine suppresses hepatitis C virus in vitro and increases the chance of a sustained virological response after liver transplantation. Liver Transpl 12: 51–57.
11. Nakagawa M, Sakamoto N, Enomoto N, Tanabe Y, Kanazawa N, et al. (2004) Specific inhibition of hepatitis C virus replication by cyclosporin A. Biochem Biophys Res Commun 313: 42–47.
12. Samonakis DN, Germani G, Burroughs AK (2012) Immunosuppression and HCV recurrence after liver transplantation. J Hepatol 56: 973–983.
13. Berenguer M, Royuela A, Zamora J (2007) Immunosuppression with calcineurin inhibitors with respect to the outcome of HCV recurrence after liver transplantation: results of a meta-analysis. Liver Transpl 13: 21–29.
14. Berenguer M, Ferrell L, Watson J, Prieto M, Kim M, et al. (2000) HCV-related fibrosis progression following liver transplantation: increase in recent years. J Hepatol 32: 673–684.
15. Ghobrial RM, Steadman R, Gornbein J, Lassman C, Holt CD, et al. (2001) A 10-year experience of liver transplantation for hepatitis C: analysis of factors determining outcome in over 500 patients. Ann Surg 234: 384–393; discussion 393–384.
16. Charlton M, Seaberg E, Wiesner R, Everhart J, Zetterman R, et al. (1998) Predictors of patient and graft survival following liver transplantation for hepatitis C. Hepatology 28: 823–830.
17. Levy G, Grazi GL, Sanjuan F, Wu Y, Muhlbacher F, et al. (2006) 12-month follow-up analysis of a multicenter, randomized, prospective trial in de novo liver transplant recipients (LIS2T) comparing cyclosporine microemulsion (C2 monitoring) and tacrolimus. Liver Transpl 12: 1464–1472.
18. Shenoy S, Hardinger KL, Crippin J, Korenblat K, Lisker-Melman M, et al. (2008) A randomized, prospective, pharmacoeconomic trial of neoral 2-hour postdose concentration monitoring versus tacrolimus trough concentration monitoring in de novo liver transplant recipients. Liver Transpl 14: 173–180.
19. Ben-Ari Z, Mor E, Bar-Nathan N, Shaharabani E, Shapira Z, et al. (2003) Comparison of tacrolimus with cyclosporin as primary immunosuppression in patients with hepatitis C virus infection after liver transplantation. Transplant Proc 35: 612–613.
20. Kim RD, Mizuno S, Sorensen JB, Schwartz JJ, Fujita S (2012) Impact of calcineurin inhibitors on hepatitis C recurrence after liver transplantation. Dig Dis Sci 57: 568–572.
21. Lai JC, Verna EC, Brown RS, Jr., O'Leary JG, Trotter JF, et al. (2011) Hepatitis C virus-infected women have a higher risk of advanced fibrosis and graft loss after liver transplantation than men. Hepatology 54: 418–424.
22. Berenguer M (2005) What determines the natural history of recurrent hepatitis C after liver transplantation? J Hepatol 42: 448–456.
23. Berenguer M, Prieto M, San Juan F, Rayon JM, Martinez F, et al. (2002) Contribution of donor age to the recent decrease in patient survival among HCV-infected liver transplant recipients. Hepatology 36: 202–210.
24. Berenguer M, Aguilera V, San Juan F, Benlloch S, Rubin A, et al. (2010) Effect of calcineurin inhibitors in the outcome of liver transplantation in hepatitis C virus-positive recipients. Transplantation 90: 1204–1209.
25. Levy G, Villamil FG, Nevens F, Metselaar HJ, Clavien PA, et al. (2014) REFINE: a randomized trial comparing cyclosporine A and tacrolimus on fibrosis after liver transplantation for hepatitis C. Am J Transplant 14: 635–646.
26. Villamil F, Levy G, Grazi GL, Mies S, Samuel D, et al. (2006) Long-term outcomes in liver transplant patients with hepatic C infection receiving tacrolimus or cyclosporine. Transplantation Proceedings 38: 2964–2967.
27. Firpi RJ, Soldevila-Pico C, Morelli GG, Cabrera R, Levy C, et al. (2010) The use of cyclosporine for recurrent hepatitis C after liver transplant: a randomized pilot study. Dig Dis Sci 55: 196–203.
28. Selzner N, Renner EL, Selzner M, Adeyi O, Kashfi A, et al. (2009) Antiviral treatment of recurrent hepatitis C after liver transplantation: predictors of response and long-term outcome. Transplantation 88: 1214–1221.
29. Barbier L, Garcia S, Cros J, Borentain P, Botta-Fridlund D, et al. (2013) Assessment of chronic rejection in liver graft recipients receiving immunosuppression with low-dose calcineurin inhibitors. J Hepatol 59: 1223–1230.
30. Dumortier J, Guillaud O, Boillot O (2013) Conversion from twice daily tacrolimus to once daily tacrolimus in long-term stable liver transplant recipients: a single-center experience with 394 patients. Liver Transpl 19: 529–533.
31. Zervos XA, Weppler D, Fragulidis GP, Torres MB, Nery JR, et al. (1998) Comparison of tacrolimus with microemulsion cyclosporine as primary

immunosuppression in hepatitis C patients after liver transplantation. Transplantation 65: 1044–1046.

32. Segev DL, Sozio SM, Shin EJ, Nazarian SM, Nathan H, et al. (2008) Steroid avoidance in liver transplantation: meta-analysis and meta-regression of randomized trials. Liver Transpl 14: 512–525.

33. Sgourakis G, Radtke A, Fouzas I, Mylona S, Goumas K, et al. (2009) Corticosteroid-free immunosuppression in liver transplantation: a meta-analysis and meta-regression of outcomes. Transpl Int 22: 892–905.

34. Foxton Mr QA, Muiesan P, Heneqhan MA, Portmann B, Norris S, Heaton ND, (2006) The impact of diabetes mellitus on fibrosis progression in patients transplanted for hepatitis C. Am J Transplant: 1922–1929.

35. Kjaergard LL, Villumsen J, Gluud C (2001) Reported methodologic quality and discrepancies between large and small randomized trials in meta-analyses. Ann Intern Med 135: 982–989.

36. Savovic J, Jones H, Altman D, Harris R, Juni P, et al. (2012) Influence of reported study design characteristics on intervention effect estimates from randomised controlled trials: combined analysis of meta-epidemiological studies. Health Technol Assess 16: 1–82.

37. Martin P, Busuttil RW, Goldstein RM, Crippin JS, Klintmalm GB, et al. (2004) Impact of tacrolimus versus cyclosporine in hepatitis C virus-infected liver transplant recipients on recurrent hepatitis: a prospective, randomized trial. Liver Transpl 10: 1258–1262.

38. wiesner RH (1998) A long-term comparison of tacrolimus versus cyclosporine in liver transplantation: A report of the United States. TRANSPLANTATION: 493–499.

39. Mueller AR, Platz KP, Blumhardt G, Bechstein WO, Steinmuller T, et al. (1995) The optimal immunosuppressant after liver transplantation according to diagnosis: cyclosporine A or FK506? Clinical Transplantation 9: 176–184.

9

Prevention of Liver Fibrosis by Intrasplenic Injection of High-Density Cultured Bone Marrow Cells in a Rat Chronic Liver Injury Model

Jie Lian⁹, Yang Lu⁹, Peng Xu, Ai Ai, Guangdong Zhou, Wei Liu, Yilin Cao, Wen Jie Zhang*

Department of Plastic and Reconstructive Surgery, Shanghai 9th People's Hospital, Shanghai Jiao Tong University School of Medicine, Shanghai Key Laboratory of Tissue Engineering, National Tissue Engineering Center of China, Shanghai, China

Abstract

Endothelial progenitor cells (EPCs) from bone marrow have proven to be functional for the prevention of liver fibrosis in chronic liver injury. However, expansion of EPCs in culture is complicated and expansive. Previously, we have established a simple method that could enrich and expand EPCs by simple seeding bone marrow cells in high density dots. The purpose of this study is to evaluate whether cells derived from high-density (HD) culture of rat bone marrow cells could prevent the liver fibrosis in a chronic liver injury rat model, induced by carbon tetrachloride (CCl_4). Flow cytometric analysis showed that cells from HD culture were enriched for EPCs, expressing high levels of EPC markers. Intrasplenic injection of HD cultured bone marrow cells in the CCl_4-induced liver injury rat showed an enhanced antifibrogenic effect compared with animals treated with cells from regular-density culture. The antifibrogenic effect was demonstrated by biochemical and histological analysis 4 weeks post-transplantation. Furthermore, cells from HD culture likely worked through increasing neovascularization, stimulating liver cell proliferation, and suppressing pro-fibrogenic factor expression. HD culture, which is a simple and cost-effective procedure, could potentially be used to expand bone marrow cells for the treatment of liver fibrosis.

Editor: Maria Cristina Vinci, Cardiological Center Monzino, Italy

Funding: This work was supported by the Major State Basic Research Development Program of China (2007CB948004, 2011CB964704), and the National Basic Research Program of China (30800231, 31170944). The funders had no role in study design, data collection and analysis, decision to publish, or preparation of the manuscript.

Competing Interests: The authors have declared that no competing interests exist.

* Email: wenjieboshi@aliyun.cn

⑨ These authors contributed equally to this work.

Introduction

The liver possesses great regenerative capacity in response to injury. However, chronic injuries caused by autoimmune hepatitis, alcohol abuse, metabolic disorders, or viral hepatitis, could disturb the regenerative process, leading to development of a common pathology known as liver fibrosis [1]. In some cases, persistent injuries progress the fibrosis and eventually lead to liver cirrhosis [1]. At this stage, the only therapeutic option is organ transplantation. Liver transplants are not widely performed because of problems such as donor shortage, surgical invasiveness, risk of immunological rejection, and medical costs [2]. Therefore, it is essential that therapeutic alternatives to liver transplantation are developed.

Recently, the emergence of stem cell research has opened new possibilities for the treatment of chronic liver diseases. Various cell populations from the bone marrow, including hematopoietic stem cells (HSCs) [3–5], mesenchymal stem cells (MSCs) [6,7], endothelial progenitor cells (EPCs) [8,9], and bone marrow mononuclear cells (BMNCs) [10], have been transplanted and have proved to be functional for the prevention of liver fibrosis in animal models, as well as in patients. The transplanted cells likely play multiple roles in the repair process. They may differentiate directly into hepatocytes, or release growth factors to protect intrinsic hepatocytes, stimulate regeneration, regulate inflammatory response, and/or decompose the extracellular matrix (ECM) [9,11–13]. Although non-cultured autologous bone marrow-derived cells have been successfully applied in patients [7,10], the use of *in vitro* culture-expanded cells for treatment could reduce the initial amount of bone marrow needed.

Expansion of stem cells in culture is still a big challenge in the field. For example, it is difficult and expensive to expand EPCs without losing their stemness and function [14]. Previously, we established a novel and simple bone marrow high-density (HD) culture system by seeding BMNCs in HD dots on tissue culture plates [15]. Pre-coating of the plates and addition of growth factors are not required using this culture technique. Cells expanded in HD culture display EPC characteristics and have high pro-angiogenic potential. In addition, the cells secrete higher levels of vascular endothelial growth factor (VEGF) and hepatocyte growth factor (HGF), compared with cells grown in regular-density (RD) culture [15]. On the basis of these advantages, we speculate that these cells might be better than cells from RD culture (which contains mainly MSCs), for the treatment of liver fibrosis. To test this hypothesis, the antifibrogenic and regenerative effects of high- and RD cultured bone marrow cells were investigated in a carbon tetrachloride (CCl_4)-induced rat chronic liver fibrosis model.

Materials and Methods

1. Animals and experimental models

Male Wistar rats (6 weeks old) weighing approximately120 g were purchased from the Shanghai Chuansha Experimental Animal Raising Farm (Shanghai, China). Animal study protocols were approved by The Animal Care and Experiment Committee of Shanghai Jiao Tong University School of Medicine. The liver injury model was created by injections of CCl_4 (Sigma, St. Louis, MO, USA) as described previously [16]. Briefly, a 10% solution of $CCl_4$was prepared in olive oil and a dose of 2 mL/kg was injected intra-peritoneally every other day over 6 weeks. After the 6-week injection course, all rats were submitted to a blood test for serum level of albumin (ALB), glutamic oxalacetic transaminase (AST), and glutamic pyruvic transaminase (ALT), to evaluate liver injury and function. Only those animals presenting blood values different from the predefined range, for all three parameters, were used in the transplantation studies.

2. Isolation and culture of bone marrow cells

Rat bone marrow cells were extracted from the femurs of 6-week-old male Wistar rats. To remove the majority of non-adherent blood cells, primary culture of bone marrow cells was performed by seeding the cells at 1.6×10^4 cells/cm^2 in Dulbecco's modified Eagle's medium (DMEM; Invitrogen, Carlsbad, CA, USA) with 10% fetal bovine serum (FBS; HyClone, Logan, UT, USA) and 0.2% penicillin/streptomycin(Sigma). Medium was changed every 3 days. After 6–7 days of culture, primary adherent cells (P0) were harvested using trypsin/EDTA (0.25% w/v trypsin, and 0.02% EDTA; Invitrogen), and were subcultured at high or regular density. For RD culture, 9×10^5 primary cultured cells were seeded evenly at a density of 1.6×10^4 cells/cm^2 in a 10-cm diameter tissue culture dish in 10 mL DMEM with 10% FBS. Cells were passaged in the same manner every 3 days. For HD culture, 9×10^5primary cells (equal to the cell number of RD culture) were suspended in 300 μL of culture medium, and then six drops (50 μL each) of cell suspension were dot-seeded separately onto a 10-cm-diameter culture dish within equal distance. The average diameter of each dot was 1 cm, resulting in a final local cell density of 2×10^5 cells/cm^2. Culture dishes were placed in an incubator for 30 min, and then 10 mL of culture medium was gently added to cover each dish. Medium was changed every 3 days. Cells were passaged in the same manner at day 7 and collected for analysis and transplantation at day 15.

3. Flow cytometric analyses

After 15 days culture, cells were trypsinized and aliquots of 2×10^5 cells were suspended in 200 μL washing buffer (PBS containing 2% FBS). Cells were then incubated on ice for 30 min with phycoerythrin (PE)- or fluorescein isothiocyanate (FITC)-conjugated antibodies. PE- and FITC-conjugated isotype matched immunoglobulins were used as controls. After staining and washing, cells were analyzed on a flow cytometer (Epics Altra; Beckman Coulter, Fullerton, CA, USA). Antibodies against the following markers were used: CD29, CD90, CD31 (BD Biosciences, San Diego, CA, USA), CD133, and KDR (Abcam, Cambridge, UK). Flow cytometric data were analyzed with CXP software (Beckman Coulter).

4. *In vitro* angiogenesis assay

One hundred μL of Matrigel (BD Biosciences) basement membrane matrix was added to 24-well plates. The plates were then incubated for 30 min to allow gel solidification. Then, 2×10^4 cells from 15-day HD or RD cultures were seeded onto the gel in 500 μL EGM-2 (Invitrogen). Twelve hours later, the plates were observed under a light microscope (Olympus, Tokyo, Japan). Nine representative fields were recorded and the average number of branch points was calculated by Image-Pro Plus software (Media Cybernetics, Atlanta, GA, USA).

5. Cell labeling and transplantation

After 15 days of HD or RD culture, cells were labeled with 1,1′-dioctadecyl-3,3,3′,3′-tetramethylindocarbocyanine dye (CM-DiL; Invitrogen) following the manufacturer's instructions, before transplantation. Rats with liver injury, induced by the 6-week injection course of CCl_4, were divided into three groups (n = 6/group): (1) HD group; (2) RD group; (3) PBS group. Two million cells from HD or RD cultures were suspended in 200 μL PBS and injected intrasplenic using a 29-G needle. Rats that received the same volume of PBS served as controls. After cell transplantation, CCl_4 injections were continuously administrated every other day for another 4 weeks. Rats were then sacrificed and all blood samples and livers were harvested. Serum ALB, AST, and ALT were measured according to standard clinical methods.

6. Histopathology

Liver tissues were fixed in 4% paraformaldehyde for 12 h, embedded in paraffin and cut into 5-μm sections. Sections were stained with hematoxylin and eosin (HE), picric acid-sirius red (PSR), and Masson, for histological structure analysis and fibrosis area analysis. Five randomly selected fields of view, from PSR- and Masson-stained sections of each sample (n = 3/group), were captured by a light microscope (Olympus, Tokyo, Japan).The fibrosis area was measured using Image-Pro Plus software (Media Cybernetics). The percentage fibrosis area was calculated by comparing the collagen stained area to the total area of the fields examined.

Immunohistochemical (IHC) staining was carried out as described previously using commercially available antibodies against collagen I, α-smooth muscle actin (α-SMA), Ki-67 (all from Abcam), and CD31 (Santa Cruz Biotechnology, Santa Cruz, CA, USA). This was followed by horseradish peroxidase-conjugated goat anti-mouse antibody (Dako, Denmark) and colorized with diaminobenzidine tetrahydrochloride (DAB, Dako) [8]. For blood vessel density analysis, five randomly selected fields, from anti-CD31 staining of each sample (n = 3/group), were captured by a light microscope (Olympus).The number of blood vessels was calculated by Image-Pro Plus software (Media Cybernetics).

7. Immunofluorescent analysis of cell distribution

To detect cell distribution in the liver after intrasplenic injection, liver tissues were harvested at 4 weeks post-transplantation, embedded in OTC compound and frozen slides were sectioned at 10 μm. Three mice from each group and three sections from each mouse, were stained with FITC-conjugated anti-collagen type I (Abcam) and DAPI (Invitrogen), and were observed under a confocal microscope (Leica, Solms, Germany). The number of CM-DiL-labeled cells was calculated from five fields of view for each sample by Image-Pro Plus software (Media Cybernetics).

8. Quantitative reverse transcription polymerase chain reaction (qRT-PCR)

Total RNA extracted from liver tissues were reverse transcribed into cDNA and subsequently amplified using a Power SYBR Green PCR master mix (2×) (Applied Biosystems) in a real-time thermal cycler (Mx3000PTM QPCR System; Stratagene). Primers are listed in Table 1. qRT-PCR was conducted in triplicate for each sample. Gene expression was normalized to glyceraldehyde-3-phosphate dehydrogenase (GAPDH) expression. Results represent three independent experiments.

9. Statistical analysis

Data were expressed as the mean ± standard deviation. Comparisons between groups were analyzed by ANOVA. A value of $p < 0.05$ was considered statistically significant.

Results

1. Identification of bone marrow cells after *in vitro* expansion

The characteristics of rat bone marrow cells after 15 days culture were identical to those previously described [15]. In HD culture, a population of small bright cells growing on top of spindle-shaped cells was observed, while cells in RD culture displayed a spindle-shaped fibroblastic morphology only (Fig. 1A).

Flow cytometric analysis showed that cells from HD culture expressed higher levels of CD34, CD133, and FLK-1(KDR) EPC markers, compared with cells from RD culture (Fig. 1B). MSC markers, CD90 and CD29, were highly expressed in both cultures. The *in vitro* tubular formation assay confirmed that cells from HD culture formed obvious tubular networks, which were absent in cells from RD culture (Fig. 1C), indicating that cells from the HD culture contained more EPCs.

2. Protective effect of cell transplantation in liver function

Rats that received 6 weeks of CCl_4 injection displayed chronic liver injury, with an increased serum level of ALT (58.6±9.56 U/L) and AST (155±10.54 U/L), and a decreased serum level of ALB (32.6±1.48 U/L) (Fig. 2). Four weeks after cell transplantation, blood samples were tested again. As shown in Fig. 2, both ALT and AST were significantly increased in the PBS-treated group, but not in the group that received HD cultured cells. ALT and AST levels in the group that received RD cultured cells were also increased but lower than those in the PBS-treated group. A decreased ALB level was observed in the PBS group but not in the other two cell-transplanted groups. These results indicate that cell transplantation could prevent liver damage to some extent, and HD cultured bone marrow cells performed better than RD cultured cells.

Table 1. Primers used in qRT-PCR analyses.

Target Gene	Primer (5'-3')	Sequence (5'-3')
α₂-procollagen	Forward	ATGTTCAGCTTTGTGGACCT
	Reverse	CAGCTGACTTCAGGGATGT
Fibronectin	Forward	AGACTGCAGTGACCACCATCC
	Reverse	CAATGTGTCCTTGAGAGCATAGAC
α-SMA	Forward	CGAAGCGCAGAGCAAGAGA
	Reverse	CATGTCGTCCCAGTTGGTGAT
TGF-β	Forward	GAAGGACCTGGGTTGGAAGT
	Reverse	CGGGTTGTGTTGGTTGTAGAG
HGF	Forward	CCTATTTCCCGTTGTGAAG
	Reverse	ACTAACCATCCACCCTACTG
VEGF-A	Forward	CCACACCACCATCGTCAC
	Reverse	CCAGAAACAAAACTCCCTAATC
VEGFR-2	Forward	GCAAATACAACCCTTCAGATTA
	Reverse	CACCCTTTCCTCAGAGTCAC
Ang-1	Forward	GCTGGCAGTACAATGACAGT
	Reverse	TCTGGAAGAATGAAAGTGTAGG
Tie-2	Forward	GATGAAGGGCAAGATGGATAG
	Reverse	AGAAGCAGGCGGTAACAGT
MMP-2	Forward	CAAGTGGGACAAGAATCAGA
	Reverse	GAGAAAAGCGTAGTGGAGTTAC
TIMP-2	Forward	CTTAGCATCACCCAGAAGAAGA
	Reverse	GTCCATCCAGAGGCACTCAT
PDGF-B	Forward	GAGGAGGAGACGGGCA
	Reverse	CACTGAACAAACGGACACT
PDGFR	Forward	TTGTCACGGATGTCACTGAGA
	Reverse	AAACCTCGCTGGTGGTCATA

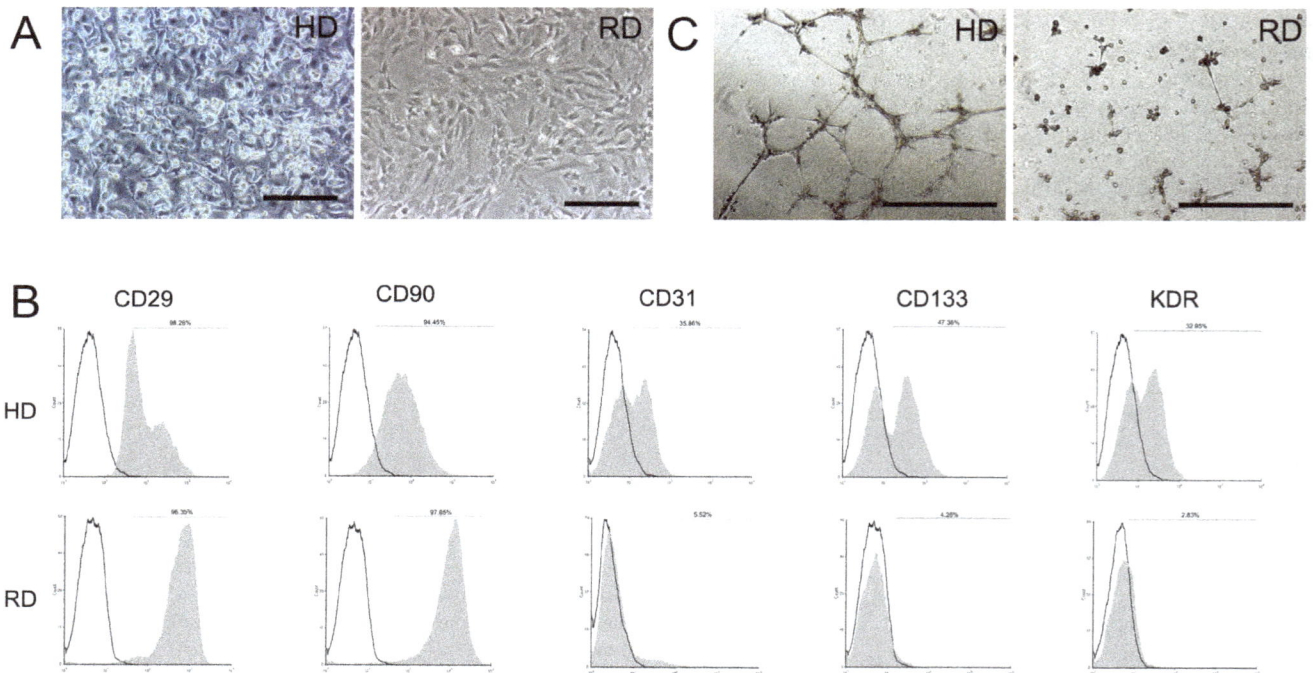

Figure 1. Endothelial progenitor cells enriched in HD cultured bone marrow cells. (A) Morphology of rat bone marrow cells in HD and RD culture. (Scale bars:100 μm). (B) Flow cytometry analyses of HD and RD cultured cells after 15 days of expansion. (C) Tube formation ability of RD and RD cultured cells on matrigel. (Scale bars:200 μm).

3. Antifibrogenic effect of cell transplantation in liver fibrosis

To evaluate the antifibrogenic effect following cell transplantation, histologic examinations were performed to detect liver structures and ECM deposition. HE staining showed that after 6 weeks of CCl_4 injection, rat liver tissues formed pseudolobules that remolded the liver morphology (Fig. 3A). After 4 more weeks of CCl_4 injection, liver structure in the PBS-treated group was further destroyed with wide formation of pseudolobules. However, less pseudolobule structures were observed in both cell-transplanted groups. Morphological changes were confirmed by PSR and Masson staining (Fig. 3A). Quantitative analyses of liver fibrosis were performed from PSR and Masson staining. The fibrotic area increased after 6 weeks of CCl_4 injection, and continuously progressed in the PBS group. However, fewer fibrotic areas were observed in the cell-transplanted groups with an enhanced antifibrogenic effect observed in the group treated with HD cultured cells (Fig. 3B).

To further confirm the antifibrogenic effect of cell transplantation, IHC staining of collagen I and α-SMA were performed. Like PSR and Masson staining, similar changes in liver structure and ECM deposition patterns were observed (Fig. 4A). Quantitative RT-PCR analyses of $α_2$-procollagen and α-SMA in liver tissues showed that gene expression levels were lower in both HD and RD groups than those in the PBS group, while the gene expression of fibronectin in HD group was lower than those in RD and PBS groups (Fig 4B). Accompany this, expression of TGF-β, a key pro-fibrogenic growth factor, was decreased in the cell-transplanted groups compared with the PBS group. However, no significant difference was observed between the HD group and the

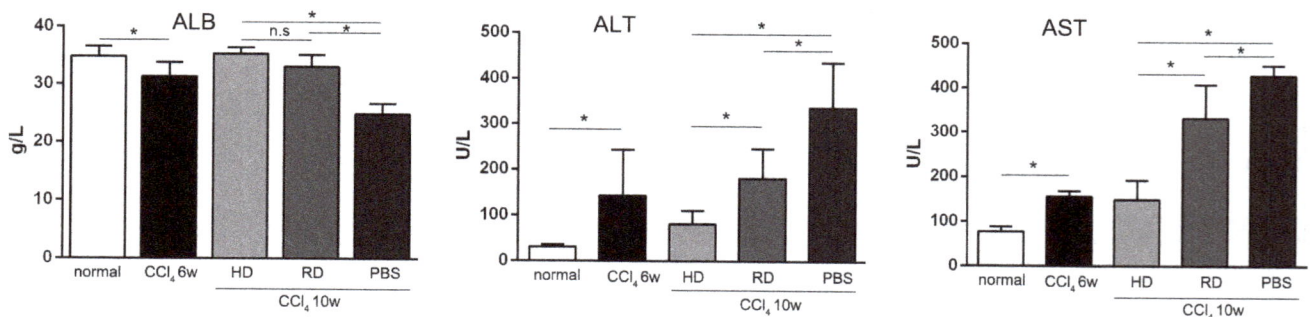

Figure 2. Protective effect of cell transplantation in liver function. Blood samples of normal and experimental rats were collected and serum levels of albumin (ALB), glutamic oxalacetic transaminase (AST) and glutamic pyruvic transaminase (ALT) were tested before (CCl_4 6w) and after (CCl_4 10w) cell transplantation. (n = 6/group; *p<0.05).

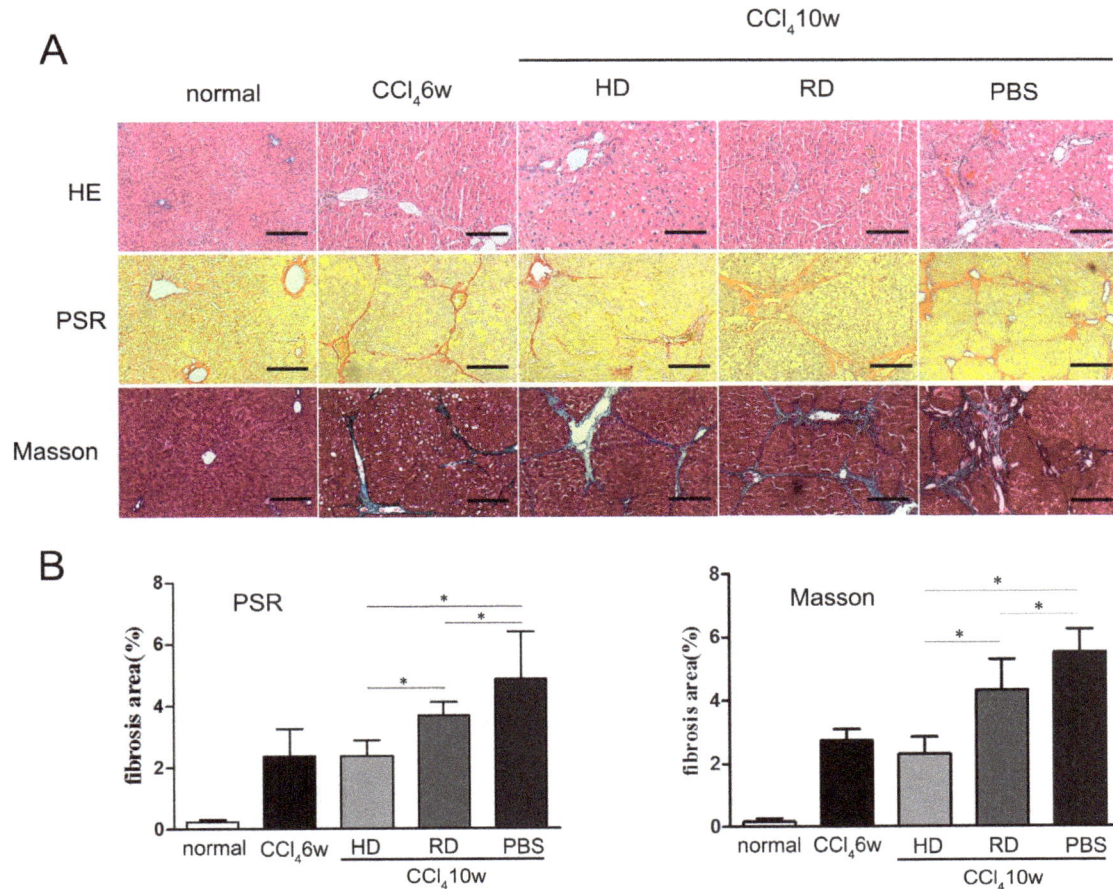

Figure 3. Antifibrogenic effect of cell transplantation in liver fibrosis. (A) Representative structural changes in livers were detected by hematoxylin & eosin (HE), picric acid-sirius red (PSR) and Masson staining (Scale bars: 100 μm). (B) Quantitative analyses of liver fibrosis were performed from PSR and Masson staining. Five views from each sample with three samples in each group were analyzed. *$p < 0.05$.

RD group (Fig. 4B). The expressions of another pro-fibrogenic growth factor, platelet-derived growth factor subunit B (PDGF-B), and its receptor (PDGFR), were also decreased in the cell-transplanted groups (Fig. 4B). Matrix metalloproteinase (MMP)-2, which relates to matrix degradation, were up-regulated in the cell-transplanted groups. While, the tissue inhibitor of metalloproteinase (TIMP)-2 were down-regulated in those groups (Fig. 4B).

4. Distribution of transplanted cells in liver

An enhanced antifibrogenic effect was observed in the group treated with HD cultured cells. To explain this phenomenon, we first detected distribution of the injected cells in the liver 4 weeks after cell transplantation. As shown in Fig. 5, CM-DiL-labeled cells were observed in the liver, with a greater number of cells observed in the HD cultured group (Fig. 5A,C), indicating that more HD cultured cells homed to the liver and survived. Interestingly, the majority of transplanted cells were observed around the portal tracts, fibrous septa, and hepatic sinusoids in both the HD and RD groups (Fig. 5B). In accordance with the IHC staining, less collagen I staining was observed in the HD group than in the RD group (Fig. 5B).

5. Promotion of liver regeneration by transplanted cells

It has been widely observed that transplanted cells stimulate liver regeneration through promoting the proliferation of resident hepatocytes. Liver weights and liver/body weight ratios measured at 4 weeks post-treatment showed a higher liver weights and liver/body weight ratios in the cell-transplanted groups compare to those in the PBS-treated group (Fig. 6A). We further performed IHC staining of Ki-67 in the liver sections. More Ki-67 positive cells were observed in the HD group compared with the RD and PBS groups (Fig. 6B). Because cells in the HD culture expressed higher levels of HGF [15], expression of HGF in the liver tissue was examined 4 weeks after cell transplantation. As expected, a higher level of HGF expression was observed in the HD group compared with the other groups (Fig. 6C).

6. Increased sinusoidal blood vessel density by transplanted cells

In many organs, neovascularization has been demonstrated to be crucial to the healing of injured tissues, which involves mature endothelial cells and EPCs. In many ways, the liver's response to injury involves neovascularization, including new vessel formation and sinusoid remodeling [17]. To measure blood vessel density after cell transplantation, anti-CD31 IHC staining of liver sections was performed. As shown in Fig. 7A, more CD31 positive blood vessels were observed in the HD group than those in the RD and PBS groups. Further qRT-PCR analysis of pro-angiogenic gene expression was consistent with the above observation, that a higher level of VEGF-A and angiopoietin-1 (Ang-1) expression were

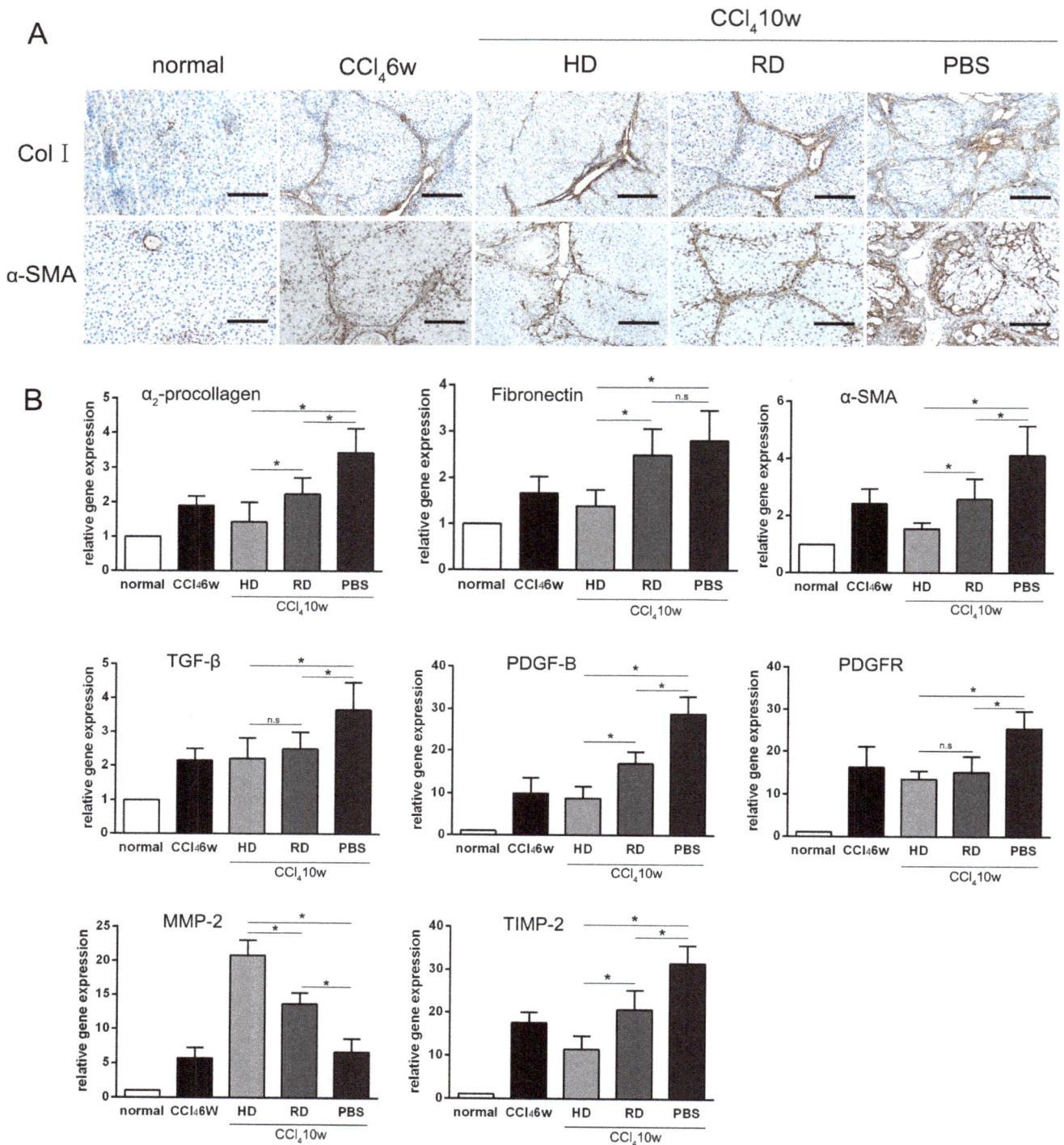

Figure 4. Antifibrogenic effect of cell transplantation measured by immunohistology and qRT-PCR analyses. (A) Immunohistochemical staining of collagen type I (Col I) and α-smooth muscle actin (α-SMA) before (CCl₄ 6w) and after (CCl₄ 10w) cell transplantation (Scale bars: 100 μm). (B) Quantitative RT-PCR analysis of fibrosis related markers α₂-procollagen, fibronectin, α-SMA, TGF-β,PDGF-B, PDGFR, MMP-2 and TIMP-2. Each sample was repeated three times with three samples from each group. *p<0.05; n.s: p>0.05.

observed in livers transplanted with HD cultured cells, accompanied with an increased expression of VEGF receptor-2 (VEGFR-2) but decreased expression of Tie-2 (Fig. 7B).

Discussion

Recent advances in stem cell research have revealed that bone marrow-derived cells, including HSCs, MSCs, EPCs, and BMNCs, could significantly protect liver function after injury

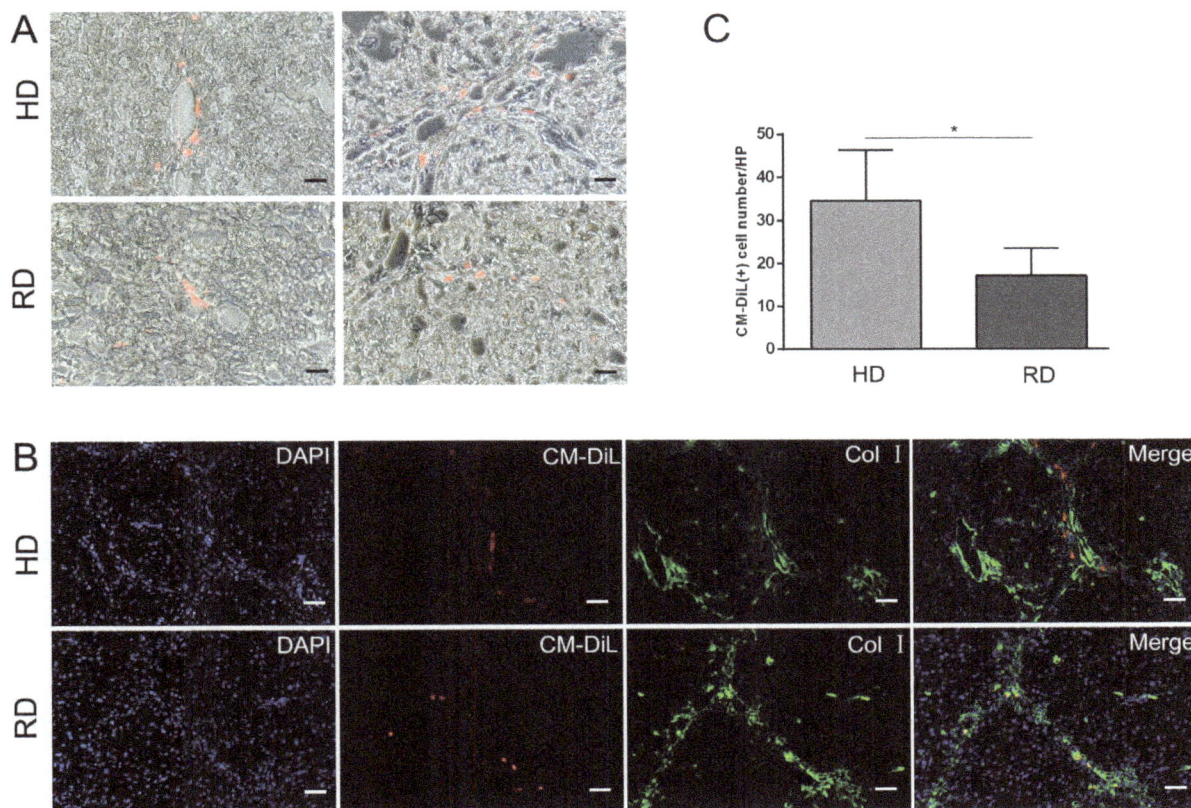

Figure 5. Distribution of transplanted cells in fibrotic liver. (A) Transplanted cells with red fluorescence of 1,1'-dioctadecyl-3,3,3',3'-tetra-methylindocarbocyanine dye (CM-DiL) were detected under confocal microscope (Scale bars: 50 μm). Positive cell were counted form five views from each sample with three samples in each group. *p<0.05. (B) Immunofluorescence staining of collagen type I (Col I) revealed that CM-DiL positive cells were located around portal vein and fibrous septa (Scale bars: 50 μm).

[11,18]. In the present study, we demonstrated that an EPC enriched population from a novel HD culture of bone marrow cells, displayed better antifibrogenic potential in the treatment of chronic liver injury. The antifibrogenic effect was determined by biochemical and histological evidence.

Previously, we demonstrated that EPCs could be expanded in HD culture without pre-coating culture dishes and addition of extra growth factors, which is a simple and cost-effective method for *in vitro* expansion of bone marrow EPCs [15]. On the contrary, the RD culture, which has been adopted widely for MSCs culture [19], could efficiently expand MSCs with loss of EPCs during cell passage (Fig. 1B,C). Although no previous reports have compared the efficacy of EPCs to MSCs in the treatment of chronic liver injury, the current work provides evidence that bone marrow cells enriched for EPCs could function better than relatively pure MSCs *in vivo*. The mechanism of action can be explained as follows: first, more cells from the HD culture homed to and survived in the injured liver after injection (Fig. 5); second, a lower level of the pro-fibrogenic factors, TGF-β and PDGF-B, were expressed in the liver of the HD group (Fig. 4B); third, matrix degradation enzyme MMP-2 were highly expression in HD group (Fig. 4B); fourth, cell proliferation was stimulated through higher expression of HGF in the HD group (Fig. 6); and finally, more blood vessels were formed, induced by higher expressions of VEGF-A and Ang-1 in the HD group (Fig. 7B). Obviously, the secretion of growth factors played a crucial role in the antifibrogenic process, which is consistent with

other reports. Interestingly, differentiation of transplanted cells into hepatocytes was not observed (data not shown), indicating that the injected cells functioned mainly through a paracrine mechanism to prevent liver fibrosis and regeneration, rather than by direct differentiation into hepatocytes.

The enhanced antifibrogenic effect of HD cultured bone marrow cells could also be explained by the natural liver repairing mechanism after injury. It is known that in many tissues, the response to injury involves angiogenesis, which requires a supply of growth factors, nutrients, and oxygen. In liver regeneration, resident sinusoidal endothelial cells, have been shown to proliferate, migrate, and reconstruct hepatic sinusoids [20–23]. As reviewed recently, following CCl4-induced injury, endothelial cells of the liver portal vein contract with lumen constriction, and liver tissue becomes ischemic and hypoxic [24,25]. Infusion of EPCs or VEGF can enhance neovascularization, relieving portal pressure and eventually ameliorating the fibrosis [26,27]. In the present research, HD culture of bone marrow cells enriched EPCs more than RD culture (Fig. 1). In addition, IHC of frozen sections confirmed that more blood vessels were formed in the liver after treatment with HD cultured cells [15]. The enhancement of capillary density was coinciding with the treatment by EPCs Prevention of liver fibrosis and liver reconstitution of DMN-treated rat liver by transplanted EPCs [28]. Interestingly, these findings are conflicting with the reports that liver fibrogenesis and angiogenesis develop in parallel during progression towards cirrhosis [29,30]. It has been reported that the drugs that

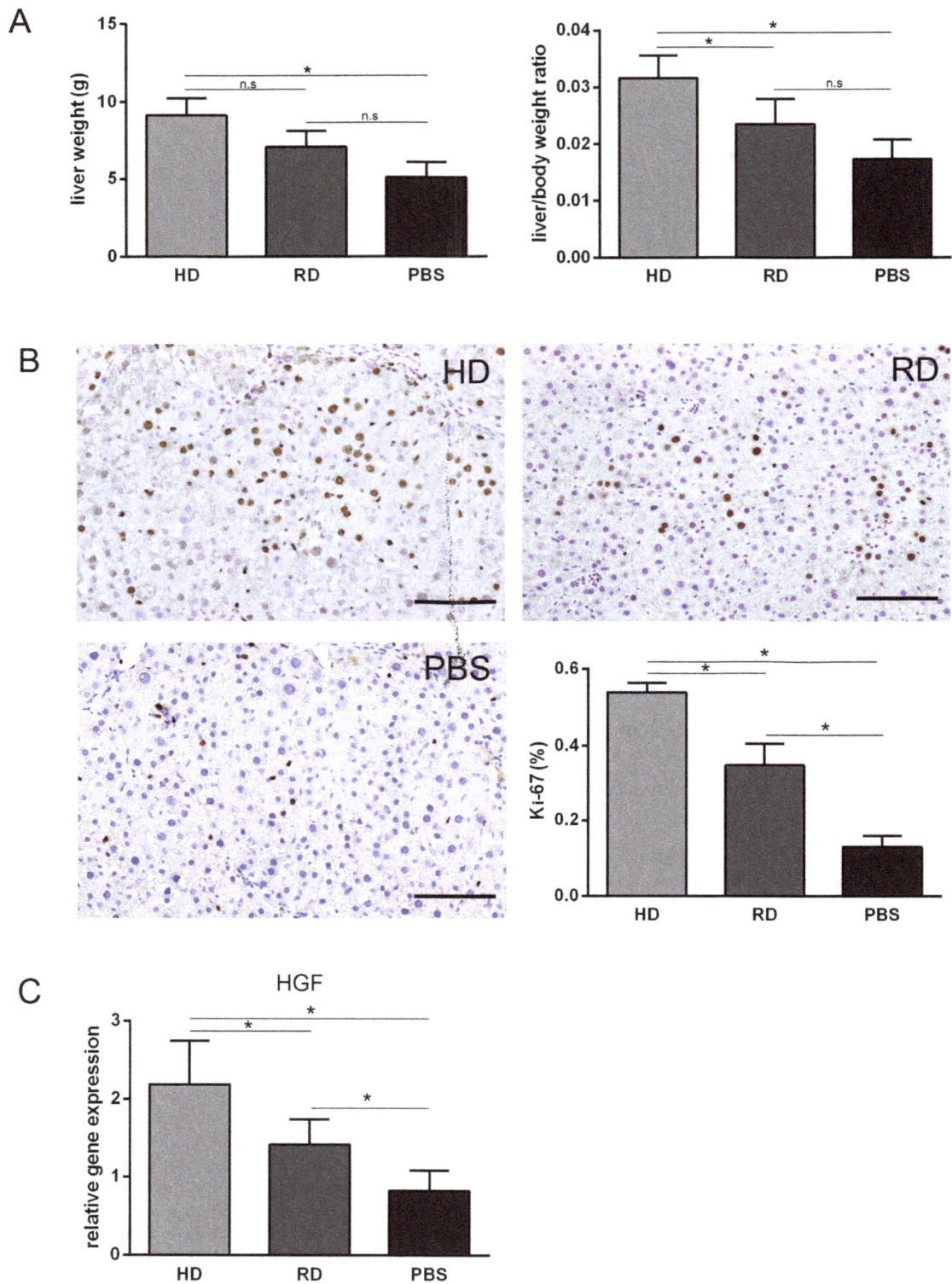

Figure 6. Promotion of liver regeneration by transplanted cells. (A) The liver weights and liver/body weight ratios at 4 weeks post-treatment. (B) Representative views of immunohistological staining of Ki-67 in HD group, RD group and PBS group (Scale bars: 150 μm). Percentage of Ki-67 positive cells calculated from immunohistological staining. Five views from each sample with three samples in each group were analyzed. (C) Expression of hepatocyte growth factor (HGF) analyzed by qRT-PCR. Each sample was repeated three times with three samples from each group. *p< 0.05.

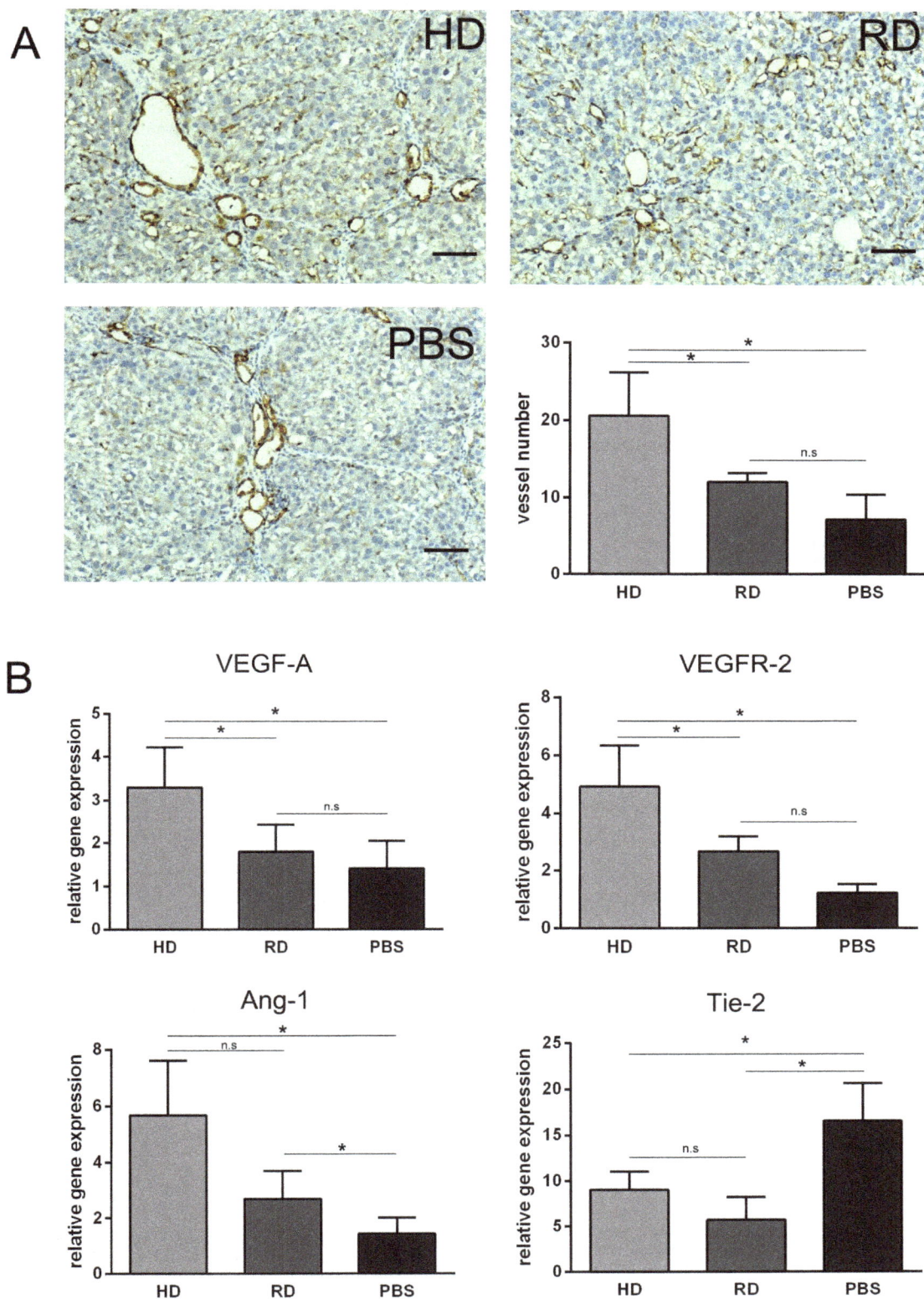

Figure 7. Increased sinusoidal blood vessel density by transplanted cells. (A) Representative views of immunohistological staining of CD31 in HD group, RD group and PBS group (Scale bars: 150 μm). Number of CD31 positive vessels counted from immunohistological staining. Five views in each sample with three samples in each group were analyzed. (B) Expression of Ang-1, Tie-2, VEGF-A and VEGFR-2 analyzed by qRT-PCR. Each sample was repeated three times with three samples from each group. *p<0.05.

specifically inhibit angiogenesis could reduce hepatic fibrosis [29,30]. However, other studies showed that an inhibition of angiogenesis could even worsen fibrosis [31,32]. Theoretically, angiogenesis is important for the tissue repair. Therefore, in this study, the enhanced blood supply could prevent injury, stimulate regeneration, and inhibit fibrosis.

The basic idea of HD culture is to maintain cell-cell interactions in culture, which is a well-known factor of the stem cell niche *in situ* [33]. Theoretically, besides EPCs, other stem cells, including HSCs and MSCs from the bone marrow, might also be expanded in this culture. The higher expression levels of CD34, CD29, and CD90 supported this (Fig. 1). The osteogenic and chondrogenic potential of HD cultured cells has been shown (unpublished data), while the hematogenic potential of these cells is still under investigation. HSCs and MSCs are cell types shown to possess antifibrogenic potential in liver injury. Comparing transplantation of purified cell populations, transplantation of a mix population can enhance tissue repair in many cell therapy models [34–36]. This is likely because of the different role of cells in one physiological and pathological process. For example, EPCs require

the presence of MSCs to enhance new blood vessel formation [37]. Therefore, it is not surprising that an enhanced antifibrogenic effect was achieved by treatment with HD cultured cells containing mixed stem cell populations. In addition, growth factors favored for liver regeneration were highly expressed in this culture, which also supports better outcome of this treatment.

Conclusions

Taken together, we demonstrated that HD cultured bone marrow cells played a more effective role in amelioration of rat liver fibrosis, functional recovery, and hepatic regeneration. This simple and cost-effective culture system provides an effective way for expansion of bone marrow cells for future clinical applications.

Author Contributions

Conceived and designed the experiments: JL YL WJZ GDZ WL YLC. Performed the experiments: JL YL WJZ PX AA. Analyzed the data: JL YL WJZ GDZ WL YLC. Contributed to the writing of the manuscript: JL. Animal experiments: JL YL PX AA. Statistical analysis: JL YL WJZ.

References

1. Schuppan D, Afdhal NH (2008) Liver cirrhosis. Lancet 371: 838–851.
2. Lee DS, Gil WH, Lee HH, Lee KW, Lee SK, et al. (2004) Factors affecting graft survival after living donor liver transplantation. Transplant Proc 36: 2255–2256.
3. Lagasse E, Connors H, Al-Dhalimy M, Reitsma M, Dohse M, et al. (2000) Purified hematopoietic stem cells can differentiate into hepatocytes in vivo. Nat Med 6: 1229–1234.
4. Wang X, Ge S, McNamara G, Hao QL, Crooks GM, et al. (2003) Albumin-expressing hepatocyte-like cells develop in the livers of immune-deficient mice that received transplants of highly purified human hematopoietic stem cells. Blood 101: 4201–4208.
5. Mallet VO, Mitchell C, Mezey E, Fabre M, Guidotti JE, et al. (2002) Bone marrow transplantation in mice leads to a minor population of hepatocytes that can be selectively amplified in vivo. Hepatology 35: 799–804.
6. Chamberlain J, Yamagami T, Colletti E, Theise ND, Desai J, et al. (2007) Efficient generation of human hepatocytes by the intrahepatic delivery of clonal human mesenchymal stem cells in fetal sheep. Hepatology 46: 1935–1945.
7. Peng L, Xie DY, Lin BL, Liu J, Zhu HP, et al. (2011) Autologous bone marrow mesenchymal stem cell transplantation in liver failure patients caused by hepatitis B: short-term and long-term outcomes. Hepatology 54: 820–828.
8. Nakamura T, Torimura T, Sakamoto M, Hashimoto O, Taniguchi E, et al. (2007) Significance and therapeutic potential of endothelial progenitor cell transplantation in a cirrhotic liver rat model. Gastroenterology 133: 91–107 e101.
9. Taniguchi E, Kin M, Torimura T, Nakamura T, Kumemura H, et al. (2006) Endothelial progenitor cell transplantation improves the survival following liver injury in mice. Gastroenterology 130: 521–531.
10. Terai S, Ishikawa T, Omori K, Aoyama K, Marumoto Y, et al. (2006) Improved liver function in patients with liver cirrhosis after autologous bone marrow cell infusion therapy. Stem Cells 24: 2292–2298.
11. Almeida-Porada G, Zanjani ED, Porada CD (2010) Bone marrow stem cells and liver regeneration. Exp Hematol 38: 574–580.
12. Sakaida I, Terai S, Yamamoto N, Aoyama K, Ishikawa T, et al. (2004) Transplantation of bone marrow cells reduces CCl4-induced liver fibrosis in mice. Hepatology 40: 1304–1311.
13. Kuo TK, Hung SP, Chuang CH, Chen CT, Shih YR, et al. (2008) Stem cell therapy for liver disease: parameters governing the success of using bone marrow mesenchymal stem cells. Gastroenterology 134: 2111–2121, 2121 e2111–2113.
14. Hur J, Yoon CH, Kim HS, Choi JH, Kang HJ, et al. (2004) Characterization of two types of endothelial progenitor cells and their different contributions to neovasculogenesis. Arterioscler Thromb Vasc Biol 24: 288–293.
15. Lu Y, Gong Y, Lian J, Wang L, Kretlow JD, et al. (2014) Expansion of Endothelial Progenitor Cells in High Density Dot Culture of Rat Bone Marrow Cells. PLoS ONE 9(9) e107127.10.1371/journal.pone.0107127
16. Carvalho AB, Quintanilha LF, Dias JV, Paredes BD, Mannheimer EG, et al. (2008) Bone marrow multipotent mesenchymal stromal cells do not reduce fibrosis or improve function in a rat model of severe chronic liver injury. Stem Cells 26: 1307–1314.
17. Lee JS, Semela D, Iredale J, Shah VH (2007) Sinusoidal remodeling and angiogenesis: a new function for the liver-specific pericyte? Hepatology 45: 817–825.
18. Couto BG, Goldenberg RC, da Fonseca LM, Thomas J, Gutfilen B, et al. (2011) Bone marrow mononuclear cell therapy for patients with cirrhosis: a Phase 1 study. Liver Int 31: 391–400.
19. Bruder SP, Jaiswal N, Haynesworth SE (1997) Growth kinetics, self-renewal, and the osteogenic potential of purified human mesenchymal stem cells during extensive subcultivation and following cryopreservation. J Cell Biochem 64: 278–294.
20. Taniguchi E, Sakisaka S, Matsuo K, Tanikawa K, Sata M (2001) Expression and role of vascular endothelial growth factor in liver regeneration after partial hepatectomy in rats. J Histochem Cytochem 49: 121–130.
21. Ross MA, Sander CM, Kleeb TB, Watkins SC, Stolz DB (2001) Spatiotemporal expression of angiogenesis growth factor receptors during the revascularization of regenerating rat liver. Hepatology 34: 1135–1148.
22. Assy N, Spira G, Paizi M, Shenkar L, Kraizer Y, et al. (1999) Effect of vascular endothelial growth factor on hepatic regenerative activity following partial hepatectomy in rats. J Hepatol 30: 911–915.
23. Shimizu H, Miyazaki M, Wakabayashi Y, Mitsuhashi N, Kato A, et al. (2001) Vascular endothelial growth factor secreted by replicating hepatocytes induces sinusoidal endothelial cell proliferation during regeneration after partial hepatectomy in rats. J Hepatol 34: 683–689.
24. Thabut D, Shah V (2010) Intrahepatic angiogenesis and sinusoidal remodeling in chronic liver disease: new targets for the treatment of portal hypertension? J Hepatol 53: 976–980.
25. Corpechot C, Barbu V, Wendum D, Kinnman N, Rey C, et al. (2002) Hypoxia-induced VEGF and collagen I expressions are associated with angiogenesis and fibrogenesis in experimental liver fibrosis. Hepatology 35: 1010–1021.
26. Ueno T, Nakamura T, Torimura T, Sata M (2006) Angiogenic cell therapy for hepatic fibrosis. Med Mol Morphol 39: 16–21.
27. Sakamoto M, Nakamura T, Torimura T, Iwamoto H, Masuda H, et al. (2013) Transplantation of endothelial progenitor cells ameliorates vascular dysfunction and portal hypertension in carbon tetrachloride-induced rat liver cirrhotic model. J Gastroenterol Hepatol 28: 168–178.
28. Nakamura T, Torimura T, Iwamoto H, Masuda H, Naitou M, et al. (2012) Prevention of liver fibrosis and liver reconstitution of DMN-treated rat liver by transplanted EPCs. Eur J Clin Invest 42: 717–728.
29. Taura K, De Minicis S, Seki E, Hatano E, Iwaisako K, et al. (2008) Hepatic stellate cells secrete angiopoietin 1 that induces angiogenesis in liver fibrosis. Gastroenterology 135: 1729–1738.
30. Yoshiji H, Kuriyama S, Yoshii J, Ikenaka Y, Noguchi R, et al. (2003) Vascular endothelial growth factor and receptor interaction is a prerequisite for murine hepatic fibrogenesis. Gut 52: 1347–1354.
31. Stockmann C, Kerdiles Y, Nomaksteinsky M, Weidemann A, Takeda N, et al. (2010) Loss of myeloid cell-derived vascular endothelial growth factor accelerates fibrosis. Proc Natl Acad Sci U S A 107: 4329–4334.
32. Patsenker E, Popov Y, Stickel F, Schneider V, Ledermann M, et al. (2009) Pharmacological inhibition of integrin alphavbeta3 aggravates experimental liver fibrosis and suppresses hepatic angiogenesis. Hepatology 50: 1501–1511.
33. Fuchs E, Tumbar T, Guasch G (2004) Socializing with the neighbors: stem cells and their niche. Cell 116: 769–778.
34. Xiao N, Zhao X, Luo P, Guo J, Zhao Q, et al. (2013) Co-transplantation of mesenchymal stromal cells and cord blood cells in treatment of diabetes. Cytotherapy 15: 1374–1384.

35. Mohammad-Gharibani P, Tiraihi T, Delshad A, Arabkheradmand J, Taheri T (2013) Improvement of contusive spinal cord injury in rats by co-transplantation of gamma-aminobutyric acid-ergic cells and bone marrow stromal cells. Cytotherapy 15: 1073–1085.

36. Muller AM, Shashidhar S, Kupper NJ, Kohrt HE, Florek M, et al. (2012) Co-transplantation of pure blood stem cells with antigen-specific but not bulk T cells augments functional immunity. Proc Natl Acad Sci U S A 109: 5820–5825.

37. Foubert P, Matrone G, Souttou B, Lere-Dean C, Barateau V, et al. (2008) Coadministration of endothelial and smooth muscle progenitor cells enhances the efficiency of proangiogenic cell-based therapy. Circ Res 103: 751–760.

10

Frequency of and Predictive Factors for Vascular Invasion after Radiofrequency Ablation for Hepatocellular Carcinoma

Yoshinari Asaoka[1], Ryosuke Tateishi[1]*, Ryo Nakagomi[1], Mayuko Kondo[1], Naoto Fujiwara[1], Tatsuya Minami[1], Masaya Sato[1], Koji Uchino[1], Kenichiro Enooku[1], Hayato Nakagawa[1], Yuji Kondo[1], Shuichiro Shiina[2], Haruhiko Yoshida[1], Kazuhiko Koike[1]

1 Department of Gastroenterology, Graduate School of Medicine, The University of Tokyo, Tokyo, Japan, 2 Department of Gastroenterology, Graduate School of Medicine, Juntendo University, Tokyo, Japan

Abstract

Background: Vascular invasion in patients with hepatocellular carcinoma (HCC) is representative of advanced disease with an extremely poor prognosis. The detailed course of its development has not been fully elucidated.

Methods: We enrolled 1057 consecutive patients with HCC who had been treated with curative intent by radiofrequency ablation (RFA) as an initial therapy from 1999 to 2008 at our department. We analyzed the incidence rate of and predictive factors for vascular invasion. The survival rate after detection of vascular invasion was also analyzed.

Results: During a mean follow-up period of 4.5 years, 6075 nodules including primary and recurrent lesions were treated by RFA. Vascular invasion was observed in 97 patients. The rate of vascular invasion associated with site of original RFA procedure was 0.66% on a nodule basis. The incidence rates of vascular invasion on a patient basis at 1, 3, and 5 years were 1.1%, 5.9%, and 10.4%, respectively. Univariate analysis revealed that tumor size, tumor number, alpha-fetoprotein (AFP), des-gamma-carboxy prothrombin (DCP), and Lens culinaris agglutinin-reactive fraction of alpha-fetoprotein were significant risk predictors of vascular invasion. In multivariate analysis, DCP was the most significant predictor for vascular invasion (compared with a DCP of ≤100 mAu/mL, the hazard ratio was 1.95 when DCP was 101–200 mAu/mL and 3.22 when DCP was >200 mAu/mL). The median survival time after development of vascular invasion was only 6 months.

Conclusion: Vascular invasion occurs during the clinical course of patients initially treated with curative intent. High-risk patients may be identified using tumor markers.

Editor: Yujin Hoshida, Icahn School of Medicine at Mount Sinai, United States of America

Funding: This work was supported by Health Sciences Research Grants of The Ministry of Health, Labour and Welfare of Japan (Research on Hepatitis). No additional external funding received for this study. The funders had no role in study design, data collection and analysis, decision to publish, or preparation of the manuscript.

Competing Interests: The authors have declared that no competing interests exist.

* Email: tateishi-tky@umin.ac.jp

Introduction

Hepatocellular carcinoma (HCC) is a leading cause of cancer death. It has a particularly high incidence in Asian countries, including Japan [1,2]. To control this disease, close surveillance using advanced diagnostic modalities including ultrasonography (US), computed tomography (CT), and gadolinium-ethoxybenzyl-diethylenetriamine pentaacetic acid-enhanced magnetic resonance imaging (EOB-MRI) in designated high-risk patients has facilitated HCC detection at a very early stage at which surgical resection, liver transplantation, and percutaneous ablative therapies are feasible [3]. Although surgical resection is usually the first-choice treatment option for early stage disease, it is not frequently indicated in patients with underlying liver function impaired by

chronic infection of hepatitis B or C virus [4]. Liver transplantation can treat both cancer and liver dysfunction; it has shown excellent survival rates in patients with early stage HCC [5]. However, in countries where cadaveric donor organs are scarce, as in Japan, the application of liver transplantation is limited.

Radiofrequency ablation (RFA) is currently considered to be the most effective first-line percutaneous ablative therapy because it has greater efficacy in terms of local cure than does ethanol injection [6]. The survival outcomes for patients who achieve a complete response by RFA are comparable with those for patients treated by hepatic resection [7,8]. However, even after locally curative resection or ablation, patients encounter frequent recurrence in the remnant liver because of intrahepatic spread of tumor cells and metachronous multicentric carcinogenesis; the rate of recurrence at 5 years is as high as 70–80% [9,10]. Although repeated resection or ablation can be performed in patients with recurrent HCC [11,12], the tumor tends to be out of control during the clinical course of frequent recurrence and retreatment. This is a major reason for the poor long-term survival after curative resection or ablation [13].

The development of vascular invasion and extrahepatic metastasis are representative events of an advanced stage of HCC [14,15]. Once tumor cells have invaded the portal vein, they progressively spread and increase the portal venous pressure, resulting in ascites and the rupture of esophageal varices. The spread also decreases portal flow into the hepatic parenchyma,

causing fatal liver failure [16–18]. Hepatic venous invasion causes tumor thrombi to form in the pulmonary arteries and lung tissue [19], and biliary invasion may cause jaundice, hemobilia, or cholangitis [20]. Previous studies have reported that patients with HCC with vascular invasion survive for only three months [15].

The detailed course of development of vascular invasion could not be fully elucidated by analyzing the cases who unfortunately encountered the advanced disease with vascular invasion at the time of the initial diagnosis. Because patients who undergo RFA are rigorously followed up for recurrence, the use of imaging modalities might allow for the identification of the early form of vascular invasion.

In this paper, we analyzed the incidence and predictive factors of vascular invasion as well as its detailed characteristics in patients with HCC treated with RFA with curative intent as the initial therapy.

Patients and Methods

Ethics statement

This retrospective study was conducted according to the ethical guidelines for epidemiological research of the Japanese Ministry of Education, Culture, Sports, Science and Technology and Ministry of Health, Labour and Welfare. The study design was included in a comprehensive protocol at the Department of Gastroenterology, The University of Tokyo Hospital and approved by the University of Tokyo Medical Research Center Ethics Committee (approval number 2058). Informed consent was waived because of the retrospective design. The following statements were posted at a website (http://gastro.m.u-tokyo.ac.jp/med/0602A.htm) and participants who do not agree to the use of their clinical data can claim deletion of them.

Department of Gastroenterology at The University of Tokyo Hospital contains data from our daily practice for the assessment of short-term (treatment success, immediate adverse events etc.) and long-term (late complications, recurrence etc.) outcomes. Obtained data were stored in an encrypted hard disk separated from outside of the hospital. When reporting analyzed data, we protect the anonymity of participants for the sake of privacy

Table 1. Patients' characteristics at initial RFA (n = 1057).

Variable	
Age in years	
Median	68.8
IQR	63.4–74.4
Male sex, n (%)	685 (64.8)
Etiology	
HBsAg-positive only, n (%)	119 (11.3)
Anti-HCVAb-positive only, n (%)	789 (74.6)
Both positive, n (%)	11 (1.0)
Both negative, n (%)	138 (13.0)
Alcohol consumption>80 g/day	154 (14.6)
Platelet count (×10⁹/L)	
Median	108
IQR	78–146
Child-Pugh classification, n (%)	
Class A	781 (73.9)
Class B	265 (25.1)
Class C	11 (1.0)
Tumor number, n (%)	
1	622 (58.8)
2–3	350 (33.1)
>3	85 (8.0)
Maximal tumor size (mm)	
Median	24
IQR	18–31
AFP, n (%)	
≤100 ng/mL	832 (78.7)
>100 and ≤200 ng/mL	72 (6.8)
>200 ng/mL	153 (14.5)
DCP, n (%)*	
≤100 mAU/mL	878 (83.6)
>100 and ≤200 mAU/mL	72 (6.9)
>200 mAU/mL	100 (9.5)
AFP-L3, n (%)	
≤10%	878 (83.1)
>10%	179 (16.9)

* Not determined in seven patients due to warfarin use.
Abbreviations: HBsAg, hepatitis B surface antigen; HCVAb, hepatitis C virus antibody; AFP, alpha-fetoprotein; AFP-L3, *Lens culinaris* agglutinin-reactive fraction of AFP; DCP, des-gamma-carboxyprothrombin; IQR, interquartile range.

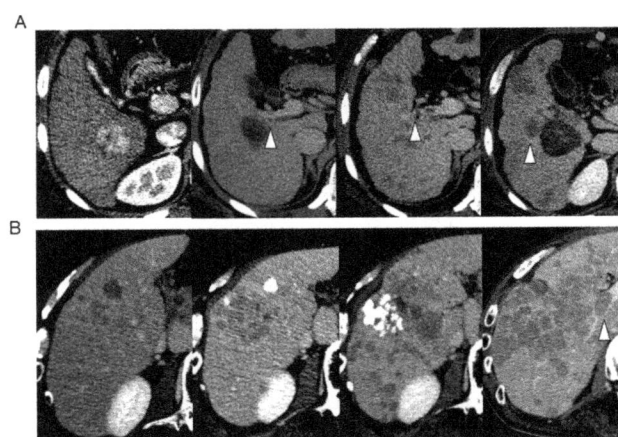

Figure 1. Images of vascular invasion developing adjacent (A) and apart (B) from the ablated area. (Case A: left panel: primary lesion before RFA, middle left panel: development of VI, middle right and right panel: evident development of VI after 4 months, Case B: left panel: multiple recurrence after RFA, middle left panel: after TACE, middle right and right panel: VI development after repeated TACE). Arrowheads denote portal venous invasion.

Table 2. Patients' characteristics at diagnosis of vascular invasion (n = 97).

Variable	
Extension of vascular invasion, n (%)	
Portal invasion within subsegmental branch	20 (20.6)
Portal invasion within segmental branch	22 (22.6)
Portal invasion within first branch	30 (30.9)
Portal invasion to main trunk	12 (12.3)
Bile duct invasion	17 (17.5)
Hepatic venous invasion	4 (4.1)
Tumor location	
Adjacent to previously ablated area, n (%)	40 (41.2)
Apart from previously ablated area, n (%)	57 (58.8)
Tumor number, n (%)	
1	10 (10.3)
2–3	8 (8.3)
4–10	14 (14.4)
>10	44 (45.4)
Undetectable*	21 (21.6)
Maximal tumor size	
Median (mm)	27.5
IQR	15.5–41.0
Diffuse/infiltrative, n (%)	36 (37.1)
Extrahepatic metastasis, n (%)	28 (28.9)
AFP, n (%)	
≤100 ng/mL	34 (35.1)
>100 and ≤200 ng/mL	9 (9.3)
>200 ng/mL	54 (55.7)
DCP, n (%)†	
≤100 mAU/mL	31 (32.3)
>100 and ≤200 mAU/mL	10 (10.4)
>200 mAU/mL	55 (57.3)
AFP-L3, n (%)	
≤10%	42 (43.3)
>10%	55 (56.7)

*Intrahepatic tumor was not clearly identified. †DCP was not measured in one patient due to warfarin use.
Abbreviations: HR, hazard ratio; HBsAg, hepatitis B surface antigen; HCVAb, hepatitis C virus antibody; AFP, alpha-fetoprotein; AFP-L3, Lens culinaris agglutinin-reactive fraction of AFP; DCP, des-gamma-carboxyprothrombin.

protection. If you do not wish the utilization of your data for the clinical study or have any question on the research content, please do not hesitate to make contact with us.

Patients

From 1999 to 2008, a total of 1057 patients with HCC underwent RFA as the initial treatment for naïve HCC. All the patients were included in this study and followed. The inclusion criteria for RFA were: 1) no prior HCC treatment other than TACE as part of sequential TACE-RFA treatment protocol; 2) three or fewer lesions of ≤3 cm in diameter; 3) a total bilirubin level of <3 mg/dL; 4) a platelet count of $\geq 50 \times 10^3/mm^3$; and 5) a prothrombin activity level of ≥50%. Exclusion criteria were: 1) portal vein tumor thrombosis; 2) refractory ascites; or 3) extrahepatic metastasis However, we also performed RFA on

patients outside these criteria if treatment was predicted to be clinically effective [21].

Diagnosis and treatment of primary HCC

HCC was diagnosed using dynamic computed tomography (CT); hyperattenuation in the arterial phase with washout in the late phase was considered to be a definitive sign of this disease [22]. Most nodules were also confirmed histopathologically via ultrasound (US)-guided biopsy. All patients underwent dynamic CT with a slice thickness of 5 mm within 1 month prior to RFA for comparison. The detailed protocol for RFA is described elsewhere [21]. Briefly, a 17-gauge, cooled tip electrode was inserted into the lesion under real-time ultrasound guidance. We started ablation at 60 W for the 3-cm exposed tip and 40 W for the 2-cm exposed tip. The power was increased to 140 W at a rate of 20 W/min. When a rapid increase in impedance was observed

A

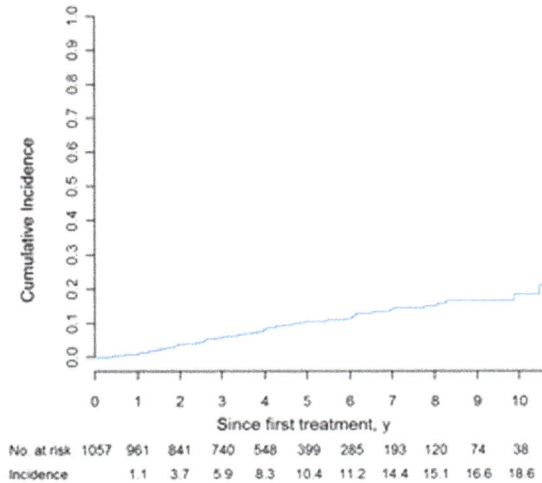

No. at risk

1057	961	841	740	548	399	285	193	120	74	38

Incidence

	1.1	3.7	5.9	8.3	10.4	11.2	14.4	15.1	16.6	18.6

B

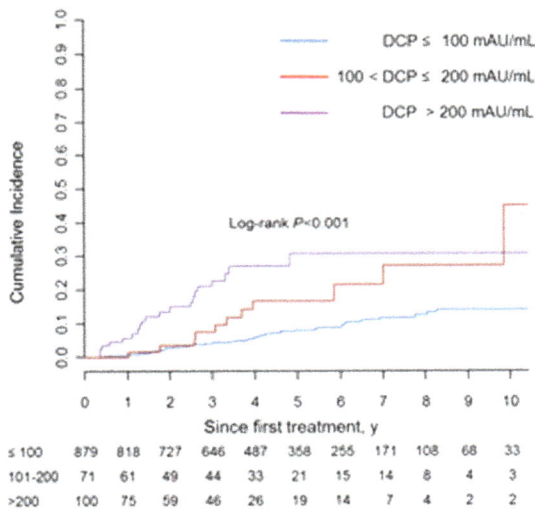

≤ 100	879	818	727	646	487	358	255	171	108	68	33
101-200	71	61	49	44	33	21	15	14	8	4	3
>200	100	75	59	46	26	19	14	7	4	2	2

C

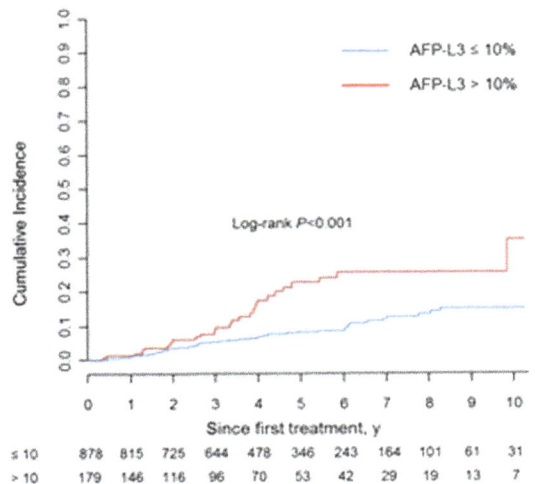

≤ 10	878	815	725	644	478	346	243	164	101	61	31
> 10	179	146	116	96	70	53	42	29	19	13	7

Figure 2. Cumulative incidence of vascular invasion after the initial treatment (A) and incidence stratified based on the DCP (B) and AFP-L3 (C) levels at the initial treatment.

during thermal ablation, we minimized the output for 15 seconds and restarted the emission at a lower output. The duration of a single ablation was 12 minutes for the 3-cm electrode and 6 minutes for the 2-cm electrode. During the treatment evaluation, a lesion was judged to be completely ablated when the nonenhanced area shown in the late phase of post-ablation CT covered the entire lesion shown in both the early and late phases of pre-ablation CT with a safety margin in the surrounding liver parenchyma. We confirmed complete ablation in all slices in which the target nodule was visualized. Patients underwent additional sessions until complete ablation was confirmed in each nodule.

Follow-up and assessment of vascular invasion

The follow-up regimen comprised blood tests to monitor tumor markers in an outpatient setting. Dynamic CT was also performed every 4 months. When HCC recurrence was identified, patients who met the same criteria used for primary HCC underwent RFA. When RFA was not indicated for the recurrent nodules due to their multiplicity, the patient underwent TACE if liver function was categorized as Child-Pugh class B or better. Those with extrahepatic tumor metastasis received systemic chemotherapy if they had well-preserved liver function and a good performance status. Vascular invasion was defined as invasion of an HCC tumor into the first and/or second branch or the main trunk of the vasculature. Vascular invasion was confirmed by demonstrating the following imaging characteristics: 1) a low-attenuation intraluminal mass that expanded the vasculature on CT, MRI, or conventional US[23,24] or 2) attenuation of portal blood flow and detection of vascularity in the thrombi by contrast-enhanced CT, MRI, or US [25,26]. The follow-up period was defined as the interval from the date of the initial RFA until the date of diagnosis of vascular invasion development, the date of death, or the end of December 2011.

Statistical analysis

Cumulative incidence of vascular invasion was calculated using the Kaplan–Meier method. Predictive factors for the development of vascular invasion were analyzed using univariate and multivariate Cox proportional hazard regression. The following factors at the initial therapy were used for the analyses: age, sex, hepatitis B surface antigen positivity, hepatitis C antibody positivity, Child-Pugh class, platelet count, alanine aminotransferase level, maximum tumor size, number of lesions, alpha-fetoprotein (AFP) level, des-gamma-carboxyprothrombin (DCP) level, and *Lens culinaris* agglutinin-reactive fraction of AFP (AFP-L3). In the multivariate analysis, stepwise variable selection based on the Akaike information criterion was used to build the final model. Scatter plots were used to assess the relationship between tumor marker values immediately before the initial treatment and at the time of diagnosis of vascular invasion. We also estimated survival rates after the development of vascular invasion using the Kaplan–Meier method. Survival curves were stratified according to the mode of vascular invasion, which was classified by the level of portal vein invasion. For the survival analysis, the follow-up was censored on 31 December 2012. Differences with a P value of < 0.05 were considered to be statistically significant. All statistical analyses were performed with R 2.13.0 (http://www.R-project. org).

Table 3. Predictors of vascular invasion after RFA (n = 1057).

Variable	Univariate Analysis		Multivariate Analysis	
	HR (95% CI)	P	HR (95% CI)	P
Age (per 1 year)	1.01 (0.98–1.03)	0.69		
Male sex	0.85 (0.55–1.30)	0.45		
HCVAb-positive	1.10 (0.69–1.75)	0.70		
HBsAg-positive	1.54 (0.93–2.55)	0.11		
Platelet count (per 10^9/L)	1.00 (0.97–1.04)	0.97		
ALT>80 U/L	0.88 (0.53–1.46)	0.62		
Child Pugh (per 1 point)	1.05 (0.87–1.26)	0.65		
Tumor size (mm)				
≤20	1		1	
21–30	1.54 (0.92–2.57)	0.098	1.30 (0.77–2.19)	0.320
>30	2.51 (1.49–4.22)	<0.001	1.74 (1.01–3.01)	0.048
Tumor number				
1	1		1	
2–3	1.59 (1.04–2.43)	0.033	1.61 (1.05–2.47)	0.029
>3	2.18 (1.13–4.20)	0.002	2.02 (1.05–3.92)	0.037
AFP (ng/mL)				
≤100	1			
101–200	1.41 (0.68–2.94)	0.36		
>200	1.93 (1.18–3.15)	0.008		
DCP (mAU/mL)				
≤100	1		1	
101–200	2.34 (1.23–4.43)	0.008	1.99 (1.03–3.84)	0.041
>200	4.33 (2.62–7.16)	<0.001	3.24 (1.90–5.51)	<0.001
AFP-L3 (%)				
≤10	1		1	
>10	2.22 (1.42–3.48)	<0.001	1.75 (1.10–2.78)	0.018

Abbreviations: HR, hazard ratio; HBsAg, hepatitis B surface antigen; HCVAb, hepatitis C virus antibody; AFP, alpha-fetoprotein; AFP-L3, *Lens culinaris* agglutinin-reactive fraction of AFP; DCP, des-gamma-carboxyprothrombin.

Results

Patient profiles and development of vascular invasion

The enrolled HCC patient cohort in this study comprised 685 males and 372 females with a median age of 68.8 years (Table 1). Approximately 75% of cases were hepatitis C-related. The median [interquartile range (IQR)] maximal tumor size was 2.4 [1.8–3.1] cm. The mean (± standard deviation) number of nodules was 1.7±1.2.

During the mean follow-up period of 4.5 years, 735 of the 1057 enrolled patients underwent 2288 RFA treatments for tumor recurrence in addition to the initial RFA. Thus, the total number of RFA treatments and target nodules were 3345 and 6075, respectively. Vascular invasion was observed in 97 patients, developing adjacent and apart from the ablated area in 40 and 57 patients, respectively (Fig. 1). Therefore, the rate of vascular invasion development associated with site of original RFA was 0.66% on a nodule basis. The detailed tumor characteristics of the patients at the time of diagnosis of vascular invasion are shown in Table 2. The sites of vascular invasion were the portal vein in 85, biliary tract in 17, and hepatic vein in 4. The cumulative incidence

rates of vascular invasion on a patient basis at 1, 3, 5, and 10 years were 1.1%, 5.9%, 10.4%, and 18.6%, respectively (Fig. 2A).

Predictive factors related to vascular invasion

Univariate Cox proportional regression revealed that the following factors were significantly associated with vascular invasion: tumor size, tumor number, AFP, DCP, and AFP-L3. Multivariate analysis with step-wise variable selection showed that the final model included tumor size, tumor number, DCP, and AFP-L3 (Table 3, Fig. 2B and C). We assessed the relationship of tumor marker values prior to ablation and at the time of diagnosis of vascular invasion. As shown in Figure 3, the sensitivities of tumor markers were higher at the time of diagnosis of vascular invasion than at the time of initial treatment: 64.9% for AFP, 67.7% for DCP, and 47.4% for AFP-L3 at the diagnosis of vascular invasion when cut-off values of 100 ng/mL, 100 mAU/mL, and 15% were adopted, respectively. Although DCP at the time of the initial treatment showed a high ability to predict vascular invasion, DCP at the initial treatment was also positive in only 23 (41.8%) of the 55 patients with a DCP of >100 mAU/mL

A

B

C

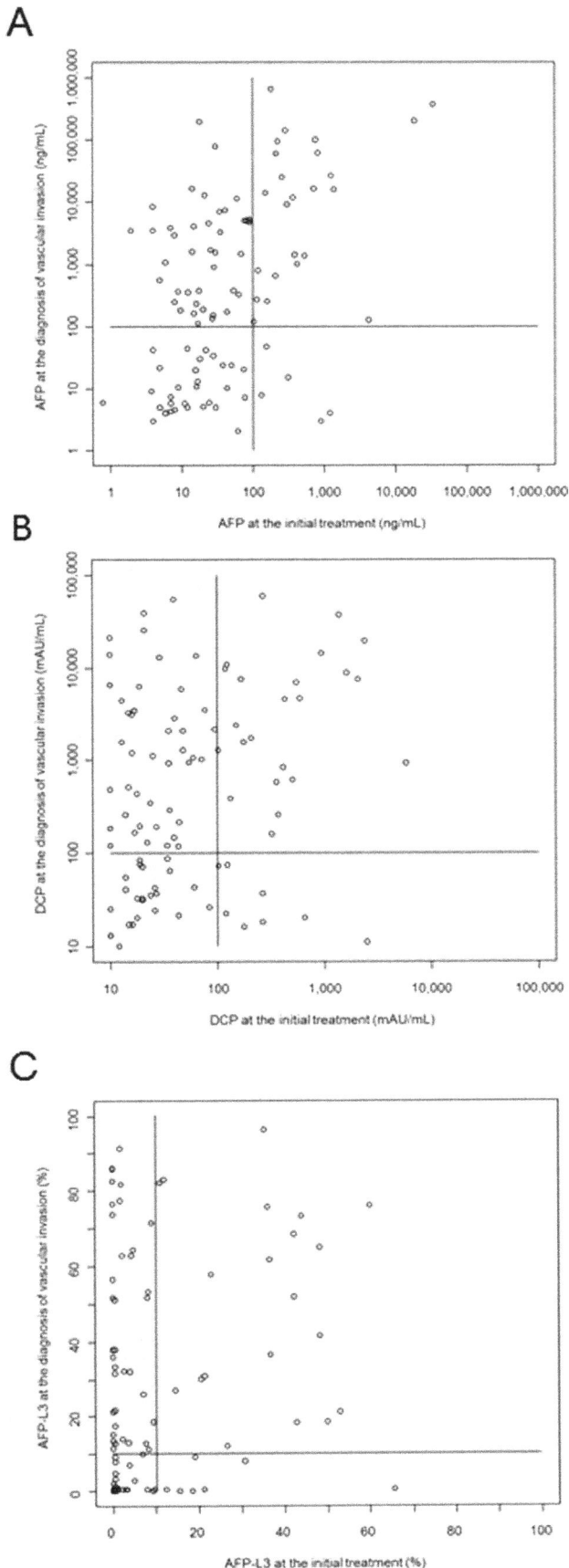

Figure 3. Scatter plots of AFP (A), DCP (B), and AFP-L3 (C) at initial treatment and at diagnosis of vascular invasion.

at the time of vascular invasion development. This result indicates that the tumor characteristics changed during the clinical course.

Treatment of vascular invasion and associated survival outcomes

Among the 97 patients diagnosed with vascular invasion, 53 (55%) underwent hepatic arterial infusion chemotherapy. Four patients underwent hepatic resection because of a localized tumor in three and tumor shrinkage due to hepatic arterial chemotherapy in one. Six patients received systemic chemotherapy including sorafenib. The remaining patients were treated with combination therapies including TACE, irradiation, and chemotherapy. Twenty-four patients (25%) received supportive therapy due to liver dysfunction or a poor performance status. The 1-, 3-, and 5-year survival rates after development of vascular invasion were 33.1%, 10.6%, and 6.4%, respectively (Fig. 4A). Survival rates differed with the severity of vascular invasion (Fig. 4B), but even in the mildest disease group with Vp1 (invasion within the second branch of the portal vein), survival was still poor (1-, 2-, and 3-year survival rates were 58.9%, 12.0%, and 6.0%, respectively). The survival rate did not change whether the vascular invasion developed adjacent to or apart from the ablated area (Fig. 4C).

Discussion

Vascular invasion is one of the most important predictors of poor survival of HCC patients [15–18]. This study showed that vascular invasion occurred in 10% of patients within 5 years when HCC was initially diagnosed at an early stage. The fact that tumor-related factors at the initial diagnosis could predict the appearance of vascular invasion as a late event may suggest that intrahepatic metastasis of primary tumors can determine overall survival. However, more than half of patients in whom a tumor marker was elevated at the diagnosis of vascular invasion were negative for the tumor marker at the initial diagnosis, which suggests that the appearance of a more aggressive tumor during the clinical course was the direct cause of vascular invasion.

Compatible with our previous report on patients with HCC treated with ethanol injection and microwave ablation, DCP was strongly related to the development of vascular invasion [27]. Some cross-sectional studies reported that DCP was correlated with microvascular invasion [28,29]. As high DCP tumors were suggested to possess invasive capacity, a high DCP level is proposed to be regarded as a contraindication for liver transplantation in several institutions in Japan [30,31]. One suggested mechanism behind the relationship between vascular invasion and DCP was that hypoxia in the tumor, which is a key trigger of epithelial-mesenchymal transition, correlates with DCP elevations [32]. It is quite reasonable that tumors with such an invasive phenotype finally develop macrovascular invasion. One concern is that patients with high DCP level may not be suitable for RFA. However, considering the fact that a high DCP level is regarded as a contraindication for liver transplantation and there is no evidence that TACE is superior to RFA in terms of local cure, it would be reasonable to consider resection in patients with good liver function[33] or to perform RFA with a wider margin in unresectable cases with deteriorated liver function when patients show a high DCP level [34].

Several reports have suggested that incomplete thermal ablation might increase tumor aggressiveness. In this study, only 0.66% of

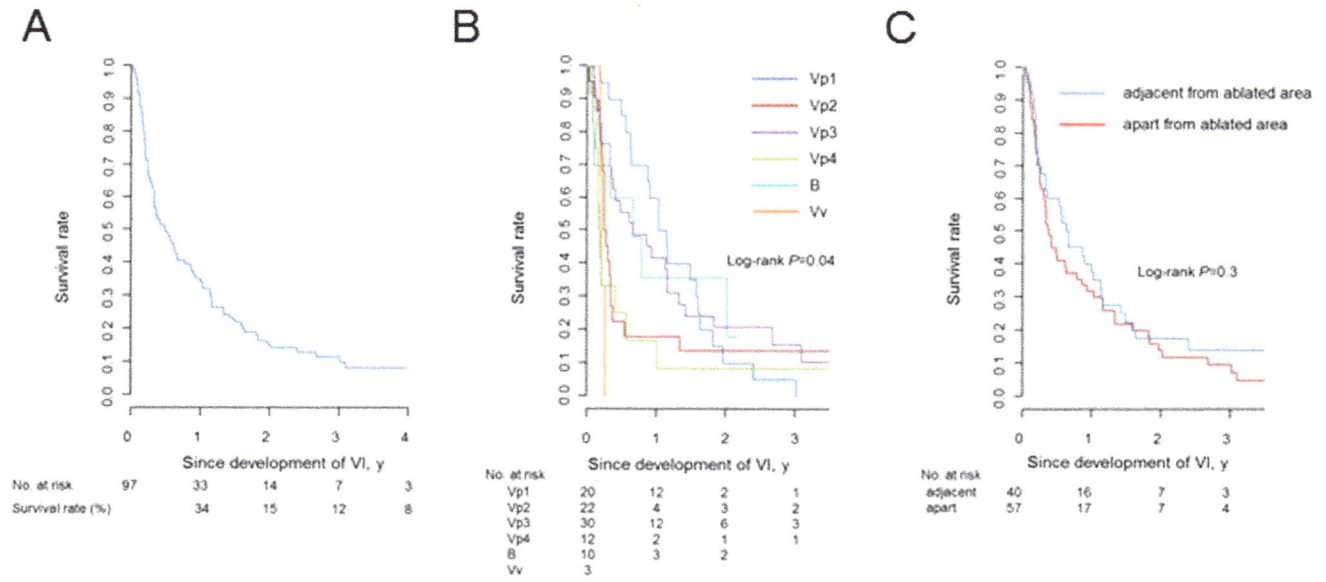

Figure 4. Overall survival rate after development of vascular invasion (A) and survival rate stratified based on severity of invasion (B). Survival rates of patients with vascular invasion developing adjacent to (blue) and apart from (red) the ablated area (C).

ablated nodules developed vascular invasion as local tumor progression [35]. This rate is acceptable considering the low mortality rate related to RFA compared with resection [36], although there is room for technical improvement. In addition, the survival rates of patients with vascular invasion adjacent to and apart from the ablated area were similar. This suggests that vascular invasion might not be a consequence of malignant transformation caused by RFA.

Vascular invasion was diagnosed in an advanced form in 52 of 97 patients, although most of them were followed closely by imaging modalities. One possible reason is that once a tumor invades the vasculature, it extends quite rapidly, probably because there is no obstacle within the lumen. Another reason would be that tumors located in the hilar region of the liver directly invaded the main trunk in some cases. This suggests that early diagnosis of vascular invasion is quite difficult. In addition, it should be noted that even when a minimal extent of portal invasion is diagnosed, the outcome is disappointing with a median survival of 1 year.

After the development of vascular invasion in this study, the therapeutic options were limited and the prognosis was poor. Surgical resection may be preferable in patients with limited tumor extension, but only four patients were indicated for resection; 25% of patients were ineligible for aggressive treatment and received best supportive care because of liver dysfunction caused by the vascular invasion itself or because of repeated recurrence and

treatment. Sorafenib is now the treatment of choice for patients with vascular invasion. However, the survival outcome is still unsatisfactory, even in patients with Child-Pugh class A [37], probably because tumors in the portal vein rarely decrease in size with the use of sorafenib and liver function may deteriorate with reduced portal blood flow.

In conclusion, vascular invasion occurs during the clinical course of patients with HCC initially treated with curative intent. The serum DCP level is the most useful predisposing parameter for the development of vascular invasion after RFA. Once vascular invasion has developed, the prognosis is poor. We must develop another strategy by which to improve the survival of these patients.

Author Contributions

Conceived and designed the experiments: YA RT KK. Analyzed the data: RT. Contributed reagents/materials/analysis tools: YA RN MK NF TM MS KU KE HN YK SS. Wrote the paper: YA RT. Critical revision of manuscript: SS HY KK.

References

1. Parkin DM, Bray F, Ferlay J, Pisani P (2005) Global cancer statistics, 2002. CA Cancer J Clin 55: 74–108.
2. Matsuda T, Marugame T, Kamo K, Katanoda K, Ajiki W, et al. (2009) Cancer incidence and incidence rates in Japan in 2003: based on data from 13 population-based cancer registries in the Monitoring of Cancer Incidence in Japan (MCIJ) Project. Jpn J Clin Oncol 39: 850–858.
3. Sato T, Tateishi R, Yoshida H, Ohki T, Masuzaki R, et al. (2009) Ultrasound surveillance for early detection of hepatocellular carcinoma among patients with chronic hepatitis C. Hepatol Int 3: 544–550.
4. Shiratori Y, Shiina S, Imamura M, Kato N, Kanai F, et al. (1995) Characteristic difference of hepatocellular carcinoma between hepatitis B- and C- viral infection in Japan. Hepatology 22: 1027–1033.

5. Mazzaferro V, Regalia E, Doci R, Andreola S, Pulvirenti A, et al. (1996) Liver transplantation for the treatment of small hepatocellular carcinomas in patients with cirrhosis. N Engl J Med 334: 693–699.
6. Lin SM, Lin CJ, Lin CC, Hsu CW, Chen YC (2004) Radiofrequency ablation improves prognosis compared with ethanol injection for hepatocellular carcinoma < or = 4 cm. Gastroenterology 127: 1714–1723.
7. Livraghi T, Meloni F, Di Stasi M, Rolle E, Solbiati L, et al. (2008) Sustained complete response and complications rates after radiofrequency ablation of very early hepatocellular carcinoma in cirrhosis: Is resection still the treatment of choice? Hepatology 47: 82–89.
8. Shiina S, Tateishi R, Arano T, Uchino K, Enooku K, et al. (2012) Radiofrequency ablation for hepatocellular carcinoma: 10-year outcome and prognostic factors. Am J Gastroenterol 107: 569–577; quiz 578.

9. Tateishi R, Shiina S, Yoshida H, Teratani T, Obi S, et al. (2006) Prediction of recurrence of hepatocellular carcinoma after curative ablation using three tumor markers. Hepatology 44: 1518–1527.

10. Okada S, Shimada K, Yamamoto J, Takayama T, Kosuge T, et al. (1994) Predictive factors for postoperative recurrence of hepatocellular carcinoma. Gastroenterology 106: 1618–1624.

11. Nagasue N, Kohno H, Hayashi T, Uchida M, Ono T, et al. (1996) Repeat hepatectomy for recurrent hepatocellular carcinoma. Br J Surg 83: 127–131.

12. Liang HH, Chen MS, Peng ZW, Zhang YJ, Zhang YQ, et al. (2008) Percutaneous radiofrequency ablation versus repeat hepatectomy for recurrent hepatocellular carcinoma: a retrospective study. Ann Surg Oncol 15: 3484–3493.

13. Ikai I, Arii S, Okazaki M, Okita K, Omata M, et al. (2007) Report of the 17th Nationwide Follow-up Survey of Primary Liver Cancer in Japan. Hepatol Res 37: 676–691.

14. Llovet JM, Bru C, Bruix J (1999) Prognosis of hepatocellular carcinoma: the BCLC staging classification. Semin Liver Dis. pp. 329–338.

15. Giannelli G, Pierri F, Trerotoli P, Marinosci F, Serio G, et al. (2002) Occurrence of portal vein tumor thrombus in hepatocellular carcinoma affects prognosis and survival. A retrospective clinical study of 150 cases. Hepatol Res 24: 50.

16. Albacete RA, Matthews MJ, Saini N (1967) Portal vein thromboses in malignant hepatoma. Ann Intern Med 67: 337–348.

17. Adachi E, Maeda T, Kajiyama K, Kinukawa N, Matsumata T, et al. (1996) Factors correlated with portal venous invasion by hepatocellular carcinoma: univariate and multivariate analyses of 232 resected cases without preoperative treatments. Cancer 77: 2022–2031.

18. Fujii T, Takayasu K, Muramatsu Y, Moriyama N, Wakao F, et al. (1993) Hepatocellular carcinoma with portal tumor thrombus: analysis of factors determining prognosis. Jpn J Clin Oncol 23: 105–109.

19. Sawabe M, Nakamura T, Kanno J, Kasuga T (1987) Analysis of morphological factors of hepatocellular carcinoma in 98 autopsy cases with respect to pulmonary metastasis. Acta Pathol Jpn 37: 1389–1404.

20. Qin LX, Tang ZY (2003) Hepatocellular carcinoma with obstructive jaundice: diagnosis, treatment and prognosis. World J Gastroenterol 9: 385–391.

21. Tateishi R, Shiina S, Teratani T, Obi S, Sato S, et al. (2005) Percutaneous radiofrequency ablation for hepatocellular carcinoma. An analysis of 1000 cases. Cancer 103: 1201–1209.

22. Torzilli G, Minagawa M, Takayama T, Inoue K, Hui AM, et al. (1999) Accurate preoperative evaluation of liver mass lesions without fine-needle biopsy. Hepatology 30: 889–893.

23. Inamoto K, Sugiki K, Yamasaki H, Miura T (1981) CT of hepatoma: effects of portal vein obstruction. AJR Am J Roentgenol 136: 349–353.

24. Van Gansbeke D, Avni EF, Delcour C, Engelholm L, Struyven J (1985) Sonographic features of portal vein thrombosis. AJR Am J Roentgenol 144: 749–752.

25. Mathieu D, Grenier P, Larde D, Vasile N (1984) Portal vein involvement in hepatocellular carcinoma: dynamic CT features. Radiology 152: 127–132.

26. Mitani T, Nakamura H, Murakami T, Nishikawa M, Maeshima S, et al. (1992) Dynamic MR studies of hepatocellular carcinoma with portal vein tumor thrombosis. Radiat Med 10: 232–234.

27. Koike Y, Shiratori Y, Sato S, Obi S, Teratani T, et al. (2001) Des-gamma-carboxy prothrombin as a useful predisposing factor for the development of portal venous invasion in patients with hepatocellular carcinoma: a prospective analysis of 227 patients. Cancer 91: 561–569.

28. Shimada M, Yonemura Y, Ijichi H, Harada N, Shiotani S, et al. (2005) Living donor liver transplantation for hepatocellular carcinoma: a special reference to a preoperative des-gamma-carboxy prothrombin value. Transplant Proc 37: 1177–1179.

29. Shirabe K, Itoh S, Yoshizumi T, Soejima Y, Taketomi A, et al. (2007) The predictors of microvascular invasion in candidates for liver transplantation with hepatocellular carcinoma-with special reference to the serum levels of des-gamma-carboxy prothrombin. J Surg Oncol 95: 235–240.

30. Ito T, Takada Y, Ueda M, Haga H, Maetani Y, et al. (2007) Expansion of selection criteria for patients with hepatocellular carcinoma in living donor liver transplantation. Liver Transpl 13: 1637–1644.

31. Hasegawa K, Imamura H, Ijichi M, Matsuyama Y, Sano K, et al. (2008) Inclusion of tumor markers improves the correlation of the Milan criteria with vascular invasion and tumor cell differentiation in patients with hepatocellular carcinoma undergoing liver resection (#JGSU-D-07-00462). J Gastrointest Surg 12: 858–866.

32. Murata K, Suzuki H, Okano H, Oyamada T, Yasuda Y, et al. (2009) Cytoskeletal changes during epithelial-to-fibroblastoid conversion as a crucial mechanism of des-gamma-carboxy prothrombin production in hepatocellular carcinoma. Int J Oncol 35: 1005–1014.

33. Kobayashi M, Ikeda K, Kawamura Y, Yatsuji H, Hosaka T, et al. (2009) High serum des-gamma-carboxy prothrombin level predicts poor prognosis after radiofrequency ablation of hepatocellular carcinoma. Cancer 115: 571–580.

34. Takahashi S, Kudo M, Chung H, Inoue T, Ishikawa E, et al. (2008) PIVKA-II is the best prognostic predictor in patients with hepatocellular carcinoma after radiofrequency ablation therapy. Oncology 75 Suppl 1: 91–98.

35. Baldan A, Marino D, M DEG, Angonese C, Cillo U, et al. (2006) Percutaneous radiofrequency thermal ablation for hepatocellular carcinoma. Aliment Pharmacol Ther 24: 1495–1501.

36. Sato M, Tateishi R, Yasunaga H, Horiguchi H, Yoshida H, et al. (2012) Mortality and morbidity of hepatectomy, radiofrequency ablation, and embolization for hepatocellular carcinoma: a national survey of 54,145 patients. J Gastroenterol 47: 1125–1133.

37. Jeong SW, Jang JY, Shim KY, Lee SH, Kim SG, et al. (2013) Practical effect of sorafenib monotherapy on advanced hepatocellular carcinoma and portal vein tumor thrombosis. Gut Liver 7: 696–703.

11

Impact of Early Reoperation following Living-Donor Liver Transplantation on Graft Survival

Yoshikuni Kawaguchi[1], Yasuhiko Sugawara[1]*, Nobuhisa Akamatsu[1], Junichi Kaneko[1], Tsuyoshi Hamada[3], Tomohiro Tanaka[2], Takeaki Ishizawa[1], Sumihito Tamura[1], Taku Aoki[1], Yoshihiro Sakamoto[1], Kiyoshi Hasegawa[1], Norihiro Kokudo[1]

1 Artificial Organ and Transplantation Surgery Division, Department of Surgery, Graduate School of Medicine, University of Tokyo, Tokyo, Japan, 2 Organ Transplantation Service, University of Tokyo, Tokyo, Japan, 3 Department of Gastroenterology, Graduate School of Medicine, University of Tokyo, Tokyo, Japan

Abstract

Background: The reoperation rate remains high after liver transplantation and the impact of reoperation on graft and recipient outcome is unclear. The aim of our study is to *evaluate the impact of early reoperation following living-donor liver transplantation* (LDLT) on graft and recipient survival.

Methods: Recipients that underwent LDLT (n = 111) at the University of Tokyo Hospital between January 2007 and December 2012 were divided into two groups, a reoperation group (n = 27) and a non-reoperation group (n = 84), and case-control study was conducted.

Results: Early reoperation was performed in 27 recipients (24.3%). Mean time [standard deviation] from LDLT to reoperation was 10 [9.4] days. Female sex, Child-Pugh class C, Non-HCV etiology, fulminant hepatitis, and the amount of intraoperative fresh frozen plasma administered were identified as possibly predictive variables, among which females and the amount of FFP were identified as independent risk factors for early reoperation by multivariable analysis. The 3-, and 6- month graft survival rates were 88.9% (95%confidential intervals [CI], 70.7–96.4), and 85.2% (95%CI, 66.5–94.3), respectively, in the reoperation group (n = 27), and 95.2% (95%CI, 88.0–98.2), and 92.9% (95%CI, 85.0–96.8), respectively, in the non-reoperation group (n = 84) (the log-rank test, p = 0.31). The 12- and 36- month overall survival rates were 96.3% (95%CI, 77.9–99.5), and 88.3% (95%CI, 69.3–96.2), respectively, in the reoperation group, and 89.3% (95%CI, 80.7–94.3) and 88.0% (95%CI, 79.2–93.4), respectively, in the non-reoperation group (the log-rank test, p = 0.59).

Conclusions: Observed graft survival for the recipients who underwent reoperation was lower compared to those who did not undergo reoperation, though the result was not significantly different. Recipient overall survival with reoperation was comparable to that without reoperation. The present findings enhance the importance of vigilant surveillance for postoperative complication and surgical rescue at an early postoperative stage in the LDLT setting.

Editor: Guy Brock, University of Louisville, United States of America

Funding: This work was supported by a Grant-in-aid for Scientific Research from the Ministry of Education, Culture, Sports, Science and Technology of Japan and from the Ministry of Health, Labor and Welfare of Japan (AIDS Research). The funders had no role in study design, data collection and analysis, decision to publish, or preparation of the manuscript.

Competing Interests: The authors have declared that no competing interests exist.

* Email: yasusugatky@yahoo.co.jp

Introduction

Continuous advances in surgical techniques, postoperative management, and immunosuppression have improved the safety of liver transplantation (LT) and patient survival [1–5]. In fact, overall survival rates in the later period of experience are reportedly better than those in the earlier period [6]. The Japanese Liver Transplantation Society reported overall survival rates for deceased-donor LT (DDLT) (n = 98) of 80.5% at 1 year, 77.8% at 3 years, and 76.0% at 5 years, and overall survival rates for living-donor LT (LDLT) (n = 6097) of 83.4% at 1 year, 79.3% at 3 years, and 76.9% at 5 years based on the data from 1998 to 2010 [7]. Similar survival rates are reported in Europe (83% at 1

year, and 71% at 5 years [1995–2000]) [8] and the United States (83.3% at 1 year [2002–2004], and 67.4% at 5 years [1997–2000]) [9].

Despite improved graft and recipient survival, the reoperation rate among LT recipients remains high, ranging from 9.2% to 34% [10–13], compared to that for liver resection, which ranges from 2.5% to 10.9% [14–16]. While several studies about the post-LT complication rates, including early reoperation, have been reported, there are few reports of the factors associated with early reoperation and the influence of early reoperation on LT recipient outcome. Recent reports indicate that early reoperation is a risk factor for impaired recipient outcome in both LDLT [12] and DDLT [10] recipients.

In the present study, we conducted a retrospective analysis investigating the incidence and cause of early reoperation, the factors associated with early reoperation, and the impact of early reoperation on graft and recipient survival among 111 consecutive adult LDLT recipients.

Patients and Methods

Patients

Between January 1996 and December 2012, 500 patients, including 77 pediatric patients, underwent LDLT at the University of Tokyo Hospital. Considering the technical standardization and establishment of criteria for reoperation, 111 consecutive adult LDLT cases between January 2007 and December 2012 were the subjects of the present study. The clinical records of these patients were retrospectively reviewed. The data of blood tests were based on the results in recipients' admission for the transplantation. All operations and reoperations were performed after obtaining informed consent from the patients and approval by the local ethics committee of the University of Tokyo.

Graft selection criteria and surgical treatment

The indication for LDLT and the type of liver graft were determined according to the ratio of the remnant liver volume to the total liver volume in living donors, and that of the graft volume to the standard liver volume (SLV) [17] in recipients [4]. Briefly, 40% of the recipient SLV was the minimum requirement for the graft and the donor remnant liver volume needed to be over 30% of total liver volume of the donor. Our detailed donor selection criteria and surgical procedures for both the donor and recipient are described elsewhere [18].

Postoperative management

All recipients were transferred to the intensive care unit with respirator support after the initial LDLT procedure. Recipients with an uneventful course were transferred to the surgical ward around postoperative day (POD) 5.

Routine postoperative investigations were as follows; blood tests (complete blood count, biochemical measurements, and coagulation profiles) were performed three or four times daily until POD 3, and twice daily between POD 4 and POD 14, chest and abdominal radiographs were examined twice daily until POD 3 and once daily between POD 4 and POD 14, Doppler ultrasonography to examine flow in the graft vessels was performed at least twice daily until POD 14 to detect abnormal flow in the hepatic artery/portal vein/hepatic vein, thrombi in the graft vessels, and intraabdominal fluid collection.

Indications for blood transfusions were as follows: red blood cell concentrate if the hemoglobin level or hematocrit was less than 6 g/dL and 15%, respectively, FFP if the prothrombin time-international normalized ratio (PT-INR) was greater than 2.00, and platelet concentrate if the platelet count was less than $3.0 \times 10^4/\mu L$.

The basic immunosuppression regimen consisted of tacrolimus and steroids for all recipients, and the doses of each drug were gradually tapered for 6 months after LDLT. Our detailed protocol of immunosuppression is described elsewhere [2].

Anticoagulation regimen after LDLT

To prevent early vascular thrombosis, anticoagulation therapy was started just after transplantation and continued until POD 14 in all recipients. The regimen was started with dalteparin (25 IU/kg/d), which was administered until POD 2. On POD 3, the anticoagulant drug was changed to heparin (unfractionated

heparin sodium, 5000 U/d), the dose of which was adjusted to achieve a targeted activated clotting time of between 130 and 160 seconds.

Definitions for early reoperation and early graft loss

Early reoperation in our study was defined as surgical intervention after LDLT between just after transplant and the day of initial discharge. Early graft loss was defined as graft loss occurring within 6 months after LDLT.

Indications for early reoperation after LDLT

Indications for early reoperation were generally divided into three categories, postoperative bleeding, vessel flow problems, and biliary complications. Reoperation for postoperative bleeding was indicated for recipients with postoperative bleeding with hemodynamic instability, hemorrhage above Grade B defined by International Study Group of Liver Surgery [19], or suspected intraabdominal hematoma infection. Vessel flow problems included hepatic arterial thrombosis, portal venous thrombosis, and decreased or hepatofugal portal flow developing during the early postoperative period, all which were detected by Doppler US. Biliary complications, which we initially attempted to treat with interventional strategies, were indicated for early reoperation in cases with massive biliary leakage resulting in biliary peritonitis or biliary obstruction with intrahepatic biliary dilatation just after LDLT.

Ethics Statement

All LDLTs were performed after individually obtaining informed consent from recipients and donors. LDLT program at the University of Tokyo Hospital has been approved by its Institutional Review Board, and all aspects of the procedures have been conducted according to the principles expressed in the Declaration of Helsinki. The current human subject research was approved as project number G3515 by Graduate School of Medicine and Faculty of Medicine, the University of Tokyo Research Ethics Committee and Human Genome, Gene Analysis Research Ethics Committee. All subjects have been properly instructed and participated by signing the appropriate informed consent paperwork. In the preparation of this manuscript, all efforts have been made to protect patient privacy and anonymity.

Statistical analysis

Continuous variables are expressed as mean values (with standard deviations). Categorical variables are expressed as number (%), and were compared between groups using Fisher's exact test or the chi-square test, as appropriate. Graft and overall survival were measured from the time of LT. Survival curves were constructed using the Kaplan-Meier method, and compared using the log-rank test. Factors with $p < 0.10$ in a Cox proportional hazard model as a univariable analysis were considered potential risk factors and were further analyzed in a multivariable Cox model. Hazard ratios (HR) and 95% confidential intervals (CI) were calculated for each factor. A p value of less than 0.05 was considered to indicate statistical significance. Statistical analysis was performed with JMP software (version 9.0.2; SAS Institute Inc., Cary, NC).

Results

Patient characteristics

The characteristics of the 111 consecutive patients are summarized in Table 1. The cohort included 50 males and 61 females (male:female, reoperation group; 7: 20, non-reoperation group; 43: 41). Mean [standard deviation (SD)] age was 51 [12] years (reoperation group; 49.9 [13.2] years, non-reoperation group; 50.7 [11.6] years). Mean [SD] Child-Pugh score was 9.3 [1.9] (reoperation group; 9.6 [1.9], non-reoperation group 9.1 [1.9]) and the mean [SD] model for end-stage liver disease score was 16.8 [7.3] (reoperation group; 17.6 [7.0], non-reoperation group; 16.6 [7.4]). There was no significant difference in the indications between the reoperation group and the non-reoperation group (Table 2). The indications for LT were liver cirrhosis caused by hepatitis C virus infection (reoperation group vs. non-reoperation group, 5 [18.5%] vs. 32 [38.1%], p = 0.052), liver cirrhosis caused by hepatitis B virus infection (2 [7.4%] vs. 13 [15.5%], p = 0.35), primary biliary cirrhosis (5 [18.5%] vs. 15 [17.8%], p>0.99), primary sclerosing cholangitis (5 [18.5%] vs. 15 [17.8%], p>0.99), alcoholic cirrhosis (2 [7.4%] vs. 5 [6.0%], p = 0.68), biliary atresia (1 [3.7%] vs. 2 [2.4%], p = 0.57), autoimmune hepatitis (1 [3.7%] vs. 2 [2.4%], p = 0.57), fulminant hepatitis (6 [22.3%] vs. 7 [8.3%], p = 0.07), and others (5 [18.5%] vs. 2 [2.4%]).

Profiles of early reoperation

Early reoperations after LDLT (reoperation group) were performed in 27 recipients (24.3%) on POD 10 [9.4]. Among them, 19 cases (70.4%) were performed within 10 days after LDLT and 5 cases (18.5%) required multiple reoperations. Table 3 lists the reasons for reoperation, which comprised mainly postoperative bleeding (n = 13, 48%), vessel problems (n = 8, 30%), and biliary complications (n = 5, 19%). One recipient underwent reoperation for strangulated bowel obstruction. Early graft loss subsequent to early reoperation occurred in 4 cases. Two recipients had graft loss subsequent to reoperation for portal venous thrombosis and simultaneous hepatic artery and portal venous thrombosis, and both underwent successful retransplantation. The remaining two recipients underwent reoperation for biliary problems, one for severe biliary leakage and the other for biliary stricture with severe cholangitis, both of which finally resulted in graft loss; only one recipient was saved by retransplantation.

Table 1. Characteristics of reoperation and non-reoperation cases after LDLT.

Variables			Total (n = 111)	Reoperation Group (n = 27, 24.3%)	Non-reoperation Group (n = 84, 75.7%)
Recipient factors					
	Age, y*		50.5 [12.0]	49.9 [13.2]	50.7 [11.6]
	Sex (female), n (%)		61 (55.0)	20 (74.1)	41 (48.8)
	Child-Pugh score, pts*		9.3 [1.9]	9.6 [1.9]	9.1 [1.9]
	MELD score, pts*		16.8 [7.3]	17.6 [7.0]	16.6 [7.4]
	Preoperative status (hospitalized), n (%)		5 (4.5)	1 (3.7)	4 (4.8)
	Preoperative blood data*				
		Albumin level, g/dL	2.9 [0.4]	2.8 [0.3]	2.9 [0.5]
		Serum creatinine, mg/dL	0.8 [0.5]	0.8 [0.3]	0.8 [0.6]
		Total bilirubin, mg/dL	8.9 [9.1]	8.9 [8.5]	9.0 [9.4]
		PT-INR	1.51 [0.68]	1.60 [0.46]	1.49 [0.74]
		Platelet count, ×10⁴/µL	8.8 [6.5]	8.9 [7.3]	8.7 [6.2]
Donors factors					
	Age, years*		39.6 [12.7]	38.6 [13.5]	39.6 [12.5]
	Sex (female), n (%)		60 (54.1)	15 (55.6)	45 (53.6)
	Graft type (LL: RL:PS)		40: 67: 4	12: 14: 1	28: 53: 3
	GV/SLV, %		45.4 [9.7]	45.5 [11.1]	45.4 [9.3]
	GV, g		528 [126]	504 [129]	536 [125]
Operative factors*					
	Operative time, min		788 [132]	801 [206]	783[99]
	Operative blood loss, L		5.5 [7.9]	7.7 [15.2]	4.8 [2.7]
	Transfusion				
		Red blood cell concentrate, U	9.5 [12.3]	13.6 [22.2]	8.2 [6.2]
		Fresh frozen plasma, U	21.2 [19.2]	29.8 [33.8]	18.4 [9.8]
		Platelet concentrate, U	24.6 [19.7]	25.9 [24.5]	24.2 [18.1]
	Biliary reconstruction, duct-to-duct, n (%)		99 (89.2)	25 (92.6)	74 (88.1)

Abbreviations: LDLT, living-donor liver transplantation; LL, left lobe; MELD, model for end-stage liver disease; PT-INR, international normalized ratio of prothrombin time; PS, posterior sector; RL, right lobe; GV, graft volume; SLV, standard liver volume.* mean [standard deviation].

Table 2. Comparison of primary disease between reoperation and non-reoperation cases after LDLT.

Variables	Total (n = 111)	Reoperation Group (n = 27, 24.3%)	Non-reoperation Group (n = 84, 75.7%)	p value
Liver cirrhosis-HCV	37 (33.4)	5 (18.5)	32 (38.1)	0.052
Liver cirrhosis-HBV	15 (13.5)	2 (7.4)	13 (15.5)	0.35
PBC	20 (18.1)	5 (18.5)	15 (17.8)	>0.99
PSC	6 (5.4)	0 (0)	6 (7.1)	0.33
Alcoholic cirrhosis	7 (6.3)	2 (7.4)	5 (6.0)	0.68
Biliary atresia	3 (2.7)	1 (3.7)	2 (2.4)	0.57
Autoimmune hepatitis	3 (2.7)	1 (3.7)	2 (2.4)	0.57
Fulminant hepatitis	13 (11.6)	6 (22.3)	7 (8.3)	0.07
Others	7 (6.3)	5 (18.5)	2 (2.4)	N.A.

Abbreviations: HCV, hepatitis C virus; HBV, hepatitis B virus; PBC, primary biliary cirrhosis, PBC; PSC, Primary sclerosing cholangitis; LDLT, living-donor liver transplantation; N.A., not applicable. n (%).

Risk factors for early reoperation

The results of analyses to identify risk factors for early reoperation in a Cox proportional hazard model were shown in Table 4. Recipient female sex (hazards ratio [HR] 2.63, 95% confidential intervals [CI] 1.17–6.72, p = 0.02), Child-Pugh class C (HR 2.27, 95% CI 1.04–5.29, p = 0.04), Non-HCV etiology (HR 2.44, 95%CI 1.00–7.28, p = 0.05), fulminant hepatitis (HR 2.78, 95%CI 1.02–6.49, p = 0.05), and the amount of fresh frozen plasma (FFP) administered (HR 1.01, 95% CI 1.00–1.02, p = 0.04) were demonstrated to be potential risk factors for early reoperation with p<0.10 in the univariable Cox model. Subsequent multivariable Cox model revealed that female sex (HR 2.90, 95% CI 1.18–8.27, p = 0.02) and the amount of FFP (HR 1.02, 95%CI 1.00–1.03, p = 0.03) were independent risk factors for early reoperation.

Graft and recipient survival in each group

Among the present cohort, early graft loss occurred in 10 cases, 4 in the reoperation group and 6 in the non-reoperation group. Mean follow-up time was 48.2 [25.9] months in the reoperation group and 50.6 [24.1] months in the non-reoperation group (p = 0.679). The 3-, 6-, 12-, and 36- month graft survival rates were 88.9% (95%CI, 70.7–96.4), 85.2%, (95%CI, 66.5–94.3), 85.2% (95%CI, 66.5–94.3), and 77.1% (95%CI, 57.4–89.4), respectively, in the reoperation group (n = 27), and 95.2% (95%CI, 88.0–98.2), 92.9% (95%CI, 85.0–96.8), 89.3% (95%CI, 80.7–94.3), and 88.1% (95%CI, 79.2–93.4), respectively, in the non-reoperation group (n = 84). The 1- and 3-year overall survival rates were 96.3% (95%CI, 77.9–99.5), and 88.3% (95%CI, 69.3–96.2), respectively, in the reoperation group, and 89.3% (95%CI,

Table 3. Reasons of reoperation after LDLT.

Variables		Number of cases (n = 27)	Early graft loss, n (%)
Postoperative bleeding		13	
	Graft surface	4	0
	Diaphragm	3	0
	Hepatic artery	3	0
	Hilar plate	1	0
	Drain insertion site	1	0
	Undetected	1	0
Vessels		8	
	HAT	2	0
	PVT	3	1(33)
	Simultaneous HAT and PVT	1	1(100)
	Regurgitant portal flow	1	0
	The portal steal phenomenon in APOLT	1	0
Biliary tract		5	
	Biliary peritonitis	4	1 (25)
	Biliary stenosis	1	1 (100)
Others		1	
	Incarcerated obstruction of the jejunum	1	0

Abbreviations: LDLT, living-donor liver transplantation; HAT, hepatic artery thrombosis; PVT, portal vein thrombosis; APOLT, auxiliary partial orthotopic liver transplantation.

Table 4. Univariable and multivariable Cox proportional hazards model analysis to identify risk factors for early reoperation.

Variables		Univariable analysis			Multivariable analysis		
		HR	95% CI	p value	HR	95% CI	p value
Recipient factors							
Age, years		0.99	0.97–1.03	0.72			
Sex, female		2.63	1.17–6.72	0.02	2.90	1.18–8.27	0.02
Child-Pugh, C vs A, B		2.27	1.04–5.29	0.04	1.47	0.61–3.67	0.39
MELD score		1.01	0.96–1.06	0.57			
Preoperative blood data							
	Albumin level, g/dL	0.87	0.37–1.99	0.75			
	Serum creatinine, mg/dL	0.71	0.22–1.47	0.43			
	Total bilirubin, mg/dL	1.00	0.95–1.04	0.97			
	PT-INR	1.17	0.67–1.62	0.50			
	Platelet count, $\times 10^4$/µL	1.00	0.94–1.06	0.87			
Primary disease							
	Non-HCV vs others	2.44	1.00–7.28	0.05	1.59	0.60–4.98	0.37
	Fulminant hepatitis vs others	2.78	1.02–6.49	0.05	2.44	0.84–6.45	0.10
Donors factors							
Age, years		0.99	0.96–1.02	0.69			
Sex, female		1.15	0.40–1.86	0.72			
GV/SLV, %		1.00	0.96–1.04	0.87			
GV, g		1.00	0.99–1.00	0.18			
Operative factors							
Operative time, min		1.00	1.00–1.003	0.58			
Operative blood loss, L		1.00	1.00–1.00004	0.16			
Transfusion							
	RCC, U	1.02	1.00–1.03	0.10			
	FFP, U	1.01	1.00–1.02	0.04			
	PC, U	1.00	0.98–1.02	0.74			
Biliary duct-to-duct		1.61	0.48–9.98	0.49	1.02	1.00–1.03	0.03

Abbreviations: LDLT, living-donor liver transplantation; MELD, model for end-stage liver disease; PT-INR, international normalized ratio of prothrombin time; GV, graft volume; SLV, standard liver volume; RCC, red blood cell concentrate; FFP, fresh frozen plasma; PC, platelet concentration.

80.7–94.3) and 88.0% (95%CI, 79.2–93.4), respectively, in the non-reoperation group. Graft and recipient survival did not differ significantly between groups (the log-rank test, p = 0.31, and 0.59, respectively) (Figure 1). A multivariable Cox proportional hazards model was applied to evaluate the risk of early reoperation for graft survival adjusting for other potential risk factors (female sex; HR 2.67, 95%CI 1.02–8.27, p = 0.05, GV/SLV; HR 1.05, 95%CI 1.00–1.09, p = 0.06) (Table 5). Reoperation was not a significant risk factor for graft survival (HR 1.28, 95% CI 0.45–3.29, p = 0.63). No significant risk factors for overall survival were identified in a Cox proportional hazards model. The duration of postoperative hospital stay was significantly longer in the reoperation group than in non-reoperation group (99 [117] vs. 52 [29]; p<0.01).

Discussion

In the present study, 24% (27/111) of LDLT recipients required early reoperation, comparable to previous reports [10–12]. The causes of reoperation, most of which were categorized as postoperative bleeding, vascular complications, and biliary complications, were also consistent with those in previous reports [10–12]. Early reoperation places additional surgical stress on each recipient, which may theoretically have a negative impact on both the graft and recipient. Previous reports have indicated an impaired graft/overall survival rate of recipients with early reoperation [10,12]. In the current study, early reoperation also tended to lead decreased graft survival rate. However, overall survival rates for recipients who underwent reoperation were comparable to those who did not, and therefore, our results

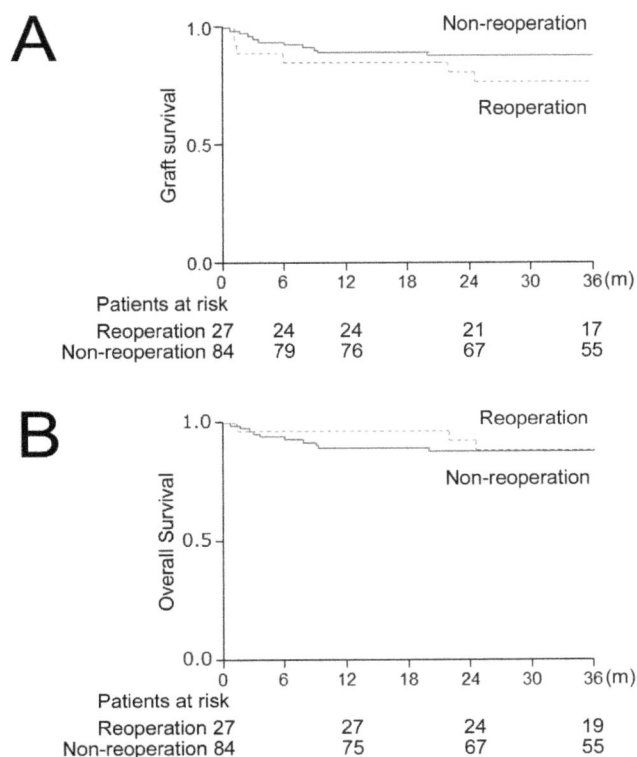

Figure 1. Graft and overall survival. (**A**) Graft survival rates for the reoperation group and the non-reoperation group. p = 0.31(the log-rank test). (**B**) Overall survival rates for the reoperation group and the non-reoperation group. p = 0.59 (the log-rank test).

enhance the importance of vigilant surveillance for early postoperative complication and early surgical rescue.

The reoperation rate after LT is reported to be high, ranging from 9.2% to 34% [10–13], while the reoperation rate after liver resection is reported to be as low as 2.5% to 10.9% [14–16]. In fact, at our institute, reoperations were performed for only 3 cases (2.7%) among 111 corresponding donors for biliary leakage (2 cases, 1.8%) and postoperative bleeding (1 case, 0.9%). The reasons for the increased rate of reoperation after LT could be attributed to poor recipient preoperative condition with hepatic failure, the administration of particular drugs such as immunosuppressants and anticoagulants, and the need for meticulous vessel reconstructions, including the hepatic vein, hepatic artery, portal vein, and bile duct [20–22]. The reoperation rate is reported to be even higher for LDLT than for DDLT [11,20,23].

Regarding risk factors for early reoperation, female sex, Child-Pugh class C, Non-HCV etiology, fulminant hepatitis, and the amount of intraoperative FFP administered were identified as possibly predictive variables, among which female sex and the amount of intraoperative FFP were identified as independent risk factors by multivariable analysis. Hendriks et al. [10] and Kappa et al. [13] reported that intraoperative blood loss predicted early reoperation. Child-Pugh class C and the amount of intraoperative FFP, which represent poor recipient liver function and have been associated with poor recipient outcome [24,25], can reasonably be associated with early reoperation after liver transplantation, although, to the best of our knowledge, this is the first report demonstrating a higher early reoperation rate in more seriously ill recipients. Although there is no previous reports supporting the reason for female sex as a predictive risk factors of reoperation in liver transplantation, in the setting of coronary stenting, there is the preponderance of evidence supporting that female had increased risk of in-hospital death and complications [26,27]. One possible reason in our study is that female recipient has significant smaller body and graft size in comparison with male (body height; female vs male, 156.6 [7.1] cm vs 170.5 [5.9] cm, p<0.01, body weight; 52.8 [8.4] kg vs 69.1 [9.9] kg, p<0.01, and graft size; 486.6 [127.7] g vs 579.4 [105.0] g, p<0.01), which might indicate the possible technical complications in smaller vessel reconstructions as reported in liver transplantation in children [28].

One concern for patients with liver failure and LT recipients is hemostatic balance [29]. While routine laboratory tests of these patients show bleeding diathesis, they are actually in hemostatic balance, because both pro- and antihemostatic factors are affected, the latter of which are not well reflected in routine coagulation testing [30]. This balance, however, can easily be tipped toward a hypo- or hypercoagulable state [31]. Our results demonstrating the high incidence of postoperative hemorrhage and vessel thrombosis as the cause for reoperation despite close monitoring with heparin administration, are representative of this situation. Further studies to investigate the ideal balance of coagulability are needed to reduce the incidence of early reoperation after LDLT.

Recently, Yoshiya et al. [12] of the Kyushu group and Hendriks et al. [10] reported that early reoperation was significantly associated with poor graft and/or recipient survival after LDLT and DDLT, respectively. In the present study, observed graft survival for the recipients who underwent reoperation was also lower compared to those who did not, though the result was not significantly different. Overall survival in the reoperation group was comparable to that in the non-reoperation group (Figure 1). These results in our study imply the importance of vigilant surveillance for early complications and early surgical interventions to improve graft/overall survival of recipients. However, the

Table 5. Univariable and multivariable Cox proportional hazards model analysis for graft survival.

Variables		Univariable analysis			Multivariable analysis		
		HR	95% CI	p value	HR	95% CI	p value
Reoperation		1.54	0.54–3.89	0.40	1.28	0.45–3.29	0.63
Recipient factors							
	Age, years	0.99	0.96–1.03	0.51			
	Sex, female	2.67	1.02–8.27	0.05	2.54	0.95–7.94	0.06
	Child-Pugh, C vs A, B	1.00	0.40–2.50	0.99			
	MELD score	1.05	0.99–1.11	0.14			
Preoperative blood data							
	Albumin level, g/dL	0.92	0.33–2.44	0.87			
	Serum creatinine, mg/dL	1.36	0.66–2.12	0.34			
	Total bilirubin, mg/dL	1.03	0.98–1.07	0.28			
	PT-INR	1.23	0.69–1.70	0.40			
	Platelet count, $\times 10^4/\mu L$	1.01	0.93–1.07	0.86			
Primary disease							
	Non-HCV vs others	1.11	0.32–2.28	0.83			
	Fulminant hepatitis vs others	2.37	0.67–6.53	0.16			
Donors factors							
	Age, years	0.95	0.38–2.38	0.90			
	Sex, female	1.15	0.40–1.86	0.72			
	GV/SLV, %	1.05	1.00–1.09	0.06	1.04	1.00–1.09	0.06
	GV, g	1.00	1.00–1.004	0.70			
Operative factors							
	Operative time, min	1.00	1.00–1.002	0.61			
	Operative blood loss, L	1.00	1.00–1.00003	0.40			
Transfusion							
	RCC, U	0.99	0.92–1.02	0.60			
	FFP, U	1.00	0.96–1.01	0.85			
	PC, U	0.99	0.97–1.02	0.64			
	Biliary duct-to-duct	0.65	0.21–2.77	0.51			

Abbreviations: LDLT, living-donor liver transplantation; MELD, model for end-stage liver disease; PT-INR, international normalized ratio of prothrombin time; GV, graft volume; SLV, standard liver volume; RCC, red blood cell concentrate; FFP, fresh frozen plasma; PC, platelet concentration.

different results between our study (4 early graft losses [14.8%] in 27 recipients with reoperation) and the Kyushu group study (10 graft losses [34.5%] in 26 recipients with reoperation) need further investigation. The learning curve, as suggested by Kyushu group, as well as the radiologic and hematologic assays used to detect early complications, and differences in the criteria for reoperation might partially explain the discrepancy.

The main limitations of our study are its retrospective nature, the small number of cases, and biases caused by learning curves of surgical techniques and postoperative management. The early reoperation group was a small inhomogenous cohort with various causes for reoperation, which may make the data inadequate to support the findings with a multivariable analysis. Further analyses with a large number of patients in a well-designed multicenter study are needed to clarify the impact of early reoperation on outcome.

In conclusion, observed graft survival for the recipients who underwent reoperation was lower compared to those who did not undergo reoperation, though the result was not significantly different. Recipient overall survival with reoperation was comparable to that without reoperation. Independent risk factors for reoperation were recipient female sex and the amount of intraoperative FFP in our study. The present findings enhance the importance of vigilant surveillance for early postoperative complication and early surgical rescue at a postoperative period in the LDLT setting.

Author Contributions

Conceived and designed the experiments: YK Y. Sugawara. Performed the experiments: NA JK TH TT. Analyzed the data: TI ST TA Y. Sakamoto. Contributed reagents/materials/analysis tools: KH. Wrote the paper: YK Y. Sugawara NK.

References

1. Starzl TE, Klintmalm GB, Porter KA, Iwatsuki S, Schroter GP (1981) Liver transplantation with use of cyclosporin a and prednisone. N Engl J Med 305: 266–269.
2. Sugawara Y, Makuuchi M, Kaneko J, Ohkubo T, Imamura H, et al. (2002) Correlation between optimal tacrolimus doses and the graft weight in living donor liver transplantation. Clin Transplant 16: 102–106.
3. Sugawara Y, Makuuchi M, Akamatsu N, Kishi Y, Niiya T, et al. (2004) Refinement of venous reconstruction using cryopreserved veins in right liver grafts. Liver Transpl 10: 541–547.
4. Kokudo N, Sugawara Y, Imamura H, Sano K, Makuuchi M (2005) Tailoring the type of donor hepatectomy for adult living donor liver transplantation. Am J Transplant 5: 1694–1703.
5. Pomposelli JJ, Verbesey J, Simpson MA, Lewis WD, Gordon FD, et al. (2006) Improved survival after live donor adult liver transplantation using right lobe grafts: program experience and lessons learned. Am J Transplant 6: 589–598.
6. Jain A, Reyes J, Kashyap R, Dodson SF, Demetris AJ, et al. (2000) Long-term survival after liver transplantation in 4,000 consecutive patients at a single center. Ann Surg 232: 490–500.
7. (2010) Liver transplantation in Japan: registry by the Japanese Liver Transplantation Society. Jap J Transpl 46: 524–536.
8. Adam R, McMaster P, O'Grady JG, Castaing D, Klempnauer JL, et al. (2003) Evolution of liver transplantation in Europe: report of the European Liver Transplant Registry. Liver Transpl 9: 1231–1243.
9. The Organ Procurement and Transplantation Network. http://optn.transplant.hrsa.gov/accessed on 2014 July 14.
10. Hendriks HG, van der Meer J, de Wolf JT, Peeters PM, Porte RJ, et al. (2005) Intraoperative blood transfusion requirement is the main determinant of early surgical re-intervention after orthotopic liver transplantation. Transpl Int 17: 673–679.
11. Freise CE, Gillespie BW, Koffron AJ, Lok AS, Pruett TL, et al. (2008) Recipient morbidity after living and deceased donor liver transplantation: findings from the A2ALL Retrospective Cohort Study. Am J Transplant 8: 2569–2579.
12. Yoshiya S, Shirabe K, Kimura K, Yoshizumi T, Ikegami T, et al. (2012) The Causes, Risk Factors, and Outcomes of Early Relaparotomy After Living-Donor Liver Transplantation. Transplantation Journal 94: 947–952.
13. Kappa SF, Gorden DL, Davidson MA, Wright JK, Guillamondegui OD (2010) Intraoperative blood loss predicts hemorrhage-related reoperation after orthotopic liver transplantation. Am Surg 76: 969–973.
14. Schroeder RA, Marroquin CE, Bute BP, Khuri S, Henderson WG, et al. (2006) Predictive indices of morbidity and mortality after liver resection. Ann Surg 243: 373–379.
15. Barbas AS, Turley RS, Mallipeddi MK, Lidsky ME, Reddy SK, et al. (2013) Examining reoperation and readmission after hepatic surgery. J Am Coll Surg 216: 915–923.
16. Imamura H, Seyama Y, Kokudo N, Maema A, Sugawara Y, et al. (2003) One thousand fifty-six hepatectomies without mortality in 8 years. Arch Surg 138: 1198–1206; discussion 1206.
17. Urata K, Kawasaki S, Matsunami H, Hashikura Y, Ikegami T, et al. (1995) Calculation of child and adult standard liver volume for liver transplantation. Hepatology 21: 1317–1321.
18. Sugawara Y, Makuuchi M, Kaneko J, Ohkubo T, Matsui Y, et al. (2003) Living-donor liver transplantation in adults: Tokyo University experience. J Hepatobiliary Pancreat Surg 10: 1–4.
19. Rahbari NN, Garden OJ, Padbury R, Maddern G, Koch M, et al. (2011) Post-hepatectomy haemorrhage: a definition and grading by the International Study Group of Liver Surgery (ISGLS). HPB (Oxford) 13: 528–535.
20. Duailibi DF, Ribeiro MA Jr (2010) Biliary complications following deceased and living donor liver transplantation: a review. Transplant Proc 42: 517–520.
21. Soong RS, Chan KM, Chou HS, Wu TJ, Lee CF, et al. (2012) The risk factors for early infection in adult living donor liver transplantation recipients. Transplant Proc 44: 784–786.
22. Arshad F, Lisman T, Porte RJ (2013) Hypercoagulability as a contributor to thrombotic complications in the liver transplant recipient. Liver Int 33: 820–827.
23. Khalaf H (2010) Vascular complications after deceased and living donor liver transplantation: a single-center experience. Transplant Proc 42: 865–870.
24. Onaca NN, Levy MF, Sanchez EQ, Chinnakotla S, Fasola CG, et al. (2003) A correlation between the pretransplantation MELD score and mortality in the first two years after liver transplantation. Liver Transpl 9: 117–123.
25. Kamath PS, Wiesner RH, Malinchoc M, Kremers W, Therneau TM, et al. (2001) A model to predict survival in patients with end-stage liver disease. Hepatology 33: 464–470.
26. Anderson ML, Peterson ED, Brennan JM, Rao SV, Dai D, et al. (2012) Short-and long-term outcomes of coronary stenting in women versus men: results from the National Cardiovascular Data Registry Centers for Medicare & Medicaid services cohort. Circulation 126: 2190–2199.
27. Peterson ED, Lansky AJ, Kramer J, Anstrom K, Lanzilotta MJ (2001) Effect of gender on the outcomes of contemporary percutaneous coronary intervention. Am J Cardiol 88: 359–364.
28. Sanada Y, Wakiya T, Hishikawa S, Hirata Y, Yamada N, et al. (2013) Risk factors and treatments for hepatic arterial complications in pediatric living donor liver transplantation. J Hepatobiliary Pancreat Sci.
29. Lisman T, Caldwell SH, Burroughs AK, Northup PG, Senzolo M, et al. (2010) Hemostasis and thrombosis in patients with liver disease: the ups and downs. J Hepatol 53: 362–371.
30. Tripodi A, Primignani M, Chantarangkul V, Dell'Era A, Clerici M, et al. (2009) An imbalance of pro- vs anti-coagulation factors in plasma from patients with cirrhosis. Gastroenterology 137: 2105–2111.
31. Lisman T, Porte RJ (2009) Hepatic artery thrombosis after liver transplantation: more than just a surgical complication? Transpl Int 22: 162–164.

12

Regulation of Coagulation Factor XI Expression by MicroRNAs in the Human Liver

Salam Salloum-Asfar[1], Raúl Teruel-Montoya[1], Ana B. Arroyo[1], Nuria García-Barberá[1], Amarjit Chaudhry[2], Erin Schuetz[2], Ginés Luengo-Gil[1], Vicente Vicente[1], Rocío González-Conejero[1]*⁹, Constantino Martínez[1]*⁹

1 Centro Regional de Hemodonación, University of Murcia, Instituto Murciano de Investigación Biosanitaria Virgen de la Arrixaca, Murcia, Spain, **2** Department of Pharmacology, St. Jude Children's Research Hospital, Memphis, Tennessee, United States of America

Abstract

High levels of factor XI (FXI) increase the risk of thromboembolic disease. However, the genetic and environmental factors regulating FXI expression are still largely unknown. The aim of our study was to evaluate the regulation of FXI by microRNAs (miRNAs) in the human liver. *In silico* prediction yielded four miRNA candidates that might regulate FXI expression. HepG2 cells were transfected with miR-181a-5p, miR-23a-3p, miR-16-5p and miR-195-5p. We used mir-494, which was not predicted to bind to *F11*, as a negative control. Only miR-181a-5p caused a significant decrease both in FXI protein and *F11* mRNA levels. In addition, transfection with a miR-181a-5p inhibitor in PLC/PRF/5 hepatic cells increased both the levels of *F11* mRNA and extracellular FXI. Luciferase assays in human colon cancer cells deficient for Dicer (HCT-DK) demonstrated a direct interaction between miR-181a-5p and 3'untranslated region of *F11*. Additionally, *F11* mRNA levels were inversely and significantly correlated with miR-181a-5p levels in 114 healthy livers, but not with miR-494. This study demonstrates that FXI expression is directly regulated by a specific miRNA, miR-181a-5p, in the human liver. Future studies are necessary to further investigate the potential consequences of miRNA dysregulation in pathologies involving FXI.

Editor: Ratna B. Ray, Saint Louis University, United States of America

Funding: This work was supported by Instituto de Salud Carlos III and Fondo Europeo de Desarrollo Regional (FEDER) [PI11/00566]: CMG, RT-M, NG-B, Instituto de Salud Carlos III, Red RIC (RD12/0042/0050): VV, RG-C, CM and NIH/NIGMS R01 GM094418: AC, ES. The funders had no role in study design, data collection and analysis, decision to publish, or preparation of the manuscript.

Competing Interests: The authors have declared that no competing interests exist.

* Email: rocio.gonzalez@carm.es (RG-C); constant@um.es (CM)

⁹ These authors contributed equally to this work.

Introduction

Although coagulation factor XI (FXI) was discovered nearly 50 years ago [1], its role in pathophysiological conditions is still not fully understood. A wide range of FXI plasma levels has been found in the healthy population [2]. The available functional data on FXI function are confusing, probably reflecting the fact that FXI might be involved not only in haemostasis but also in pathologic processes as inflammation or innate immunity [3,4]. Epidemiological and animal model studies have associated FXI levels with the risk of thrombotic disease (for review see [5,6]) or septic survival advantage [7]. On the other hand, FXI deficiency does not usually lead to spontaneous bleeding, but it is associated with an increased risk of bleeding when the haemostatic system is challenged [6,8]. Moreover, FXI inhibition has been proposed as a novel approach to developing new anti-thrombotic therapies to achieve an improved benefit-risk ratio [9,10].

In this framework, several groups have been engaged in an intensive study of the influence of genetic and environmental factors on FXI plasma levels in an attempt to understand whether the heterogeneous values found in the healthy population confer a pro- or anti-thrombotic phenotype. Although some of these studies

have identified the involvement of common single nucleotide polymorphisms in the structural *F11* gene and alterations in other genes that might indirectly regulate plasma levels of this factor [11–13], the molecular mechanisms of FXI regulation are still largely unknown.

MicroRNAs (miRNAs), which are small non-coding RNAs that regulate protein expression [14], have been involved in the regulation of many complex mechanisms or physiological conditions, including the haemostatic system. Available predictive algorithms estimate that a third of the human mRNAs may contain a single or multiple binding sites for miRNAs [15]. As such, a single miRNA can potentially target hundreds of genes, or a single gene could be targeted by many different miRNAs [15–18]. However, it has been shown that overexpression of miRNAs only provokes a mild repression of both mRNA [19] and protein [20].

During the last four years, several groups including ours, have evaluated the role of miRNAs in the regulation of haemostasis [21]. Coagulation factors like fibrinogen [22] or tissue factor have been described as interacting with miRNAs, which may have an impact on the thrombotic etiology associated with pathologies such as antiphospholipid syndrome or systemic lupus erythematosus [23]. Recently, PAI-1 [24] and protein S [25] have also been shown to be directly regulated by miRNAs. In the current study, we investigated the potential relevance of miRNAs aiming to discover new elements that may modulate FXI in the liver. *In silico* predictions together with *in vitro* experiments showed that only miR-181a-5p caused a slight although significant decrease both in FXI protein and *F11* mRNA levels. Luciferase assays helped us to demonstrate a direct interaction between miR-181a-5p and 3′ untranslated region (3′UTR) of *F11*. Importantly, *F11* mRNA levels were inversely and significantly correlated with miR-181a-5p levels in 114 healthy livers. This study demonstrates that FXI expression in the human liver is directly regulated by a specific miRNA, miR-181a-5p, opening up new prospects in a better understanding of the pathophysiology of haemostatic diseases where FXI is involved and in the development of miRNA-based therapeutic technologies.

Results

A microarray and *in silico* target search yielded four miRNAs that could potentially bind to *F11* mRNA

In order to select miRNAs with the potential to bind to *F11* mRNA, two criteria were established (i) the miRNA expression cut-off in liver had to be >500 arbitrary units (au) (see array in Table S1) and (ii) the miRNA binding had to be anticipated in 4 or more of the prediction algorithms of miRNA targets used (n = 8). Such filtering allowed the selection of four miRNAs: miR-181a-5p (liver expression = 1233 au; 6 prediction algorithms), miR-23a-3p (liver expression = 6052 au; 5 prediction algorithms), miR-16-5p (liver expression = 3513 au; 4 prediction algorithms), and miR-195-5p (liver expression = 3046 au; 4 prediction algorithms) (see Table 1 and Table S1). Additionally, a negative control miRNA (miR-494; see Table 1), which was not predicted to bind to *F11* mRNA (only 2 prediction algorithms) and with a liver expression >500 au, was also investigated (Table 1). Putative binding sites for miRNAs are shown in Figure 1. Whereas miR-181a-5p and miR-23a-3p bind to two closely located sites, miR-16-5p and miR-195-5p share the same binding site located ~200 bp downstream of the miR-23a-3p seed (Figure 1).

In vitro studies suggested miR-181a-5p as a direct inhibitor of FXI and *F11* mRNA expression

To test which miRNAs may inhibit FXI expression, we employed HepG2 cells, expressing lower levels of these miRNAs than the liver (Figure S1A). Transfection of HepG2 cells with the different miRNA mimics showed that only miR-181a-5p mimic provoked a significant reduction of endogenous *F11* mRNA levels of almost 30% (100% *vs.* 71±9%; p = 0.03; N = 3) compared with non-specific scrambled negative control (SCR) transfection (Figure 2A). No inhibition was found when transfecting HepG2 with the other selected miRNAs or with miR-494 (Figure 2A). In fact, miR-181a-5p caused a significant decrease (~30%) in the levels of extracellular FXI (100% *vs.* 71±7%; p = 0.04; N = 3) (Figure 2B).

In addition, when the intracellular levels of FXI in cells transfected with miR-181a-5p were evaluated an almost 50% decrease was observed compared with cells transfected with SCR (100% *vs.* 53±16%; p = 0.02; N = 3) (Figure 2C).

Next, we tested the effect of a miR-181a-5p inhibitor in another hepatic cell line where miR-181a-5p expression levels were similar to those reported in the liver (Figure S1B), PLC/PRF/5 hepatic cell line. Our results indicated that inhibition of miR-181a-5p increased both the levels of *F11* mRNA (100% *vs.* 121±3%; p = 0.006; N = 3) (Figure 2D) and of extracellular FXI (100% *vs.*

Table 1. *In silico* Prediction Results.

Human miRNA	RNAhybrid[A]	TargetScan[B]	miRSVR[C]	DIANAmT[D]	miRDB[D]	PITA[D]	RNA22[D]	PICTAR5[D]	Total prediction algorithms	Liver Expression (arbitrary units)
miR-181a-5p	1 (−19.70)	1 (−0.05)	1 (−0.36)	1	1	1	-	-	6	1233
miR-23a-3p	1 (−14.70)	1 (−0.07)	1 (−0.67)	1	-	1	-	-	5	6052
miR-16-5p	1 (−15.00)	1 (−0.13)	1 (−0.13)	1	-	-	-	-	4	3513
miR-195-5p	1 (−8.00)	1 (−0.13)	1 (−0.14)	1	-	-	-	-	4	3046
miR-494	-	-	1 (−0.03)	-	-	1	-	-	2	1395

The presence of the selected miRNA in the target prediction tool is recognized in the table by number "1".
A: RNA hybrid minimum free energy (MFE; kcal/mol) [42], B: TargetScan (context + score) [43], C: miRSVR score[44], D: algorithms included in miRWalk.

$116 \pm 6\%$; $p = 0.038$; $N = 3$) (Figure 2E) further supporting a physiological regulation of FXI by miR-181a-5p.

Whether the lower levels of *F11* mRNA observed in transfected HepG2 were due to an indirect effect of miR-181a-5p or to mRNA decay was further investigated. Co-transfection of HCT-DK cells with a luciferase reporter vector containing the 3′UTR of *F11* and miR-181a-5p showed a significant decrease of ~30% of the luciferase activity in comparison with SCR ($100 \pm 17\%$ *vs.* $71 \pm 27\%$; $p = 0.04$; $N = 3$). This inhibition was not observed when using a mutated vector which lacked the binding site of miR-181a-5p (Figure 3).

F11 mRNA and FXI levels were inversely correlated with miR-181a-5p in human livers

In order to establish the potential physiological significance of the above results, we measured *F11* mRNA and miR-181a-5p levels in samples from a cohort of healthy livers that had been used for liver transplant. Using a linear regression model, *F11* mRNA levels were found to be inversely and significantly related to miR-181a-5p levels ($r = -0.184$; $p < 0.05$) (Figure 4A). To confirm the specificity of this result, we compared levels of *F11* mRNA with those of miR-494 (that showed no *in silico* or *in vitro* effect on FXI expression) and we found no association between these two molecules ($r = -0.033$; $p = 0.727$) (Figure 4B).

Previous studies have shown that FXI plasma antigenic levels are correlated with those of FIX [2]. In this study, we observed a strong correlation between *F9* and *F11* mRNA levels (Figure 4C), which supported the described correlation in plasma. Aiming to further confirm the specificity of *F11* mRNA: miR-181a-5p interaction, we investigated a potential correlation between miR-181a-5p and *F9* mRNA levels. As expected, our results demonstrated that miR-181a-5p had no influence on *F9* mRNA levels in healthy livers ($p = 0.115$) (Figure 4D).

Next, we investigated the dynamic range of expression of *F11* mRNA in hepatocytes, finding that it was larger than that described for plasma levels of FXI [26]. More specifically, there was a three-fold difference in *F11* mRNA values between the 75th and 25th percentiles (Figure 5A). Interestingly, we also observed a wide range of expression of miR-181a-5p among individuals. In fact, miR-181a-5p expression in liver samples with *F11* mRNA levels below 15th percentile was two-fold higher than in the samples above the 85th percentile (Figure 5B).

Discussion

It has been consistently reported that miRNAs may regulate haemostatic proteins such as fibrinogen [22], tissue factor [23], PAI-1[24] or antithrombin [21], while variations in the levels of miRNAs [23] or in the efficacy of the miRNA: mRNA interaction [27] might have an impact on the development of thrombotic diseases. In the present study, we provide new evidence that miRNAs fine-regulates the expression of FXI in human hepatocytes, which in turn opens an alternative regulation pathway that may be exploited for future studies.

The *in silico* results were the starting point in our work. Bearing in mind that approximately 70% of all *in silico* predictions are thought to be false-positive [28], this encouraged us to more accurately establish filters to select the candidate miRNAs to be studied. Our filters led to the selection of 4 candidate miRNAs with potential to bind to *F11* mRNA and, even then, we observed 75% false positives. The effective prediction of miRNA: mRNA pairs in animal systems is still a challenge because of the complexity of this interaction [29]. Future studies to unravel these issues will probably help identify a more selective *in silico* search method for additional miRNAs which target FXI and other haemostatic factors.

In a second step consisting in performing an *in vitro* validation, only miR-181a-5p was potentially a direct regulator of *F11* expression, which enabled it to induce a significant decrease in both extra- and intracellular FXI and *F11* mRNA levels. As expected, and in accord with other studies describing that the effect of a given miRNA on its target is generally modest [19,20,28] and that it is the total of various miRNA interactions that would determine the effect as a whole, we found that the effect of miR-181a-5p on FXI expression was mild. Future studies will determinate additional miRNAs that may act in conjunction with miR-181a-5p to regulate FXI expression. In this sense, we found that a neutral miRNA (miR-494) neither interacted nor correlated with *F11* mRNA (Figure 4B). Moreover, the lack of correlation found between miR-181a-5p and *F9* mRNA further supported our hypothesis that miR-181a-5p has a specific effect on FXI expression.

Next, we investigated the physiological relevance of FXI regulation by miR-181a-5p. Given our inability to test this hypothesis *in vivo*, we performed *ex vivo* analysis in livers from healthy donors that had been used for transplant. Our data showed that levels of miR-181a-5p and *F11* mRNA were correlated in human livers (Pearson's coefficient $= -0.184$, $p<$

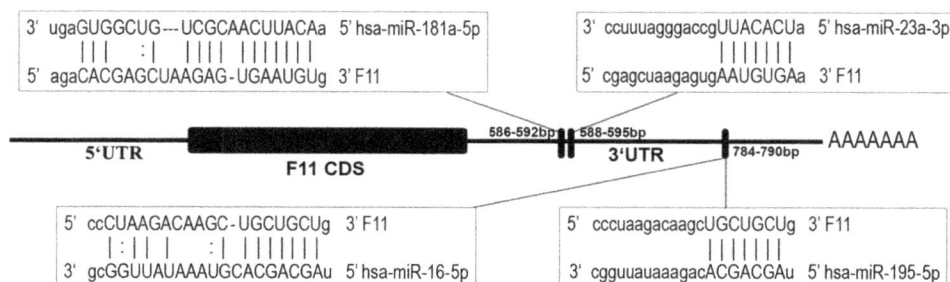

Figure 1. Schematic representation of predicted target sites of miRNAs in *F11* 3′UTR. The predicted binding sites of miR-181a-5p, miR-23a-3p, miR-16-5p, and miR-195-5p are indicated in the *F11* 3′UTR (1,060 bp). The first nucleotide after the stop codon of *F11* is defined as "+1", and the start- and end-positions of the complementary sequence between *F11* and miRNAs are indicated. Complementarities between the seed region (7 nucleotides) of miRNAs and 3′UTR of *F11* mRNA target site are shown in parentheses. MiR-16-5p and miR-195-5p share the same binding site. MiRNA: mRNA interactions are represented by upper-case letters (provided by mirSVR algorithm).

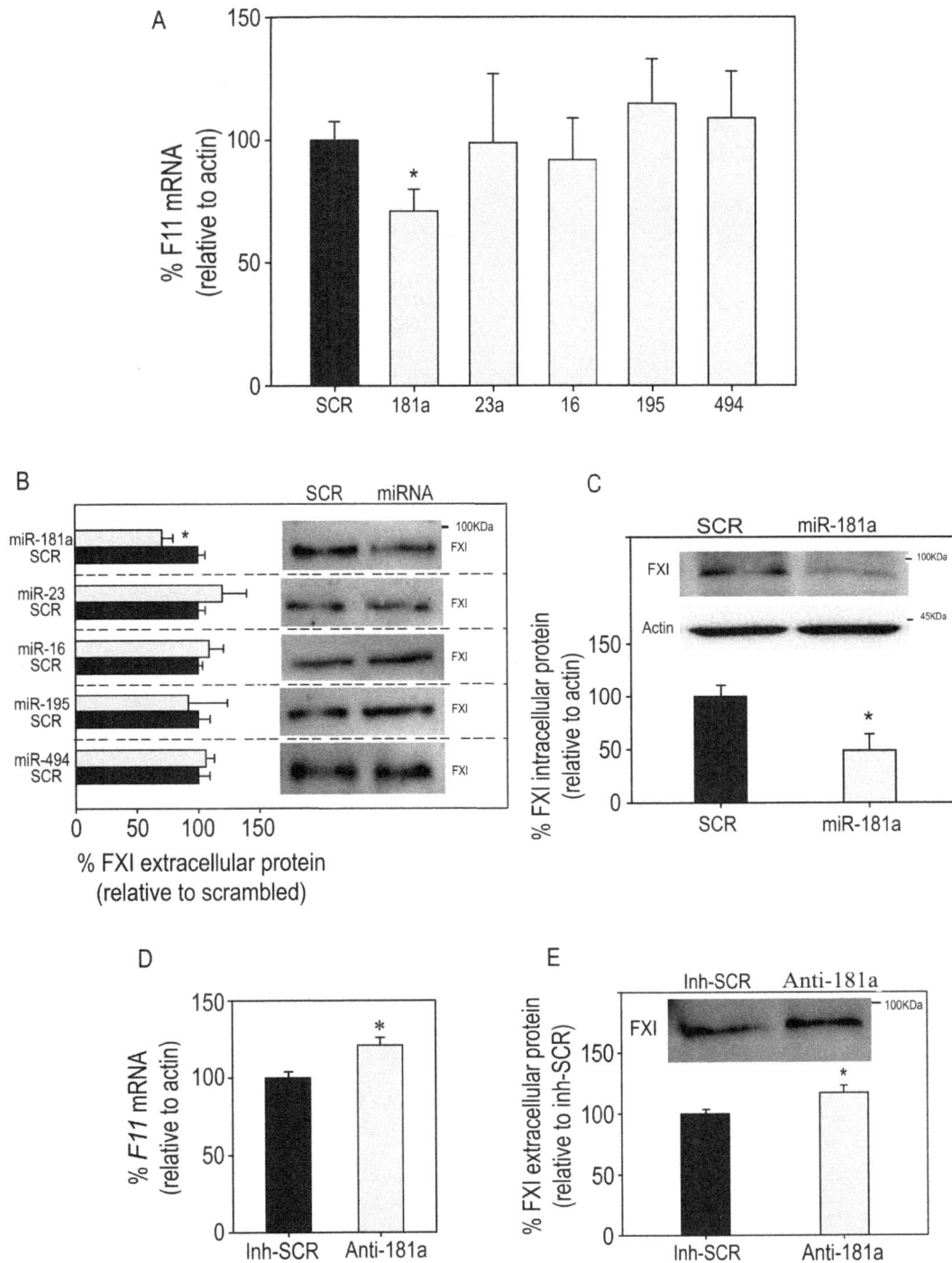

Figure 2. Effect of miRNAs on FXI expression. HepG2 cells were transfected with 100 nM mimic precursors miR-181a-5p (181a), miR-23a-3p (23a), miR-16-5p (16), miR-195-5p (195), miR-494 (494) or SCR. Protein lysate, total RNA and extracellular media were obtained after 48 h incubation and analyzed. (A) qRT-PCR analysis of *F11* mRNA expression. (B) Densitometric analysis of FXI extracellular protein expression with a representative Western blot. (C) Densitometric analysis of FXI intracellular protein expression with a representative Western blot in cells transfected with SCR and 181a. (D) qRT-PCR analysis of *F11* mRNA expression in PLC/PRF/5 cells transfected with 100 nM miR-181a-5p inhibitor or SCR inhibitor. (E) Densitometric analysis of FXI extracellular protein expression with a representative Western blot in PLC/PRF/5 cells transfected with miR-181a-5p inhibitor (anti-181a) or SCR inhibitor (Inh-SCR). Results are represented as mean ± SD of three replicates from three independent experiments. The normalized data were expressed as changes relative to the data of the cells transfected with SCR mimic or SCR inhibitor and set as 100%. *$P < 0.05$. Student's t-test was calculated in mimic precursors *vs.* SCR.

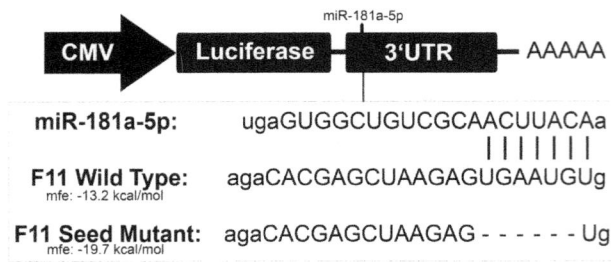

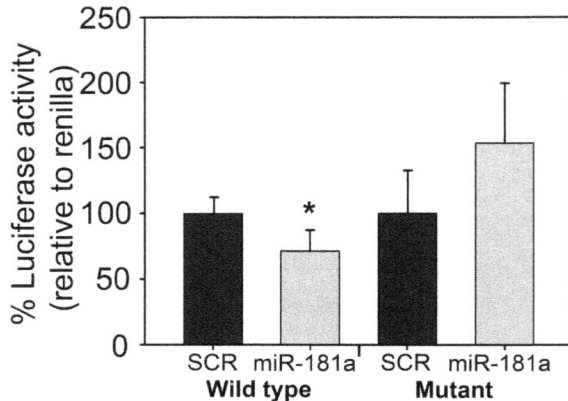

Figure 3. Luciferase reporter assays. Schematic diagram of the luciferase reporter plasmids including *F11* WT 3'UTR or *F11* mutant 3'UTR in which the seven nucleotides forming the seed region of miR-181a-5p were deleted. HCT-DK cells, that do not express miR-181a-5p nor other Dicer-dependent miRNAs that may interfere in miRNA overexpression experiments, were transfected with either *F11* WT 3'UTR or *F11* mutant 3'UTR along with 100 nM miR-181a-5p precursor. A SCR precursor was used as control. Luciferase activities were normalized to renilla activities. Results are represented as mean ± SD of three replicates from three independent experiments. The normalized data were expressed as changes relative to the data of the cells transfected with SCR mimic and set as 100%. *P<0.05. Student's t-test was calculated in mimic precursors vs. SCR.

0.05). In fact, the *in vitro* study demonstrated that the decrease of both target *F11* mRNA and protein levels was proportional and therefore we speculate that the *ex vivo* correlation may be extrapolated. Together with the fact that protein levels are determined by additional tightly modulating processes including protein degradation rates, the final effect of a miRNA on an mRNA is very difficult to predict [30]. In this sense, we found a three-fold difference in *F11* mRNA values between the 75th and 25th percentiles in healthy livers, whereas only a 1.3-fold difference in plasma between the same percentiles has previously been found [26]. Therefore, translational, post-translational, and degradation processes, together with the regulation of the secretory pathway (involving both miRNAs and target genes), may act to adjust the final amount of FXI in plasma.

Many observations of miRNA-mediated regulation in mammalian cells considered them as fine-tuners of gene expression [31]. Indeed, miRNA expression can be regulated by the same genetic alterations that modulate protein coding genes [32] as well as by environmental factors [6]. Specifically, miR-181a-5p has been shown to be regulated by dopamine [33] and TGF-β [34]. Our data showed a surprising heterogeneity of miR181a-5p expression in human liver samples (Figure 5A). We observed a 2.5-fold

difference in miRNA values between the 75th and 25th percentiles, which reached more than 12-fold when the 90th and 10th percentiles were compared. Interestingly, recently Mendell and Olson suggested that miRNA deficiency or overexpression may have an important impact under pathophysiological stress conditions [35] while, in physiological conditions, miRNAs may only play a modest role in regulating their target.

Overall, our *in vitro* and *ex vivo* results establish miRNAs as new modulators of FXI, opening up new prospects for the regulation of FXI by miRNAs that deserves further attention and confirmation. However, our *in vitro* experimental conditions did not allow us to test the effect of miR-181a-5p on functional activity of FXI. Additional studies are necessary to fully understand this new FXI regulation and to test the possibility that it is regulated by other miRNAs in an indirect way. It would also be useful to further investigate the association of miR-181a-5p expression with the development of thromboembolic disease. In this sense, FXI is seen as a potential therapeutic target since its inhibition prevents thrombosis without bleeding episodes [10]. Indeed, the use of several miRNA-based therapies in the liver is under investigation. The most advanced is the use of anti-miR-122 in the treatment of hepatitis C [36]. On the other hand, it has already been shown that antisense oligonucleotides inhibit factor XI expression *in vivo* [37], and a clinical phase 2 trial is currently ongoing (http://www. isispharm.com/Pipeline/Therapeutic-Areas/Cardiovascular.htm #ISIS-FXIRx) using a drug antisense in patients with total knee arthroplasty. Therefore, the characterization of miR-181a-5p that regulates FXI expression may be seen as an opportunity to start envisaging the potential use of miRNA precursors as an antithrombotic drug.

Materials and Methods

Cell line and tissue samples

HepG2 (American Type Culture Collection, Manassas, VA), PLC/PRF/5 (kind gift of Fernando Corrales, CIMA, Pamplona, Spain. Original commercial source: American Type Culture Collection, Manassas, VA), and human colon cancer cell line deficient for Dicer [38,39] (HCT-DK) were conventionally cultured. Briefly, HepG2 and PLC/PRF/5 were cultured in DMEM (Life Technologies, Madrid, Spain) and HCT-DK in McCoy's 5A (Sigma-Aldrich, Madrid, Spain). All media were supplemented with 0.1mM non-essential amino acids, 2 mM Glutamax I, and with 10% fetal calf serum (Life Technologies, Madrid, Spain). Cells were grown at 37°C under 5% CO_2. Liver samples from Caucasian donors (n = 114) were kindly provided by the Biobanc CIBERehd [40] (La Fe Hospital, Valencia, Spain) (n = 19) and by St. Jude Children's Research Hospital Liver Resource (Liver Tissue Procurement and Distribution System (NIH Contract #N01-DK-9-2310) and the Cooperative Human Tissue Network) [41] (n = 95) (Table S2). All donors gave a written informed consent that was recorded following the procedures of each Biobanc. Human liver studies were further approved by Local Ethics Committee from Hospital Universitario Morales Meseguer in Murcia (#ESTU-19/12).

MiRNA array and *in silico* identification of miRNA binding sites in *F11* mRNA

To identify miRNAs expressed in healthy liver, we performed expression arrays including 1,898 human mature miRNAs (LCSciences, Houston, TX; Sanger mirBase Release 18.0 and 19.0) using total RNA extracted from 4 healthy human liver samples (Table S1). Raw miRNA microarray data are available in public archives under corresponding author name (GSE61219).

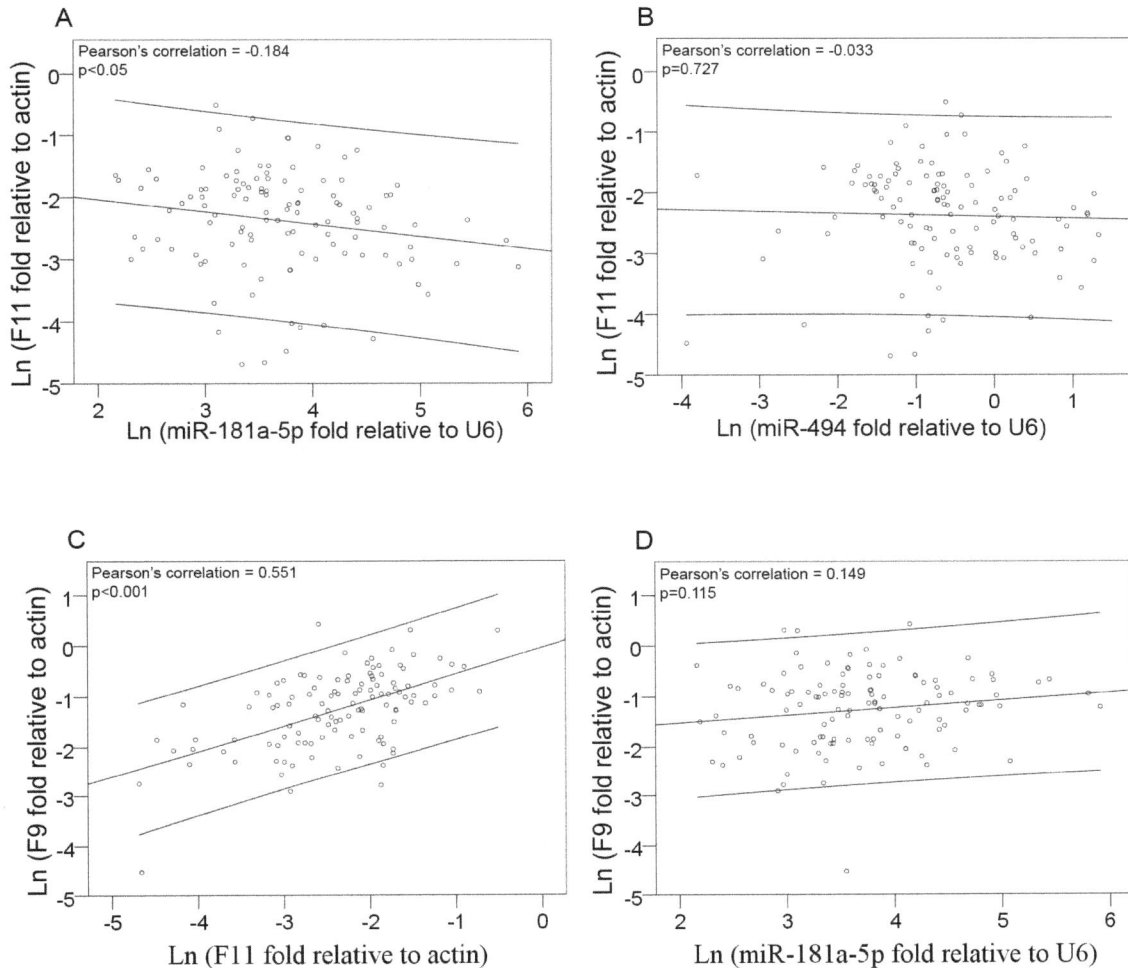

Figure 4. *Ex vivo* **expression of** *F11* **mRNA and mature miRNAs.** Linear regression analysis between endogenous mature miRNAs (miR-181a-5p and miR-494) levels and *F11* mRNA (A & B respectively). (C) Linear regression between *F11* and *F9* mRNAs and (D) between miR-181a-5p and *F9* mRNA. qRT-PCR were performed in total RNA purified from healthy livers (n = 114). Statistical significance was taken as p<0.05. The results are presented as Ln fold change with respect to the normalization standard.

For the determination of mature hepatic miRNAs potentially regulating human *F11* 3′UTR, we used four miRNA prediction algorithms.

Cell transfection

To validate *in silico* experiments, we performed transfection assays in cell lines mentioned above. Briefly, cells were seeded twenty four hours before transfection in complete medium without antibiotics and transfected with 100 nM of chemically modified double-stranded RNAs that mimic endogenous miRNAs (mimic), 100 nM miRNA inhibitors (miRCURY LNA microRNA Inhibitor from Exiqon, Vedbaek, Denmark) or 100 nM SCR from Life Technologies (Madrid, Spain) as previously described [40]. Transfection efficiency was >90% (Figure S2). After 48 h, supernatants and cells were collected for subsequent mRNA and protein analyses.

MiRNA and mRNA expression levels

Total RNA was isolated from both fresh livers and transfected cells using Trizol Reagent (Life Technologies, Madrid, Spain).

RNA (400 ng) and SuperScript III First-Strand Synthesis System (Life Technologies, Madrid, Spain) were used for reverse transcription (RT) reactions. *F11* and *ACTB* (as endogenous reference control) genes expression were quantified by qRT-PCR (Hs01030011_m1 and Hs99999903_m1, respectively, from Life Technologies, Madrid, Spain).

Commercial assays for miR-181a-5p, miR-23a-3p, miR-16-5p, miR-195-5p, miR-494, and U6 snRNA (endogenous reference control) (Life Technologies, Madrid, Spain) were used to quantify expression levels of miRNAs in human cell lines and/or hepatocytes.

Western blot

Proteins from the lysate of transfected HepG2 cells (60 μg) or liver (50 μg) were blotted and immunostained with anti-human FXI polyclonal antibody (Enzyme Research Laboratories, Swansea, UK) and anti-human β-actin monoclonal antibody (Sigma-Aldrich, Madrid, Spain). Additionally, we collected and lyophilized 500 μL supernatants from HepG2 and PLC/PRF/5 using CentriVap Concentrator (Labconco, Kansas, MO) and 24 μL

A

B

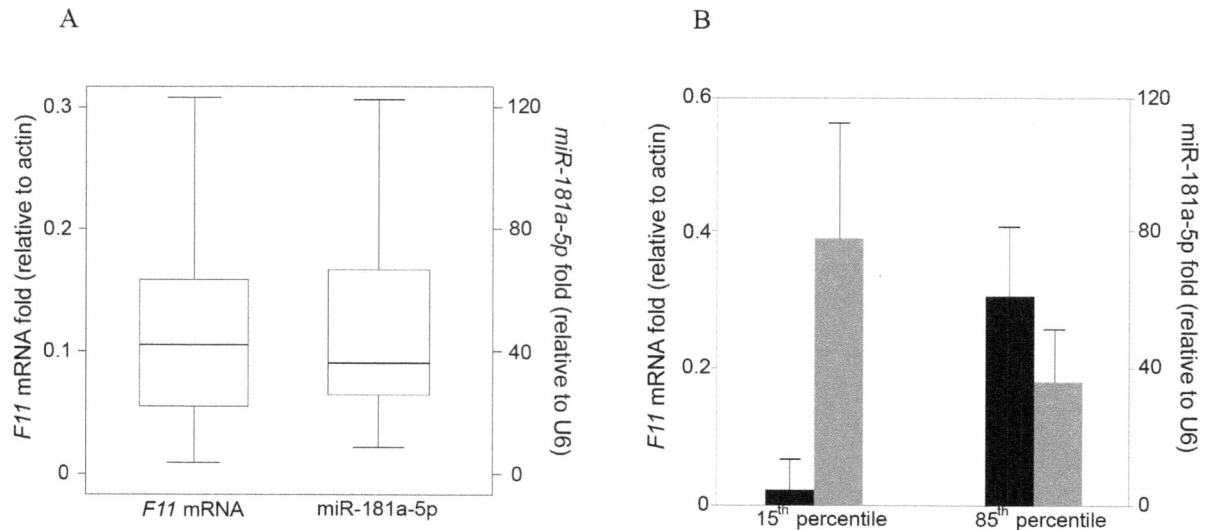

Figure 5. Expression range of miR-181a-5p and *F11* mRNA in healthy livers. (A) Box plot of *F11* mRNA and miR-181a-5p levels in livers. The upper and lower bars are the 90th and 10th percentiles, respectively. (B) Levels of miR-181a-5p (black) in livers corresponding to 15th and 85th percentiles of *F11* mRNA expression (grey), mean ± SD.

were blotted and immunostained with anti-human FXI polyclonal antibody. FXI and β-actin were immunodetected with the appropriate secondary antibody labeled with peroxidase (GE Healthcare, Barcelona, Spain). Detection was performed using ECL Prime Western Blotting Detection Kit (GE Healthcare, Barcelona, Spain) and ImageQuant LAS 4000 Imager. Densitometric analysis was performed with ImageJ software (http://rsb. info.nih.gov/ij/). Data were expressed as changes relative to the values of the cells transfected with SCR, taken as 100%.

Luciferase reporter assay

In order to test if the regulation of F11 by miRNAs is done through a direct interaction between both molecules, we performed luciferase reporter assays, as described below.

Plasmid construction. PCR product (1,060 bp) containing the F11 3'UTR from human genomic DNA (NM_000128), obtained using primers *F11*-3'UTR_F and *F11*-3'UTR_R, was cloned into the pCR 2.1 vector (Life Technologies, Madrid, Spain) (Table S3). Positive clones were digested with SpeI and MluI (New England Biolabs, Ipswich, MA) and the insert was subcloned into luciferase reporter plasmid pMIR-REPORT (Life Technologies, Madrid, Spain) previously digested with SpeI and MluI. Insertion of *F11* 3'UTR was checked by sequencing (ABI3130 XL, Life Technologies Corporation, Carlsbad, CA). All sequence analyses and alignments were performed with the SeqmanPro program (Lasergene version 7.1, DNASTAR, Madison, WI).

To generate mutations in the predicted target site for miR-181a-5p, seven nucleotides (TGAATGT) located in the seed sequence were deleted using the QuikChange site-directed mutagenesis kit (Agilent Technologies, Santa Clara, CA). *In silico* prediction, using RNAHybrid, of miR-181a-5p binding to the mutated sequence showed a 33% decrease in the minimum free energy value (not shown) indicating that miR-181a-5p: *F11* mRNA interaction was completely suppressed. Sequencing was performed to check for the deletion of the seed sequence. The primers used (del_181_AS and Del_181_S) are detailed in Table S3.

Luciferase vector transfection. HCT-DK cells, that do not express miR-181a-5p, were seeded at a density of 80,000 cells/well in 24-well plates with complete McCoy's 5A supplemented with 10% fetal calf serum without antibiotics. The following day, cells were co-transfected with miR-181a-5p (both pMIR-REPORT plasmids -1000 ng/well- wild type or mutated for the miR-181a-5p seed site) or SCR precursor, and 100 ng/well of renilla luciferase control plasmid (pRL-TK; Promega, Madison, WI) using Lipofectamine LTX (Life Technologies, Madrid, Spain) according to the manufacturer's instructions. Luciferase assays were performed as previously described [40]. The enzymatic activities of renilla and firefly luciferases were quantified in a Synergy 2 luminometer (Biotek, Winooski, VT). Each combination of pMIR-REPORT (wild-type and mutated 3'UTR) and pRL-TK was tested in triplicate in five independent experiments. Firefly luciferase activity was normalized to renilla luciferase activity for each transfected well. The normalized data were expressed as changes relative to the data of the cells transfected with 100 nM miR-181a-5p mimic, SCR was taken as 100%.

Statistical Analysis

Comparisons between groups were performed by the unpaired t-test. Data are given as mean ± SD. Linear regression tests were performed; β regression coefficient (r) and r^2 were calculated. Results were considered statistically significant for $p<0.05$. Analyses were carried out using Statistical Package for Social Science (version 21.0; SPSS, Chicago, IL).

Supporting Information

Figure S1 Levels of miRNAs in human liver and cell lines. Levels of miRNAs were Quantified by qRT-PCR. (A) Levels of miRNAs in HepG2 relative to human liver. (B) Levels of miR181a-5p in HepG2 and PLC/PRF/5 relative to human liver. Results are represented as mean ± SD of three replicates from two independent experiments.

Figure S2 miRNA inhibitor transfection efficiency. miRCURY LNA microRNA Inhibitor Negative Control (100 nM) labeled with fluorescein (Exiqon, Vadbaek, Denmark) were transfected into PLC/PRF/5 cells with siPORTTM NeoFXTM (Life TechnologiesTM, Madrid, Spain), following manufacturer's instructions. After 6 hours transfection, cells were harvested and washed with PBS. Flow cytometry was performed using a BD FACSCalibur flow cytometer (BD Biosciences, Madrid, Spain) and samples were run through the flow cytometer until 2,000 events were collected. The mean ± SD of transfection efficiency for three replicates was 92.1%±0.3%. X-axis represents the intensity of fluorescence for FL1 channel in log scale and Y-axis the numbers of cells. We defined transfection efficiency as a percentage of cells positive for FL1 (dotted lines), taken as background signal the non-LNA transfected cells signal (solid lines).

Acknowledgments

The authors thank Dr Renato Baserga, Department of Cancer Biology, Thomas Jefferson University, for kindly providing us HCT116-Dicer KO cells and Dr Fernando Corrales, CIMA, Pamplona, Spain for kindly providing us PLC/PRF/5 cells.

Author Contributions

Conceived and designed the experiments: SS-A RG-C CM. Performed the experiments: SS-A RT-M ABA NG-B. Analyzed the data: SS-A RG-C CM. Contributed reagents/materials/analysis tools: AC ES. Wrote the paper: SS-A RG-C CM. Performed statistical analyses: GL. Critically read the manuscript: VV.

References

1. Rosenthal RL, Dreskin OH, Rosenthal N (1953) New hemophilia-like disease caused by deficiency of a third plasma thromboplastin factor. Proc Soc Exp Biol Med 82: 171–174.
2. Van Hylckama Vlieg A, Callas PW, Cushman M, Bertina RM, Rosendaal FR (2003) Inter-relation of coagulation factors and d-dimer levels in healthy individuals. J Thromb Haemost 1: 516–522.
3. Itakura A, Verbout NG, Phillips KG, Insall RH, Gailani D, et al. (2011) Activated factor XI inhibits chemotaxis of polymorphonuclear leukocytes. J Leukoc Biol 90: 923–927.
4. Tucker EI, Verbout NG, Leung PY, Hurst S, McCarty OJ, et al. (2012) Inhibition of factor XI activation attenuates inflammation and coagulopathy while improving the survival of mouse polymicrobial sepsis. Blood 119: 4762–4768.
5. Seligsohn U (2007) Factor XI in haemostasis and thrombosis: past, present and future. Thromb Haemost 98: 84–89.
6. He R, Chen D, He S (2012) Factor XI: hemostasis, thrombosis, and antithrombosis. Thromb Res 129: 541–550.
7. Tucker EI, Gailani D, Hurst S, Cheng Q, Hanson SR, et al. (2008) Survival advantage of coagulation factor XI-deficient mice during peritoneal sepsis. J Infect Dis 198: 271–274.
8. Kravtsov DV, Matafonov A, Tucker EI, Sun MF, Walsh PN, et al. (2009) Factor XI contributes to thrombin generation in the absence of factor XII. Blood 114: 452–458.
9. Salomon O, Steinberg DM, Zucker M, Varon D, Zivelin A, et al. (2011) Patients with severe factor XI deficiency have a reduced incidence of deep-vein thrombosis. Thromb Haemost 105: 269–273.
10. Muller F, Gailani D, Renne T (2011) Factor XI and XII as antithrombotic targets. Curr Opin Hematol 18: 349–355.
11. Bezemer ID, Bare LA, Doggen CJ, Arellano AR, Tong C, et al. (2008) Gene variants associated with deep vein thrombosis. JAMA 299: 1306–1314.
12. Li Y, Bezemer ID, Rowland CM, Tong CH, Arellano AR, et al. (2009) Genetic variants associated with deep vein thrombosis: the F11 locus. J Thromb Haemost 7: 1802–1808.
13. Sabater-Lleal M, Martinez-Perez A, Buil A, Folkersen L, Souto JC, et al. (2012) A genome-wide association study identifies KNG1 as a genetic determinant of plasma factor XI Level and activated partial thromboplastin time. Arterioscler Thromb Vasc Biol 32: 2008–2016.
14. Bartel DP (2009) MicroRNAs: target recognition and regulatory functions. Cell 136: 215–233.
15. Lewis BP, Burge CB, Bartel DP (2005) Conserved seed pairing, often flanked by adenosines, indicates that thousands of human genes are microRNA targets. Cell 120: 15–20.
16. Bartel DP (2004) MicroRNAs: genomics, biogenesis, mechanism, and function. Cell 116: 281–297.
17. Grimson A, Farh KK, Johnston WK, Garrett-Engele P, Lim LP, et al. (2007) MicroRNA targeting specificity in mammals: determinants beyond seed pairing. Mol Cell 27: 91–105.
18. Lai EC (2002) Micro RNAs are complementary to 3′UTR sequence motifs that mediate negative post-transcriptional regulation. Nat Genet 30: 363–364.
19. Lim LP, Lau NC, Garrett-Engele P, Grimson A, Schelter JM, et al. (2005) Microarray analysis shows that some microRNAs downregulate large numbers of target mRNAs. Nature 433: 769–773.
20. Selbach M, Schwanhausser B, Thierfelder N, Fang Z, Khanin R, et al. (2008) Widespread changes in protein synthesis induced by microRNAs. Nature 455: 58–63.
21. Teruel R, Corral J, Perez-Andreu V, Martinez-Martinez I, Vicente V, et al. (2011) Potential role of miRNAs in developmental haemostasis. PLoS One 6: e17648.
22. Fort A, Borel C, Migliavacca E, Antonarakis SE, Fish RJ, et al. (2010) Regulation of fibrinogen production by microRNAs. Blood 116: 2608–2615.
23. Teruel R, Perez-Sanchez C, Corral J, Herranz MT, Perez-Andreu V, et al. (2011) Identification of miRNAs as potential modulators of tissue factor expression in patients with systemic lupus erythematosus and antiphospholipid syndrome. J Thromb Haemost 9: 1985–1992.
24. Marchand A, Proust C, Morange PE, Lompre AM, Tregouet DA (2012) miR-421 and miR-30c inhibit SERPINE 1 gene expression in human endothelial cells. PLoS One 7: e44532.
25. Tay JW, Romeo G, Hughes QW, Baker RI (2013) Micro-Ribonucleic Acid 494 regulation of protein S expression. J Thromb Haemost 11: 1547–1555.
26. Meijers JC, Tekelenburg WL, Bouma BN, Bertina RM, Rosendaal FR (2000) High levels of coagulation factor XI as a risk factor for venous thrombosis. N Engl J Med 342: 696–701.
27. Chen Z, Nakajima T, Tanabe N, Hinohara K, Sakao S, et al. (2010) Susceptibility to chronic thromboembolic pulmonary hypertension may be conferred by miR-759 via its targeted interaction with polymorphic fibrinogen alpha gene. Hum Genet 128: 443–452.
28. Baek D, Villen J, Shin C, Camargo FD, Gygi SP, et al. (2008) The impact of microRNAs on protein output. Nature 455: 64–71.
29. Witkos TM, Koscianska E, Krzyzosiak WJ (2011) Practical Aspects of microRNA Target Prediction. Curr Mol Med 11: 93–109.
30. Whichard ZL, Motter AE, Stein PJ, Corey SJ (2011) Slowly produced microRNAs control protein levels. J Biol Chem 286: 4742–4748.
31. Mukherji S, Ebert MS, Zheng GX, Tsang JS, Sharp PA, et al. (2011) MicroRNAs can generate thresholds in target gene expression. Nat Genet 43: 854–859.
32. Agirre X, Martinez-Climent JA, Odero MD, Prosper F (2012) Epigenetic regulation of miRNA genes in acute leukemia. Leukemia 26: 395–403.
33. Saba R, Storchel PH, Ksoy-Aksel A, Kepura F, Lippi G, et al. (2012) Dopamine-regulated microRNA MiR-181a controls GluA2 surface expression in hippocampal neurons. Mol Cell Biol 32: 619–632.
34. Taylor MA, Sossey-Alaoui K, Thompson CL, Danielpour D, Schiemann WP (2013) TGF-beta upregulates miR-181a expression to promote breast cancer metastasis. J Clin Invest 123: 150–163.
35. Mendell JT, Olson EN (2012) MicroRNAs in stress signaling and human disease. Cell 148: 1172–1187.
36. Janssen HL, Reesink HW, Lawitz EJ, Zeuzem S, Rodriguez-Torres M, et al. (2013) Treatment of HCV infection by targeting microRNA. N Engl J Med 368: 1685–1694.
37. Zhang H, Lowenberg EC, Crosby JR, MacLeod AR, Zhao C, et al. (2010) Inhibition of the intrinsic coagulation pathway factor XI by antisense oligonucleotides: a novel antithrombotic strategy with lowered bleeding risk. Blood 116: 4684–4692.
38. Nagalla S, Shaw C, Kong X, Kondkar AA, Edelstein LC, et al. (2011) Platelet microRNA-mRNA coexpression profiles correlate with platelet reactivity. Blood 117: 5189–5197.
39. Cummins JM, He Y, Leary RJ, Pagliarini R, Diaz LA Jr, et al. (2006) The colorectal microRNAome. Proc Natl Acad Sci U S A 103: 3687–3692.
40. Perez-Andreu V, Teruel R, Corral J, Roldan V, Garcia-Barbera N, et al. (2012) Mir-133a regulates VKORC1, a key protein in vitamin K cycle. Mol Med 2013 18: 1466–1472

41. Lamba V, Panetta JC, Strom S, Schuetz EG (2010) Genetic predictors of interindividual variability in hepatic CYP3A4 expression. J Pharmacol Exp Ther 332: 1088–1099.
42. Rehmsmeier M, Steffen P, Hochsmann M, Giegerich R (2004) Fast and effective prediction of microRNA/target duplexes. RNA 10: 1507–1517.
43. Friedman RC, Farh KK, Burge CB, Bartel DP (2009) Most mammalian mRNAs are conserved targets of microRNAs. Genome Res 19: 92–105.
44. Betel D, Koppal A, Agius P, Sander C, Leslie C (2010) Comprehensive modeling of microRNA targets predicts functional non-conserved and non-canonical sites. Genome Biol 11: R90.

13

Association between Single Nucleotide Polymorphisms in the *ADD3* Gene and Susceptibility to Biliary Atresia

Shuaidan Zeng[1,2], Peng Sun[1,2], Zimin Chen[2], Jianxiong Mao[2], Jianyao Wang[2], Bin Wang[2]*, Lei Liu[1,2]*

1 Zhuhai Campus of Zunyi Medical College, Zhuhai, Guangdong, China, **2** Department of General Surgery, Shenzhen Children's Hospital, Shenzhen, Guangdong, China

Abstract

Background and Objectives: Based on the results of previous studies, the *ADD3* gene, located in the 10q24.2 region, may be a susceptibility gene of biliary atresia (BA). In this study, two single nucleotide polymorphisms (SNPs) in the *ADD3* gene, rs17095355 C/T and rs10509906 G/C, were selected to investigate whether there is an association between these SNPs and susceptibility to BA in a Chinese population.

Methods: A total of 752 Han Chinese (134 BA cases and 618 ethnically matched healthy controls) were included in the present study. The *ADD3* gene polymorphisms were genotyped using a TaqMan genotyping assay.

Results: Positive associations were found for the SNP rs17095355 in the codominant model; specifically, the frequencies of the CT and TT genotypes and the T allele were higher in the cases than the controls, demonstrating a significant risk for BA (odds ratio [OR] = 1.62, 95% confidence interval [CI] = 1.02–2.58; OR = 2.89, 95% CI = 1.72–4.86; and OR = 1.75, 95% CI = 1.34–2.29, respectively). Regarding rs10509906, the per-C-allele conferred an OR of 0.70 (95% CI = 0.49–1.00) under the additive model. A greater risk of BA was associated with the T_a-G_b (a for rs17095355 and b for rs10509906) haplotype (OR = 1.82, 95% CI = 1.27–2.61) compared with the C_a-C_b haplotype.

Conclusion: This study suggests that the *ADD3* gene plays an important role in BA pathogenesis and reveals a significant association between two SNPs, rs17095355 and rs10509906, and BA.

Editor: Xiaoping Miao, MOE Key Laboratory of Environment and Health, School of Public Health, Tongji Medical College, Huazhong University of Science and Technology, China

Funding: The authors have no support or funding to report.

Competing Interests: The authors have declared that no competing interests exist.

* Email: szwb1967@126.com (BW); liulei3322@aliyun.com (LL)

Introduction

Biliary atresia (BA) is a devastating disease of infancy that invariably leads, if left untreated, to cirrhosis, liver failure, and death. Similar to North America and Western Europe, the incidence in the UK is approximately 1 in 16,000 neonates; the incidence is much higher in parts of Asia, including Japan and, most likely, China, estimated at approximately 1 in 10,000 neonates. Conjugated jaundice, pale acholic stools, and dark urine are the primary clinical manifestations of BA [1]. The initial treatment for BA, Kasai radical surgery, needs to be performed within the first 3 months of life to achieve a better outcome. If the surgery fails to reconstruct a new biliary system, the patient will die at approximately 1 year of age due to liver failure and other serious complications. Liver transplantation is a potential solution, but only a few patients can receive a new liver because of the insufficient liver source in China. The etiology of BA is still unknown, but several hypotheses have been considered, including perinatal virus infection, congenital and acquired immune injury, maternal microchimerisms in the liver that cause a graft-vs-host reaction, the inherited pathogenic factor hypothesis, and ductal plate malformation [2–8]. Moreover, genetic factors are strongly suggested to play an important role in BA. In the past 10 years, researchers have identified a number of genes associated with BA,

such as the migration inhibitory factor (*MIF*), *CD14*, intercellular adhesion molecule-1 (*ICAM-1*), adiponectin (*APM1*), and ITGB2 (*CD18*) [9–13].

In 2010, a Chinese population-based genome-wide association study (GWAS) was performed by Garcia-Barceló et al. [14]. Rs17095355, which maps to the intergenic region between *ADD3* (adducin 3) and *XPNPEP1* (X-prolyl aminopeptidase 1), was identified in a GWAS of 200 patients and 481 controls. This finding was supported by the replication genotyping of the 10 most BA-associated SNPs in 124 cases and 90 controls, with the strongest overall association found in 10q24.2 ($P = 6.94 \times 10^{-9}$). This SNP was subsequently replicated in the Thai population ($P < 0.002$) [15].

However, Cheng et al. [16] accomplished a fine-mapping study of the BA-associated region in 2013 in a Han Chinese population. This study revealed a common risk haplotype composed of 5 tag SNPs, including rs17095355, rs10509906, rs2501577, rs6584970, and rs7086057; rs10509906 on the common protective haplotype CCATA was also independently associated with BA. Moreover, they also found that the BA-associated potentially regulatory SNPs correlated with *ADD3* gene expression in bioinformatics and *in vivo* genotype-expression investigations.

With the aim of investigating the association between the *ADD3* gene polymorphisms and susceptibility to BA, we conducted a case-control study to verify the effects of rs17095355 and rs10509906 in an independent Chinese sample.

Materials and Methods

1. Study Population

From 2010 to 2013, 134 unrelated children were diagnosed with BA by laparoscopic cholangiography and a biopsy of the liver and the extrahepatic biliary tree at the Shenzhen Children's Hospital. Parental written consent was given. This study included 66 males and 68 females with an average age of 72 days (range 46–123) at the time of surgery. None of the patients had any other associated congenital malformations. All patients underwent the Roux-en-Y hepaticojejunostomy reconstruction successfully, and no serious postoperative complications were noted during hospitalization.

For the controls, 618 individuals (303 males and 315 females) of southern Chinese origins without a diagnosis of BA, congenital disease, or liver disease were included. Written informed consent to take blood samples from the children was obtained from all the subjects and the legal guardians of every child. The study protocol conformed to the ethical guidelines of the 1975 Declaration of Helsinki and was approved by the Ethics Committee on Human Research of the Faculty of the Shenzhen Children's Hospital.

2. Genotyping

The genomic DNA was extracted from peripheral blood leukocytes or liver tissue collected during the surgery of the BA children and from peripheral blood leukocytes of the healthy controls using a DNeasy Blood & Tissue Kit (Qiagen, Hilden, Germany). The genomic DNA samples were stored at $-20°C$ for further analysis. The genotypes of rs17095355 and rs10509906 were determined using a TaqMan SNP Genotyping Assay (Applied Biosystems, Foster City, CA, USA). Polymerase chain reaction (PCR) was carried out in a 384-well GeneAmp PCR System 9700 (Applied Biosystems) with mixtures consisting of 1 µl of DNA (10 ng/µl), 2.5 µl of TaqMan genotyping master mix, 0.125 µl of TaqMan MGB probes (containing distinct fluorescent dyes and a PCR primer pair), and ddH$_2$O, with a final volume of 5 µl. The thermal cycling conditions were as follows: denaturation at 95°C for 10 min, followed by 50 cycles of denaturation at 92°C for 15 s and annealing and extension at 60°C for 90 s. After PCR,

the TaqMan assay plates were transferred to the ABI PRISM 7900 Sequence Detection System (Applied Biosystems), where the endpoint fluorescence intensity in each well of the plate was read. The allelic-specific fluorescence data from each plate were analyzed using the SDS v2.4 software (Applied Biosystems) to automatically determine each genotype.

3. Statistical Analysis

The χ^2 test was performed to estimate the differences in the variables and the distributions of the genotypes between the cases and controls. Hardy-Weinberg equilibrium was evaluated using the goodness-of-fit χ^2 test in the controls, and a value of $P<0.05$ was considered to indicate significant disequilibrium. The association between the case-control status and each SNP was assessed by the odds ratio (OR) and the corresponding 95% confidence interval (CI). To avoid the assumption of genetic models, codominant, dominant, recessive, and additive models were all analyzed. A stepwise procedure was performed to control the false discovery rate (FDR), which was applied for multiple comparison correction. The linkage disequilibrium (LD) of the candidate SNPs and the haplotype frequencies were estimated using HaploView V4.2 and PHASE V2.0 software, respectively. The r^2 value was used to measure the degree of linkage disequilibrium. The ORs and 95% CIs, adjusted by gender, were calculated with an unconditional logistic regression. The statistical analyses were performed using SPSS software V.20.0 (SPSS, Chicago, Illinois, USA); a $P<0.05$ was considered statistically significant.

Results

1. Population characteristics

A total of 134 incident cases of BA and 618 controls were enrolled in this study. The genotype distributions of rs17095355 and rs10509906 in the controls were in Hardy-Weinberg equilibrium ($P=0.24$ and $P=0.27$). The male to female ratios of the cases and controls were 0.97 (66/68) and 0.96 (303/315), respectively, and there was no significant difference in gender distribution between the patients and controls ($P=0.962$). Genotyping was successful in a total of 133 cases (99%) for rs17095355, 129 cases (96%) for rs10509906, and all of the controls.

Table 1. Associations between rs17095355 and BA risk in a Chinese population.

	Controls (%)	Cases (%)	$P^{\#}$	OR (95% CI)	P^{+}	P_{FDR}*
rs17095355	618	133				
CC	231(37.4)	31(23.3)		1.00(reference)		
CT	281(45.5)	61(45.9)		1.62(1.02–2.58)	0.043	0.043
TT	106(17.2)	41(30.8)	<0.001	2.89(1.72–4.86)	6.50×10^{-5}	1.95×10^{-4}
Dominant model	387(62.6)	102(76.7)	0.002	1.97(1.27–3.03)	2.00×10^{-3}	2.40×10^{-3}
Recessive model	512(82.8)	92(69.2)	<0.001	2.15(1.41–3.29)	3.82×10^{-4}	5.73×10^{-4}
Allele C	743(60.1)	123(46.2)		1.00(reference)		
Allele T	493(39.9)	143(53.8)	<0.001	1.75(1.34–2.29)	3.70×10^{-5}	2.22×10^{-4}
Additive model				1.70(1.31–2.21)	7.20×10^{-5}	1.44×10^{-3}

$^{\#}P$ values were computed by the Pearson chi-square test.
$^{+}$Data were calculated by logistic regression after adjusting for gender.
*P values were modified by the FDR correction for multiple comparisons.

2. Association analysis

Regarding the two SNPs investigated, after correction for multiple comparisons by FDR, rs17095355 showed a significant association with BA in all of the models, while rs10509906 exhibited no significant association with BA under every model. The detailed genotype frequencies of rs17095355 among the 618 controls and 133 cases are shown in Table 1. In the unconditional logistic regression analysis, the individuals with CT and TT genotypes had a significantly increased risk of BA ($P_{FDR} = 0.043$, OR = 1.62, 95% CI = 1.02–2.58; $P_{FDR} = 1.95 \times 10^{-4}$, OR = 2.89, 95% CI = 1.72–4.86, respectively) compared with those with the CC homozygote genotype. The dominant and recessive models were analyzed, and the genotypic models (CT plus TT vs CC) and (TT vs CC plus CT) showed a significant association with BA ($P_{FDR} = 2.40 \times 10^{-3}$, OR = 1.97, 95% CI = 1.27–3.03; $P_{FDR} = 5.73 \times 10^{-4}$, OR = 2.15, 95% CI = 1.41–3.29, respectively). The C and T allele frequencies of the controls were 60.1% and 39.9%, respectively, and the T allele was also found to be associated with an increased risk for BA ($P_{FDR} = 2.22 \times 10^{-4}$, OR = 1.75, 95% CI = 1.34–2.29). Similarly, a positive result was found in the additive model, with a per-T-allele OR of 1.70 (95% CI = 1.31–2.20, $P_{FDR} = 1.44 \times 10^{-3}$).

When comparing the cases with controls, we observed no statistically significant differences in genotype ($P = 0.062$) or allele ($P = 0.053$) distributions of rs10509906 (Table 2). Additionally, the C allele seems to reduce the risk for BA ($P_{FDR} = 0.108$, OR = 0.72, 95% CI = 0.51–1.00). An independent effect of rs10509906 was formally test by the logistic regression analysis of the two SNPs to verify significance of the rs10509906 after inclusion of the rs17095355, however, no significant difference was found in each model.

3. Haplotypes and risk of BA

We did not observe LD between rs17095355 and rs10509906 ($r^2 = 0.173$). The *ADD3* haplotypes in the cases and controls were constructed and the results are shown in Table 3. The distribution of haplotype frequencies was significantly different between the cases and controls ($P < 0.001$). Compared with the low-risk C_a-C_b (a for rs17095355 and b for rs10509906) haplotype, the adjusted ORs for the T_a-C_b and C_a-G_b haplotypes were 0.65 (95% CI = 0.08–4.91) and 1.04 (95% CI = 0.71–1.54), respectively. The last haplotype containing the high-risk alleles T_a and G_b was associated with an increased risk for BA (OR = 1.82, 95% CI = 1.27–2.61) ($P_{trend} < 0.001$).

Discussion

In the current study, we investigated the association of rs17095355 with BA risk. Our results suggested that the rs17095355 SNP was significantly associated with an enhanced BA risk under the genotypic, dominant, recessive, and additive models, while the other SNP, rs10509906, only presented a significant protective effect under the additive model. In the haplotype analysis, we found that these two SNPs had a certain interaction within a haplotype to influence the risk of BA; specifically, the T_a-G_b haplotype was associated with an increased risk of BA compared with the C_a-C_b haplotype.

The etiology and pathogenesis of BA are currently unknown. While other hypotheses remain, with the development of genotyping technologies and the discovery of inherited pathogenic factors in BA, increasingly more researchers are focusing on the genes and SNPs that are associated with BA. The GWAS, as reported by Garcia-Barcelo et al., revealed a relationship between rs17095355, located in 10q24, and BA; this conclusion was a

Table 2. Associations between rs10509906 and BA risk in a Chinese population.

	Controls (%)	Cases (%)	P#	OR (95% CI)	P+	P*FDR	ORb (95% CI)	Pb+	P*FDR
rs10509906	618	129							
GG	350(56.6)	82(63.6)		1.00(reference)			1.00(reference)		
CG	237(38.3)	46(35.7)		0.83(0.56–1.23)	0.353	0.353	1.15(0.74–1.79)	0.541	0.901
CC	31(5.0)	1(0.8)	0.062	0.14(0.02–1.02)	0.053	0.159	0.23(0.03–1.75)	0.155	0.388
Dominant model	268(43.4)	47(36.4)	0.147	0.75(0.51–1.11)	0.148	0.178	0.91(0.60–1.38)	0.649	0.811
Recessive model	587(95.0)	128(99.2)	0.030	6.84(0.92–50.57)	0.060	0.090	5.67(0.77–42.23)	0.089	0.445
Allele G	937(75.8)	210(81.4)		1.00(reference)					
Allele C	299(24.2)	48(18.6)	0.053	0.72(0.51–1.01)	0.054	0.108	0.97(0.66–1.42)	0.869	0.869
Additive model				0.70(0.49–1.00)	0.047	0.282			

#P values were computed by the Pearson chi-square test.
+Data were calculated by logistic regression after adjusting for gender.
b: Logistic regression analysis of the independent effect of rs10509906 after inclusion of the rs17095355.
*P values were modified by the FDR correction for multiple comparisons.

Table 3. Risk estimates for the extended *ADD3* haplotypes in the BA cases and controls.

Haplotype	Controls (n = 618) No. of chromosomes (%)	Cases (n = 134) No. of chromosomes (%)	$P^{\#}$	OR (95% CI)	P^{+}
C_a-C_b	289(23.4)	47(17.5)		1.00(reference)	
T_a-C_b	10(0.8)	1(0.4)		0.62(0.08–4.91)	0.646
C_a-G_b	454(36.7)	77(28.7)		1.04(0.71–1.54)	0.831
T_a-G_b	483(39.1)	143(53.4)	<0.001	1.82(1.27–2.61)	<0.001
P for trend				<0.001	

a: rs17095355 b: rs10509906.
$^{\#}P$ values were computed by the Pearson chi-square test.
$^{+}$Data were calculated by logistic regression after adjusting for gender.

milestone in this field. Because rs17095355 has been shown to fall within the intergenic region of the *ADD3* and *XPNPEP1* genes, Garcia-Barceló et al. further tried to determine whether the SNP most associated with BA regulated the *ADD3* or *XPNPEP1* genes. The results revealed that the C>T transition at rs17095355 did not appear to have a functional effect, and no evidence linked the other BA-associated SNPs with the regulation of *ADD3* or *XPNPEP1* [14].

Cheng, et al. conducted a fine-mapping study that revealed a common haplotype in 10q24.2 that was associated with BA risk. Rs10509906 had a significant effect $(P = 7.97 \times 10^{-4})$ and was detected in the common protective haplotype CCATA. This study revealed that the risk alleles were associated with a reduced *ADD3* expression level in BA livers and that the genotype-*ADD3*-expression correlation only existed in BA livers, not in the non-BA livers. *ADD3* was also found to be expressed in biliary epithelia. Therefore, *ADD3* may play a role in managing biliary epithelia and its deregulation; this most likely result in a congenital bile duct defect, which can biologically influence BA. Additionally, they reported that the risk haplotype was correlated with *ADD3* but not with *XPNPEP1* [16]. In addition, a replication of the GWAS was conducted in a Caucasian population by Tsai et al. [17], and the expression data in this study suggested that only *ADD3* is differentially expressed in BA patients.

Due to the difference in expression that only exists for the *ADD3* gene, we considered *ADD3* to be the key gene in the development of BA. *ADD3* encodes adducin 3, which is a member of the membrane skeletal proteins that are involved in the assembly of the spectrin-actin network in erythrocytes and is found at the sites of cell-cell contact in epithelial tissues [18], including the liver and bile ducts; it is also more abundantly expressed in the fetal liver than in the adult liver. Contractions of the bile canalicular membrane are controlled by actin-myosin interactions, and damage to these interaction mechanisms causes cholestasis. Increased actin and myosin deposition around the bile canaliculi has been observed in BA patients with bile discharge mechanism dysfunction after surgery. Additionally, the smooth muscle actin expression intensity influences the degree of fibrosis in patients with BA [14,19–21].

Our study verified the results of the GWAS regarding rs17095355. The C and T allele frequencies of the controls are similar to the Chinese data in HapMap (58.3% and 41.7%). In the logistic regression analysis, the CT and TT genotypes of the dominant model (CT plus TT) and the T allele of rs17095355 were all associated with a more significant risk for BA than the wild-type homozygous CC genotype. This result means that individuals carrying the risk allele of rs17095355 have a higher susceptibility to BA. In the additive model, we observed that each T allele of rs17095355 increased the OR value of the risk for BA. As for rs10509906, our minor C allele frequency in the controls was 24.2%, which was similar to MAF 16.7% from HapMap. The C allele, the heterogeneous mutation CG, and the homozygous mutation CC of rs10509906 were associated with a non-significantly reduced risk for BA (Table 2), possibly because of our small sample size. However, we found that an additional C allele of rs10509906 marginally decreased the risk of BA. Furthermore, the results of the logistic regression analysis of the two SNPs showed that, even the rs10509906 was adjusted by the rs17095355, it still presented a negative effect on BA risk, which means there is no independent effect of the rs10509906 in our study. Nevertheless, the tendency yielded by the additive model and the marginal effect, yielded by the recessive model imply that the polymorphism rs10509906 may play a protective role in BA, similar to the results of the fine-mapping study conducted by Cheng, et al.

To understand how the haplotypes rs17095355 and rs10509906 contribute to the risk of BA, we conducted a haplotype analysis. The results showed that carriers of the T_a-G_b haplotype had a 2-fold increased risk for BA compared with non-carriers. However, the two SNPs were not in LD ($r^2 = 0.16$ in the HapMap database; $r^2 = 0.173$ in our study). Based on the conclusion of the research conducted by Cheng, et al. [16], namely, that the risk allele was associated with a reduced expression level of *ADD3*, we hypothesized that the T allele of rs17095355 may play an integral role in BA susceptibility and *ADD3* transcription. In other words, we hypothesized that the T allele may be associated with decreased *ADD3* transcription, which in turn produces lower levels of the *ADD3* protein in the CT and TT genotypes or in the T_a-G_b haplotype carriers than in the non-carriers; thus, the insufficient *ADD3* protein levels lead to the BA phenotype. However, we did not have a large enough sample size to estimate whether the C allele of the rs10509906-containing haplotype, as a protective allele carried by individuals, might enhance the transcriptional activity of *ADD3* and thus prevent the phenotype that usually results from a low level of *ADD3*. Therefore, the haplotype construction may suggest that the two SNPs together tag a third, untyped, SNP associated to BA, to some extent, probably revealed increased risk in the BA susceptibility. Above all, these results suggested that the *ADD3* gene was associated with the pathogenesis and development of BA.

However, several limitations should be noted in our study. The sample size was relatively small. BA is a complex trait resulting from both environmental and genetic factors. The environmental factors and rare genetic variations associated with BA have not yet been identified, which limited further investigation of the gene-environment interactions. In the absence of functional experiments, it is unclear whether these two SNPs are causally related to BA. Hence, fine-mapping of 10q24.2 region and functional experiments is warranted to identify causal variant.

In conclusion, the results from our study in a Chinese population verified the effective role of rs17095355 in BA susceptibility and suggested that the variant of rs17095355 was also associated with an increased BA risk. The haplotype analysis revealed that the T_a-G_b haplotype in *ADD3* may be a genetic BA susceptibility factor.

Acknowledgments

We would like to show our gratitude to all the children with BA, the healthy controls and their families, and all the doctors who participated in this study. We also acknowledge the Department of Epidemiology and Biostatistics, Huazhong University of Science and Technology, for providing laboratory and equipment support.

Author Contributions

Conceived and designed the experiments: LL. Performed the experiments: SZ PS. Analyzed the data: SZ PS. Contributed reagents/materials/analysis tools: LL. Wrote the paper: SZ. Collected samples: BW JM JW ZC.

References

1. Puri P, Höllwarth M (2009) Pediatric Surgery Diagnosis and Management. Springer-Verlag Berlin Heidelberg. 537–540 p.
2. Fischler B, Ehrnst A, Forsgren M, Orvell C, Nemeth A (1998) The viral association of neonatal cholestasis in Sweden: a possible link between cytomegalovirus infection and extrahepatic biliary atresia. J Pediatr Gastroenterol Nutr 27(1):57–64.
3. Tyler KL, Sokol RJ, Oberhaus SM, Le M, Karrer FM, et al. (1998) Detection of reovirus RNA in hepatobiliary tissues from patients with, extrahepatie biliary atresia and choledochal cysts. Hepatology 27(6):1475–1482.
4. Chuang JH, Chou MH, Wu CL, Du YY (2006) Implication of Innate Immunity in the Pathogenesis of Biliary Atresia. Chang Gung Med J 29(3):240–250.
5. Silveira TR, Salzano FM, Donaldson PT, Mieli-Vergani G, Howard ER, et al. (1993) Association between HLA and extrahepatic biliary atresia. J Pediatr GastroenteroJ Nutr 16(2):114–117.
6. Suskin DL, Rosenthal P, Heyman MB, Kong D, Magrane G, et al. (2004) Maternal microchimefism in the Iivers of patients with Biliary atresia. BMC Gastroenterol 4:14.
7. Smith BM, Laberge JM. Schreiber R, Weber AM, Blanchard H (1991) Familial biliary atresia in three siblings including twins. J Pediatr Surg 26(11):1331–1333.
8. Vijayan V, TarI EC (2000) Computer-generated three-dimensional morphology of the hepatic hilar bile ducts in biliary atresia. J Pediatr Surg 35(8):1230–1235.
9. Arikan C, Berdeli A, Ozgenc F, Tumgor G, Yagci RV, et al. (2006) Positive association of macrophage migration inhibitory factor gene-173G/C polymorphism with biliary atresia. J Pediatr Gastroenterol Nutr 42:77–82.
10. Shih HH, Lin TM, Chuang JH, Eng HL, Juo SH, et al. (2005) Promoter polymorphism of the CD14 endotoxin receptor gene is associated with biliary atresia and idiopathic neonatal cholestasis. Pediatrics 116(2):437–441.
11. Arikan C, Berdeli A, Kilic M, Tumgor G, Yagci RV, et al. (2008) Polymorphisms of the ICAM-1 gene are associated with biliary atresia. Dig Dis Sci 53:2000–2004.
12. Udomsinprasert W, Tencomnao T, Honsawek S, Anomasiri W, Vejchapipat P, et al. (2012) +276 G/T single nucleotide polymorphism of the adiponectin gene is associated with the susceptibility to biliary atresia. World J Pediatr 8(4):328–334.
13. Zhao R, Song Z, Dong R, Li H, Shen C, et al. (2013) Polymorphism of ITGB2 gene 3′-UTR+145C/A is associated with biliary atresia. Digestion 88:65–71.
14. Garcia-Barceló MM, Yeung MY, Miao XP, Tang CS, Cheng G, et al. (2010) Genome-wide association study identifies a susceptibility locus for biliary atresia on 10q24.2. Hum Mol Genet 19(14):2917–2925.
15. Kaewkiattiyot S, Honsawek S, Vejchapipat P, Chongsrisawat V, Poovorawan Y (2011) Association of X-prolyl aminopeptidase 1 rs17095355 polymorphism with biliary atresia in Thai children. Hepatol Res 41:1249–1252.
16. Cheng G, Tang CS, Wong EH, Cheng WW, So MT, et al. (2013) Common genetic variants regulating *ADD3* gene expression alter biliary atresia risk. J Hepatol 59(6):1285–91.
17. Tsai EA, Grochowski CM, Loomes KM, Bessho K, Hakonarson H, et al. (2014) Replication of a GWAS signal in a Caucasian population implicates ADD3 in susceptibility to biliary atresia. Hum Genet 133:235–243.
18. Naydenov NG, Ivanov AI (2010) Adducins regulate remodeling of apical junctions in human epithelial cells. Mol Biol Cell 21:3506–3517.
19. Oshio C, Phillips MJ (1981) Contractility of bile canaliculi: implications for liver function. Science 212:1041–1042.
20. Segawa O, Miyano T, Fujimoto T, Watanabe S, Hirose M, et al. (1993) Actin and myosin deposition around bile canaliculi: a predictor of clinical outcome in biliary atresia. J Pediatr Surg 28:851–856.
21. Shteyer E, Ramm GA, Xu C, White FV, Shepherd RW (2006) Outcome after portoenterostomy in biliary atresia: pivotal role of degree of liver fibrosis and intensity of stellate cell activation. J Pediatr Gastroenterol Nutr 42:93–99.

14

Urinary Neutrophil Gelatinase-Associated Lipocalin: A Useful Biomarker for Tacrolimus-Induced Acute Kidney Injury in Liver Transplant Patients

Ayami Tsuchimoto[1ɔ], Haruka Shinke[1ɔ], Miwa Uesugi[1], Mio Kikuchi[1,2], Emina Hashimoto[1], Tomoko Sato[1], Yasuhiro Ogura[3¤a], Koichiro Hata[3], Yasuhiro Fujimoto[3], Toshimi Kaido[3], Junji Kishimoto[4], Motoko Yanagita[5], Kazuo Matsubara[1], Shinji Uemoto[3], Satohiro Masuda[1*¤b]

1 Department of Clinical Pharmacology and Therapeutics, Kyoto University Hospital, Kyoto, Japan, 2 Department of Pharmacy, Kagawa University Hospital, Kagawa, Japan, 3 Division of Hepatobiliary-Pancreatic Surgery and Transplantation, Department of Surgery, Graduate School of Medicine, Kyoto University, Kyoto, Japan, 4 Department of Research and Development of Next Generation Medicine, Faculty of Medical Sciences, Kyushu University, Fukuoka, Japan, 5 Department of Nephrology, Graduate School of Medicine, Kyoto University, Kyoto, Japan

Abstract

Tacrolimus is widely used as an immunosuppressant in liver transplantation, and tacrolimus-induced acute kidney injury (AKI) is a serious complication of liver transplantation. For early detection of AKI, various urinary biomarkers such as monocyte chemotactic protein-1, liver-type fatty acid-binding protein, interleukin-18, osteopontin, cystatin C, clusterin and neutrophil gelatinase-associated lipocalin (NGAL) have been identified. Here, we attempt to identify urinary biomarkers for the early detection of tacrolimus-induced AKI in liver transplant patients. Urine samples were collected from 31 patients after living-donor liver transplantation (LDLT). Twenty recipients developed tacrolimus-induced AKI. After the initiation of tacrolimus therapy, urine samples were collected on postoperative days 7, 14, and 21. In patients who experienced AKI during postoperative day 21, additional spot urine samples were collected on postoperative days 28, 35, 42, 49, and 58. The 8 healthy volunteers, whose renal and liver functions were normal, were asked to collect their blood and spot urine samples. The urinary levels of NGAL, monocyte chemotactic protein-1 and liver-type fatty acid-binding protein were significantly higher in patients with AKI than in those without, while those of interleukin-18, osteopontin, cystatin C and clusterin did not differ between the 2 groups. The area under the receiver operating characteristics curve of urinary NGAL was 0.876 (95% confidence interval, 0.800–0.951; P<0.0001), which was better than those of the other six urinary biomarkers. In addition, the urinary levels of NGAL at postoperative day 1 (p = 0.0446) and day 7 (p = 0.0006) can be a good predictive marker for tacrolimus-induced AKI within next 6 days, respectively. In conclusion, urinary NGAL is a sensitive biomarker for tacrolimus-induced AKI, and may help predict renal event caused by tacrolimus therapy in liver transplant patients.

Editor: Martin H. de Borst, University Medical Center Groningen and University of Groningen, Netherlands

Funding: This work was supported in part by a Grant-in-Aid for Scientific Research (KAKENHI) from the Ministry of Education, Science, Culture, Sports, and Technology of Japan (MEXT); a grant-in-aid for Research on Biological Markers for New Drug Development and Health and Labour Sciences Research Grants from the Ministry of Health, Labour, and Welfare of Japan (08062855); and a funding program for Next Generation World-Leading Researchers (NEXT Program: LS073 to SM) initiated by the Council for Science and Technology Policy of the Japan Society for the Promotion of Science. The funders had no role in study design, data collection and analysis, decision to publish, or preparation of the manuscript.

Competing Interests: The authors have declared that no competing interests exist.

* Email: satomsdb@pharm.med.kyushu-u.ac.jp

¤a Current address: Transplantation Surgery, Nagoya University Hospital, Nagoya, Japan
¤b Current address: Department of Pharmacy, Kyushu University Hospital, Fukuoka, Japan

ɔ These authors contributed equally to this work.

Introduction

Tacrolimus, a calcineurin inhibitor, is widely used as an immunosuppressant in patients undergoing liver transplantation. Although therapeutic drug monitoring helps maintain the blood concentration of tacrolimus within a narrow therapeutic range (5–15 ng/mL), preventing adverse reactions such as nephrotoxicity and neurotoxicity, adverse reactions do occur in patients with greater blood concentrations of tacrolimus [1]. One such severe adverse reaction is nephrotoxicity. Acute kidney injury (AKI) is a frequent complication of liver transplantation and its incidence has been reported to range between 36% and 78% [2–4]. Postoperative AKI has been reported to cause high mortality in the recipients [3,4], and one of the main risk factors for acute renal failure after liver transplantation is calcineurin inhibitor toxicity [5,6]. Thus, tacrolimus nephrotoxicity is a serious problem for liver transplant recipients.

Although serum creatinine (Scr) is a commonly used marker for renal function, it fails as a marker for renal injury due to the following reasons: Scr level increases after changes in glomerular

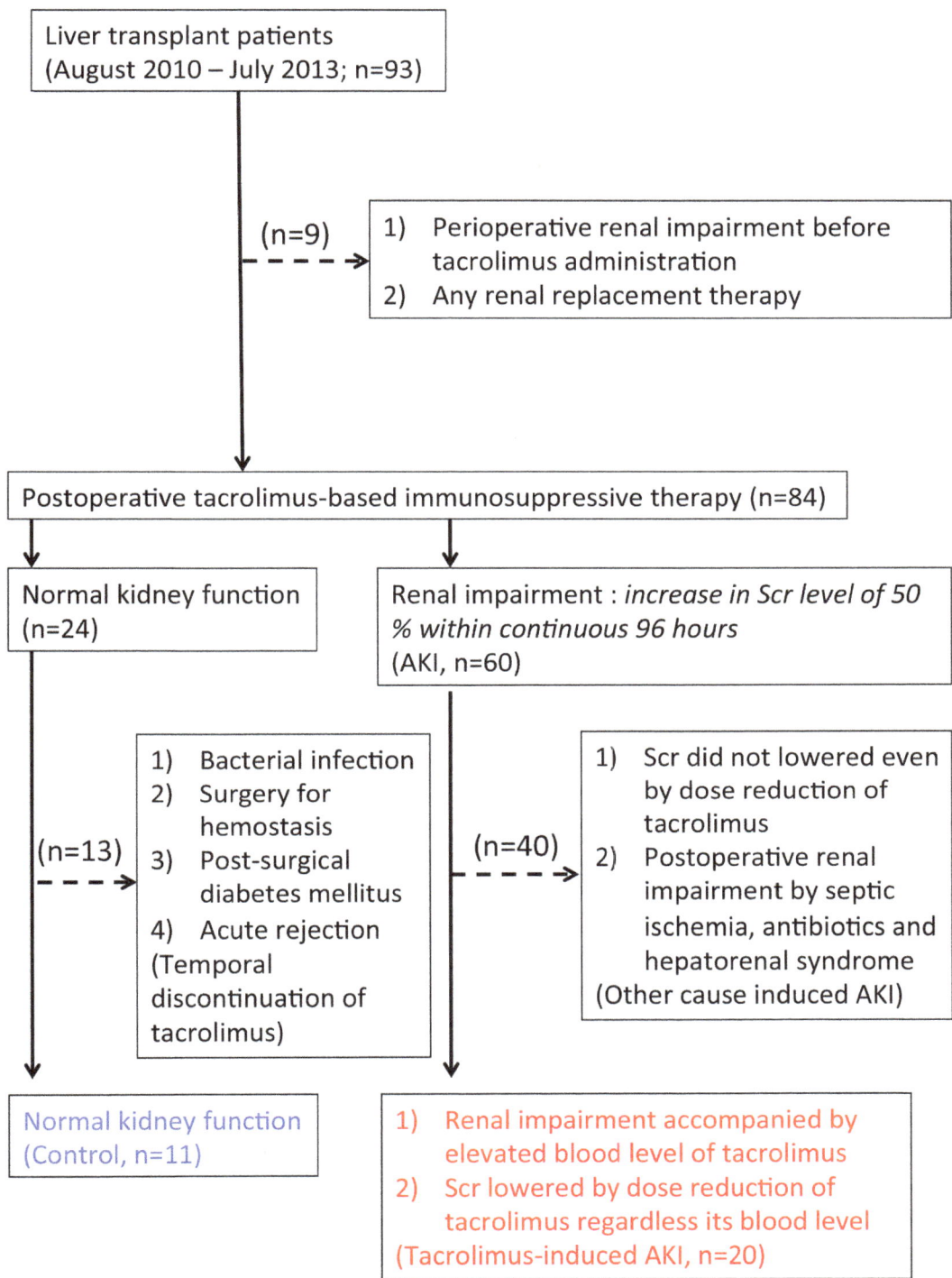

Figure 1. Diagnostic algorithm of tacrolimus-induced AKI in the patients after liver transplantation. Between August 2010 and July 2013, 93 patients were enrolled with the written informed consent. Nine patients with perioperative renal impairment before the administration of tacrolimus-based posttransplant immunosuppressive treatment and patients with any renal replacement therapy were excluded. Patients with renal impairment by some other causes including septic ischemia, antibiotics and hepatorenal syndrome were also excluded from this study. In addition, the patients of renal impairment with low tacrolimus levels, whose Scr levels were not changed even by the decrease of tacrolimus dosage, were also excluded indicating other causes-derived renal impairment such as tubular necrosis post-surgery. Among 24 patients with normal kidney function, 13 patients with post-transplant infectious disease, surgery for hemostasis, post-surgical diabetes mellitus and acute rejection episode were excluded for the temporal discontinuation of tacrolimus administration. Finally, the clinical data of the 11 control patients and 20 patients with tacrolimus-induced AKI were used.

filtration, and hence is thought to be a delayed marker for decreased renal function [7]. In addition, Scr is affected by non-renal factors such as age, sex, body weight, muscle mass, total body volume, and protein intake [8,9]. Therefore, more sensitive and specific biomarkers are needed to detect AKI at an early stage.

Until now, various biomarkers for AKI have been identified, such as neutrophil gelatinase-associated lipocalin (NGAL), and liver-type fatty acid-binding protein (L-FABP). In clinical practice, NGAL serves as a good biomarker for AKI in emergency room patients [10], during septic shock [11], and after cardiac surgery [12,13] and liver transplantation [14,15]. L-FABP is also a good biomarker for renal damage following cisplatin-induced nephrotoxicity [16], contrast-induced nephrotoxicity [17], and septic shock induced AKI [18].

In 2007, the Acute Kidney Injury Network (AKIN) criteria for the classification and staging of AKI was published [19]. According to these criteria, an absolute increase in Scr levels of at least 0.3 mg/dL or a percentage increase of more than or equal to 50% within 48 h is defined as AKI. However, in some liver transplant recipients, the changes in Scr are gradual and cannot be evaluated according to the AKIN criteria. Therefore, new and reliable diagnostic methods for the detection of tacrolimus-induced AKI are needed. In this light, here, we attempt to identify urinary biomarkers for the early detection of tacrolimus-induced AKI in patients undergoing living-donor liver transplantation (LDLT).

Experimental Procedures

Patients and urine samples

A total of 21 adult patients (7 men and 14 women) who underwent LDLT at Kyoto University Hospital between August 2010 and March 2012, were enrolled in a pilot study after obtaining written informed consent. We performed power analysis using the patients who developed AKI within 14 days after liver transplantation. Among the 21 patients, 14 were diagnosed with AKI. Additionally, the patients were classified into 2 groups according to the urinary NGAL levels. The number of patients with NGAL levels lower than the cut-off value (62.0 ng/mg creatinine) was 4 among AKI-free patients and 1 among AKI patients. The power of this study was calculated as 0.606. For a power greater than 0.8, a sample size of 30 would be required.

Based on the results of the preliminary study, we extended the observation period to add 10 more patients. A total of 93 patients (45 men and 48 women; age, >18 years) who underwent LDLT at Kyoto University Hospital between August 2010 and July 2013, were enrolled in the present study after obtaining written informed consent. Nine patients with perioperative renal impairment before the administration of tacrolimus-based posttransplant immuno-suppressive treatment, patients with renal impairment by some other causes including septic ischemia, antibiotics and hepatorenal syndrome, and patients with any renal replacement therapy were also excluded from this study. In addition, the patients of renal impairment with low tacrolimus levels, whose Scr levels were not

Table 1. Patient characteristics.

	Healthy (n = 8)	AKI-free (n = 11)	AKI (n = 20)	P value
Age (years)	33.6±11.2	43.6±10.0	48.7±14.0	0.026
Sex (male/female)	8/0	4/7	8/12	
Body weight (kg)	65.1±9.8	61.0±12.4	54.7±10.2	NS
Primary disease (n)				
Biliary atresia		2	2	
Primary biliary cirrhosis		1	6	
Hepatitis C virus-related liver cancer		1	5	
Other		7	7	
ABO blood group match				
Identical		6	14	
Compatible		2	2	
Incompatible		3	4	
Child Pugh score	-	8.5±2.3	10.5±2.2	0.037
MELD score	-	15.0±6.9	18.3±5.2	NS
Donor (Living/Cadaveric), n	-	10/1	18/2	
Preoperative Scr (mg/dL)	0.78±0.06	0.61±0.19	0.69±0.24	0.024
Preoperative BUN (mg/dL)	12.6±4.8	13.6±5.8	17.1±7.0	NS
Preoperative eGFR (mL/minute/1.73 m²)	94.9±9.4	96.8±28.0	86.6±26.7	NS
Total dose of tacrolimus between POD 1 and 21 (mg)	-	67.8±41.5	58.5±35.3	NS
Mean blood levels of tacrolimus during the 21-day postoperative period (ng/mL)	-	8.65±1.97	8.51±1.79	NS

NOTE: The results are given as mean ± standard deviation. Statistical analysis was performed using the Mann-Whitney U test and Kruskal-Wallis test.
Abbreviations: BUN, blood urea nitrogen; eGFR, estimated glomerular filtration rate; MELD, Model for End-stage Liver Disease; Scr, serum creatinine; POD, postoperative day.

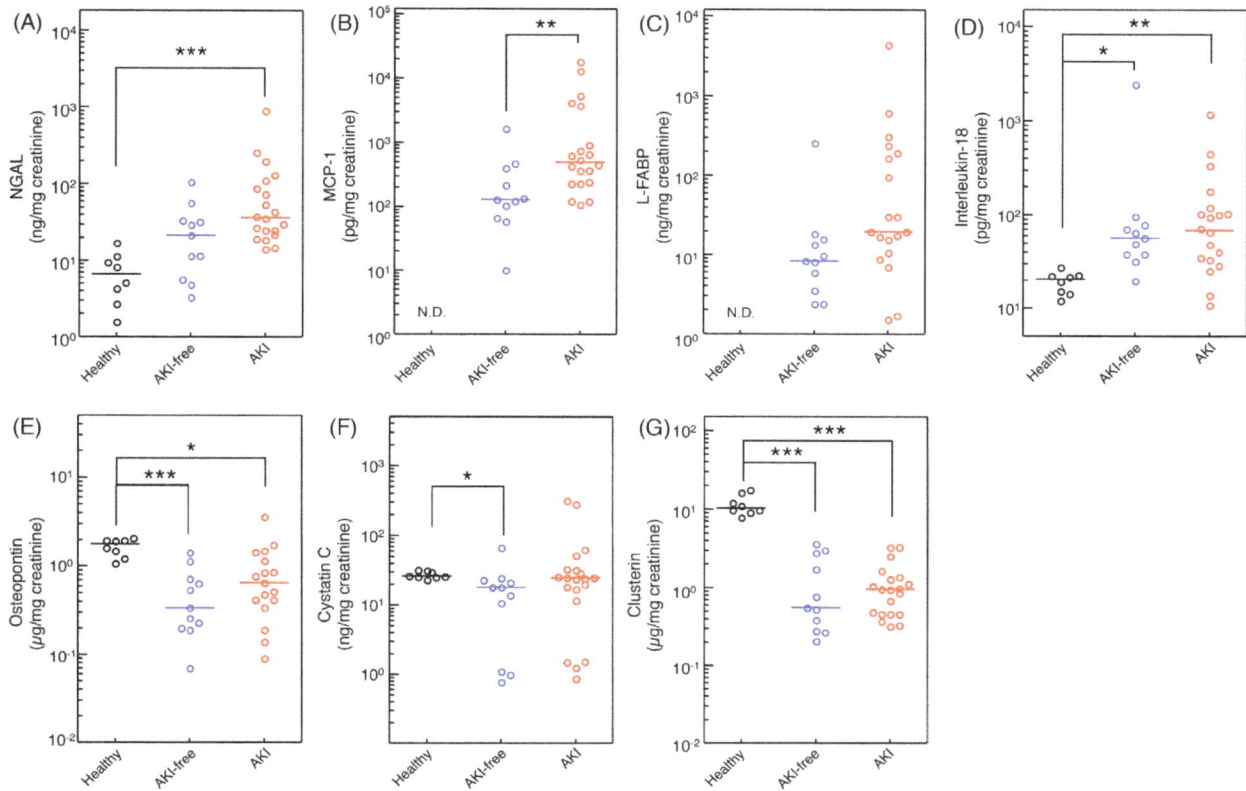

Figure 2. Comparison of the urinary levels of NGAL (A), MCP-1 (B), L-FABP (C), IL-18 (D), osteopontin (E), cystatin C (F), and clusterin (G) among healthy volunteers (8 measurements of 8 subjects), AKI-free group (11 measurements of 11 subjects) and AKI group (20 measurements of 20 subjects). Data were from urinary samples on postoperative day 1 immediately before the administration of tacrolimus in liver transplant patients (AKI-free group and AKI group). Data were normalized to urinary creatinine concentration and plotted on a logarithmic Y axis. Statistical analyses were performed using the Mann-Whitney U test and Kruskal-Wallis test. *<0.05, **P<0.01, ***P<0.001. NGAL, neutrophil gelatinase-associated lipocalin; MCP-1, monocyte chemotactic protein-1; L-FABP, liver-type fatty acid-binding protein; IL-18, interleukin-18, N.D., not detected.

changed even by the decrease of tacrolimus dosage, were also excluded from this study indicating other causes-derived renal impairment such as tubular necrosis post-surgery. Among them, the clinical data of the 31 liver transplant patients (12 men and 19 women) were retrospectively analyzed in the present study (Fig. 1). For comparison, 8 healthy male volunteers were also recruited with written informed consent. This study was conducted in accordance with the Declaration of Helsinki and its amendments, and was approved by the Ethics Committee of Kyoto University Graduate School and Faculty of Medicine. All patients provided written informed consent.

In all liver transplant patients, postoperative immunosuppressive therapy using tacrolimus was initiated on the morning after surgery (postoperative day 1). The blood concentration of tacrolimus was measured using a chemiluminescent enzyme immunoassay (ARCHITECT, Abbott). The daily oral dose of tacrolimus was adjusted to achieve target trough blood concentrations of 10–15 ng/mL during the first 2 weeks following surgery, approximately 10 ng/mL during the next 2 weeks, and 5–7 ng/mL thereafter [20]. Spot urine samples were collected immediately before the administration of tacrolimus on postoperative day 1 as the control urine lacking tacrolimus. After the initiation of tacrolimus therapy, urine samples were collected on postoperative days 7, 14, and 21. In patients who experienced AKI during postoperative day 21, additional spot urine samples were

collected on postoperative days 28, 35, 42, 49, and 58. The 8 healthy volunteers, whose renal and liver functions were normal, were asked to collect their blood and spot urine samples. All urine samples were stored at −80°C with protease inhibitor cocktail tablets (Complete Mini, Roche Diagnostics, Mannheim, Germany).

Urinary creatinine was determined according to the Jaffé reaction by using the LabAssay Creatinine kit (Wako Pure Chemical Industries Ltd., Osaka, Japan). The biomarker candidates were measured using commercially available ELISA kits, according to the manufacturer's instructions. NGAL, monocyte chemotactic protein-1 (MCP-1), osteopontin, and cystatin C were measured using ELISA kits purchased from R&D Systems (Minneapolis, MN). L-FABP level was determined using ELISA kits from CMIC Co., Ltd (Tokyo, Japan). Interleukin-18 (IL-18) was assessed using ELISA kits from Medical & Biological Laboratories Co. Ltd (Nagoya, Japan). Clusterin was measured using kits from AdipoGen Inc. (Incheon, Korea). The level of each urinary biomarker was normalized to urinary creatinine levels to adjust for changes in urine concentration.

Diagnostic criteria of tacrolimus-induced AKI and data collection

Tacrolimus-induced AKI was diagnosed by the attending physicians or nephrologists, and not fully according to the AKIN

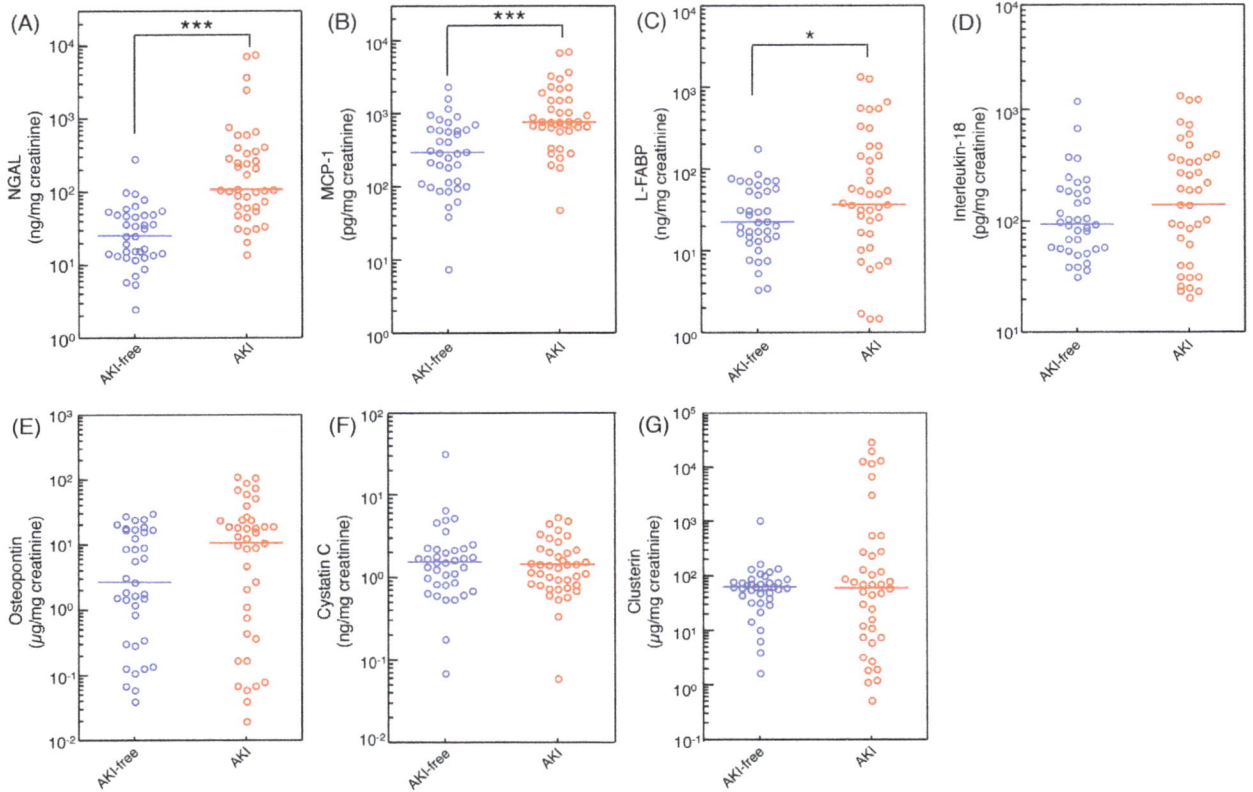

Figure 3. Comparison of the urinary levels of NGAL (A), MCP-1 (B), L-FABP (C), IL-18 (D), osteopontin (E), cystatin C (F), and clusterin (G) between AKI-free group (37 measurements of 11 subjects) and AKI group (40 measurements of 20 subjects). Data were from urinary samples in the post-transplant tacrolimus therapy. Data were normalized to urinary creatinine concentration and plotted on a logarithmic Y axis. Statistical analyses were performed using the Mann-Whitney U test and Kruskal-Wallis test. *P<0.05, ***P<0.001. NGAL, neutrophil gelatinase-associated lipocalin; MCP-1, monocyte chemotactic protein-1; L-FABP, liver-type fatty acid-binding protein; IL-18, interleukin-18, N.D., not detected.

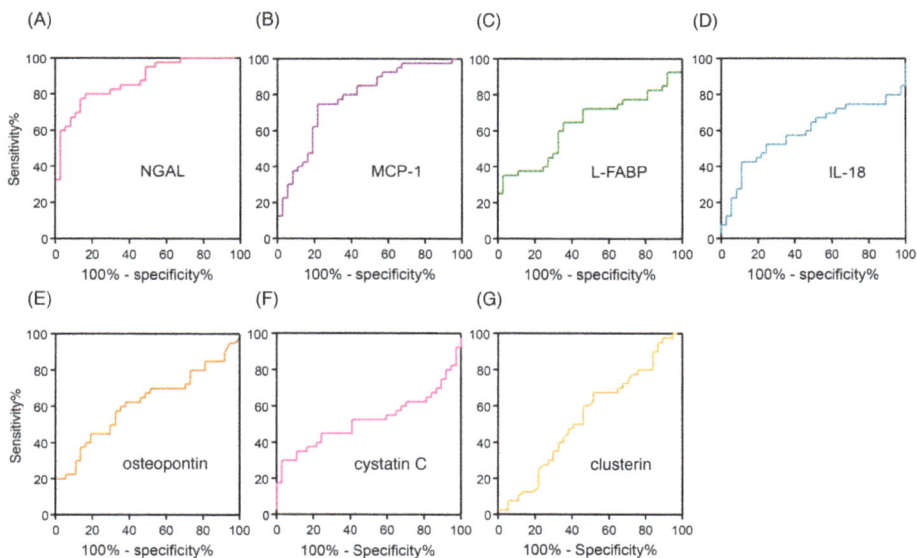

Figure 4. Receiver operating characteristic curve analysis of urinary NGAL (A), MCP-1 (B), L-FABP (C), IL-18 (D), osteopontin (E), cystatin C (F), and clusterin (G). Urinary biomarker levels were corrected using urinary creatinine concentrations. NGAL, neutrophil gelatinase-associated lipocalin; MCP-1, monocyte chemotactic protein-1; L-FABP, liver-type fatty acid-binding protein; IL-18, interleukin-18.

Table 2. Characteristics of the urinary biomarkers.

	AUC (95% CI)	Cut-off value	Sensitivity (95% CI)	Specificity (95% CI)	Positive predictive value	Negative predictive value	Positive likelihood ratio	Negative likelihood ratio	P value
NGAL (ng/mg creatinine)	0.876 (0.800–0.951)	61.0	0.78 (0.62–0.89)	0.86 (0.71–0.95)	0.83	0.74	5.57	0.26	<0.0001
MCP-1 (pg/mg creatinine)	0.781 (0.677–0.885)	642.0	0.75 (0.59–0.87)	0.78 (0.62–0.90)	0.79	0.69	3.41	0.32	<0.0001
L-FABP (ng/mg creatinine)	0.635 (0.509–0.762)	91.3	0.35 (0.21–0.52)	0.97 (0.86–1.00)	0.93	0.55	11.7	0.67	0.041
IL-18 (pg/mg creatinine)	0.595 (0.463–0.726)	268.9	0.43 (0.27–0.59)	0.89 (0.75–0.97)	0.67	0.56	3.91	0.64	0.153
Osteopontin (μg/mg creatinine)	0.618 (0.491–0.745)	17.6	0.45 (0.29–0.62)	0.81 (0.65–0.92)	0.6	0.55	2.37	0.68	0.075
Cystatin C (ng/mg creatinine)	0.511 (0.379–0.643)	13.6	0.35 (0.21–0.51)	0.89 (0.75–0.97)	0.41	0.21	3.18	0.73	0.866
Clusterin (μg/mg creatinine)	0.521 (0.392–0.650)	1.63	0.65 (0.49–0.79)	0.49 (0.32–0.66)	0.50	0.46	1.27	0.71	0.746

Abbreviations: AUC, area under the curve; CI, confidence interval; IL-18, interleukin-18; L-FABP, liver-type fatty acid-binding protein; MCP-1, monocyte chemotactic protein-1; NGAL, neutrophil gelatinase-associated lipocalin.

criteria. They diagnosed renal impairment basically defined as an increase in Scr level of 50% within continuous 96 hours regardless the blood levels of tacrolimus was higher and/or lower than the target range. Retrospectively, the renal impairment was also diagnosed in the patients when their elevated Scr levels were lowered by the decrease of tacrolimus dosage. The AKI group comprised patients who had developed AKI, while the AKI-free group comprised patients who had not developed renal disease during the 35-day postoperative period. The clinical information, treatment process, and laboratory data of all patients were obtained from electronic medical records. The preoperative estimated glomerular filtration rate (eGFR) was calculated according to the eGFR equation for the Japanese:

$$eGFR = 194 \times Age{-}0.287 \times Scr{-}1.094 \ (\times 0.739, \text{ if female}) \ [21].$$

Statistical analyses

All statistical analyses were performed using Prism version 5.02 (GraphPad Software, Inc., San Diego, CA). Mann-Whitney U-test and Kruskal-Wallis test were used to compare the differences between urinary biomarker levels in AKI patients, AKI-free patients, and healthy volunteers. To compare categorical variables, we used the chi-square test or Fisher's exact test. We determined receiver operating characteristic (ROC) curves and calculated the area under the curve, 95% confidence intervals (CI), sensitivity, specificity, positive predictive value, negative predictive value, positive likelihood ratio, and negative likelihood ratio. For ROC curve analysis, all the collected data of AKI-free group after administration of tacrolimus and those between the initiation and termination of diagnosis as renal impairment in AKI group were used. A value of $P<0.05$ was considered statistically significant. Probability analysis was performed according to the Kaplan-Meier method, and the outcome was compared between the subgroups by using a log-rank test. The cut-off point was examined by Youden Index [22].

Results

Patient characteristics

Of the 31 patients who underwent LDLT, 20 (64.5%) developed tacrolimus-induced AKI during the 35-day postoperative period. The primary diseases observed are listed in Table 1. The Child-Pugh score and model for end-stage liver disease score were significantly higher in AKI group patients than in AKI-free group patients. Because the healthy volunteers had higher muscle mass, preoperative Scr levels were significantly different between the 3 groups. Age, sex, body weight, preoperative blood urea nitrogen level, preoperative eGFR level, total dose of tacrolimus between postoperative days 1 and 21, and average blood levels of tacrolimus during the 21-day postoperative period did not differ significantly between the AKI and AKI-free groups.

Diagnostic ability of urinary biomarkers

Seven urinary biomarkers were measured in the urine samples which were collected immediately before the administration of tacrolimus on postoperative day 1 of AKI and AKI-free patients, and healthy volunteers (Fig. 2). Urinary level of NGAL in the AKI group was significantly higher than that in the healthy volunteers (Fig. 2A). Basement urinary levels of IL-18 and MCP-1 were significantly higher in the patients receiving liver transplantation immediately before administration of tacrolimus on postoperative day 1 compared to healthy volunteers. Urinary levels of biomarkers during AKI (40 measurements of 20 AKI patients)

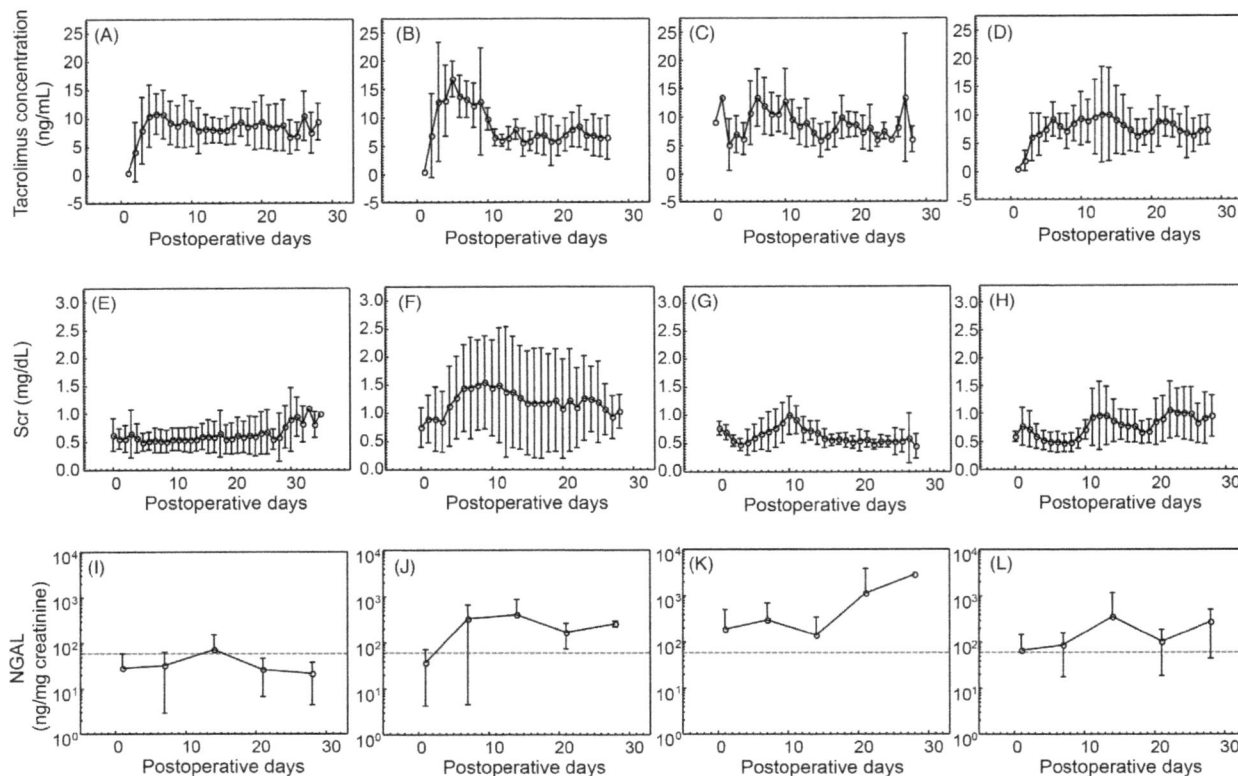

Figure 5. Time-dependent changes tacrolimus concentration, Scr levels and urinary NGAL concentrations. The average ± SD values of tacrolimus trough concentrations, Scr levels and urinary NGAL concentrations in the liver transplant patients who experienced AKI during the period of postoperative day 1–5 (B, F, J), during the postoperative day 6–10 (C, G, K), after the postoperative day 11 (D, H, L) and AKI-free patients (A, E, I) are summarized. The cut-off values of urinary NGAL calculated from ROC analysis were 61.0 ng/mg creatinine (red dotted line).

and all measurements of 11 AKI-free patients (37 measurements) were summarized (Fig. 3). Urinary levels of NGAL, MCP-1 and L-FABP in AKI patients were significantly higher than those in AKI-free patients during the posttransplant course with administration of tacrolimus. However, urinary levels of IL-18, osteopontin, cystatin C, and clusterin did not differ between the AKI and AKI-free groups. To determine the specificity and sensitivity of urinary biomarkers in the diagnosis of tacrolimus-induced AKI, we performed ROC analysis (Fig. 4). The area under the curve (AUC) for ROC curve of each urinary biomarker, sensitivity, and specificity are summarized in Table 2. Based on these results, we focused on the urinary concentrations of NGAL as useful biomarker to detect tacrolimus-induced AKI in liver transplant patients.

The changes of serum and urinary markers

Next, we tried to find out the association between the concentrations of tacrolimus, Scr levels and urinary concentrations of NGAL with AKI development. In Fig. 5, the time-dependent changes of each parameter are shown. A large variation of tacrolimus concentrations and Scr was found both in AKI-free and AKI patients. Urinary concentrations of NGAL tended to be higher than the cut-off value (61.0 ng/mg creatinine) in the AKI group, but not in AKI-free group.

Predictability of urinary NGAL

Because the urinary level of NGAL was found to have the highest sensitivity and specificity in detecting tacrolimus-induced

AKI in liver transplant patients, we examined whether the urinary level of NGAL could predict the occurrence of tacrolimus-induced AKI in patients after LDLT. The 20 patients who developed AKI during the 35 days after surgery were categorized into the 3 groups based on the time of diagnosis of tacrolimus-induced AKI: 8 patients developed tacrolimus-induced AKI within 7 postoperative days (AKI 1–7), 5 developed it between postoperative days 8 and 14 (AKI 8–14), and the remaining 7 developed it after postoperative day 15. The relationship between urinary level of NGAL at postoperative day 1 and the development of AKI in next 6 days was assessed. Although no statistically significant difference was found in the urinary NGAL levels at postoperative day 1 between the AKI 1–7 and AKI-free groups (Fig. 6A), the urinary NGAL levels at postoperative day 7 of the AKI 8–14 group was markedly higher than that of the AKI-free group (Fig. 6B). After dividing the samples by using the threshold values by ROC curves, the probability of tacrolimus-induced AKI was examined based on the urinary NGAL levels before AKI development, according to the Kaplan-Meier method. As shown in Figs. 6C and 6D, high urinary levels of NGAL at postoperative day 1 and 7, respectively, were correlated with the probability of AKI.

Discussion

In this study, we examined various candidate urinary biomarkers for the early detection and/or prediction of tacrolimus-induced AKI in patients who had received LDLT. Thus far, similar studies were conducted in patients with ischemic AKI that developed after cardiovascular surgery and or in patients with severe infectious

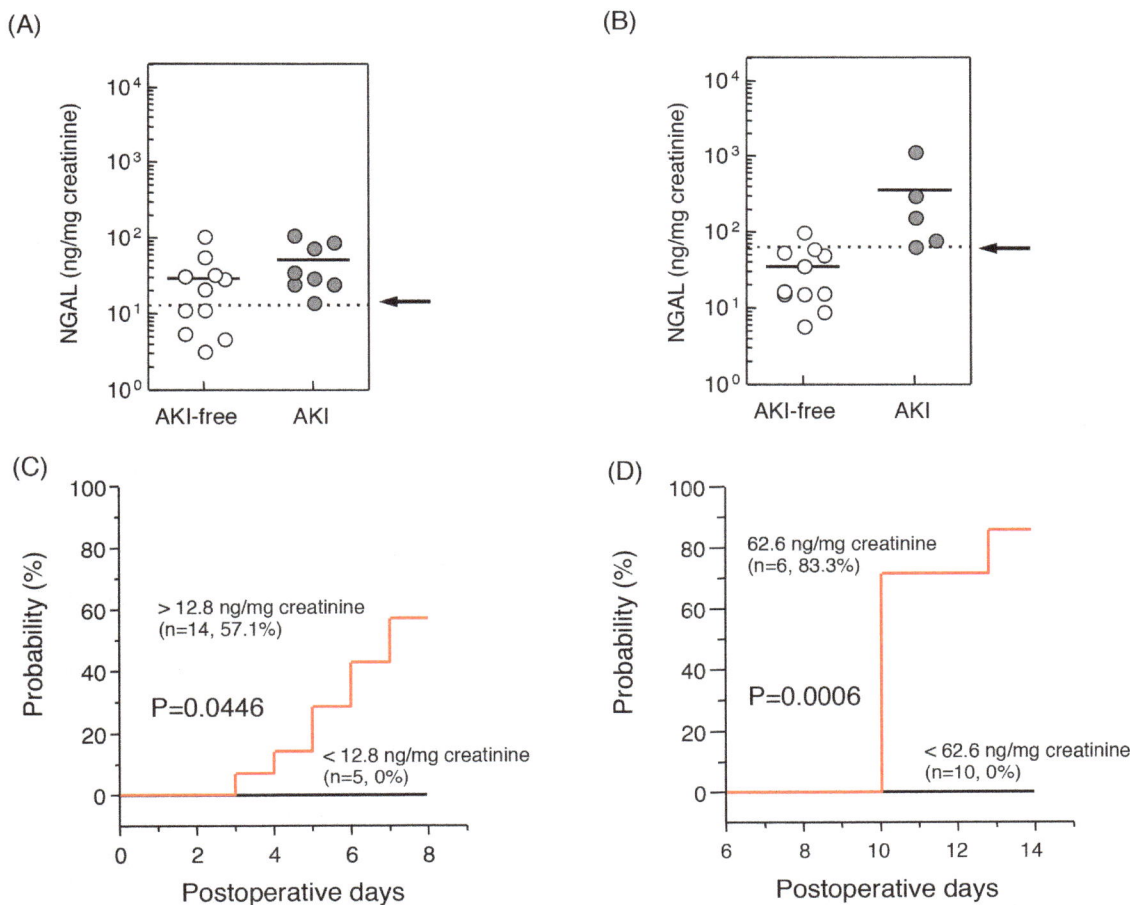

Figure 6. Urinary levels of NGAL in AKI and AKI-free patients. The cut-off values of urinary NGAL at postoperative day 1 (A, dotted line: 12.8 ng/mg creatinine) and postoperative day 7 (B, dotted line: 62.6 ng/mg creatinine) were evaluated using ROC curve analysis. Although the urinary level of NGAL in the AKI group was similar to that of the AKI-free group at postoperative day 1 (**A**), that at postoperative day 7 was markedly higher in the AKI group than in the AKI-free group (**B**). The probability of AKI developing between postoperative days 1 and 7 (**C**) and between postoperative days 8 and 14 (**D**) was examined using Kaplan-Meier analysis and a log-rank test. Statistical analysis was performed using the Mann-Whitney U test. **P<0.01. NGAL, neutrophil gelatinase-associated lipocalin.

AKI [8,23,24]. Recently, on the basis of microarray analysis with isolated renal proximal tubules, we found that urinary levels of MCP-1 could serve as sensitive and specific biomarkers for cisplatin-induced nephrotoxicity in rats [25]. Cisplatin-induced renal toxicity has been found to initiate at the proximal straight tubules, gradually transducing into glomerular damage, tubular apoptosis, and interstitial damage [26]. However, the molecular mechanisms underlying tacrolimus-induced nephrotoxicity remain unclear, although they are considered different from that of cisplatin [27,28]. In the present study, urinary level of NGAL was found to be a useful biomarker for tacrolimus-induced nephrotoxicity in LDLT patients.

In patients with end-stage liver disease, many complications in addition to hepatic dysfunction have been reported, such as renal impairment due to hepatorenal syndrome, respiratory failure due to hepatopulmonary syndrome, coagulation disorder, edema, and consciousness disorder due to hepatic coma. In addition, the surgical procedure of LDLT is highly invasive with respect to renal function. McCauley et al. [29] reported that the peak level of Scr, which was higher than 3 mg/dL, carried a significant risk of death in liver transplant patients. Fraley et al. [30] showed that the mortality of patients with post-liver transplant AKI was 41%,

whereas that of patients without post-liver transplant AKI was 5%. In the present study, the urinary levels of MCP-1 and L-FABP in AKI-free patients were markedly higher than those of healthy subjects. However, the urinary L-FABP levels between AKI-free patients and patients of AKI group were not significantly different. Among 7 biomarker candidates, only urinary level of NGAL in AKI-free patients was similar with that of healthy subjects and significantly lower than those of AKI group, suggesting that urinary NGAL level rapidly decreased in the control prior to the administration of tacrolimus by the morning of postoperative day 1. Taken together, urinary NGAL would be sensitive biomarkers for the detection of tacrolimus-induced AKI in patients after LDLT. Because power analysis showed that the r-value of 0.369 in the present study was relatively moderate in the examination of urinary NGAL, further analysis in future with larger sample size should be examined to find the accuracy of the present results.

NGAL, a 25-kDa protein, was purified from human neutrophils [31], and is expressed at very low concentrations in the bone marrow and several human tissues, such as those of the trachea, kidney, lung, and stomach [32]. NGAL is one of the most upregulated genes and overexpressed proteins after renal ischemia, and urinary levels of NGAL increase soon after ischemic renal injury in mouse and rat models [33]. The Ngal: siderophore: Fe complex upregulates heme oxygenase-1 to preserve proximal tubules and prevent cell death [34]. NGAL has been reported to be a useful marker for renal ischemic injury such as that occurring after cardiac surgery [12,13] and liver transplantation [14,15], and for acute tubular injury such as cisplatin-induced AKI [35] and contrast-induced nephropathy [36]. Calcineurin inhibitor causes structural damage to the straight segment of the proximal tubule [37] and renal vasoconstriction, which is mediated by the renal sympathetic nervous system [38]. Thus, these findings suggest that NGAL is upregulated and detected in the urine of patients with tacrolimus-induced vasoconstriction and structural renal damage.

Urinary levels of NGAL at postoperative day 7 in the AKI 8–14 group were significantly higher than those in the AKI-free group, indicating that the urinary levels of NGAL at postoperative day 7 can be a good predictive marker for tacrolimus-induced AKI. Wagener et al. [15] reported that urinary level of NGAL/urine creatinine ratio could predict postoperative AKI between 3 and 18 h after liver transplantation [15]. At postoperative day 1, urinary levels of NGAL may reflect renal injury caused by the liver transplant operation. However, of the 7 urinary biomarkers examined, NGAL, osteopontin, and clusterin are synthesized in the proximal as well as distal tubules [8]. On the other hand, MCP-1, L-FABP, and IL-18 are specifically synthesized in the proximal tubules. In a histological examination, Morgan et al. [39] reported that tacrolimus-induced nephrotoxicity caused interstitial fibrosis. In addition, excess expression of transforming growth factor beta 1 has been shown to be related to the interstitial fibrosis caused by tacrolimus-induced nephrotoxicity [40,41]. These findings suggest that the origin of urinary NGAL might be the proximal as well as distal tubules. Therefore, a biomarker synthesized at both the proximal and distal tubules such NGAL could associate well with renal vasoconstriction and interstitial fibrosis caused by tacrolimus-induced nephrotoxicity.

In conclusion, the urinary level of NGAL can serve as a sensitive and predictive biomarker for tacrolimus-induced AKI, and urinary NGAL-based monitoring of renal functions in liver transplant recipients may be a convenient and effective way of managing tacrolimus-induced AKI. However, further studies on larger populations of patients, healthy volunteers, and/or other organ transplant patients are required.

Acknowledgments

We thank Yumeko Nishino and Yoko Noguchi (Kyoto University Hospital) for excellent technical assistance.

Author Contributions

Conceived and designed the experiments: MY SU SM. Performed the experiments: AT HS EH MU MK TS. Analyzed the data: AT HS TK JK MY SM. Contributed reagents/materials/analysis tools: EH YO KH YF TK SU KM. Wrote the paper: AT HS MU SM. Critically revised the manuscript: HS SM.

References

1. Masuda S, Inui K (2006) An up-date review on individualized dosage adjustment of calcineurin inhibitors in organ transplant patients. Pharmacol Ther 112: 184–198.
2. Barri YM, Sanchez EQ, Jennings LW, Melton LB, Hays S, et al. (2009) Acute Kidney Injury Following Liver Transplantation: Definition and Outcome. Liver Transplantation 15: 475–483.
3. Lima EQ, Zanetta DMT, Castro I, Massarollo PCB, Mies S, et al. (2003) Risk factors for development of acute renal failure after liver transplantation. Renal Failure 25: 553–560.
4. O'Riordan A, Wong V, McQuillan R, McCormick PA, Hegarty JE, et al. (2007) Acute renal disease, as defined by the RIFLE criteria, post-liver transplantation. American Journal of Transplantation 7: 168–176.
5. Cabezuelo JB, Ramirez P, Rios A, Acosta F, Torres D, et al. (2006) Risk factors of acute renal failure after liver transplantation. Kidney International 69: 1073–1080.
6. McCauley J, Vanthiel DH, Starzl TE, Puschett JB (1990) Acute and Chronic-Renal-Failure in Liver-Transplantation. Nephron 55: 121–128.
7. Vaidya VS, Ferguson MA, Bonventre JV (2008) Biomarkers of acute kidney injury. Annual Review of Pharmacology and Toxicology 48: 463–493.
8. Bonventre JV, Vaidya VS, Schmouder R, Feig P, Dieterle F (2010) Next-generation biomarkers for detecting kidney toxicity. Nature Biotechnology 28: 436–440.
9. Chariton MR, Wall WJ, Ojo AO, Gines P, Textor S, et al. (2009) Report of the First International Liver Transplantation Society Expert Panel Consensus Conference on Renal Insufficiency in Liver Transplantation. Liver Transplantation 15: S1–S34.
10. Nickolas TL, O'Rourke MJ, Yang J, Sise ME, Canetta PA, et al. (2008) Sensitivity and specificity of a single emergency department measurement of urinary neutrophil gelatinase-associated lipocalin for diagnosing acute kidney injury. Annals of Internal Medicine 148: 810–U821.
11. Wheeler DS, Devarajan P, Ma D, Harmon K, Monaco M, et al. (2008) Serum neutrophil gelatinase-associated lipocalin (NGAL) as a marker of acute kidney injury in critically ill children with septic shock. Critical Care Medicine 36: 1297–1303.
12. Bennett M, Dent CL, Ma Q, Dastrala S, Grenier F, et al. (2008) Urine NGAL predicts severity of acute kidney injury after cardiac surgery: A prospective study. Clinical Journal of the American Society of Nephrology 3: 665–673.
13. Mishra J, Dent C, Tarabishi R, Mitsnefes MM, Ma Q, et al. (2005) Neutrophil gelatinase-associated lipocalin (NGAL) as a biomarker for acute renal injury after cardiac surgery. Lancet 365: 1231–1238.
14. Niemann CU, Walia A, Waldman J, Davio M, Roberts JP, et al. (2009) Acute Kidney Injury During Liver Transplantation as Determined by Neutrophil Gelatinase-Associated Lipocalin. Liver Transplantation 15: 1852–1860.
15. Wagener G, Minhaz M, Mattis FA, Kim M, Emond JC, et al. (2011) Urinary neutrophil gelatinase-associated lipocalin as a marker of acute kidney injury after orthotopic liver transplantation. Nephrology Dialysis Transplantation 26: 1717–1723.
16. Negishi K, Noiri E, Sugaya T, Li S, Megyesi J, et al. (2007) A role of liver fatty acid-binding protein in cisplatin-induced acute renal failure. Kidney Int 72: 348–358.
17. Manabe K, Kamihata H, Motohiro M, Senoo T, Yoshida S, et al. (2012) Urinary liver-type fatty acid-binding protein level as a predictive biomarker of contrast-induced acute kidney injury. Eur J Clin Invest 42: 557–563.
18. Nakamura T, Sugaya T, Koide H (2009) Urinary liver-type fatty acid-binding protein in septic shock: effect of polymyxin B-immobilized fiber hemoperfusion. Shock 31: 454–459.
19. Mehta RL, Kellum JA, Shah SV, Molitoris BA, Ronco C, et al. (2007) Acute Kidney Injury Network: report of an initiative to improve outcomes in acute kidney injury. Critical Care 11.
20. Uesugi M, Kikuchi M, Shinke H, Omura T, Yonezawa A, et al. (2014) Impact of cytochrome P450 3A5 polymorphism in graft livers on the frequency of acute cellular rejection in living-donor liver transplantation. Pharmacogenet Genomics 24: 356–366.
21. Matsuo S, Imai E, Horio M, Yasuda Y, Tomita K, et al. (2009) Revised Equations for Estimated GFR From Serum Creatinine in Japan. American Journal of Kidney Diseases 53: 982–992.
22. Fluss R, Faraggi D, Reiser B (2005) Estimation of the Youden Index and its associated cutoff point. Biom J 47: 458–472.
23. Devarajan P (2011) Biomarkers for the early detection of acute kidney injury. Curr Opin Pediatr 23: 194–200.
24. Ferguson MA, Vaidya VS, Bonventre JV (2008) Biomarkers of nephrotoxic acute kidney injury. Toxicology 245: 182–193.
25. Nishihara K, Masuda S, Shinke H, Ozawa A, Ichimura T, et al. (2013) Urinary chemokine (C-C motif) ligand 2 (monocyte chemotactic protein-1) as a tubular injury marker for early detection of cisplatin-induced nephrotoxicity. Biochem Pharmacol in press.
26. Pabla N, Dong Z (2008) Cisplatin nephrotoxicity: mechanisms and renoprotective strategies. Kidney Int 73: 994–1007.
27. Peralta CA, Katz R, Bonventre JV, Sabbisetti V, Siscovick D, et al. (2012) Associations of Urinary Levels of Kidney Injury Molecule 1 (KIM-1) and Neutrophil Gelatinase-Associated Lipocalin (NGAL) With Kidney Function Decline in the Multi-Ethnic Study of Atherosclerosis (MESA). American Journal of Kidney Diseases 60: 904–911.
28. Gijsen VM, Madadi P, Dube MP, Hesselink DA, Koren G, et al. (2012) Tacrolimus-induced nephrotoxicity and genetic variability: a review. Ann Transplant 17: 111–121.
29. McCauley J, Van Thiel DH, Starzl TE, Puschett JB (1990) Acute and chronic renal failure in liver transplantation. Nephron 55: 121–128.

30. Fraley DS, Burr R, Bernardini J, Angus D, Kramer DJ, et al. (1998) Impact of acute renal failure on mortality in end-stage liver disease with or without transplantation. Kidney International 54: 518–524.

31. Kjeldsen L, Johnsen AH, Sengelov H, Borregaard N (1993) Isolation and Primary Structure of Ngal, A Novel Protein Associated with Human Neutrophil Gelatinase. Journal of Biological Chemistry 268: 10425–10432.

32. Cowland JB, Borregaard N (1997) Molecular characterization and pattern of tissue expression of the gene for neutrophil gelatinase-associated lipocalin from humans. Genomics 45: 17–23.

33. Mishra J, Ma Q, Prada A, Mitsnefes M, Zahedi K, et al. (2003) Identification of neutrophil gelatinase-associated lipocalin as a novel early urinary biomarker for ischemic renal injury. Journal of the American Society of Nephrology 14: 2534–2543.

34. Mori K, Lee HT, Rapoport D, Drexler IR, Foster K, et al. (2005) Endocytic delivery of lipocalin-siderophore-iron complex rescues the kidney from ischemia-reperfusion injury. Journal of Clinical Investigation 115: 610–621.

35. Gaspari F, Cravedi P, Mandala M, Perico N, de Leon FR, et al. (2010) Predicting Cisplatin-Induced Acute Kidney Injury by Urinary Neutrophil Gelatinase-Associated Lipocalin Excretion: A Pilot Prospective Case-Control Study. Nephron Clinical Practice 115: C154–C160.

36. Hirsch R, Dent C, Pfriem H, Allen J, Beekman RH III, et al. (2007) NGAL is an early predictive biomarker of contrast-induced nephropathy in children. Pediatric Nephrology 22.

37. Whiting PH, Thomson AW, Blair JT, Simpson JG (1982) Experimental Cyclosporin a Nephrotoxicity. British Journal of Experimental Pathology 63: 88–94.

38. Murray BM, Paller MS, Ferris TF (1985) Effect of Cyclosporine Administration on Renal Hemodynamics in Conscious RATS. Kidney International 28: 767–774.

39. Morgan C, Sis B, Pinsk M, Yiu V (2011) Renal interstitial fibrosis in children treated with FK506 for nephrotic syndrome. Nephrol Dial Transplant 26: 2860–2865.

40. Ogutmen B, Tuglular S, Cakalagaoglu F, Ozener C, Akoglu E (2006) Transforming growth factor-beta1, vascular endothelial growth factor, and bone morphogenic protein-7 expression in tacrolimus-induced nephrotoxicity in rats. Transplant Proc 38: 487–489.

41. Shihab FS, Bennett WM, Tanner AM, Andoh TF (1997) Mechanism of fibrosis in experimental tacrolimus nephrotoxicity. Transplantation 64: 1829–1837.

15

MiR-152 May Silence Translation of CaMK II and Induce Spontaneous Immune Tolerance in Mouse Liver Transplantation

Yan Wang[1][9], Yang Tian[1][9], Yuan Ding[2][9], Jingcheng Wang[1], Sheng Yan[2], Lin Zhou[1], Haiyang Xie[1], Hui Chen[1], Hui Li[1], Jinhua Zhang[1], Jiacong Zhao[1], Shusen Zheng[2]*

1 Key Laboratory of Combined Multi-organ Transplantation, Ministry of Public Health, First Affiliated Hospital, Zhejiang University School of Medicine, Hangzhou, China, 2 Division of Hepatobiliary and Pancreatic Surgery, First Affiliated Hospital, Zhejiang University School of Medicine, Hangzhou, China

Abstract

Spontaneous immune tolerance in mouse liver transplantation has always been a hotspot in transplantation-immune research. Recent studies revealed that regulatory T cells (Tregs), hepatic satellite cells and Kupffer cells play a potential role in spontaneous immune tolerance, however the precise mechanism of spontaneous immune tolerance is still undefined. By using Microarray Chips, we investigated different immune regulatory factors to decipher critical mechanisms of spontaneous tolerance after mouse liver transplantation. Allogeneic (C57BL/6-C3H) and syngeneic (C3H-C3H) liver transplantation were performed by 6-8 weeks old male C57BL/6 and C3H mice. Graft samples (N = 4 each group) were collected from 8 weeks post-operation mice. 11 differentially expressed miRNAs in allogeneic grafts (Allografts) vs. syngeneic grafts (Syngrafts) were identified using Agilent Mouse miRNA Chips. It was revealed that 185 genes were modified by the 11 miRNAs, furthermore, within the 185 target genes, 11 of them were tightly correlated with immune regulation after Gene Ontology (GO), Kyoto Encyclopedia of Genes and Genomes (KEGG) analysis and Genbank data cross-comparison. Verified by real-time PCR and western blot, our results indicated that mRNA expression levels of IL-6 and TAB2 were respectively down regulated following miR-142-3p and miR-155 augment. In addition, increased miR-152 just silenced mRNA of CaMK II and down-regulated translation of CaMK II in tolerated liver grafts, which may play a critical role in immune regulation and spontaneous tolerance induction of mouse liver transplantation.

Editor: Kwan Man, The University of Hong Kong, Hong Kong

Funding: This work was supported by: 1. National High Technology Research and Development Program of China (863 program. No. 2012AA020501-2); 2. National Natural Science Foundation of China (Grant No. 81372626); 3. Natural Science Foundation of Zhejiang Province, China (LQ13H030001). The funders had no role in study design, data collection and analysis, decision to publish, or preparation of the manuscript.

Competing Interests: The authors have declared that no competing interests exist.

* Email: shusenzheng@zju.edu.cn

9 These authors contributed equally to this work.

Introduction

Liver transplantation is an established therapeutic option for acute and chronic end-stage liver diseases, metabolic diseases and early hepatocellular carcinoma [1]. However, donor shortage and side effects of immunosuppressants are the two major issues that hamper the progress of liver transplantation. Donor shortage has forced transplant teams to explore new methods to increase the potential donor pool [2]. On the other hand, immunosuppressant is still needed for recipients, meanwhile, the side effects and complications such as infection and tumor recurrence have always been the vexing challenges for clinical physicians [3].

The ability to produce a tolerant state after transplantation would potentially obviate long-term immunosuppressant usage. For decade of years, researches have been done to demonstrate the mechanisms of graft dysfunction and immune tolerance. Qian demonstrated hepatic satellite cells have potent immunoregulatory activity via B7-H1-mediated induction of apoptosis in activated T cells [4]. Ye Y. and colleagues provided new evidence of the

potential regulatory effects of galectin-1 in allogeneic immune responses in a murine model of liver transplantation [5]. Tregs control immune responses to foreign and allo-antigens and could induce tolerance [6]. Rapamycin has beneficial effects on Tregs' biology compared with calcineurin inhibitor in potentially attaining host hyporesponsiveness to an allograft [7,8]. And the concept "clinical operational tolerance" is proposed and used clinically in recent years, and biopsies are designed to study markers of operational tolerance and to monitor for subclinical events [9–11]. However, the exact mechanisms involved in the complicated immune system to achieve tolerance remain unclear, and the results of clinical operational tolerance are still unpersuasive.

MicroRNAs (miRNAs), an abundant class of approx 22-nucleotide small RNAs that control gene expression at the posttranscriptional level, may impact lymphocyte development or function and play important roles in transplant immunology. Recent studies revealed that miRNAs might participate in the regulation of the HLA-G gene expression through a putative

Table 1. Primers of 11 predicted target genes for quantitate RT-PCR.

Genes		Primers
IL-6	Forward	TACCACTTCACAAGTCGGAGGC
	Reverse	CTGCAAGTGCATCATCATCGTTGTTC
CaMK II	Forward	AGCCATCCTCACCACTATGCTG
	Reverse	GTGTCTTCGTCCTCAATGGTGG
TAB2	Forward	CATTCAGCATCTCACAGACCCG
	Reverse	CTTTGAAGCCGTTCCATCCTGG
IL-1 beta	Forward	TGGACCTTCCAGGATGAGGACA
	Reverse	GGTCATCTCGGAGCCTGTAGTG
UCP2	Forward	TAAAGGTCCGCTTCCAGGCTCA
	Reverse	ACGGGCAACATTGGGAGAAGTC
RAB9b	Forward	GGAGGTAGATGGACGCTTTGTG
	Reverse	CCACACTGAAGGTTAGCAGGCA
Cyclin M4	Forward	GAGATCCTCGATGAGTCGGACA
	Reverse	GAAGCGATGAGCAGCCAGAAGA
AKT	Forward	GGACTACTTGCACTCCGAGAAG
	Reverse	CATAGTGGCACCGTCCTTGATC
P53	Forward	CCTCAGCATCTTAATCCGAGTGG
	Reverse	TGGATGGTGGTACAGTCAGAGC
TLR3	Forward	GTCTTCTGCACGAACCTGACAG
	Reverse	TGGAGGTTCTCCAGTTGGACCC
RIP140	Forward	AGCCAAGCAGAGTCTCCCATCA
	Reverse	TGCCTTTCGTGAGGTCCATACAG

miRNA binding site at its 3' UTR region [12]. Specific miRNAs could govern expression of genes relevant to allograft rejection, tolerance induction and post-transplant infection [13]. Besides, they were also monitored as biomarkers in organ quality, ischemia-reperfusion injury, acute rejection, tolerance and chronic allograft dysfunction [14].

In murine model, MHC-mismatched liver grafts could be spontaneously accepted and reach immune tolerance without immunosuppressant [5,15], which provides us an ideal model to investigate the mechanisms of spontaneous immune tolerance. However, the changes of miRNA in tolerated mouse liver graft are still unprofiled.

In this study, we illuminated miRNA changes in mouse tolerant liver transplantation model by using microarray chip and further identified the important spots of miRNAs and their target genes in inducing tolerance of liver graft. Our observations offer novel findings about potential mechanism of spontaneous immune tolerance for clinic application.

Materials and Methods

Mice

6–8 weeks old male inbred C57BL/6 (H2^b) and C3H (H2^k) mice were purchased from the Animal Research Institution of Zhejiang Province (Hangzhou, China). Mice were housed under a standard SPF environment with a 12h dark-light cycle and free access to water and food. All animal experiments were conducted in accordance with the Guidelines for the Care and Use of Laboratory Animals and were approved by the Animal Ethics Review Committees of Zhejiang University.

Orthotropic liver transplantation and Sample Collection

C57BL/6 or C3H mice weighing 23~25g were used as donors and C3H mice weighing 24~26 g were used as recipients for allogeneic or syngeneic liver transplantation, respectively. Isoflurane was administrated as a general inhalation anesthetic in all case. All surgical processing was performed by two surgeons who have license for animal surgery using a combined cuff and suture technique as described in previous study [16]. The hepatic artery was not reconstructed. The warm ischemia/cold ischemia time was strictly controlled to eliminate the deviation caused by ischemia-reperfusion injury. After the postoperative restoration of temperature and rehydration, mice were sent to individual ventilated cages for housing. 8 weeks post-transplantation, allografts and syngrafts as well as normal liver of C57BL/6, C3H mice (N = 4 for each group) were collected and stored in ultra-low temperature refrigerator.

Total RNA Isolation and Quality Control

Total RNA of graft samples were extracted and purified using mirVanaTM Isolation Kit (Cat#AM1560,Ambion,Austin,TX,USA) following the manufacturer's instructions and checked for a RIN number to inspect RNA integration by an Agilent Bioanalyzer 2100 (Santa Clara,CA,USA).

Microarray Chip Analysis

Isolated RNA was analyzed on Agilent mouse miRNA (8*15K; ID: 21828) V12.0 Chips. Briefly, miRNA molecular in total RNA was labeled and hybridized with 100 ng Cy3-labeled RNA by miRNA Complete Labeling and Hyb Kit (Santa Clara, CA, USA) in hybridization Oven (Santa Clara, CA, USA) at 55°C, 20rpm for

A   Differentially expressed miRNA

8   3   23

Allograft vs. Syngraft   C57Bl/6 vs. C3H normal liver

B

technologies, Santa Clara, CA, US). Slides were scanned by Agilent Microarray Scanner and Feature Extraction software 10.7 with default settings. Raw data were normalized by Quantile algorithm, Gene Spring Software 11.0 (Agilent technologies, Santa Clara, CA, US).

All the detailed miRNA microarray information was displayed in the public database of SBC Analysis System (http://sas.ebioservice.com/). Data was available through username BH2010658 with password 091912. Differentially expressed miRNAs were defined by fold changes of detected signals.

GO and KEGG pathway analysis for predicted gene targets of differentially expressed miRNAs

The online software—TargetScanMouse 6.0 was used for microRNA target prediction (http://www.targetscan.org/mmu_61/) in conjunction with miRanda (http://www.microrna.org/microrna)and miRbase (http://www.mirbase.org/). The target genes of differentially expressed miRNA were predicted with total context score > -0.40 and then the targets were analyzed in terms of their GO categories and KEGG pathways, by using the online tool named "Database for Annotation, Visualization and Integrated Discover" (http://david.abcc.ncifcrf.gov/).

Quantitate RT-PCR

Frozen sample of grafts were the same with microarray analysis. 2 ug of total RNA extracted by Trizol (Invitrogen, USA) was used to be reverse-transcribed into cDNA using AMV Reverse Transcriptase Kit (Promega, USA); cDNA, SYBR green PCR Kit and Primers were all added to PCR plate (Axygen Inc, USA). All of the operations are in line with the manufacturer's instructions. Real-time PCR was performance on Applied Biosystems 7500 Real-Time PCR System (California, USA), $2^{-\triangle\triangle Ct}$ was calculated to represent the mRNA expression level of predicted target genes of graft samples. The gene-specific primers used in quantitate RT-PCR were shown in Table 1.

Western Blot Analysis

To investigate the expression of putative targets of mmu-miR-152, total protein fractions were purified from allografts and syngrafts as well as normal C3H mice liver. Anti-CaMK II (Cell signaling, USA) and anti-beta-actin (Dawen Biotec, Hangzhou, China) antibody were used for western blot analysis. Equal

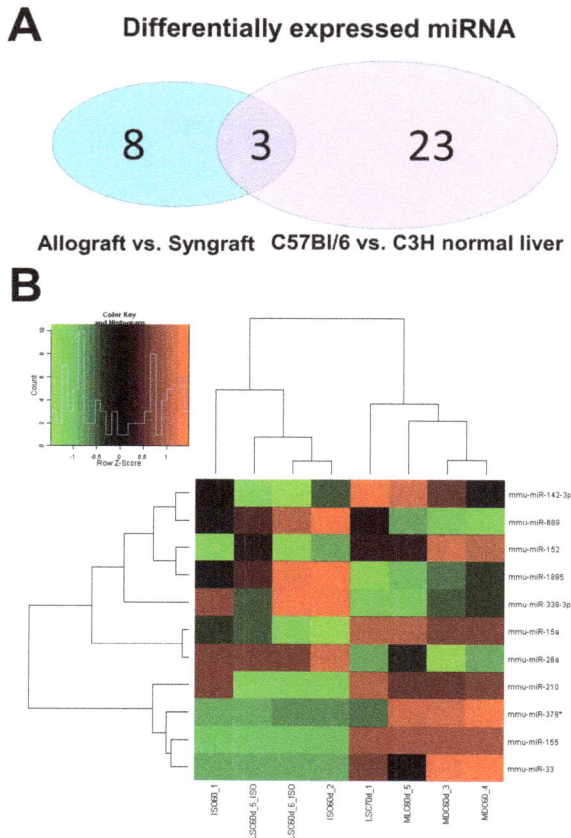

Figure 1. Expression profiles of miRNAs in allo-/syngeneic liver grafts. A: Comparison of observed miRNA in allografts vs. syngrafts and normal C57BL/6 vs. C3H mouse liver. B: miRNA expression profile between allografts and syngrafts. Clustering of the microarray showed the statistically significant (*p<0.05) miRNAs. The columns and rows represent samples and particular miRNAs.

20 hours. After hybridization, slides were washed in staining dishes (Cat# 121, Thermo Shandon, and Waltham, MA, USA) with Gene Expression Wash Buffer Kit (Cat# 5188-5327, Agilent

Table 2. Differentially expressed miRNAs in allografts vs. syngrafts.

Different miRNAs in allografts vs. syngrafts		
Systematic Name	**P values**	**Fold change**
mmu-miR-142-3p	0.039284	2.096914
mmu-miR-152	0.015278	1.152798
mmu-miR-155	1.25E-09	33.95233
mmu-miR-15a	0.007636	1.427048
mmu-miR-1895	0.018199	0.582312
mmu-miR-210	0.033868	6.880669
mmu-miR-26a	0.009468	0.876999
mmu-miR-33	0.009303	20.795
mmu-miR-338-3p	0.02321	0.363475
mmu-miR-378	0.038569	22.05339
mmu-miR-689	0.03978	0.654757

Table 3. Differentially expressed miRNAs in normal C57BL/6 vs. C3H mouse livers.

Different miRNAs in normal liver of B6 vs. C3H

Systematic Name	Log2 Fold change
mmu-let-7e	1.0795035
mmu-miR-1187	4.6175737
mmu-miR-1198	4.7325196
mmu-miR-125a-5p	8.1163
mmu-miR-142-5p	7.888199
mmu-miR-1895*	−1.3780842
mmu-miR-200b	6.960029
mmu-miR-210*	4.649441
mmu-miR-290-3p	−7.272381
mmu-miR-296-5p	−2.1873841
mmu-miR-29b	4.3295603
mmu-miR-29c	4.5762167
mmu-miR-301a	5.3840694
mmu-miR-30c-2	4.6977553
mmu-miR-31	−7.4403687
mmu-miR-33*	4.537604
mmu-miR-340-5p	7.2943954
mmu-miR-342-3p	8.638982
mmu-miR-362-3p	−1.4627097
mmu-miR-423-5p	4.777275
mmu-miR-425	6.8487062
mmu-miR-455	−7.3192835
mmu-miR-702	−6.9172764
mmu-miR-712	−2.3940206
mmu-miR-802	8.667955
mmu-miR-99b	5.4394116

* MiRNAs differentially expressed both in allografts vs. syngrafts and C57BL/6 vs. C3H normal livers.

Table 4. Main functions of the differentially expressed miRNAs in allografts/syngrafts.

miRNA	Biological Function
miR-142-3p	Cytokine-cytokine receptor interaction,Jak-STAT signaling pathway,Adherens junction,Fc gamma R-mediated phagocytosis,Regulation of actin cytoskeleton,Pathogenic Escherichia coli infection,Focal adhesion,ECM-receptor interaction,Cell adhesion molecules,Regulation of actin cytoskeleton
miR-152	Glycerophospholipid metabolism,Phosphatidylinositol signaling system,RNA degradation,ABC transporters,ABC transporters,Endocytosis,membrane associated guanylate kinase,Neuroactive ligand-receptor interaction
miR-15	Apoptosis,Neuroactive ligand-receptor interaction,muscle contraction,Aldosterone-regulated sodium reabsorption,Toll-like receptor signaling pathway,RIG-I-like receptor signaling pathway,Nucleotide excision repair,Melanogenesis,Lysine degradation,Tight junction,Cardiac muscle contraction,Focal adhesion
miR-155	MAPK signaling pathway,Toll-like receptor signaling pathway,NOD-like receptor signaling pathway
miR-210	Oxidative phosphorylation,O-Glycan biosynthesis,Axon guidance,Glycerophospholipid metabolism
miR-26b	Cytokine-cytokine receptor interaction,Focal adhesion,Renal cell carcinoma,Melanoma,Lysine degradation,Oocyte meiosis,mTOR signaling pathway,Long-term potentiation,Progesterone-mediated oocyte maturation
miR-33	ABC transporters,Lysine degradation,Cell cycle,Cytokine-cytokine receptor interaction,Endocytosis,Focal adhesion,Gap junction,Regulation of actin cytoskeleton,Pathways in cancer,Colorectal cancer,Glioma,Prostate cancer,Melanoma
miR-338-3p	SNARE interactions in vesicular transport
miR-378	Axon guidance,ErbB signaling pathway,Dorso-ventral axis formation,Focal adhesion,Gap junction,Natural killer cell mediated cytotoxicity,T cell receptor signaling pathway,Fc epsrilon RI signaling pathway

Table 5. 185 predicted target genes of the 11 differentially expressed miRNAs in allografts/syngrafts.

Mature miRNA Name	Predicted target protein
mmu-miR-142-3p	FMN1,FYCO1,PRLR,RAB2A,WASL,EGFL6,NPSR1,GORAB,DBX2,BC016423,ITGA8,ESYT3, 2210010C04RIK,ZFP943,DCAF12L1,RNF219,RAB12,CTSM,FAM114A1,IL6
mmu-miR-152	OSBPL11,DCP2,MEOX2,BCL2L11,PHACTR2,DCUN1D3,SGCB,ABCA1,EIF2C4,PLAA,ARL6IP1,EPS15, USP32,SGMS1,ARPP19,MAGI1,CDS1,B4GALT5,ABCB7,UCP3,ATP8A1,MNT,INO80,MED12L,ARRDC3, ARHGAP21,S1PR1,QK,TMEM9B,FBN1,SIK1,CAMK IIA
mmu-miR-155	RUFY2,GPD1L,TSHZ3,ODZ3,TAB2,IL1BETA
mmu-miR-15a	ZBTB34,CPEB2,RAB9B,ATP7A,ACTR2,PAPPA,C20ORF46,PRKAR2A,DCAF7,EPT1,ZNRF2,PPPDE2, GRID1,ASH1L,ZDHHC22,HTR4,KL,PWWP2B,MYT1L,KCNK10,TRAF3,CCNE1,PDK3,TLK1,ARL2,CAPZA2, COL12A1,LRP6,RASGEF1B,SPTBN2,FGF2,NUP210,SLC20A2,ATP1B4,MGAT4A,ZMYM2,GPATCH8,ITGA2, FZD10,N4BP1,CACNB1,FBXO21,DCLK1,PHF19,LUZP1,KIF23,FAM59A,WNT3A,RS1,ZYX,CLSPN,ABTB2,ODZ2, PLEKHA5,EIF3A,RAD23B,UNCOUPLING PROTEIN-2
mmu-miR-1895	CNNM4,SUPT16H,FBXL16,FAM53C,MNT,NTM,ESPN
mmu-miR-210	GPD1L,C6ORF136,B4GALT5,ELFN2,SYNGAP1,ISCU,KCMF1,NEUROD2,EFNA3,NDUFA4,BDNF,MLL2,AKT,P53
mmu-miR-26a	FAM98A,ZDHHC20,STRADB,HGF,RPS6KA6,LARP1,KIAA1737,TNRC6B,PLOD2,NAP1L5,CHFR,NAB1, ST6GAL2,DNAJC24,SLC25A16,LLPH,SLC25A36,TLR3
mmu-miR-33	ABCA1,SLC12A5,HMGA2,ZNF281,DCUN1D5,PDGFRA,CDK6,SLC25A25,SETD7,RIP140
mmu-miR-338-3p	SETD7,SNAP29,SH2D4A,MTUS1,PRRC2C,TRIM33,ZNF238,ARHGEF10L,HERPUD2
mmu-miR-378	EFNA5,KCND1,DYRK1A,KCNIP2,ARRDC2,QSER1,GRB2,TEX261,GRSF1,PURB,TFCP2L1,SRSF3,GOLT1A

amounts of protein (40 ug/lane) were resolved by 12% sodium dodecyl sulfate polyacrylamide gel electrophoresis and transferred onto a nitrocellulose membrane. After blocking of non-specific binding sites, membranes were incubated overnight at 4°C with anti-CaMK II antibody (1:2000), and anti-beta-actin antibody (1:4000) followed by the corresponding horseradish peroxidase-conjugated secondary antibodies (1:5000; Dawen Biotec).Then the membranes were developed in the ECL Western detection reagents (Amersham–Pharmacia Biotech, Piscataway, NJ, USA), according to the manufacturer's protocol. The gray value of each band was analyzed and auto-calculated by AlphaView SA software (Alpha Innotech, USA).

Statistical Analysis

All the data was analyzed using GraphPad Prism 5.0.1 software (GraphPad Prism Software Inc., San Diego, CA) and presented as Mean ± SEM. Student's t test was applied to assess data between different groups and $P<0.05$ was considered statistically significant.

Results

Microarray analysis of differentially expressed miRNAs in allo-/syngeneic grafts

650 mature miRNAs were accessed by the miRNA Chips V12.0 expression profiles. Different miRNAs expressed in allografts/syngrafts, normal liver of C57BL/6 and C3H mice were shown in Figure 1A. 11 different miRNAs from liver transplantation grafts were identified (Table 2), while 26 miRNAs were expressed differently in normal C57BL/6 and C3H mouse liver (Table 3). Among them, 3 miRNAs were both differentially expressed in grafts and normal livers, which meant the other 8 identified miRNAs might be specifically expressed in allografts after liver transplantation.

Different miRNAs identified by microarray chips with P values and/or Fold-change were listed separately in Table 2. Fold-change>1 means miRNA was up-regulated, while fold-change<1 indicates a downregulated miRNA. A dendrogram of a hierar-chical clustering analysis of differentially expressed miRNAs between allografts/syngrafts was shown in Figure 1B.

Biological Function Analysis of Identified miRNAs between Allografts and Syngrafts

Table 4 showed the main biological functions of the 11 differentially expressed miRNAs between allografts and syngrafts. Some miRNAs had important biological functions in transplantation immunology. For example, miR-142-3p could regulate cytokine-cytokine receptor interaction and Fc gamma R mediated phagocytosis, while miR-152 played a role in endocytosis and membrane associated granulate kinase. Regulation of lymphoid development, apoptosis, Toll-like receptor signaling pathway and nucleotide excision repair was modified by miR-15 and miR-155. The mTOR signaling pathway was correlated with miR-26b, while miR-378 mediated natural killer cell cytotoxicity and TCR signaling pathway. These miRNAs were all related with pro- and anti-apoptotic proteins.

Target Gene Prediction of Differentially Expressed miRNAs

Target gene prediction of all the differentially expressed miRNAs between grafts were performed using the online software and databases. In total, there were 185 target genes predicted for the 11 identified miRNAs (Table 5). MiR-689 was not matched in the database of TargetscanMouse 6.0. Then, we consulted abundant references and performed plenty of information retrieval work. Among all the 185 predicted target genes, 11 of them had an intense relationship with immune regulation of transplantation and were listed in Table 6 with their target protein, gene ID in NICB, along with their correspondent miRNA.

GO and KEGG Pathway Analyses of the Predicted Target Genes

In order to have a better understanding of biological function of these identified miRNAs, we performed GO and KEGG pathway analyses for all the predicted target genes. By using Functional

Table 6. List for the 11 predicted target genes which had an intense relationship with transplant immune regulation.

miRNA Name	Target Gene	Predicted Protein
mmu-miR-142-3p	NC_000007.13	IL-6
mmu-miR-152	NC_000084.5	CaMK II
mmu-miR-155	NC_000076.5	TAB2
	NC_000068.6	IL-1 beta
mmu-miR-15a	NC_000073.5	UCP2
	NC_000086.6	RAB9b
mmu-miR-1895	NC_000067.5	Cyclin M4
mmu-miR-210	NC_000078.5	AKT
	NC_000077.5	P53
mmu-miR-26a	NC_000074.5	TLR3
mmu-miR-33	NC_000082.5	RIP140

Annotation Tool of "Database for Annotation, Visualization and Integrated Discover", biological functions and effects of these identified miRNAs and their target genes were annotated. The top 19 annotation clusters among the predicted target genes of these differentially expressed miRNAs were shown in Figure 2. GO analyses revealed that 34% of these predicted target genes had important biological functions in binding (protein-protein binding, DNA-protein binding), 21% of them regulated cellular process including DNA binding, transcription regulation and protein synthesis, 10% mainly were involved in cation transport, metal ion transport and protein transport.

As was shown in Table 7, KEGG pathway analysis annotated pathways of all the predicted target genes. Mmu-miR-142-3p was involved in cytokine-cytokine receptor interaction, JAK-STAT signaling pathway, and chemokine signaling pathway, Fc gamma R-mediated phagocytosis and cell adhesion molecules. Mmu-miR-152 could modify RNA degradation, endocytosis, sphingolipid metabolism and phosphatidylinositol signaling system. Mmu-miR-15 family was associated with apoptosis, lysine degradation, calcium signaling pathway, Toll-like receptor signaling pathway, p53 signaling pathway and multiple pathways related with melanoma, prostate cancer, small cell lung cancer, colorectal cancer, basal cell carcinoma. Mmu-miR-155, mmu-miR-26 and mmu-miR-33 played important roles in immune reaction and response (involved in Toll-like receptor signaling pathway) and signal pathway induction (involved in MAPK signaling pathway, mTOR signaling pathway, calcium signaling pathway). Among the targets for differentially expressed miRNAs, mmu-miR-378 had important roles in immune function (involved in natural killer cell mediated cytotoxicity, T cell receptor and B cell receptor signaling pathway in miR-497), signal pathway induction (involved in the calcium signaling pathway, ErbB signaling pathway, MAPK signaling pahtway), and nutrition metabolism (involved in GnRH signaling pathway and the insulin signaling pathway).

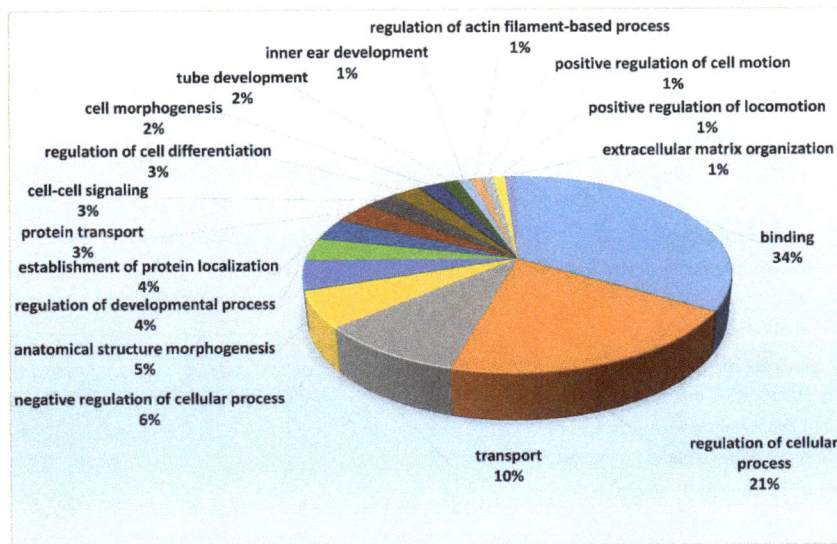

Figure 2. Pie charts showing the distribution of GO categories for the 185 predicted target genes of differentially expressed miRNAs in allografts compared with syngrafts.

Table 7. KEGG pathway analysis of the targets of the differentially expressed miRNAs in allografts/syngrafts.

miRNA	KEGG Pathways	Target Protein
mmu-miR-142-3p	Cytokine-cytokine receptor interaction	PRLR
	Chemokine signaling pathway	WASL
	Focal adhesion	ITGA8
	Cell adhesion molecules	-
	Jak-STAT signaling pathway	-
	Fc gamma R-mediated phagocytosis	-
mmu-miR-15	Nucleotide excision repair	RAD23B
	Wnt signaling pathway	WNT3A,NPSR1,HTR4,SGCB,EFNA3,FZD10
	N-Glycan biosynthesis	ST6GAL2,B4GALT5,ZDHHC22,ZDHHC20,MGAT4A
	Focal adhesion	ITGA2
	MAPK signaling pathway	FGF2
	Lysine degradation	MLL2,SETD7,ASH1L
	Calcium signaling pathway	NPSR1,FZD10,SGCB,SLC20A2,HTR4
mmu-miR-152	RNA degradation	DCP2
	ABC transporters	ABCA1,SLC25A16,SLC25A36,ABCB7
	Endocytosis	EPS15
	Sphingolipid metabolism	ST6GAL2,SGMS1
	Tight junction	MAGI1
	Glycerophospholipid metabolism	EPT1,CDS1
	Neuroactive ligand-receptor interaction	S1PR1
	Phosphatidylinositol signaling system	-
mmu-miR-155	MAPK signaling pathway	RNF219,ZDHHC20,GPATCH8,FYCO1,TAB2
	Toll-like receptor signaling pathway	-
	NOD-like receptor signaling pathway	-
mmu-miR-210	Glycerophospholipid metabolism	GPD1L
	O-Glycan biosynthesis	MGAT4A,ST6GAL2,ZDHHC22,ZDHHC20, EPT1,GOLT1A,NPSR1,B4GALT5
	Axon guidance	EFNA5,NTM,FZD10,EFNA3
	Oxidative phosphorylation	NDUFA4
	MAPK signaling pathway	BDNF
mmu-miR-26	Toll-like receptor signaling pathway	TLR3
	Cytokine-cytokine receptor interaction	HGF
	MAPK signaling pathway	SIK1,TLK1,DYRK1A,DCLK1,PKD3,CDK6,STRADB,RPS6KA6
	Lysine degradation	PLOD2
mmu-miR-33	ABC transporters	ABCA1
	MAPK signaling pathway	PDGFRA
	Cell cycle	TLK1,DYRK1A,SIK1,RPS6KA6,CDK6
	Lysine degradation	ASH1L,SETD7
mmu-miR-338-3p	SNARE interactions in vesicular transport	SNAP29
mmu-miR-378	Axon guidance	EFNA3,NTM,EFFNA5
	MAPK signaling pathway	GRB2
	ErbB signaling pathway	-
	Natural killer cell mediated cytotoxicity	-
	T cell receptor signaling pathway	-
	B cell receptor signaling pathway	-
	Insulin signaling pathway	-
	GnRH signaling pathway	-

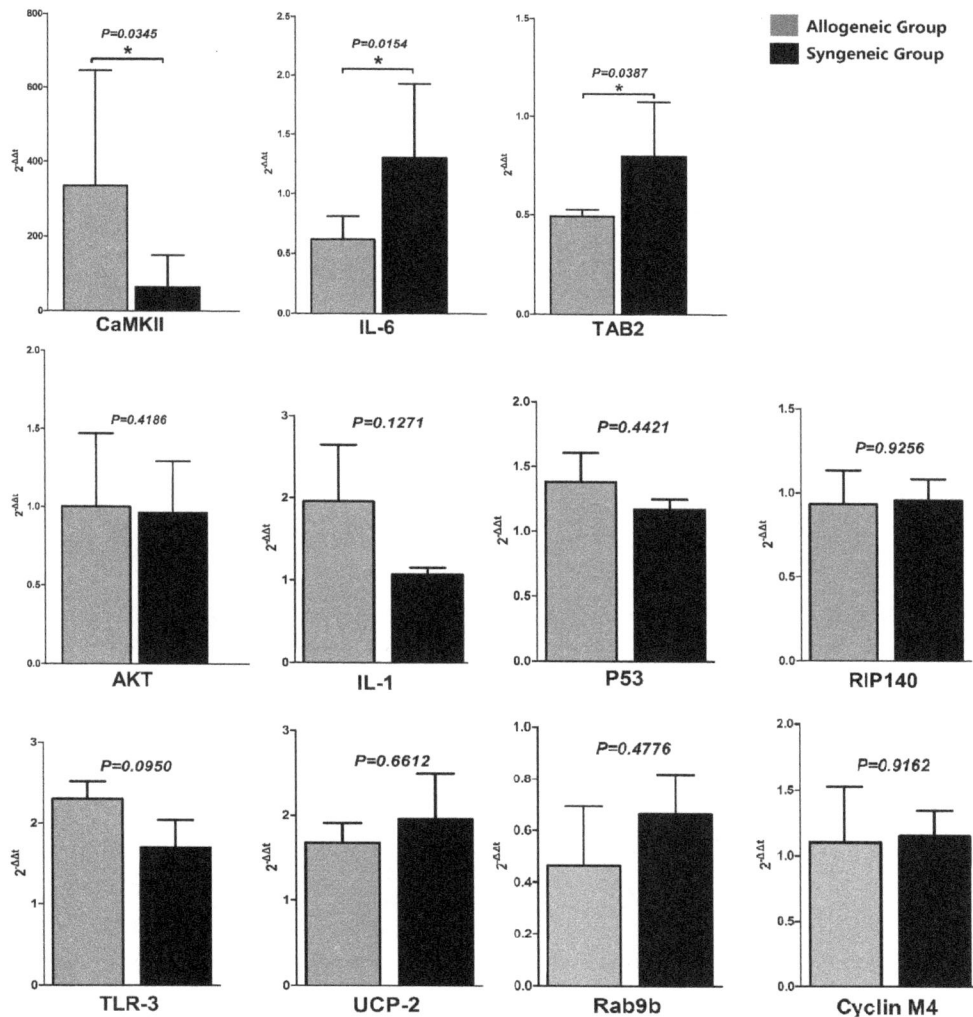

Figure 3. mRNA expression levels of 11 target genes regulated by identified miRNAs. Among them, mRNAs of CaMK II, IL-6 and TAB2 were significantly changed in allografts compared with syngrafts, whose p values was 0.0345, 0.0154 and 0.0387, respectively. mRNAs of IL-6 and TAB2 was down regulated by increased mmu-miR-142-3p and mmu-miR-15, while mmu-miR-152 and mRNA of CaMK II was both increased in allografts compared with syngrafts.

Quantitate RT-PCR Analysis of Potential Target Genes

We validated the expression of the identified miRNA correlated well with those of the microarray by quantitate RT-PCR using the same RNA sample for microarray chips. Afterwards, we selected the 11 predicted genes which might have a potential effect on immune tolerance of liver graft and assayed their mRNA level to verify whether the target genes were also significantly changed or not. To our surprise, there were only 3 predicted target genes had a significant change in mRNA level (CaMK II, IL-6, TAB2), while the others were not (AKT, IL-1, P53, RIP140, TLR3, UCP-2, RAB9b, CYCLIN M4), as was shown in Figure 3. The mRNAs levels of IL-6 and TAB2 were down-regulated by increased mmu-miR-142-3p and mmu-miR-155 in allogeneic grafts compared with syngeneic grafts. While highly expressed mmu-miR-152 didn't degrade mRNA of CaMK II. Since the mRNA level of CaMK II was higher in allografts, to verify the exact relationship of mmu-miR-152 and CaMK II, we applied western blot to verify the exact relationship of mmu-miR-152 and CaMK II.

Western Blot Analysis of CaMK II Expression

The protein expression of CaMK II in allogeneic grafts was down-regulated significantly compared with syngeneic grafts 8 weeks post-transplantation. The gray-values of normal C3H livers, allografts and syngrafts was 1.000 ± 0.1548, 0.3309 ± 0.08488 and 0.8330 ± 0.06698, respectively. Our previous study showed that the expression of CaMK II in allografts was significantly higher than syngrafts 2 weeks after transplantation, with obvious inflammation intra liver grafts. While at 4 weeks post-transplant, there was no difference in expression of CaMK II between allogeneic and syngeneic grafts, as was shown in Figure 4.

Discussion

Since the phenomenon of "spontaneous immune tolerance" without immunosuppressant was firstly reported by Qian et al, mouse liver transplantation has always been regarded as the ideal model in tolerance research [17,18]. Li W. et al revealed the increased Foxp3(+)CD25(+)CD4(+) T cells in liver grafts and recipient spleens, along with enhanced CTLA4 expression, was

A

B

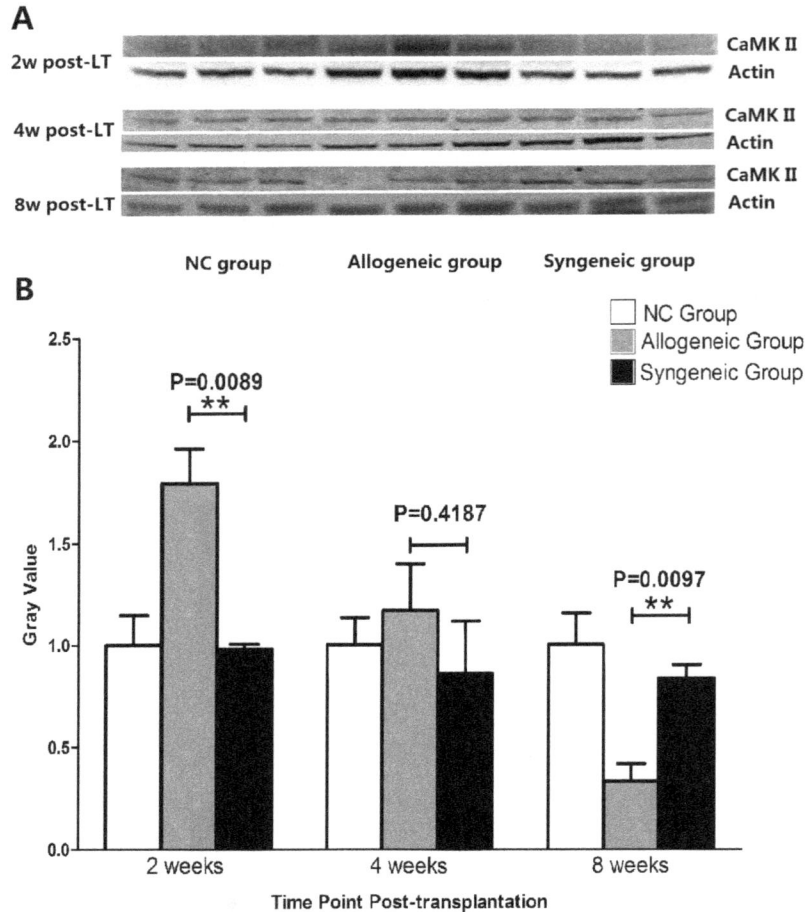

Figure 4. Western blot results showed CaMK II was decreased generally from 2 weeks to 8 weeks post-transplantation. A. Western blot bands of CaMK II and actin in normal livers, allografts and syngrafts at different time point post-transplantation. B. Gray value analysis of bands for CaMK II expression.

critical for murine liver transplant tolerance induction [19,20]. However, Steger et al. provided evidence that Tregs was more likely the result of sustained exposure to donor allo-antigens in vivo [21]. Other studies indicated liver sinusoidal endothelial cells were capable of regulating a polyclonal population of T cells with direct allo-specificity through the Fas/Fas ligand pathway [22,23]. Meanwhile, the underlying mechanisms of spontaneous tolerance still remain to be clarified. To date, no studies have ever reported the expression profile changes and biological functions of miRNAs in tolerated mouse liver grafts.

Our previous study of murine liver transplantation model revealed lymphocytes began to infiltrate into liver grafts during the first week post-operation, the number of infiltrating cells would reach peak in 14 days, and decreased gradually afterwards, immune tolerance would be reached 2 months post-transplantation. Thus, to investigate possible mechanisms involved in tolerated mouse liver graft, allografts and syngrafts 2 months post-transplantation were chosen as our study objects.

By using high-throughput technology of microarray chips, we successfully identified 11 miRNAs which changed in tolerated liver grafts. The profiles of normal C57BL/6 vs. C3H were used to exclude miRNA changes caused by species discrepancy. It means that among the 11 identified miRNAs, mmu-miR-1895, mmu-miR-210 and mmu-miR-33 could be caused by species discrep-

ancy. However, whether they are involved in immune tolerance of mouse liver transplantation requires further investigation. GO and KEGG analysis indicated the potential functions of these identified miRNAs were mainly involved in cytokine-cytokine receptor interaction, immune response, metabolism, and cell cycle and differentiation. Among them, miR-142-3p was involved in Fc gamma R-mediated phagocytosis. IL-6 was predicted to be targeted by miR-142-3p. It may play a critical and specific role in regulating IL-6 production by the dendritic cells (DCs) after LPS stimulation [24]. In vivo delivery of a miR-142-3p regulated transgene could induce antigen-specific regulatory T cells and promoted immunologic tolerance [25,26]. MiR-155 was reported to have a relationship with inflammation and CD56[+], CD14[+] monocytes or the development of DCs. It can promote the secretion of pro-inflammatory cytokines, such as IL-1, IL-2, IL-6, IFN, CXCL1 and CXCL9 [27–29]. MiR-15 family was reported to be involved in cell cycle, apoptosis and nucleotide excision repair. It could regulate multiple cellular pathways such as calcium signaling, Toll-like receptor signaling pathway, p53 signaling pathway, Wnt signaling pathway and MAPK signaling pathway [30,31]. While miR-33, which has been reported to have a protective effect on macrophage induced in inflammation, could regulate the processes of endocytosis, gap junction, focal adhesion, lysine degradation and cytokine-cytokine receptor interaction

[32,33]. MiR-152 was involved in phosphatidylinositol signaling system, and could regulate gene of CaMK II. It was reported that mmu-miR-152 combined with CaMK II alpha to inhibit innate immune response induced by DCs, and down-regulated the synthesis of IL-12, IL-6, TNF-alpha and IFN-beta to impede the maturity of DCs and activation of T cells [34-36]. MiR-378 was reported to be involved in regeneration of stem cells and KEGG analysis revealed it may play an important role in natural killer cells mediated cytotoxicity, T cell, B cell receptor signaling pathways [37-39].

After validation of the identified miRNAs, we chose 11 target genes mostly related with immune regulation to verify whether the mRNAs were changed. The mRNA levels of IL-6, TAB2 were down regulated and mRNA of CaMK II was up regulated in the tolerated allogeneic liver grafts. Since miR-142-3p (target protein IL-6), miR-155(target protein TAB2) and miR-152 (target protein CaMK II) were increased in allografts, we could speculate that miR-142-3p and miR-155 may combine with mRNAs of IL-6 and TAB2 and induce their degradation. TAB2 was proved to be essential for B cell activation leading to Ag-specific Ab responses, as well as B1 and marginal zone B cell development [40], Xu and his colleagues had already provided evidence that miR-155 regulates immune modulatory properties by targeting TAB 2 [41]. On the other hand, IL-6 have been studied for decades of years. It was proved to be pro-inflammatory cytokine that can be observed in many pathogenesis conditions such as systemic sclerosis, ankylosing spondylitis as well as in organ or cell transplantation [42-44]. While other studies revealed that IL-6 was correlated with immunosuppressive effects of ESCs and MSCs. What's more, IL-6 gene expression changes were involved in eight different immune response pathway [45]. The role of IL-6 in liver tolerance might be non-specific.

Thus, we focused our study on miR-152 and CaMK II. To clarify the relationship of miR-152 and mRNA of CaMK II, we displayed western bolt to check expression of CaMK II at protein level. As shown in Figure 4, protein of CaMK II was down regulated compared with syngeneic liver graft, thus, we could presume that mediated by the sequence complementarity, miR-152 bind to 3′-UTR of mRNA of CaMK II to inhibit the initiation of protein translation by connecting the cap of mRNA or lead to post-initiation inhibition by nascent protein degradation and ribosome drop-off [46,47]. In this potential manner, miR-152 silenced the translation of CaMK II instead of degrading its mRNA. Our previous study showed that expression of CaMK II was down regulated gradually post-transplantation (Figure 4). Two months later, the expression of CaMK II was even lower than normal C3H mouseÐ Our study were anastomotic with Liu's results and confirmed a critical role of mmu-miR-152, which combined with CaMK II to induce immune tolerance in liver grafts of murine model.

Our study firstly revealed the expression changes of miRNAs in tolerated mouse liver graft and their biological functions. IL-6, TAB2 and CaMK II may have important effect in tolerance induction. Especially the change of CaMK II was accordant with the progress of mouse liver graft from rejection to tolerance post-transplantation.

Conclusion

In summary, our present study revealed substantially a remarkable miRNA profiles differentially expressed in tolerated liver grafts and their biological functions. GO and KEGG analyses indicated their predicted target gene may be involved in cell cycle, nutritional metabolism, immune response and signal induction. Validated by quantitate RT-PCR and western blot, we proclaimed that increased mmu-miR-142-3p and mmu-miR-155 down regulated mRNA of IL-6 and TAB2, while highly expressed mmu-miR-152 could silence mRNA of CaMK II and down regulate the translation of CaMK II, which may play an important role in tolerance induction, indicating it could be a potential spot for clinic application. But how CaMK II play a part in tolerance induction and how we can use it for clinic treatment still require further investigations.

Acknowledgments

We thank Xinyi Zhao and Chunyang Xing for assistance with database cross-comparison and references retrieval work.

Author Contributions

Conceived and designed the experiments: ZSS. Performed the experiments: WY TY DY WJC CH LH ZJH ZJC. Analyzed the data: TY DY. Contributed reagents/materials/analysis tools: WY YS ZL XHY. Wrote the paper: WY TY.

References

1. Otto G (2013) Liver transplantation: an appraisal of the present situation. Dig Dis 31: 164–169.

2. Neyrinck A, Van Raemdonck D, Monbaliu D (2013) Donation after circulatory death: current status. Curr Opin Anaesthesiol 26: 382-390.

3. Calmus Y (2009) [Immunosuppression after liver transplantation]. Presse Med 38: 1307–1313.

4. Charles R, Chou HS, Wang L, Fung JJ, Lu L, et al. (2013) Human hepatic stellate cells inhibit T-cell response through B7-H1 pathway. Transplantation 96: 17–24.

5. Ye Y, Yan S, Jiang G, Zhou L, Xie H, et al. (2013) Galectin-1 prolongs survival of mouse liver allografts from Flt3L-pretreated donors. Am J Transplant 13: 569–579.

6. Shalev I, Selzner N, Shyu W, Grant D, Levy G (2012) Role of regulatory T cells in the promotion of transplant tolerance. Liver Transpl 18: 761–770.

7. Akimova T, Kamath BM, Goebel JW, Meyers KE, Rand EB, et al. (2012) Differing effects of rapamycin or calcineurin inhibitor on T-regulatory cells in pediatric liver and kidney transplant recipients. Am J Transplant 12: 3449–3461.

8. Miroux C, Morales O, Ghazal K, Othman SB, de Launoit Y, et al. (2012) In vitro effects of cyclosporine A and tacrolimus on regulatory T-cell proliferation and function. Transplantation 94: 123–131.

9. Demetris AJ, Isse K (2013) Tissue biopsy monitoring of operational tolerance in liver allograft recipients. Curr Opin Organ Transplant 18: 345–353.

10. Pons JA, Revilla-Nuin B, Ramirez P, Baroja-Mazo A, Parrilla P (2011) [Development of immune tolerance in liver transplantation]. Gastroenterol Hepatol 34: 155–169.

11. Pons JA, Revilla-Nuin B, Baroja-Mazo A, Ramirez P, Martinez-Alarcon L, et al. (2008) FoxP3 in peripheral blood is associated with operational tolerance in liver transplant patients during immunosuppression withdrawal. Transplantation 86: 1370–1378.

12. Veit TD, Chies JA (2009) Tolerance versus immune response — microRNAs as important elements in the regulation of the HLA-G gene expression. Transpl Immunol 20: 229–231.

13. Harris A, Krams SM, Martinez OM (2010) MicroRNAs as immune regulators: implications for transplantation. Am J Transplant 10: 713–719.

14. Mas VR, Dumur CI, Scian MJ, Gehrau RC, Maluf DG (2013) MicroRNAs as biomarkers in solid organ transplantation. Am J Transplant 13: 11–19.

15. Thai NL, Qian S, Fu F, Li Y, Sun H, et al. (1995) Mouse liver transplantation tolerance: the role of hepatocytes and nonparenchymal cells. Transplant Proc 27: 509–510.

16. Morita M, Fujino M, Jiang G, Kitazawa Y, Xie L, et al. (2010) PD-1/B7-H1 interaction contribute to the spontaneous acceptance of mouse liver allograft. Am J Transplant 10: 40–46.

17. Norris S (2001) Transplant tolerance—the holy grail. Transplantation 71: 711–713.

18. Qian S, Fung JJ, Demetris AJ, Starzl TE (1991) Allogeneic orthotopic liver transplantation in mice: a preliminary study of rejection across well-defined MHC barriers. Transplant Proc 23: 705–706.

19. Li W, Kuhr CS, Zheng XX, Carper K, Thomson AW, et al. (2008) New insights into mechanisms of spontaneous liver transplant tolerance: the role of Foxp3-expressing CD25+CD4+ regulatory T cells. Am J Transplant 8: 1639–1651.

20. Li W, Zheng XX, Kuhr CS, Perkins JD (2005) CTLA4 engagement is required for induction of murine liver transplant spontaneous tolerance. Am J Transplant 5: 978–986.

21. Steger U, Kingsley CI, Karim M, Bushell AR, Wood KJ (2006) CD25+CD4+ regulatory T cells develop in mice not only during spontaneous acceptance of liver allografts but also after acute allograft rejection. Transplantation 82: 1202–1209.

22. Onoe T, Ohdan H, Tokita D, Shishida M, Tanaka Y, et al. (2005) Liver sinusoidal endothelial cells tolerize T cells across MHC barriers in mice. J Immunol 175: 139–146.

23. Diehl L, Schurich A, Grochtmann R, Hegenbarth S, Chen L, et al. (2008) Tolerogenic maturation of liver sinusoidal endothelial cells promotes B7-homolog 1-dependent CD8+ T cell tolerance. Hepatology 47: 296–305.

24. Sun Y, Varambally S, Maher CA, Cao Q, Chockley P, et al. (2011) Targeting of microRNA-142-3p in dendritic cells regulates endotoxin-induced mortality. Blood 117: 6172–6183.

25. Myrvang H (2012) Transplantation: miR-142-3p expression correlates with operational tolerance. Nat Rev Nephrol 8: 194.

26. Danger R, Pallier A, Giral M, Martinez-Llordella M, Lozano JJ, et al. (2012) Upregulation of miR-142-3p in peripheral blood mononuclear cells of operationally tolerant patients with a renal transplant. J Am Soc Nephrol 23: 597–606.

27. Kurowska-Stolarska M, Alivernini S, Ballantine LE, Asquith DL, Millar NL, et al. (2011) MicroRNA-155 as a proinflammatory regulator in clinical and experimental arthritis. Proc Natl Acad Sci U S A 108: 11193–11198.

28. Malmhall C, Alawieh S, Lu Y, Sjostrand M, Bossios A, et al. (2013) MicroRNA-155 is essential for T2-mediated allergen-induced eosinophilic inflammation in the lung. J Allergy Clin Immunol.

29. Terlou A, Santegoets LA, van der Meijden WI, Heijmans-Antonissen C, Swagemakers SM, et al. (2012) An autoimmune phenotype in vulvar lichen sclerosus and lichen planus: a Th1 response and high levels of microRNA-155. J Invest Dermatol 132: 658–666.

30. Liu LF, Wang Y (2012) [Cellular function of microRNA-15 family]. Sheng Li Xue Bao 64: 101–106.

31. Yan Z, Shah PK, Amin SB, Samur MK, Huang N, et al. (2012) Integrative analysis of gene and miRNA expression profiles with transcription factor-miRNA feed-forward loops identifies regulators in human cancers. Nucleic Acids Res 40: e135.

32. Zhao GJ, Tang SL, Lv YC, Ouyang XP, He PP, et al. (2013) Antagonism of betulinic acid on LPS-mediated inhibition of ABCA1 and cholesterol efflux through inhibiting nuclear factor-kappaB signaling pathway and miR-33 expression. PLoS One 8: e74782.

33. Ho PC, Chang KC, Chuang YS, Wei LN (2011) Cholesterol regulation of receptor-interacting protein 140 via microRNA-33 in inflammatory cytokine production. FASEB J 25: 1758–1766.

34. Liu X, Zhan Z, Xu L, Ma F, Li D, et al. (2010) MicroRNA-148/152 impair innate response and antigen presentation of TLR-triggered dendritic cells by targeting CaMKIIalpha. J Immunol 185: 7244–7251.

35. Zheng X, Chopp M, Lu Y, Buller B, Jiang F (2013) MiR-15b and miR-152 reduce glioma cell invasion and angiogenesis via NRP-2 and MMP-3. Cancer Lett 329: 146–154.

36. Zhu C, Li J, Ding Q, Cheng G, Zhou H, et al. (2013) miR-152 controls migration and invasive potential by targeting TGFalpha in prostate cancer cell lines. Prostate 73: 1082–1089.

37. Fei B, Wu H (2012) MiR-378 inhibits progression of human gastric cancer MGC-803 cells by targeting MAPK1 in vitro. Oncol Res 20: 557–564.

38. Wang P, Gu Y, Zhang Q, Han Y, Hou J, et al. (2012) Identification of resting and type I IFN-activated human NK cell miRNomes reveals microRNA-378 and microRNA-30e as negative regulators of NK cell cytotoxicity. J Immunol 189: 211–221.

39. Song G, Sharma AD, Roll GR, Ng R, Lee AY, et al. (2010) MicroRNAs control hepatocyte proliferation during liver regeneration. Hepatology 51: 1735–1743.

40. Ori D, Kato H, Sanjo H, Tartey S, Mino T, et al. (2013) Essential roles of K63-linked polyubiquitin-binding proteins TAB2 and TAB3 in B cell activation via MAPKs. J Immunol 190: 4037–4045.

41. Xu C, Ren G, Cao G, Chen Q, Shou P, et al. (2013) miR-155 regulates immune modulatory properties of mesenchymal stem cells by targeting TAK1-binding protein 2. J Biol Chem 288: 11074–11079.

42. Muangchant C, Pope JE (2013) The significance of interleukin-6 and C-reactive protein in systemic sclerosis: a systematic literature review. Clin Exp Rheumatol 31: 122–134.

43. Rajalingham S, Das S (2012) Antagonizing IL-6 in ankylosing spondylitis: a short review. Inflamm Allergy Drug Targets 11: 262–265.

44. Le Luduec JB, Condamine T, Louvet C, Thebault P, Heslan JM, et al. (2008) An immunomodulatory role for follistatin-like 1 in heart allograft transplantation. Am J Transplant 8: 2297–2306.

45. Chan CK, Wu KH, Lee YS, Hwang SM, Lee MS, et al. (2012) The comparison of interleukin 6-associated immunosuppressive effects of human ESCs, fetal-type MSCs, and adult-type MSCs. Transplantation 94: 132–138.

46. Stefani G, Slack FJ (2008) Small non-coding RNAs in animal development. Nat Rev Mol Cell Biol 9: 219–230.

47. Esteller M (2011) Non-coding RNAs in human disease. Nat Rev Genet 12: 861–874.

16

Quality Assessment of Clinical Practice Guidelines on the Treatment of Hepatocellular Carcinoma or Metastatic Liver Cancer

Yingqiang Wang[1,2], Qianqian Luo[3], Youping Li[1]*, Haiqing Wang[4], Shaolin Deng[5], Shiyou Wei[5], Xianglian Li[1]

1 The Chinese Evidence-based Medicine center/The Chinese Cochrane Centre, West China Hospital, Sichuan University, Chengdu, China, 2 Department of Medical Administration, 363 Hospital, Chengdu, China, 3 National Chengdu Center for Safety Evaluation of Drugs, West China Hospital, Sichuan University, Chengdu, China, 4 Institute of Preventive Medicine, Yichun University, Yichun, China, 5 West China Medical School, West China Hospital, Sichuan University, Chengdu, China

Abstract

Objectives: To assess the quality of the currently available clinical practice guidelines (CPGs) for hepatocellular carcinoma, and provide a reference for clinicians in selecting the best available clinical protocols.

Methods: The databases of PubMed, MEDLINE, Web of Science, Chinese Biomedical Literature database (CBM), China National Knowledge Infrastructure (CNKI), WanFang, and relevant CPGs websites were systematically searched through March 2014. CPGs quality was appraised using the Appraisal of Guidelines for Research & Evaluation (AGREE) II instrument, and data analysis was performed using SPSS 13.0 software.

Results: A total of 20 evidence-based and 20 expert consensus-based guidelines were included. The mean percentage of the domain scores were: scope and purpose 83% (95% confidence interval (CI), 81% to 86%), clarity of presentation 79% (95% CI, 73% to 86%), stakeholder involvement 39% (95% CI, 30% to 49%), editorial independence 58% (95% CI, 52% to 64%), rigor of development 39% (95% CI, 31% to 46%), and applicability 16% (95% CI, 10% to 23%). Evidence-based guidelines were superior to those established by consensus for the domains of rigor of development ($p<0.001$), clarity of presentation ($p = 0.01$) and applicability ($p = 0.021$).

Conclusions: The overall methodological quality of CPGs for hepatocellular carcinoma and metastatic liver cancer is moderate, with poor applicability and potential conflict of interest issues. The evidence-based guidelines has become mainstream for high quality CPGs development; however, there is still need to further increase the transparency and quality of evidence rating, as well as the recommendation process, and to address potential conflict of interest.

Editor: Christian Gluud, Copenhagen University Hospital, Denmark

Funding: This paper was supported by National Technology Support Program (2011BAI14B01). The funders had no role in the study design, data collection and analysis, decision to publish, or preparation of the manuscript.

Competing Interests: The authors have declared that no competing interests exist.

* Email: yzmylab@hotmail.com

Introduction

Hepatocellular carcinoma (HCC) is the seventh most common cancer worldwide [1], and the third most common cause of death from cancer with an overall mortality-to-incidence ratio of 0.93[2]. Most of the burden is in developing countries, where almost 85% of cases occur [1,2]. The annual cost of HCC in the United States is $454.9 million, with an average cost per patient of $32,907. Healthcare costs and lost productivity account for 89.2% and 10.8% of the total, respectively [3]. A survey showed that the cost for patients with HCC is approximately 6 to 8 fold higher than for those without this cancer, with the mean per-patient-per-month (PPPM) cost of $7,863 for cases and $1,243 for controls [4]. It is estimated that the number of disability-adjusted life years (DALYs) lost and medical costs due to HCC will gradually increase as the incidence of HCC rises in younger people.

The Institute of Medicine (IOM) has established the definition of clinical practice guidelines (CPGs) as "systematically developed statements to assist practitioner and patient decisions about appropriate health care for specific clinical circumstances" [5]. This will provide doctors with detailed and authoritative recommendations and alter their customary or outdated clinical methods, which will improve healthcare consistency, promote health service equity and reduce healthcare costs for the government [6]. Currently, although the quantity and quality of CPGs have been improved, the differences among guidelines formulated by various institutes or researchers still differ widely. Therefore, a rigorous evaluation of the quality of CPGs is urgently needed. Appraisal of Guidelines for Research & Evaluation (AGREE II) is recognized as a preferred tool for the quality appraisal of guidelines [7,8]. This can provide a methodological strategy for the development of guidelines, and inform authors on the type of information and the manner in which the information should be reported in the guidelines, thereby ultimately improving the level of healthcare [9].

Schmidt *et al* [10] evaluated the quality of 32 guidelines on the diagnosis and treatment of HCC in 2011. They concluded that most guidelines lacked appropriate methodological quality. However, all guidelines they included were published before 2010 and were assessed using the original four-point scale of the AGREE instrument published in 2003, which is not in compliance with current methodological standards of health measurement design. In particular, this noncompliance might threaten the performance and reliability of the instrument [8]. The aim of the present study is to systematically assess the quality of current available CPGs for HCC or metastatic liver cancer using the AGREE II instrument, and provide a reference for clinicians in selecting the best clinical protocols.

Materials and Methods

Inclusion criteria

The available guidelines on the treatment of primary or metastatic liver cancer published in English or Chinese were included.

Exclusion criteria

a) HCC guidelines for diagnosis (i.e., ultrasound, enhanced computerized tomography (CT)); b) The Chinese version or other versions of oversea CPGs; c) Quality improvement guidelines, position statements or guideline summaries; d) National Institute for Health and Excellence interventional procedure guidance (NICE IPG) or overview; e) Conference abstracts, overviews, primary studies, systematic reviews or letters.

Guideline sources and search strategy

The electronic databases of PubMed, MEDLINE, Web of Science, Chinese Biomedical Literature database (CBM), China National Knowledge Infrastructure (CNKI), and WanFang were systematically searched through March 2014. The MeSH terms with free-text terms were as follows: (Liver Neoplasms OR Carcinoma, Hepatocellular) AND (Guideline OR Practice Guideline OR Consensus). We also searched the relevant CPG websites, including Guideline-International Network (G-I-N), National Guideline Clearinghouse (NGC), Clinical Practice Guideline Network (CPGN), National electronic Library for Medicines (NeLM), and NICE.

Selection of Guidelines

The PRISMA (preferred reporting items for systematic reviews and meta-analyses) statement was followed to search and select guidelines [11]. Two reviewers (WYQ, WSY) independently screened guidelines by browsing title and abstract based on predefined inclusion and exclusion criteria. Primary screening of the guidelines was undertaken by two reviewers who carefully read the full text to determine their eligibility for inclusion in the study. Discrepancies between the two reviewers were resolved by discussion or with a third person (LYP).

If a guideline has clearly stated the quality of evidence on which a recommendation is based or grading for recommendation and statements, then the guideline is judged as evidence-based. If a guideline is developed based on consensus (i.e., consensus meeting or expert panel), without illustrating the source of evidence and grade of recommendation, the guideline is judged as consensus-based.

Quality appraisal

Three appraisers (WYQ, WSY and WHQ) independently rated the included CPGs using the AGREE II instrument that consisted of 23 key items organized within six quality domains followed by two global rating items ("Overall Assessment"). Each of the items was rated on a 7-point scale (1-strongly disagree to 7-strongly agree). The appraisers scored each guideline independently using the rating scale. If the three appraisers rated items with a difference of more than two points, a consensus discussion was held to obtain the final rating [10]. Observed scores of individual items in a domain were calculated by summing up all scores of the three appraisers, and each domain score was standardized as a percentage according to the following formula [9]:

$$\text{The scaled domain score} = \frac{\text{Observed score} - \text{Minimum possible score}}{\text{Maximum possible score} - \text{Minimum possible score}} \times 100.$$

[Maximum possible score = 7 (strongly agree) × No. of items within a domain × No. of appraisers; Minimum possible score = 1 (strongly disagree) × No. of items within a domain × No. of appraisers].

A domain score of 60% was considered a threshold value of the AGREE instrument for rating the overall quality of CPGs. A guideline was 'strongly recommended' if the majority of domains (more than five) were scored above 60%. A guideline was 'weakly recommended' if more than four domains were scored above 30%. A guideline was 'not recommended' if more than three domains were scored below 30% [10].

Statistical analysis

The mean score and 95% confident intervals (CI) were calculated for each domain using AGREE II. Kendall's coefficient of concordance [12] was applied for estimating the reliability among appraisers. The independent sample Student's t-test was applied if a result of Levene's test was p>0.05. Data and graphics were performed using SPSS version 13.0 for Windows (LEAD Technologies, Inc., IL, USA) and SigmaPlot version 12.0 for Windows (Systat Software, Inc., Chicago, IL), respectively. A p-value of less than 0.05 was considered significant.

Results

Search results

A total of 1,686 records were obtained after systematically searching the database and relevant websites. After an initial screening, 99 records of potential interest were identified. Of these, 59 were removed after viewing the full texts for the following reasons: a) Twelve were guidelines for non-HCC or only for diagnosis of HCC; b) Twelve were primary studies or systematic reviews; c) Ten were guidelines written in French, Korean, Spanish, etc; d) Eight were guideline summaries or letters; e) Seven were quality improvement guidelines or position statements; and f) Five were NICE IPGs or overviews. Finally, 40 guidelines published between 1999 and 2013 were included, of which 20 were evidence-based [13–32] and 20 were consensus-based [33–52] (see Figure 1 and 2 for details).

The number of guidelines has risen dramatically over the years, and the proportions of consensus-based guidelines are rising in 2010 and 2011.However, evidence-based guidelines are predominant in 2012 (Figure 2).

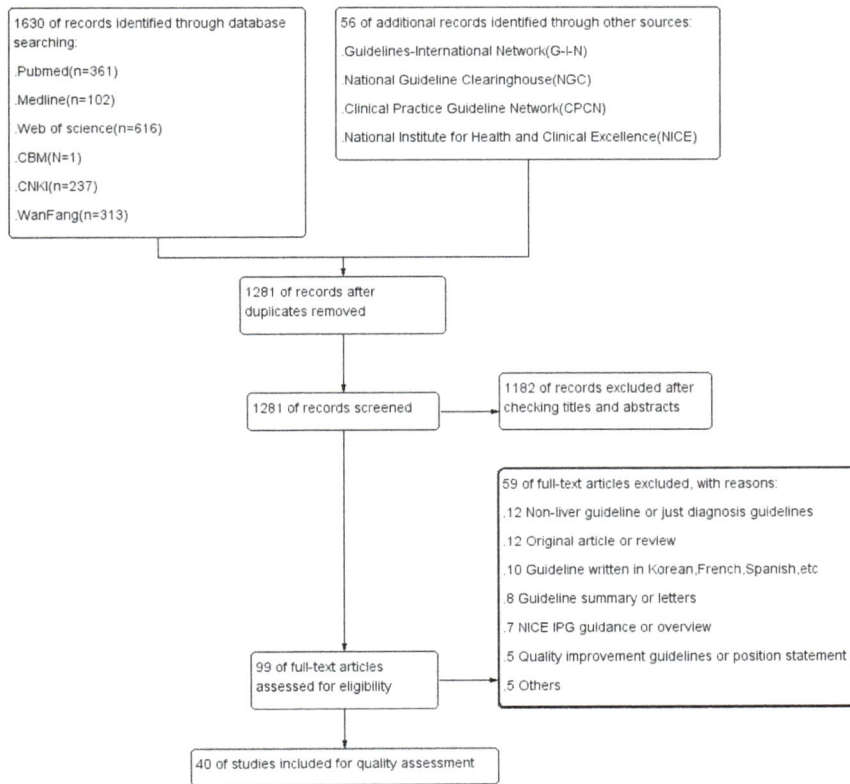

Figure 1. PRISMA flowchart of searching and selecting guidelines.

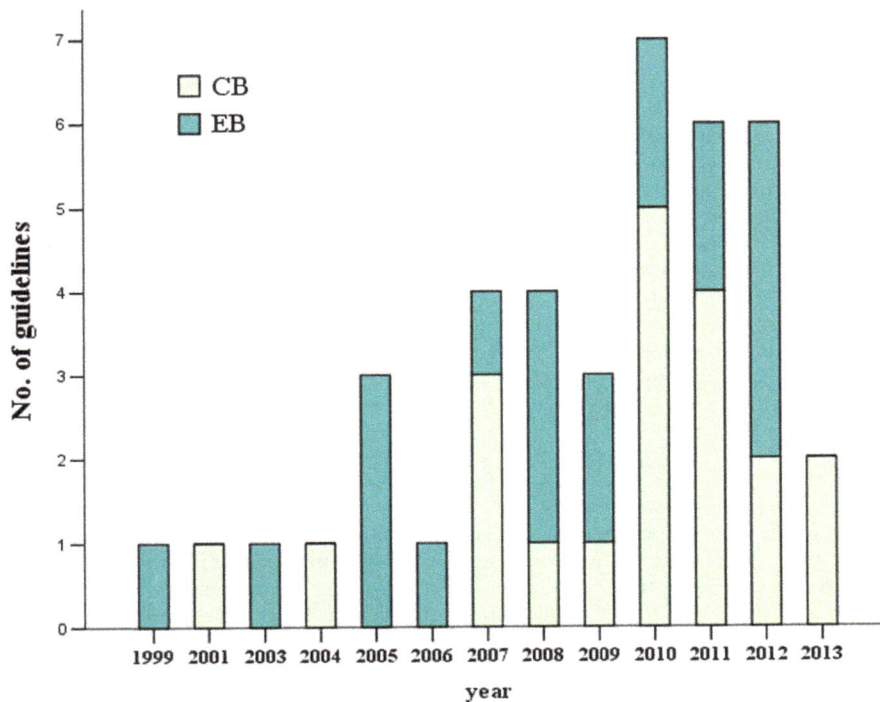

Figure 2. Bibliometric map of guidelines on the treatment of HCC or metastatic liver cancer.

Baseline characteristics of included guidelines

Among the 40 guidelines, 30 (75%) were developed for HCC [13–29,33–38,43–45,48–51], seven for colorectal liver metastases (CLM) [30–32,42,46,47,53], and four for digestive (neuro) endocrine liver metastasis [39–41,49]. Twenty guidelines (50%) were evidence-based, and twenty were consensus-based. Seven guidelines were focused on a single treatment [13,16,19,26,27,50,52]. For instance, the guidelines established by Devlin et al [13] and O'Grady et al [17] were applicable to adults or HIV-infected patients undergoing a liver transplantation. While those developed by Knox et al [19], Kaneko et al [38], and NICE [26] were guidelines on the use of sorafenib for patients with advanced HCC, the guideline conducted by Kennedy et al [39] mainly recommended yttrium-90 (Y90) microsphere brachyther-apy for treating malignant liver tumors. The other 33 guidelines all provided comprehensive recommendations of treatments for HCC, which are mainly liver resection, liver transplantation, ablation, transcatheter arterial chemoembolization (TACE)/trans-catheter arterial embolization (TAE), systematic chemotherapy or supportive care (Table 1).

Appraisal of guidelines

Guideline evaluation results using the AGREE II instrument are detailed in Table 2. Three appraisers independently evaluated these guidelines with a mean Kendall's coefficient of concordance of 0.935 (95% CI, 0.928 to 0. 941), which indicates a high level of reliability among evaluators.

Among the six domains of AGREE II, 40 guidelines were scored ≥60% with a mean of 79% to 83% for two domains, namely scope and purpose, and clarity of presentation. Sixteen guidelines were scored ≥60% for the stakeholder involvement domain and the remaining twenty-four had scores ranging from 33% to 59%. For the rigor of development domain, eight guidelines were scored ≥60% with a range of 63% to 90%, sixteen were scored 30% to 59% and the last sixteen were scored 3% to 22%. For the domain of applicability, only three guidelines were scored ≥60% with a range of 64% to 76%, and four others ranged from 39% to 53%, with 33 being scored below 30%. For the domain of editorial independence, nine guidelines were scored from 61% to 100%, and thirteen ranged from 33% to 58%, while the other eighteen were scored below 30%. Therefore, five guidelines were 'strongly recommended' according to AGREE II including three for HCC [20,25,28] and two for CLM [30,31], and 27 additional guidelines were 'weakly recommended'. Eight guidelines were not recommended because of poor quality [33,34,36,40,41,46,48,49].

Evidence-based guidelines were superior to those established by consensus for the domains of rigor of development (p<0.001), clarity of presentation (p = 0.01), and applicability (P = 0.021). However, there was no significant difference for the other three domains (p>0.05) (Figure 3).

Discussion

There has been a sharp increase in the number of CPGs worldwide since the 1980s [54]. As of June 2013, Guideline International Network (G-I-N) contains more than 6,400 guide-lines, evidence reports and related documents (http://www.g-i-n. net/library), and the National Guideline Clearinghouse (NGC) currently includes 2,549 individual guideline summaries (http://www.guideline.gov). However, there is a great discrepancy among guidelines established by varied governments, associations, and companies or other organizations, especially with respect to their quality [6,55,56]. A systematic review conducted by Alonso-Coello

et al [54] has analyzed the quality of published CPGs from 1980-2010, which showed that the quality scores measured with the AGREE instrument were moderate to low.

Zheng et al [57] and Chen et al [58] have analyzed the status of Chinese CPG development, and have concluded that considerable progress has been achieved for Chinese CPGs over time; however, all domain scores were lower than the world average, especially in rigor of development and editorial independence. There is no doubt that recommendation from low quality CPGs may mislead clinical decisions, resulting in harm to the patient. Therefore, screening for high quality CPGs is particularly vital to guide clinical practice.

In this study, it was found that the domain scores that received the highest marks as measured with AGREE II were 'scope and purpose' (mean 83%; 95% CI, 81% to 86%) and 'clarity of presentation' (mean 79%; 95% CI, 73% to 86%), which is similar to the research of Schmidt et al [10]. Furthermore, evidence-based guidelines are superior to consensus-based ones in terms of language, structure and layout. Because evidence-based guidelines have combined level of clinical evidence with strength of recommendations, these guidelines are more accurate and reflect a higher scientific standard.

However, there were some disappointing results regarding evidence-based guidelines in the domain of 'stakeholder involve-ment'. Although the average quality score measured with AGREE II is 58%, there were 24 guidelines (60%), including eleven evidence-based guidelines that were scored less than 60%, which reflected the dearth of multidisciplinary teams and lack of accounting for views and experiences of the targeted patient population during the development of these guidelines [54]. There were various stakeholders involved, including those in steering groups, research groups involved in selecting and rating the evidence, individuals involved in formulating final recommenda-tions, public and private funding bodies, managers, healthcare professionals, patients, employers and manufactures, but not independent individuals involved externally in reviewing the guideline[9,59]. Their engagement of the latter group is required for various reasons such as including overlooked evidence, transparency and democracy principles, ownership, and potential policy implications [59]. Therefore, they play a vital role during guideline development, review and modification, but their involvement can also be very complex, and it needs to be inclusive, equitable, and sufficiently resourced [59].

The quality of a guideline largely depends on whether or not its methodology is rigorous and scientific. However, most guidelines received a lower score (39%) for the domain of 'rigor of development'. Five consensus-based guidelines scored less than 30% for this domain. Although evidence-based guidelines are superior to consensus-based ones with respect to evidence gathering, quality assessment or strength of recommendations, there are still 12 evidence-based guidelines which were only scored between 30% and 60%. It is common that guidelines include references to published studies, but few of them clearly describe the searching strategy, the methodology used to formulate the final recommendations, or the dates on which guidelines were updated [10]. One reason may be the lack of methodological experts in guideline developing teams, the lack of resources needed to search for high-quality systematic reviews, or the poor reported quality of guidelines [54].

The domain of applicability mainly evaluates implementation barriers, cost factors, and monitoring criteria [9]. However, most guidelines included in this study neither discussed this field nor highlighted the tools required for facilitating or promoting guidelines, resulting in the lowest average domain scores (16%),

Table 1. General information of guidelines included in our analysis.

Organization, year	Cancer	Type	Treatment strategies Liver resection	Liver transplantation	Ablative therapy	TACE/TAE	Hormonal therapy	Systematic therapy	Radiotherapy /Radioembolization	Support care
BSG,1999[13]	HCC	EB		◎						
BSG,2003[14]	HCC	EB	◎	◎	◎	◎	◎	◎		
AASLD,2005a[15]	HCC	EB	◎	◎	◎	◎	◎	◎	◎	
AASLD,2005b[16]	HCC	EB		◎						
British HIV Association,2005[17]	HCC	EB		◎						
ESMO,2008[18]	HCC	EB	◎	◎	◎	◎		◎		◎
CCO,2008[19]	HCC	EB						◎		
JMH,2008[20]	HCC	EB	◎	◎	◎	◎		◎	◎	◎
AOS,2009[21]	HCC	EB	◎	◎	◎	◎		◎		
NCCN,2009[22]	HCC	EB	◎	◎	◎	◎			◎	◎
ESMO,2010[23]	HCC	EB	◎	◎	◎			◎		◎
APASL,2010[24]	HCC	EB	◎	◎	◎	◎		◎		
AASLD,2011[25]	HCC	EB	◎	◎	◎	◎		◎	◎	
NICE,2012[26]	HCC	EB				◎		◎		
AAGH,2012[27]	HCC	EB								
EASL-EORTC,2012[28]	HCC	EB	◎	◎	◎	◎	◎	◎		◎
SASLT/SOS,2012[29]	HCC	EB	◎	◎	◎	◎		◎	◎	
AUGS, et al, 2006[30]	CLM	EB	◎	◎	◎			◎		◎
Netherlands,2007 [31]	CLM	EB	◎		◎			◎		
CMA,2011[32]	CLM	EB	◎	◎	◎	◎		◎	◎	◎
EASL,2001[33]	HCC	CB	◎	◎	◎	◎	◎	◎		
BASL,2004[34]	HCC	CB	◎	◎	◎	◎	◎	◎	◎	
JSH,2007[35]	HCC	CB	◎	◎	◎	◎		◎	◎	◎
CSLCCO, et al, 2009[36]	HCC	CB	◎	◎	◎	◎		◎	◎	◎
JSH,2010a[37]	HCC	CB	◎	◎	◎			◎		
JSH,2010b[43]	HCC	CB	◎	◎	◎	◎		◎		◎
JSH,2010c[44]	HCC	CB	◎	◎	◎	◎		◎		◎
WGOGG,2010[48]	HCC	CB	◎		◎	◎		◎		◎
JSH,2011[45]	HCC	CB	◎	◎	◎	◎		◎		◎
ICC,2011[50]	HCC	CB		◎						
France,2011[51]	HCC	CB		◎						
SGNLCT,2012[38]	HCC	CB						◎		
EANM,2011[49]	HCC/LM	CB							◎	

Table 1. Cont.

Organization, year	Cancer	Type	Liver resection	Liver transplantation	Ablative therapy	TACE/TAE	Hormonal therapy	Systematic therapy	Radiotherapy /Radioembolization	Support care
REBOC,2007[39]	LM	CB				◎				
ENETS,2008[40]	LM	CB	◎	◎	◎	◎		◎	◎	
ENETS,2012[41]	LM	CB	◎	◎	◎			◎	◎	
ICO,2007[46]	CLM	CB	◎					◎		◎
CMA,2010[42]	CLM	CB	◎		◎			◎	◎	
AHPBA,2013a[47]	CLM	CB	◎		◎			◎	◎	
AHPBA,2013b[52]	CLM	CB						◎		
Total	30(HCC) 7(CLM) 4(LM)	20(EB) 20(CB)	28	26	27	21	5	30	13	13

EB: Evidence-based. CB: Consensus-based. HCC: Hepatocellular carcinoma; CLM: Colorectal liver metastases; LM: liver metastases; HM: Hepatic Malignancy; TACE/TAE: Transarterial chemoembolization/Transarterial embolization;BSG:British Society of Gastroenterology;AASLD:American Association for the study of Liver Disease;ESMO: European Society for Medical Oncology; CCO: Cancer Care Ontario;JMH: Japanese Ministry of Health;AOS: Asian Oncology Summit;NCCN: National Comprehensive Cancer Network; APASL: Asian Pacific Association for the study of the Liver; NICE: National Institute for Health and Clinical Excellence;AAGH: Austrian Association of Gastroenterology and Hepatology;EASL-EORTC: European Association for Study of Liver—European Organization for Research and Treatment of Cancer;SASLT/SOS: Saudi Association for the Study of Liver diseases and Transplantation/Saudi Oncology Society;AUGS: Association of Upper Gastrointestinal Surgeons;CMA: Chinese Medical Association;BASL: Belgian Association for the study of the Liver;JSH: Japan Society of Hepatology;CSLCCO: Chinese Societies of Liver Cancer and Clinical Oncology;WGOGG: World Gastroenterology Organization Global Guideline;ICC: International Consensus Conference;SGNLCT: Study Group on New Liver Cancer Therapies; EANM, European Association of Nuclear Medicine;REBOC: Radioembolization Brachytherapy Oncology Consortium;ENETS: European Neuroendocrine Tumor Society;ICO: Institute of Catalan Oncology.AHPBA:Americas Hepatopancreato-Biliary Association,

Table 2. Assessment of hepatocellular and metastatic liver cancer guidelines with the AGREE II instrument.

Organization, Reference	Type	Kendall's coefficient of concordance (W)	Domain score in %						Overall recommendation*
			Scope and purpose	Stakeholder involvement	Rigor of development	Clarity of presentation	Applicability	Editorial independence	
JMH,2008[20]	EB	0.933	100	93	90	94	64	25	Strongly
AASLD,2011[25]	EB	0.931	87	61	74	98	11	86	Strongly
EASL-EORTC,2012[28]	EB	0.925	94	94	72	100	28	50	Strongly
AUGS, et al, 2006[30]	EB	0.935	96	70	81	100	29	86	Strongly
Netherlands,2007[31]	EB	0.935	89	63	86	96	71	14	Strongly
BSG,1999[13]	EB	0.953	96	83	40	100	6	14	Weakly
BSG,2003[14]	EB	0.950	96	87	63	96	6	17	Weakly
AASLD,2005a[15]	EB	0.949	91	80	47	98	21	44	Weakly
AASLD,2005b[16]	EB	0.938	80	74	63	96	21	19	Weakly
British HIV Association, 2005[17]	EB	0.892	83	59	31	96	43	33	Weakly
ESMO,2008[18]	EB	0.930	81	33	40	87	1	50	Weakly
CCO,2008[19]	EB	0.939	87	57	56	61	6	100	Weakly
AOS,2009[21]	EB	0.932	85	46	56	93	39	53	Weakly
NCCN,2009[22]	EB	0.924	69	43	36	69	39	89	Weakly
ESMO,2010[23]	EB	0.931	76	39	45	87	0	50	Weakly
APASL,2010[24]	EB	0.929	74	50	49	100	1	0	Weakly
NICE,2012[26]	EB	0.905	74	59	59	93	76	39	Weakly
AAGH,2012[27]	EB	0.934	85	52	43	85	0	50	Weakly
SASLT/SOS,2012[29]	EB	0.942	89	54	67	96	6	3	Weakly
CMA,2011[32]	EB	0.962	80	33	19	63	6	47	Weakly
JSH,2010a[37]	CB	0.951	81	54	46	91	8	6	Weakly
JSH,2010b[43]	CB	0.957	78	59	3	76	7	86	Weakly
JSH,2010c[44]	CB	0.962	85	56	5	78	6	69	Weakly
JSH,2011[45]	CB	0.971	87	67	10	74	14	78	Weakly
SGNLCT,2012[38]	CB	0.922	83	80	46	85	0	6	Weakly
REBOC,2007[39]	CB	0.879	78	80	58	85	53	89	Weakly
JSH,2007[35]	CB	0.944	87	59	30	78	11	61	Weakly
CMA,2010[42]	CB	0.952	83	70	42	87	3	22	Weakly
ICC,2011[50]	CB	0.960	81	37	22	69	6	58	Weakly
France,2011[51]	CB	0.925	83	33	10	52	6	50	Weakly
AHPBA,2013a[47]	CB	0.948	85	33	9	70	3	56	Weakly
AHPBA,2013b[52]	CB	0.923	76	37	10	59	7	56	Weakly
EASL,2001[33]	CB	0.945	87	80	22	78	7	14	Not Recommend

Table 2. Cont.

Organization, Reference	Type	Kendall's coefficient of concordance (W)	Domain score in %						Overall recommendation*
			Scope and purpose	Stakeholder involvement	Rigor of development	Clarity of presentation	Applicability	Editorial independence	
BASL,2004[34]	CB	0.942	76	69	21	83	7	11	Not Recommend
CSLCCO, et al,2009[36]	CB	0.943	85	76	20	81	18	22	Not Recommend
ENETS,2008[40]	CB	0.942	83	43	16	81	3	3	Not Recommend
ENETS,2012[41]	CB	0.925	72	50	21	80	6	0	Not Recommend
ICO,2007[46]	CB	0.918	83	33	16	20	6	6	Not Recommend
WGOGG,2010[48]	CB	0.898	70	33	8	30	7	6	Not Recommend
EANM,2011[49]	CB	0.910	83	37	8	9	7	6	Not Recommend
Mean (95%CI)		0.935(0.928–0.941)	83(81–86)	58(52–64)	39(31–46)	79(73–86)	16(10–23)	39(30–49)	

*The overall recommendations are based on the AGREE II evaluations according to references [9] and [10]. This recommendation should be seen as a recommendation between the currently available guidelines rather than a quality stamp of the individual guideline. Please see discussion.

especially for 15 evidence-based guidelines, which were scored less than 30%.

Similarly, the domain of editorial independence addresses whether the recommendations are impacted by the funding body and conflict of interests (COIs) issues which may arise from within the guideline-developing organization [9]. Potential COIs may greatly impact the content of guidelines and the recommendations. COIs was highly prevalent (150/288, 52%) among guidelines established by Canadian specialty and US specialty societies, but a large proportion of guidelines did not publicly disclose COIs [60]. A study published by Choudhry et al [61] showed that 87% of guideline developers had some form of interaction with a pharmaceutical company, 58% of whom had received funding support to conduct their research, and 38% of whom had served as employees or consultants in the pharmaceutical industry. In our study, 20 (50%) guidelines did not publicly disclose COIs, and 18 (45%), including seven evidence-based guidelines were scored less than 30% for this domain. Three of the five guidelines that we 'strongly recommend' all reported the COIs of authors in detail. In the EASL-EORTC guideline, the authors have reported the COIs at the end of guideline, however, number of affiliated authors have received research support and/or lecture fees and/or took part in clinical trials for Bayer (a pharmaceutical company)[28], which may lead certain bias for the independence of their recommendations and reliability of guideline to some extent. Therefore, recommendations based on the AGREE II 'strongly recommend' guidelines still need to be revised and updated according to the conclusions of properly conducted systematic reviews.

We based our recommendations of the guidelines on the AGREE II instrument as previously described [9,10]. However, we would like to question the validity of this approach. First, such recommendations may lead clinicians to depend too much on and believe in the individual recommendations of guidelines that have achieved 'strongly recommend'. Second, such recommendation may falsely overrate the evidence because the bar is set too low according to our experience. In short, even the 'strongly recommend' guidelines are not sufficiently evidence based. Thirdly, we lack evidence of any patient benefits by adopting such coarse recommendations. Therefore, the recommendations should be seen as a consequence of adopting the AGREE II methodology rather than a quality stamp on some of the guidelines as being of high methodological quality. If it is a quality stamp, it is relative to the guidelines that achieved lower ratings.

The ultimate goal of the present guideline evaluation is to recognize the faults of existing guidelines so that the necessary steps are taken to improve their quality. We found that most authors had increasingly emphasized evidence gathering and synthesis, and formulated the final recommendations when they developed their guidelines. The evidence-based guideline has become a mainstream for high quality guideline development. However, the transparency of guidelines in aspects of quality appraisal of evidence, formulation of recommendations, and the COI of authors are still insufficient, and this has become a prominent problem affecting the quality of guidelines. Some guidelines have simply classified evidence according to the study design, ignoring quality assessment of evidence, therefore making it difficult to know on which one or type of specific evidence the recommendation was based.

Although some guidelines use GRADE (the Grading of Recommendations Assessment, Development and Evaluation) as a tool for evaluating the quality of evidence and formulating the final recommendations, GRADE evidence profiles and summary of finding (SoF) tables were not presented or linked in the guidelines. Therefore, the GRADE working group has suggested

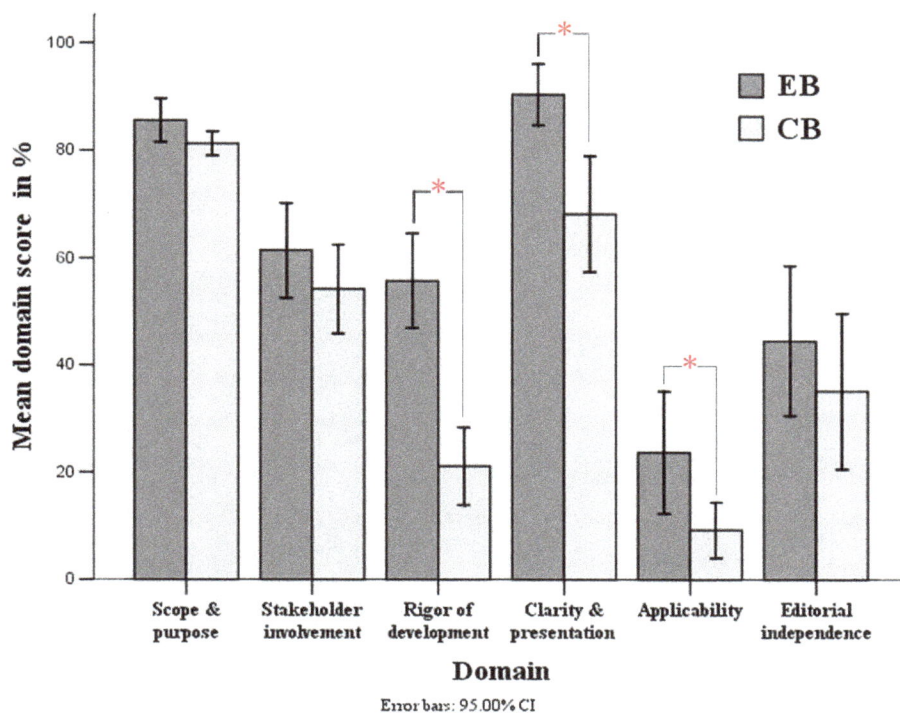

Figure 3. Comparison the difference between evidence-based (EB) and consensus-based (CB) guidelines in each domain. There were significantly difference between groups in domain of rigor of development, clarity & presentation and applicability with p<0.05. However, the other domains showed no significant difference between groups. *: p<0.05.

that the guideline-developing committee should summarize evidence in simple, transparent and informative SoF tables and evidence profiles that provide detailed information about the reason for the quality of evidence rating [62].

Before developing a guideline, it is necessary to limit funding sources coming from industries or other institutions, or provide a formal process for discussion and public disclosure of financial COIs for authors [61,63,64]. When developing or updating guidelines, the AGREE II instrument is a tool that provides the methodological strategy and standard procedure [9]. When considering guideline recommendations, however, high-quality evidence (i.e., RCTs) should not always be blindly pursued [53]. Patient and societal values or preferences should be considered and incorporated with the evidence to formulate final recommendations [53,62].

Limitations

The study is based on published guidelines in Chinese and English journals. However, most institutions have local guidelines or rely on national guidelines (i.e., those published in books, pamphlets and government documents), none of which is published. Thus the quality of guidelines used in most clinical settings might be of lower quality than published guidelines, hence causing some degree of selection bias. The AGREE II tool mainly focuses on methodology and quality of reporting, but not on the nature of the supporting evidence. Therefore, the quality of evidence on which the recommendations are based in the 'strongly recommended' guidelines still needs to be systematically reviewed and amended accordingly.

Conclusion

Although much progress has been achieved with respect to the quality of HCC and metastatic liver cancer guidelines, the overall methodological quality is moderate with poor applicability and potential conflict of interests (COIs). The evidence-based guidelines has become mainstream for high quality guideline development, such as the Japanese Ministry of Health (JMH) guideline, American Association for the Study of Liver Disease (AASLD), and European Association for the Study of Liver/European Organization for Research and Treatment of Cancer (EASL-EORTC) guideline; however, there is still a need to further increase transparency, quality of evidence rating, and the recommendation process and to address COIs issues.

Acknowledgement

The authors thanks Dr. Glund Christian for reviwing and modifying this work.

Author Contributions

Conceived and designed the experiments: YQW YPL SLD. Analyzed the data: YQW QQL HQW YPL SYW XLL. Wrote the paper: YQW QQL YPL HQW SYW.

References

1. Ferlay J, Shin HR, Bray F, Forman D, Mathers C, et al. (2010) GLOBOCAN 2008 v2.0,Cancer Incidence and Mortality Worldwise:IARC cancerBase No. 10[Internet]. http://globocan.iarc.fr. Accessed November 24, 2012.

2. Ferlay J, Shin HR, Bray F, Forman D, Mathers C, et al. (2010) Estimates of worldwide burden of cancer in 2008: GLOBOCAN 2008. *Int J Cance*;127(12):2893–2917.

3. Lang K, Danchenko N, Gondek K, Shah S, Thompson D (2009) The burden of illness associated with hepatocellular carcinoma in the United States. *J Hepatol* 50(1):89–99.

4. White LA, Menzin J, Korn JR, Friedman M, Lang K, et al. (2012) Medical care costs and survival associated with hepatocellular carcinoma among the elderly. *Clin Gastroenterol Hepatol* 10(5):547–554.

5. Field MJ, Lohr KN, eds. (1990) Clinical Practice Guidelines:directions for a new program. Washington,D.C.: Institute of Medicine.National Academy Press.

6. Woolf SH, Grol R, Hutchinson A, Eccles M, Grimshaw J (1999) Clinical guidelines: potential benefits, limitations, and harms of clinical guidelines. *BMJ* 318(7182):527–530.

7. Burls A.(2010) AGREE II-improving the quality of clinical care. *Lancet* 376(9747):1128–1129.

8. Brouwers MC, Kho ME, Browman GP, Burgers JS, Cluzeau F, et al. (2010) AGREE II: advancing guideline development, reporting, and evaluation in health care. *Prev Med* 51(5):421–424.

9. AGREE Next Steps Consortium (2009) The AGREE II Intrument [Electronic version]. http://www.agreetrust.org.

10. Schmidt S, Follmann M, Malek N, Manns MP, Greten TF (2011) Critical appraisal of clinical practice guidelines for diagnosis and treatment of hepatocellular carcinoma. *J Gastroenterol Hepatol* 26(12):1779–1786.

11. Moher D, Liberati A, Tetzlaff J, Altman DG (2009) Preferred reporting items for systematic reviews and meta-analyses: the PRISMA statement. *PLoS Med* 6(7):e1000097.

12. Field AP (2005) Kendall's Coefficient of Concordance. *Encyclopedia of Statistics in Behavioral Science*: John Wiley & Sons, Ltd.

13. Devlin J, O'Grady J (1999) Indications for referral and assessment in adultliver transplantation: a clinical guideline. *Gut* 45:1–22.

14. Ryder SD (2003) Guidelines for the diagnosis and treatment of hepatocellular carcinoma (HCC) in adults. *Gut* 52 Suppl 3:iii1–8.

15. Bruix J, Sherman M (2005) Management of hepatocellular carcinoma. *Hepatology* 42(5):1208–1236.

16. Murray KF, Carithers RL (2005) AASLD practice guidelines: Evaluation of the patient for liver transplantation. *Hepatology* 41(6):1407–1432.

17. O'Grady J, Taylor C, Brook G (2005) Guidelines for liver transplantation in patients with HIV infection(2005). *HIV Med* 6:149–153.

18. Parikh P, Malhotra H, Jelic S (2008) Hepatocellular carcinoma: ESMO clinical recommendations for diagnosis, treatment and follow-up. *Ann Oncol* 19 Suppl 2:ii27–28.

19. Knox J, Cosby R, Chan K, Sherman M (2008) Sorafenib for Advanced Hepatocellular Carcinoma. Toronto: Cancer Care Ontario (CCO).

20. Makuuchi M, Kokudo N, Arii S, Futagawa S, Kaneko S,et al. (2008) Development of evidence-based clinical guidelines for the diagnosis and treatment of hepatocellular carcinoma in Japan. *Hepatol Res* 38(1):37–51.

21. Poon D, Anderson BO, Chen LT, Tanaka K,Lau WY, et al. (2009) Management of hepatocellular carcinoma in Asia: consensus statement from the Asian Oncology Summit 2009. *Lancet Oncol* 10(11):1111–1118.

22. Benson AB 3rd, Abrams TA, Ben-Josef E, Bloomston PM, Botha JF, et al. (2009) NCCN clinical practice guidelines in oncology: hepatobiliary cancers. *J Natl Compr Canc Netw* 7(4):350–391.

23. Jelic S, Sotiropoulos GC (2010) Hepatocellular carcinoma: ESMO Clinical Practice Guidelines for diagnosis, treatment and follow-up. *Ann Oncol* 21 Suppl 5:v59–64.

24. Omata M, Lesmana LA, Tateishi R, Chen PJ, Lin SM, et al. (2010) Asian Pacific Association for the Study of the Liver consensus recommendations on hepatocellular carcinoma. *Hepatol Int* 4(2):439–474.

25. Bruix J, Sherman M (2011) Management of hepatocellular carcinoma: an update. *Hepatology* 53(3):1020–1022.

26. National Institute for Health and Clinical Excellence (2012) NICE technology appraisal guidance 189: Sorafenib for the treatment of advanced hepatocellular carcinoma. London.

27. Peck-Radosavljevic M, Sieghart W, Kolblinger C, Reiter M, Schindl M, et al. (2012) Austrian Joint OGGH-OGIR-OGHO-ASSO position statement on the use of transarterial chemoembolization (TACE) in hepatocellular carcinoma. *Wiener Klinische Wochenschrift* 124(3–4):104–110.

28. Llovet JM, Ducreux M, Lencioni R, Di Bisceglie AM, Galle PR, et al. (2012) EASL-EORTC Clinical Practice Guidelines: Management of hepatocellular carcinoma. *J Hepatol* 56(4):908–943.

29. Abdo AA, Hassanainh M, AlJumah A, Al Olayan A, Sanai FM, et al. (2012) Saudi Guidelines for the Diagnosis and Management of Hepatocellular Carcinoma: Technical Review and Practice Guidelines. *Ann Saudi Med* 32(2):174–199.

30. Garden OJ, Rees M, Poston GJ, Mirza D, Saunders M, et al. (2006) Guidelines for resection of colorectal cancer liver metastases. *Gut* 55 Suppl 3:iii1–8.

31. Bipat S, van Leeuwen MS, Ijzermans JN, Comans EF, Planting AS, et al. (2007) Evidence-based guideline on management of colorectal liver metastases in the Netherlands. *Neth J Med* 65(1):5–14.

32. Xu J, Qin X, Wang J, Zhang S, Zhong Y, et al. (2011) Chinese guidelines for the diagnosis and comprehensive treatment of hepatic metastasis of colorectal cancer. *J Cancer Res Clin Oncol* 137(9):1379–1396.

33. Bruix J, Sherman M, Llovet JM, Beaugrand M, Lencioni R, et al. (2001) Clinical management of hepatocellular carcinoma. Conclusions of the Barcelona-2000 EASL conference. European Association for the Study of the Liver. *J Hepatol* 35(3):421–430.

34. Van Vlierberghe H, Borbath I, Delwaide J, Henrion J, Michielsen P, et al. (2004) BASL guidelines for the surveillance, diagnosis and treatment of hepatocellular carcinoma. *Acta Gastroenterol Belg* 67(1):14–25.

35. Kudo M, Okanoue T (2007) Management of hepatocellular carcinoma in Japan: Consensus-based clinical practice manual proposed by the Japan Society of Hepatology. *Oncology* 72:2–15.

36. Ye SL (2009) [Expert consensus on standardization of the management of primary liver cancer][Article in Chinese]. *Zhonghua Gan Zang Bing Za Zhi* 17(6):403–410.

37. Arii S, Sata M, Sakamoto M, Shimada M, Kumada T, et al. (2010) Management of hepatocellular carcinoma: Report of Consensus Meeting in the 45th Annual Meeting of the Japan Society of Hepatology (2009). *Hepatol Res* 40(7):667–685.

38. Kaneko S, Furuse J, Kudo M, Ikeda K, Honda M, et al. (2012) Guideline on the use of new anticancer drugs for the treatment of Hepatocellular Carcinoma 2010 update. *Hepatol Res* 42(6):523–542.

39. Kennedy A, Nag S, Salem R, Murthy R, McEwan AJ, et al. (2007) Recommendations for radioembolization of hepatic malignancies using yttrium-90 microsphere brachytherapy: a consensus panel report from the radioembolization brachytherapy oncology consortium. *Int J Radiat Oncol Biol Phys* 68(1):13–23.

40. Steinmuller T, Kianmanesh R, Falconi M, Scarpa A, Taal B, et al. (2008) Consensus guidelines for the management of patients with liver metastases from digestive (neuro)endocrine tumors: foregut, midgut, hindgut, and unknown primary. *Neuroendocrinology* 87(1):47–62.

41. Pavel M, Baudin E, Couvelard A, Krenning E, Oberg K, et al. (2012) ENETS Consensus Guidelines for the Management of Patients with Liver and Other Distant Metastases from Neuroendocrine Neoplasms of Foregut, Midgut, Hindgut, and Unknown Primary. *Neuroendocrinology* 95(2):157–176.

42. Chinese Medical Association of Gastrointestinal and Colorectal Surgery Group, Chinese Anti-Cancer Association of Colorectal Cancer. (2010)Guidelines for the diagnosis and management of colorectal cancer liver metastases (V2010) [Article in Chinese]. *Chin J Gastrointest Surg* 13(6):457–470.

43. Izumi N (2010) Diagnostic and treatment algorithm of the Japanese society of hepatology: a consensus-based practice guideline. *Oncology* 78 Suppl 1:78–86.

44. Kudo M (2010) Real practice of hepatocellular carcinoma in Japan: conclusions of the Japan Society of Hepatology 2009 Kobe Congress. *Oncology* 78 Suppl 1:180–188.

45. Kudo M, Izumi N, Kokudo N, Matsui O, Sakamoto M, et al. (2011) Management of hepatocellular carcinoma in Japan: Consensus-Based Clinical Practice Guidelines proposed by the Japan Society of Hepatology (JSH) 2010 updated version. *Dig dis* 29(3):339–364.

46. Abad A, Figueras J, Valls C, Carrato A, Pardo F, et al. (2007)mGuidelines for the detection and treatment of liver metastases of colorectal cancer. *Clin transl oncol* 9(11):723–730.

47. Abdalla EK, Bauer TW, Chun YS, D'Angelica M, Kooby DA, et al. (2013) Locoregional surgical and interventional therapies for advanced colorectal cancer liver metastases: expert consensus statements. *HPB(Oxford)* 15(2):119–130.

48. Ferenci P, Fried M, Labrecque D, Bruix J, Sherman M, et al. (2010) World Gastroenterology Organisation Guideline. Hepatocellular carcinoma (HCC): a global perspective. *J gastrointestin liver dis* 19(3):311–317.

49. Giammarile F, Bodei L, Chiesa C, Flux G, Forrer F, et al. (2011) EANM procedure guideline for the treatment of liver cancer and liver metastases with intra-arterial radioactive compounds. *Eur J Nucl Med Mol Imaging* 38(7):1393–1406.

50. Prasad KR, Young RS, Burra P, Zheng SS, Mazzaferro V, et al. (2011) Summary of candidate selection and expanded criteria for liver transplantation for hepatocellular carcinoma: a review and consensus statement. *Liver transpl* 17 Suppl 2:S81–89.

51. Samuel D, Colombo M, El-Serag H, Sobesky R, Heaton N (2011) Toward optimizing the indications for orthotopic liver transplantation in hepatocellular carcinoma. *Liver transpl* 17 Suppl 2:S6–13.

52. Schwarz RE, Berlin JD, Lenz HJ, Nordlinger B, Rubbia-Brandt L, et al. (2013) Systemic cytotoxic and biological therapies of colorectal liver metastases: expert consensus statement. *HPB(Oxford)* 15(2):106–115.

53. McAlister FA, van Diepen S, Padwal RS, Johnson JA, Majumdar SR (2007) How evidence-based are the recommendations in evidence-based guidelines? *PLoS Med* 4(8):e250.

54. Alonso-Coello P, Irfan A, Sola I, Gich I, Delgado-Noguera M, et al. (2010) The quality of clinical practice guidelines over the last two decades: a systematic review of guideline appraisal studies. *Qual Saf Health Care* 19(6):e58.

55. Grilli R, Magrini N, Penna A, Mura G, Liberati A (2000) Practice guidelines developed by specialty societies: the need for a critical appraisal. *Lancet* 355(9198):103–106.

56. Rosenfeld RM, Shiffman RN, Robertson P (2013) Clinical practice guideline development manual, third edition: a quality-driven approach for translating evidence into action. *Otolaryngol Head Neck Surg* 148(1 Suppl):S1–S55.

57. Zheng ZH, Cui SQ, Lu XQ, Zakus D, Liang WN, et al. (2012) Analysis of the status of Chinese clinical practice guidelines development. *BMC Health Serv Res* 12:218.

58. Chen YL, Yao L, Xiao XJ, Wang Q, Wang ZH, et al. (2012) Quality assessment of clinical guidelines in China: 1993–2010. *Chin Med J (Engl)* 125(20):3660–3664.

59. Cluzeau F, Wedzicha JA, Kelson M, Corn J, Kunz R, et al. (2012) Stakeholder Involvement: How to Do It Right: Article 9 in Integrating and Coordinating Efforts in COPD Guideline Development. An Official ATS/ERS Workshop Report. *Proc Am Thorac Soc* 9(5):269–273.

60. Neuman J, Korenstein D, Ross JS, Keyhani S (2011) Prevalence of financial conflicts of interest among panel members producing clinical practice guidelines in Canada and United States: cross sectional study. *BMJ* 343:d5621.

61. Choudhry NK, Stelfox HT, Detsky AS (2002) Relationships between authors of clinical practice guidelines and the pharmaceutical industry. *JAMA* 287(5):612–617.

62. Guyatt G, Oxman AD, Akl EA, Kunz R, Vist G, et al. (2011) GRADE guidelines: 1. Introduction-GRADE evidence profiles and summary of findings tables. *J Clin Epidemiol* 64(4):383–394.

63. Campbell EG (2010) Public disclosure of conflicts of interest: moving the policy debate forward. *Arch Intern Med* 170(8):667.

64. Scott IA, Guyatt GH (2011) Clinical practice guidelines: the need for greater transparency in formulating recommendations. *Med J Aust* 195(1):29–33.

17

Longitudinal Brain White Matter Alterations in Minimal Hepatic Encephalopathy before and after Liver Transplantation

Wei-Che Lin[1], Kun-Hsien Chou[2], Chao-Long Chen[3], Hsiu-Ling Chen[1,4], Cheng-Hsien Lu[5], Shau-Hsuan Li[6], Chu-Chung Huang[4], Ching-Po Lin[2,4], Yu-Fan Cheng[1]*

1 Department of Diagnostic Radiology, Kaohsiung Chang Gung Memorial Hospital and Chang Gung University College of Medicine, Kaohsiung, Taiwan, 2 Brain Research Center, National Yang-Ming University, Taipei, Taiwan, 3 Department of Surgery, Kaohsiung Chang Gung Memorial Hospital and Chang Gung University College of Medicine, Kaohsiung, Taiwan, 4 Department of Biomedical Imaging and Radiological Sciences, National Yang-Ming University, Taipei, Taiwan, 5 Department of Neurology, Kaohsiung Chang Gung Memorial Hospital and Chang Gung University College of Medicine, Kaohsiung, Taiwan, 6 Department of Internal Medicine, Kaohsiung Chang Gung Memorial Hospital and Chang Gung University College of Medicine, Kaohsiung, Taiwan

Abstract

Cerebral edema is the common pathogenic mechanism for cognitive impairment in minimal hepatic encephalopathy. Whether complete reversibility of brain edema, cognitive deficits, and their associated imaging can be achieved after liver transplantation remains an open question. To characterize white matter integrity before and after liver transplantation in patients with minimal hepatic encephalopathy, multiple diffusivity indices acquired via diffusion tensor imaging was applied. Twenty-eight patients and thirty age- and sex-matched healthy volunteers were included. Multiple diffusivity indices were obtained from diffusion tensor images, including mean diffusivity, fractional anisotropy, axial diffusivity and radial diffusivity. The assessment was repeated 6–12 month after transplantation. Differences in white matter integrity between groups, as well as longitudinal changes, were evaluated using tract-based spatial statistical analysis. Correlation analyses were performed to identify first scan before transplantation and interval changes among the neuropsychiatric tests, clinical laboratory tests, and diffusion tensor imaging indices. After transplantation, decreased water diffusivity without fractional anisotropy change indicating reversible cerebral edema was found in the left anterior cingulate, claustrum, postcentral gyrus, and right corpus callosum. However, a progressive decrease in fractional anisotropy and an increase in radial diffusivity suggesting demyelination were noted in temporal lobe. Improved pre-transplantation albumin levels and interval changes were associated with better recoveries of diffusion tensor imaging indices. Improvements in interval diffusion tensor imaging indices in the right postcentral gyrus were correlated with visuospatial function score correction. In conclusion, longitudinal voxel-wise analysis of multiple diffusion tensor imaging indices demonstrated different white matter changes in minimal hepatic encephalopathy patients. Transplantation improved extracellular cerebral edema and the results of associated cognition tests. However, white matter demyelination may advance in temporal lobe.

Editor: Elizabeth J. Coulson, University of Queensland, Australia

Funding: Chang Gang Memorial Hospital (Chang Gang Medical Research Project CMRPG870482 to W.-C. Lin) and from the National Science Council (NSC 97-2314-B-182A-104-MY3 to W.-C. Lin). The funders had no role in study design, data collection and analysis, decision to publish, or preparation of the manuscript.

Competing Interests: The authors have declared that no competing interests exist.

* Email: cheng.yufan@msa.hinet.net

Introduction

Hepatic encephalopathy (HE) is frequently associated with a wide range of neuropsychiatric abnormalities in liver cirrhosis, and has been classified as a continuum from minimal HE (MHE) to different grades of overt HE. [1] It is believed that cerebral edema is the common pathogenic mechanism for cognitive impairment in MHE and overt HE. [2,3] Although patients with MHE present as essentially normal, such patients perform abnormally on psychometric tests and have an increased risk of motor vehicle accidents. Liver transplantation (LT) can correct liver function, resulting in an improvement symptom of MHE. [4] However, at least during the first 2 years after LT, some cognitive defects seem to persist to some degree. [5] Thus, whether complete reversibility of brain edema, cognitive deficits, and their associated imaging can be achieved remains an open question.

The MHE patients can experience persistent cognitive deficits after LT. [6] In addition, permanent brain injury with volume atrophy has been found in those with previous episode of overt HE. [6] Each of these observations suggests that cirrhosis may cause brain damage that persists after LT. Some prospective imaging studies have shown improvement in HE related brain edema [7,8] after treatment, with such improvement being primarily due to removal of interstitial type brain edema. [8] However, it is also common for cirrhotic patients to experience acute liver failure or overt HE accompanied by irreversible cytotoxic cerebral edema. [9] The interaction or evolution between two forms of cerebral edema complicates the interpretation of their effects on cognition outcomes after LT, a subject which has not been studied in depth before.

Diffusion tensor imaging (DTI) provides information about different direction of water mobility, as well as information about tissue microstructure and organization, through different quantitative DTI metrics. In quantitative terms, mean diffusivity (MD), an index of averaged diffusivity across three-dimensional space, and fractional anisotropy (FA), an index of the microstructural integrity of the brain's white matter (WM), have been widely used as quantitative metrics in previous studies. [10] Recently, the directional diffusivities, axial diffusivity ($D_{ax} = \lambda_1$) and radial diffusivity [$D_{rad} = (\lambda_2 + \lambda_3)/2$], have been used to demonstrate the advantage of obtaining additional information about the potential underlying pathophysiology of WM changes. Alterations in D_{ax} suggest the presence of axonal damage and/or Wallerian degeneration in the primary fiber orientation, [11] while increased D_{rad} implies demyelination or dysmyelination. [12] The widely used DTI indices, FA and MD, are associated with cognitive impairment in MHE patients before LT. [8,13] However, there are no reports of longitudinal neuro-imaging studies investigating changes in WM in MHE patients before and after LT through the use of multiple diffusion indices. There is a paucity of knowledge regarding the associations between clinical evaluations and the characteristics of WM integrity evolution in MHE patients receiving LT.

To elucidate the underlying WM microstructural changes occurring in MHE patients, we used voxel-wise analysis of multiple diffusivity indices before and after LT in this longitudinal study, and compared the results with data from healthy volunteers. We sought to determine (1) whether MHE patients show deterioration of WM integrity after LT by assessing multiple DTI indices (2) whether changes in WM integrity either affected by baseline or interval changes in liver functions after LT and (3) whether there is any correlation between WM integrity and cognitive performance before and after LT.

Materials and Methods

1. Participants

A consecutive series of patients with liver cirrhosis who were evaluated for LT were recruited to the study. The project was approved by Chang Gung Memorial Hospital's Institutional Review Committee on Human Research, and all subjects gave written informed consent before participating. All participants were informed that the study was designed to evaluate manifestations of MHE both before and at 6 to 12 months after LT.

The diagnosis of liver cirrhosis was based on a consistent clinical history, radiological studies, and liver biopsy when available. [8] Patient functional status was assessed using the Child-Pugh scoring system. [14] According to Ferenci's report, [15] MHE was evaluated by the Wechsler Adult Intelligence Scale III (WAIS-III) subtests, including the digit-symbol and block design subtests. [16] A test result was considered abnormal for the digit-symbol and block design subtests if it was 2 standard deviations below the mean score of normal subjects. Thirty age- and sex-matched normal subjects (19 men, 11 women; 52.80±9.77 years) without any medical history of neurological disease served as the control group and were recruited by advertisement within the hospital. The mean digit-symbol score for the normal controls was 57.28±13.52 and the block design score was 40.50±10.86. Therefore, cirrhotic patients with a digit-symbol score of 30 or lower or with a block design score lower than 19 were recognized as having MHE.

Laboratory screening, MRI scans, and neuropsychiatric tests were performed on the same day for all patients. Initially, 70 cirrhotic patients who completed the neuropsychological evaluation and MRI examinations were enrolled in the study. Participants were excluded if they were diagnosed with overt HE or produced normal neuropsychological tests results. Any history of drug abuse, psychiatric or neurological illness, head injury, or poor image quality with severe distortion and metallic artifacts that might compromise diffusion tensor image analysis was also grounds for exclusion.

Finally, 28 adult cirrhotic patients with MHE (24 men, 4 women; 51.14±8.38 years) were included in this study, and 42 patients were excluded (normal neuropsychiatric test results, $n = 29$; overt HE, $n = 9$; poor image quality, $n = 4$).

2. Neuropsychological tests

A battery of neuropsychological tests, which focused on attention, executive function, speech and language function, and visuo-construction function, was performed. Different domains of neuropsychological evaluations were measured by subtests from Cognitive Ability Screening Instrument (CASI), [17] WAIS-III [18] and Wisconsin Card Sorting Test (WCST-64, Computer Version Scoring Program). [19].

3. MRI data acquisition

Images were obtained using a 3.0-T whole body GE MR system (Signa, General Electric Healthcare, Milwaukee, WI, USA) with a standard eight-channel phase-array head coil. Participant head movement inside the coil was minimized immobilization with cushions. Whole brain DTI images were acquired using an axial single-shot spin-echo diffusion-weighted echo-planer imaging sequence, with array spatial sensitivity encoding to reduce susceptibility and eddy-current distortions. The DTI imaging parameters were as follows: repetition time (TR)/echo time (TE) = 15800/77 ms, number of excitations (NEX) = 3, field of view (FOV) = 256 mm^2, slice thickness = 2.5 mm, matrix dimensions = 128×128, 55 slices without gaps, b-value = 1000 s/mm^2, 13 non-collinear diffusion directions and a non-diffusion-weighted T2 images (b-value = 0 s/mm^2). The DTI session design was based on the balancing of diffusion gradients to minimize eddy-current artifacts.

Structural images were acquired using standard T1-weighted three-dimensional fluid-attenuated inversion recovery fast spoiled gradient-recalled echo pulse sequence with the following imaging parameters: TR/TE/TI = 9.5/3.9/450 ms; flip angle = 15 degrees; NEX = 1; field of view = 240*240 mm^2; slice thickness = 1.3 mm; matrix size = 512*512; voxel size = 0.47*0.47*1.3 mm^3 and 110 contiguous slices that aligned to the anterior commissure-posterior commissure.

Additional whole brain axial T2-weighted, and fluid-attenuated inversion-recovery fast-spin-echo sequences were applied to define anatomical details. One author blinded to participant status visually checked all MRI scans to confirm that the participants were free from morphological abnormalities. The total MRI scanning time was approximately 23 min for each participant. The mean duration between MRI acquisition at baseline and follow up for the patient group was 8.43 months (range: 6.5 to 12 months).

4. DTI data preprocessing and voxel-wise WM microstructure investigations

Image data was analyzed by a researcher with 8 years of experience in MRI research using FSL v5.0.4 (Functional

Table 1. Demographics, clinical characteristics, and cognitive test results of minimal hepatic encephalopathy patients and healthy controls.

	Control	Pre-transplantation	Post-transplantation	p-value	p-value	p-value
				NC vs Pre-LT	NC vs Post-LT	Pre-LT vs Post-LT
Number of subjects	30	28	28			
Age (years)	52.8±9.8	51.1±8.4	51.1±8.4	0.49	0.49	
Gender (male/female)	19/11	24/4	24/4	0.91	0.91	
Education (years)	11.6±4.1	10.7±3.4	10.7±3.4	0.34	0.34	
Previous hepatic encephalopathy (n)	–	15	15	–	–	
Child-Pugh's class: A/B/C (n)	–	0/17/9	0/17/9	–	–	
Biochemical parameters						
Prothrombin time (seconds)	–	13. 1±3.1	10.4±2.2	–	–	**<0.001**
Albumin (mg/dL)	–	3.4±0.5	4.2±0.5	–	–	**<0.001**
International Normalized Ratio (INR)	–	1.2±0.2	1.1±0.1	–	–	**<0.001**
AST(IU/L)	–	65.8±65.1	64.9±29.5	–	–	0.97
ALT(IU/L)	–	48.5±46.4	47.8±38.4	–	–	0.19
Total Bilirubin (mg/dL)	–	3.0±4.2	1.5±1.7	–	–	**0.04**
Direct Bilirubin (mg/dL)	–	1.6±2.9	0.7±0.2	–	–	0.13
Venous ammonia (μg/dL)	–	125.0±65.5	56.5±48.1	–	–	**<0.001**
Neuro-psychiatric tests						
Attention						
Mental control (CASI)	9.0±1.3	8.5±2.5	9.2±2.2	0.36	0.68	**0.03**
Attention (CASI)	7.7±0.7	7.4±0.8	7.6±0.7	0.10	0.43	0.16
Orientation (CASI)	17.8±0.5	16.8±2.5	17.8±0.6	0.06	0.89	0.05
Executive function						
Digit symbol (WAIS)	57.3±13.5	18.3±5.6	26.7±4.9	**0.004***	**0.010**	**0.006***
Abstraction (CASI)	10.7±1.4	8.7±1.8	9.1±2.2	**<0.001***	**0.001***	0.30
Number correct (WCST)	39.7±11.6	36.6±13.5	41.0±14.5	0.44	0.72	**0.018**
Total error (WCST)	24.4±11.6	27.4±13.5	23.0±14.5	0.44	0.72	**0.018**
Perseverative response (WCST)	12.0±6.2	15.0±11.7	13.0±13.9	0.24	0.73	0.16
Perseverative error (WCST)	11.4±5.4	12.6±8.9	11.2±10.2	0.53	0.93	0.24
Non-perseverative error (WCST)	14.3±10.0	14.5±12.0	11.8±10.9	0.98	0.34	0.10
Conceptual level responses (WCST)	43.6±22.4	44.2±27.7	40.20±35.2	0.85	0.77	**0.04**
Category (WCST)	2.2±1.4	2.0±1.6	2.3±1.6	0.61	0.68	0.10
Memory function						
Long-term memory (CASI)	9.9±0.4	9.6±2.5	9.7±1.3	0.52	0.31	0.88
Short-term memory (CASI)	10.8±1.5	10.1±1.9	10.3±2.5	0.13	0.48	0.69
Speech and Language function						
Language(CASI)	10.1±1.5	9.9±0.4	9.7±1.1	0.40	0.26	0.42
Verbal fluency (CASI)	8.5±1.6	8.2±2.1	8.0±2.3	0.56	0.26	0.43
Visuospatial function						
Picture completion (WAIS)	15.6±5.4	13.2±5.8	14.7±5.9	0.12	0.54	**0.007***
Letter number search (WAIS)	65.2±22.0	49.6±21.3	60.7±19.7	**0.01**	0.40	**<0.001***
Block design (WAIS)	40.5±10.9	29.3±12.0	37.3±11.2	**0.04**	0.36	**0.009***
Drawing (CASI)	9.6±1.4	9.6±1.0	9.4±2.0	0.98	0.85	0.69
CASI total score	94.2±4.6	88.9±11.4	91.1±11.5	**0.02**	0.16	**0.02**

Demographic data, including age and sex, were compared among the study groups using the two-sample Student's *t* test, Pearson's chi-squared test, and paired *t* test, where appropriate, and are reported as means ± standard deviation (SD).
Abbreviations: WASI, Wechsler Abbreviated Scale of Intelligence; CASI, Cognitive Ability Screening Instrument.
Statistical threshold was set at *p*<0.05 (Boldface).
*Stand for the appropriate test passed the statistical criteria set at corrected P$_{false-discovery-rate}$ <0.05.

Magnetic Resonance Imaging software obtained from the Brain Software Library; http://fsl.fmrib.ox.ac.uk/fsl/fslwiki/). [20]

Each diffusion-weighted image was affine registered to the non-diffusion-weighted image to correct the head motion and eddy-

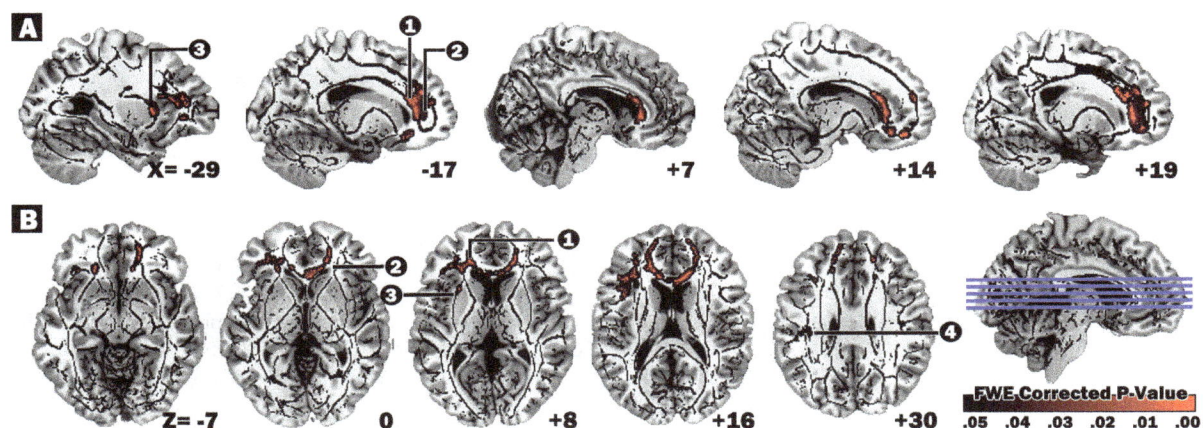

Figure 1. Regions showing significant reductions in axial diffusivity in follow-up scan compared with baseline scan. Regions with decreased axial diffusivity after LT (threshold-free cluster enhancement corrected for multiple comparisons at $P_{FWE} <.05$). Number 1, Left anterior cingulate; number 2, Right anterior cingulate; number 3, Left claustrum; number 4, Left Postcentral Gyrus; Red maps indicate the degree of the corrected p-value. Anatomical changes are superimposed on the mean WM skeleton and on the T1 template located in MNI space in (A) sagittal and (B) axial views. We used the tbss_fill script to aid visualization. The numbers in the lower right corner of each image represent the MNI (A) x- and (B) z-coordinates respectively. Abbreviations: FWE, family-wise error; MNI, Montreal Neurological Institute.

current distortion. To further minimize motion effects in DTI estimation, each applied gradient direction of the diffusion-weighted image was reoriented to the corresponding transformation matrix that described the rotation parameters of subject motion. [21] After skull stripping, diffusion indices were calculated by fitting a tensor model using FMRIB's Diffusion Toolbox. Longitudinal voxel-wise analysis of WM microstructure was performed using Tract-based Spatial-Statistic (TBSS), [22] which has been described in detail in previous study. [23] First, all subjects' FA maps were non-linearly warped to the Montreal Neurological Institute (MNI) space FMRIB58_FA template using FMRIB's nonlinear registration tool. Next, MNI space FA maps were averaged and thinned to generate a mean FA skeleton; we defined the WM skeleton threshold at an FA value greater than 0.2 to further reduce the partial volume effects. Each individual's MNI space FA map was projected onto the mean threshold skeleton and the resulting data were subsequently fed into the statistical analysis framework. The same registration procedures were applied to MD, D_{ax}, and D_{rad}. An experienced neuroradiologist visually checked all warped indices to ensure the accuracy of the whole automatic image-preprocessing pipeline.

5. Group comparisons of T1 DARTEL VBM

T1 voxel based morphometry (VBM) with the diffeomorphic anatomical registration through exponentiated lie algebra (DARTEL) registration scheme was used for investigating gray matter (GM) volume changes between study groups. [24,25] Individual T1 scan were analyzed with the VBM8 toolbox (http://dbm. neuro.uni-jena.de) with default settings under Statistical Parametric Mapping (SPM8; Wellcome Institute of Neurology, University College London, UK). The detailed T1 DARTEL VBM pipeline was the same with previous published study from our groups. [26] In briefly, T1 structural scans were bias-corrected, tissue segmented [segmented into GM, WM and cerebrospinal fluid (CSF) compartments], and spatial normalized to MNI space using affine and high dimensional DARTEL registration approach. To conserve the total amount of GM before and after spatial normalization, the nonlinear deformation parameters of the spatial normalization procedure were used to modulate the GM tissue segments and resized voxel sizes to $1.5 \times 1.5 \times 1.5$ mm^3. This

non-linear only modulation procedure allow us to make inferences on regional GM volume measurements rather than tissue density (concentration) and further ensure that statistical comparisons are made on relative (controlling for overall brain size) rather than absolute volumes. The resultant MNI space modulated GM segments were smoothed with a Gaussian kernel of 8 mm full-width Gaussian kernel at half-maximum (FWHM) and served as inputs for further voxel-wised group comparisons in GM volume.

The longitudinal T1 DARTEL VBM preprocessing module with default setting in the VBM8 toolbox was used for investigating the longitudinal GM volume changes before and after liver transplantation in patients with cirrhotic. The following preprocessing steps were used in this analysis: (1) the follow-up measurement scan was registered to the baseline measurement scan for each participants; (2) the mean T1 anatomical scan were calculated from the realigned images from previous step of each participant and served as a reference image for subsequent spatial registration; (3) intra-subject bias correction for each time-point realigned T1 anatomical scans were performed with regard to the reference mean image; (4) the bias-corrected mean anatomical scan and realigned scans were segmented into GM, WM and CSF respectively; (5) spatial normalization parameter of DARTEL registration algorithm were estimated using the tissue segments (GM and WM) of the bias-corrected mean anatomical scan; (6) the DARTEL normalization parameters were applied to the GM tissue segments of bias-corrected realigned anatomical scan for each time-point. Finally, the resulting MNI space GM tissue segments were smoothed with 8 mm FWHM Gaussian kernel which was also used in the previous cross-sectional analysis.

6. Statistical analysis

All statistical analyses of demographic data were performed using the SPSS (version 12, SPSS Inc., Chicago, IL, USA) with appropriate tests. Age and sex were compared between the study groups by the independent t-test and Pearson's Chi-square test. Laboratory data were compared between the patient groups before and after LT by the pair t-test. The neuropsychological tests were compared between groups by using independent t-test or the pair t-test with correcting the multiple comparison problem using

Table 2. Regions of longitudinal changes in white matter microstructure between baseline and follow-up scan in MHE patients.

Decreased D_{ax} in follow up vs. baseline scan

| MNI atlas coordinates | | | Voxels size | White matter tract | Corresponding cortical area | D_{ax} mean (SD) | | Z_{max} | Other DTI indices (follow up–baseline) | | |
X	Y	Z				Baseline	Follow up		FA	MD	D_{rad}
-18	36	10	1716	Left Limbic Lobe, Anterior Cingulate	Anterior Cingulate, BA32	1.27 (0.08)	1.24 (0.08)	4.32	0.00	-25	-18
19	38	4	1050	Right Frontal Lobe, Corpus Callosum	Anterior Cingulate, BA32	1.18 (0.09)	1.12 (0.07)	4.32	0.00	**-27***	-15
-28	13	5	63	Left Sub-lober, Extra-Nuclear	Claustrum	1.26 (0.06)	1.20 (0.06)	5.55	0.00	**-35***	-23
-36	-23	27	35	Left Sub-lober, Extra-Nuclear	Postcentral Gyrus, BA2	1.47 (0.05)	1.42 (0.05)	4.81	0.00	**-27***	-17

Mean D_{ax} values were directly obtained from clusters showing significant changes between baseline and follow-up scan. Z_{max} values represent TFCE FWE-corrected clusters (p<.05). Multiple brain atlases implemented in FSL were used to define anatomical regions of significant clusters after statistical comparisons. Diffusivity values corresponding to each cluster with significant longitudinal changes are represented as differences (baseline – follow up) in MD and D_{rad} (mm²/s) multiplied by a factor of 10⁶. Boldfaced diffusivity values with "*" represent significant differences (P<.05, Bonferroni-adjusted) between baseline and follow-up scans.
Abbreviations: FA, fractional anisotropy; MNI, Montreal Neurological Institute; SD, standard deviation; DTI, diffusion-tensor imaging; D_{ax}, axial diffusivity; MD, mean diffusivity; D_{rad}, radial diffusivity; BA, Brodmann area; TFCE, threshold-free cluster enhancement; FWE, family-wise error.

false discovery rate (FDR). The statistical significant level for neuropsychological tests were set as corrected P_{FDR} <0.05.

Group comparisons of diffusion tensor index. For image-based voxel-wise analysis, non-parametric permutation-based statistical analyses were performed to investigate regional WM changes between baseline and follow-up scans of the patient and control group (analysis of covariance model with age and sex as covariates of no interest), and the longitudinal changes before and after LT in the MHE group (paired t test). 5000 permutations were used for each possible statistical contrast, and the results were corrected for multiple comparisons across space using a threshold-free cluster enhancement (TFCE) approach with family wised error (FWE) corrected P value <0.05. [27] Mean DTI indices representing each significant cluster were calculated for each participant and further correlated to clinical evaluations. Data was adjusted for age and sex, and the relationships between regional diffusivity indices, cognitive function, and laboratory test results were investigated using partial Pearson correlation analysis. After Bonferroni correction for the number of ROIs, the significance threshold for the two-tailed partial correlation tests was set to a p-value of less than 0.05 (the p-values were adjusted for the number of regions by a factor of 5, similar to an uncorrected p = 0.05/5).

Group comparisons of gray matter volume. To ensure that statistical thresholds in T1 DARTEL VBM and DTI TBSS analysis were comparable, the smoothed modulated GM segments were also analyzed using the same statistical design and statistical criteria with a framework of permutation-based non- parametric testing using FSL v5.0.4. The cluster-wised statistic with TFCE clustering approach which used in the DTI-TBSS analysis was used again to determine clusters with significant GM volume changes, and FWE corrected *P value* <0.05 was used to correct for multiple comparisons across space.

Results

1. Clinical characteristics

LT significantly corrected liver function in MHE patients, including prothrombin time (p<0.001), International Normalized Ratio ratio (p<0.001), concentration of albumin (p<0.001), total bilirubin (p = 0.04), and venous ammonia (p<0.001) (Table 1).

2. Neuropsychological performance

2.1 Differences in cognition performance between MHE and controls before LT. The MHE patient group exhibited significantdisturbances in executive function (Digit symbol, p = 0.004; Abstraction, p<0.001). We also found a worse performance of visuospatial function (Letter-number search, p = 0.01; Block design, p = 0.04) and the CASI global performance score (p = 0.02) but was not survived with correcting for multiple comparisons (FDR<0.05). The group also displayed a trend of lower attention, memory, and language function scores.

2.2 Differences in cognition performance between MHE and controls after LT. After LT, the MHE patients presented with poorer executive function in the abstraction test (p = 0.001) compared to healthy subjects. The MHE group also had a trend of lower memory and language function.

2.3 Longitudinal changes of cognition performance in MHE patients. Longitudinal comparison after LT showed significant improvements in executive function (digit-symbol test, p = 0.006), and visuospatial function (picture completion, p = 0.007; letter-number search p<0.001; block design, p = 0.009).

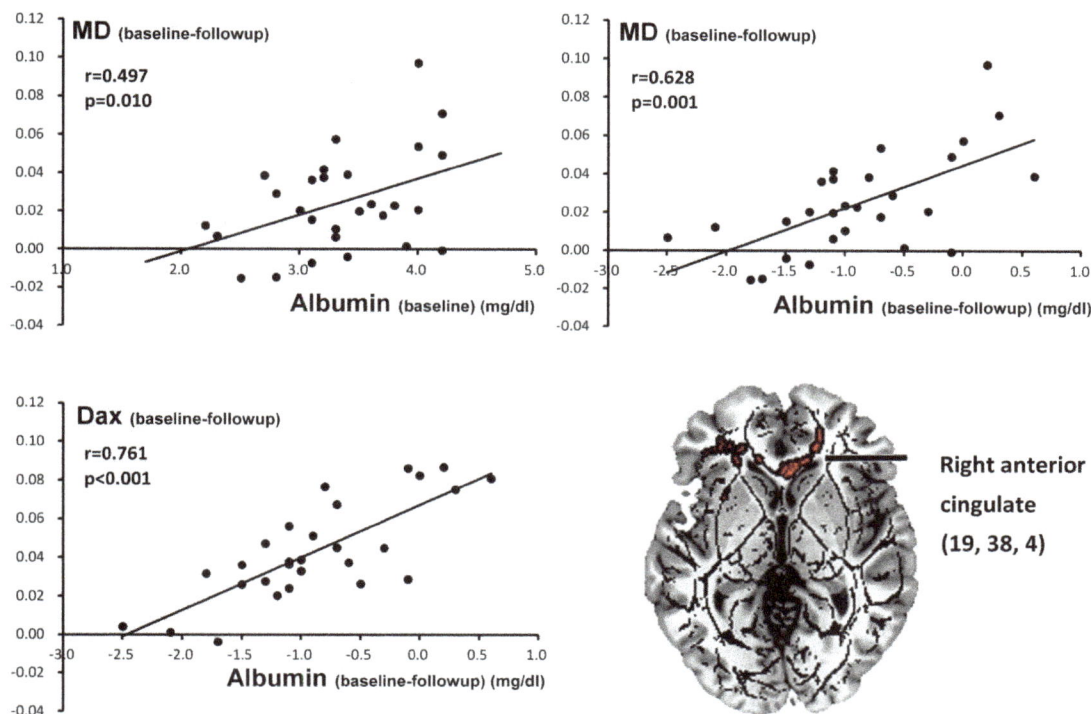

Figure 3. Correlation between albumin level and DTI indices before and after LT. Pearson correlation between interval albumin changes and diffusivity values [D_{ax} and MD, $(mm^2/s) \times 10^6$] of clusters derived from the comparison of MHE before and after LT. Abbreviations: D_{ax}, axial diffusivity; MD, mean diffusivity.

In the present study, we interpreted decreased FA and increased D_{rad} in the temporal lobe, without changes in D_{ax}, as demyelination and gliosis, consistent with histological findings. [31] The WM in MHE patients might present with mixed effects, [30] from longstandingvasogenic edema secondary to cirrhosis, episodic acute cytotoxic edema, secondary to hyperammonemic decompensation and/or neurotoxicity effect from immunosuppressive agent.

In the present study, the changes in WM integrity were as subtle as the cognition deficits in MHE patients when compared with healthy subjects. The healthy condition in patients with minimal HE is quite good showing limited cognitive decline before operation. This is somewhat reasonable that we could not find any difference between the patient group and healthy controls with the conservative statistical threshold. We reported more strictly statistical criteria which may increase specificity, but also reduces the sensitivity necessary for detecting subtle temporal changes in WM. In addition, cerebrovascular small-vessel degeneration in the temporal lobe and other WM could not be totally excluded in MHE [39] because an interval-imaging study was not performed on the normal groups, however, changes in the WM of healthy participants over a short duration can be limited.

Conclusions

Our longitudinal voxel-wise multiple DTI indices study revealed various WM changes, including improvement of the extracellular cerebral edema and of the demyelination of vulnerable WM that occur in MHE patients accepting liver transplantation. DTI may be useful for investigating the pathogenesis of MHE for adequate interpretation of cognitive impairment and for assessing the

efficacy of therapeutic measures focused on correcting this disorder.

Supporting Information

Figure S1 Regions showing significant gray matter volume changes between cirrhotic patients before/after liver transplantation, and healthy subjects. Different color maps show the cluster-level statistics with the FWE-corrected p values of the corresponding group comparison using TFCE approach. (a), (b) and (c) shows regions of significant gray matter volume changes in cirrhotic patients before/after liver transplantation compared with the NC group. (d) and (e) shows regions of significant longitudinal gray matter volume changes between cirrhotic patients before and after liver transplantation. All of the above results are displayed at the MNI T1 template. Abbreviation: FWE: family-wise error; L: left; MNI: Montreal Neurological Institute; NC: normal control; R: right; TFCE: threshold-free cluster enhancement.

Acknowledgments

The authors acknowledge MR support from the MRI Core Facility in Kaohsiung Chang Gung Memorial Hospital and all subjects who participated in this study.

Author Contributions

Conceived and designed the experiments: WCL YFC CLC. Performed the experiments: WCL HLC CHL. Analyzed the data: WCL KHC CCH. Contributed reagents/materials/analysis tools: CLC SHL. Contributed to the writing of the manuscript: WCL CPL YFC.

References

1. Bajaj JS, Wade JB, Sanyal AJ (2009) Spectrum of neurocognitive impairment in cirrhosis: Implications for the assessment of hepatic encephalopathy. Hepatology 50: 2014–2021.
2. Donovan JP, Schafer DF, Shaw BW, Jr., Sorrell MF (1998) Cerebral oedema and increased intracranial pressure in chronic liver disease. Lancet 351: 719–721.
3. Lin WC, Hsu TW, Chen CL, Wu CW, Lu CH, et al. (2012) Connectivity of default-mode network is associated with cerebral edema in hepatic encephalopathy. PLoS One 7: e36986.
4. Mattarozzi K, Stracciari A, Vignatelli L, D'Alessandro R, Morelli MC, et al. (2004) Minimal hepatic encephalopathy: longitudinal effects of liver transplantation. Arch Neurol 61: 242–247.
5. Mattarozzi K, Cretella L, Guarino M, Stracciari A (2012) Minimal hepatic encephalopathy: follow-up 10 years after successful liver transplantation. Transplantation 93: 639–643.
6. Garcia-Martinez R, Rovira A, Alonso J, Jacas C, Simon-Talero M, et al. (2011) Hepatic encephalopathy is associated with posttransplant cognitive function and brain volume. Liver Transpl 17: 38–46.
7. Rovira A, Grive E, Pedraza S, Alonso J (2001) Magnetization transfer ratio values and proton MR spectroscopy of normal-appearing cerebral white matter in patients with liver cirrhosis. AJNR Am J Neuroradiol 22: 1137–1142.
8. Kale RA, Gupta RK, Saraswat VA, Hasan KM, Trivedi R, et al. (2006) Demonstration of interstitial cerebral edema with diffusion tensor MR imaging in type C hepatic encephalopathy. Hepatology 43: 698–706.
9. Saksena S, Rai V, Saraswat VA, Rathore RS, Purwar A, et al. (2008) Cerebral diffusion tensor imaging and in vivo proton magnetic resonance spectroscopy in patients with fulminant hepatic failure. J Gastroenterol Hepatol 23: e111–119.
10. Basser PJ (1995) Inferring microstructural features and the physiological state of tissues from diffusion-weighted images. NMR Biomed 8: 333–344.
11. Song SK, Sun SW, Ju WK, Lin SJ, Cross AH, et al. (2003) Diffusion tensor imaging detects and differentiates axon and myelin degeneration in mouse optic nerve after retinal ischemia. Neuroimage 20: 1714–1722.
12. Song SK, Yoshino J, Le TQ, Lin SJ, Sun SW, et al. (2005) Demyelination increases radial diffusivity in corpus callosum of mouse brain. Neuroimage 26: 132–140.
13. Kumar R, Gupta RK, Elderkin-Thompson V, Huda A, Sayre J, et al. (2008) Voxel-based diffusion tensor magnetic resonance imaging evaluation of low-grade hepatic encephalopathy. J Magn Reson Imaging 27: 1061–1068.
14. Pugh RN, Murray-Lyon IM, Dawson JL, Pietroni MC, Williams R (1973) Transection of the oesophagus for bleeding oesophageal varices. Br J Surg 60: 646–649.
15. Ferenci P, Lockwood A, Mullen K, Tarter R, Weissenborn K, et al. (2002) Hepatic encephalopathy–definition, nomenclature, diagnosis, and quantification: final report of the working party at the 11th World Congresses of Gastroenterology, Vienna, 1998. Hepatology 35: 716–721.
16. Das A, Dhiman RK, Saraswat VA, Verma M, Naik SR (2001) Prevalence and natural history of subclinical hepatic encephalopathy in cirrhosis. J Gastroenterol Hepatol 16: 531–535.
17. Teng EL, Hasegawa K, Homma A, Imai Y, Larson E, et al. (1994) The Cognitive Abilities Screening Instrument (CASI): a practical test for cross-cultural epidemiological studies of dementia. Int Psychogeriatr 6: 45–58; discussion 62.
18. Wechsler D (1981) Wechsler adult intelligence scale. New York: Psychological Cooperation.
19. Nyhus E, Barcelo F (2009) The Wisconsin Card Sorting Test and the cognitive assessment of prefrontal executive functions: a critical update. Brain Cogn 71: 437–451.
20. Jenkinson M, Beckmann CF, Behrens TE, Woolrich MW, Smith SM (2012) Fsl. Neuroimage 62: 782–790.
21. Leemans A, Jones DK (2009) The B-matrix must be rotated when correcting for subject motion in DTI data. Magn Reson Med 61: 1336–1349.
22. Smith SM, Jenkinson M, Johansen-Berg H, Rueckert D, Nichols TE, et al. (2006) Tract-based spatial statistics: voxelwise analysis of multi-subject diffusion data. Neuroimage 31: 1487–1505.
23. Barrick TR, Charlton RA, Clark CA, Markus HS (2010) White matter structural decline in normal ageing: a prospective longitudinal study using tract-based spatial statistics. Neuroimage 51: 565–577.
24. Ashburner J (2007) A fast diffeomorphic image registration algorithm. Neuroimage 38: 95–113.
25. Ashburner J, Friston KJ (2000) Voxel-based morphometry–the methods. Neuroimage 11: 805–821.
26. Yang FC, Chou KH, Fuh JL, Lee PL, Lirng JF, et al. (2014) Altered hypothalamic functional connectivity in cluster headache: a longitudinal resting-state functional MRI study. J Neurol Neurosurg Psychiatry.
27. Smith SM, Nichols TE (2009) Threshold-free cluster enhancement: addressing problems of smoothing, threshold dependence and localisation in cluster inference. Neuroimage 44: 83–98.
28. Guevara M, Baccaro ME, Gomez-Anson B, Frisoni G, Testa C, et al. (2011) Cerebral magnetic resonance imaging reveals marked abnormalities of brain tissue density in patients with cirrhosis without overt hepatic encephalopathy. J Hepatol 55: 564–573.
29. Lin WC, Chou KH, Chen CL, Chen CH, Chen HL, et al. (2012) Significant volume reduction and shape abnormalities of the basal ganglia in cases of chronic liver cirrhosis. AJNR Am J Neuroradiol 33: 239–245.
30. Chavarria L, Alonso J, Garcia-Martinez R, Aymerich FX, Huerga E, et al. (2011) Biexponential analysis of diffusion-tensor imaging of the brain in patients with cirrhosis before and after liver transplantation. AJNR Am J Neuroradiol 32: 1510–1517.
31. Matsusue E, Kinoshita T, Ohama E, Ogawa T (2005) Cerebral cortical and white matter lesions in chronic hepatic encephalopathy: MR-pathologic correlations. AJNR Am J Neuroradiol 26: 347–351.
32. Lawrence AD, Watkins LH, Sahakian BJ, Hodges JR, Robbins TW (2000) Visual object and visuospatial cognition in Huntington's disease: implications for information processing in corticostriatal circuits. Brain 123 (Pt 7): 1349–1364.
33. Sort P, Navasa M, Arroyo V, Aldeguer X, Planas R, et al. (1999) Effect of intravenous albumin on renal impairment and mortality in patients with cirrhosis and spontaneous bacterial peritonitis. N Engl J Med 341: 403–409.
34. Marlin AE, Wald A, Hochwald GM, Malhan C (1976) On the movement of fluid through the brain of hydrocephalic cats. Neurology 26: 1159–1163.
35. Gupta RK, Yadav SK, Saraswat VA, Rangan M, Srivastava A, et al. (2012) Thiamine deficiency related microstructural brain changes in acute and acute-on-chronic liver failure of non-alcoholic etiology. Clin Nutr 31: 422–428.
36. Gale SD, Hopkins RO (2004) Effects of hypoxia on the brain: neuroimaging and neuropsychological findings following carbon monoxide poisoning and obstructive sleep apnea. J Int Neuropsychol Soc 10: 60–71.
37. Bartynski WS, Grabb BC, Zeigler Z, Lin L, Andrews DF (1997) Watershed imaging features and clinical vascular injury in cyclosporin A neurotoxicity. J Comput Assist Tomogr 21: 872–880.
38. Truwit CL, Denaro CP, Lake JR, DeMarco T (1991) MR imaging of reversible cyclosporin A-induced neurotoxicity. AJNR Am J Neuroradiol 12: 651–659.
39. Rovira A, Minguez B, Aymerich FX, Jacas C, Huerga E, et al. (2007) Decreased white matter lesion volume and improved cognitive function after liver transplantation. Hepatology 46: 1485–1490.

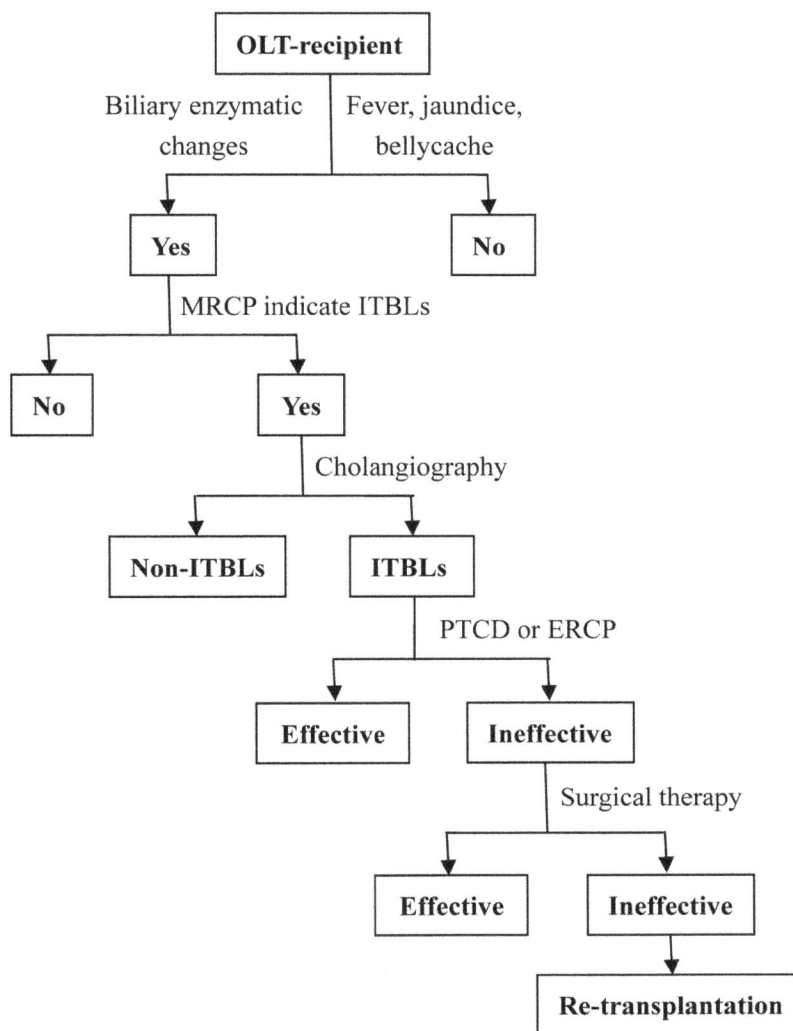

Figure 1. Algorithm for the diagnosis and treatment of ITBLs after OLT in the control group. ERCP, endoscopic retrograde cholangio-pancreatography; ITBLs, ischemic-type biliary lesion; MRCP, magnetic resonance cholangiopancreatography; OLT, orthotopic liver transplantation; PTCD, percutaneous transhepatic cholangiodrainage.

infection in the EDIM group compared with the control group (28.6% vs. 48.6%, $P = 0.04$).

Survival of Transplanted Livers and Hosts

The liver function improved after interventional and/or surgical therapy in 18 patients in the control group and 20 patients in the EDIM group. Repeat transplantation after failure of the above interventions was required in 11 patients in the control group and six patients in the EDIM group. Eight patients in the control group and two patients in the EDIM group died before re-transplantation was performed. The 1- and 3-year graft survival rates were 78.4% and 53.2% in the control, and 92.9% and 78.6% in the EDIM group. The graft survival rate was significantly poorer in the control group than in the EDIM group ($P = 0.008$ Figure 5). The mean time of graft loss was significantly longer in the EDIM group (24±9.6 months, range 11–41 months) than in the control group (17±12.3 months; range 6–44 months) ($P = 0.02$).

Discussion

ITBLs after OLT are difficult to diagnose and treat. Currently, the diagnosis of ITBLs after OLT depends mainly on cholangiography during investigations such as MRCP, ERCP and PTCD [5,6,10–12]. MRCP is a non-invasive investigation that is becoming the first choice for diagnosis of ITBLs [13–15]. Borasci et al. reported that MRCP had a sensitivity of 93%, specificity of 92%, positive predictive value of 86%, and negative predictive value of 96% for the the diagnosis of biliary complications after OLT [13]. MRCP can detect tortuosity and deformity of the biliary tree, cholangiectasis of the intrahepatic ducts, accumulation of biliary sludge and destruction of the bile ducts. However, these changes do not occur until the advanced stages of ITBLs, after the optimal period for therapeutic intervention. ERCP and PTCD are currently the gold standard methods for diagnosing ITBLs. However, ERCP and PTCD are both invasive and can cause pancreatitis or bleeding [16,17], and are therefore not suitable for early monitoring and diagnosis of ITBLs after OLT. It is

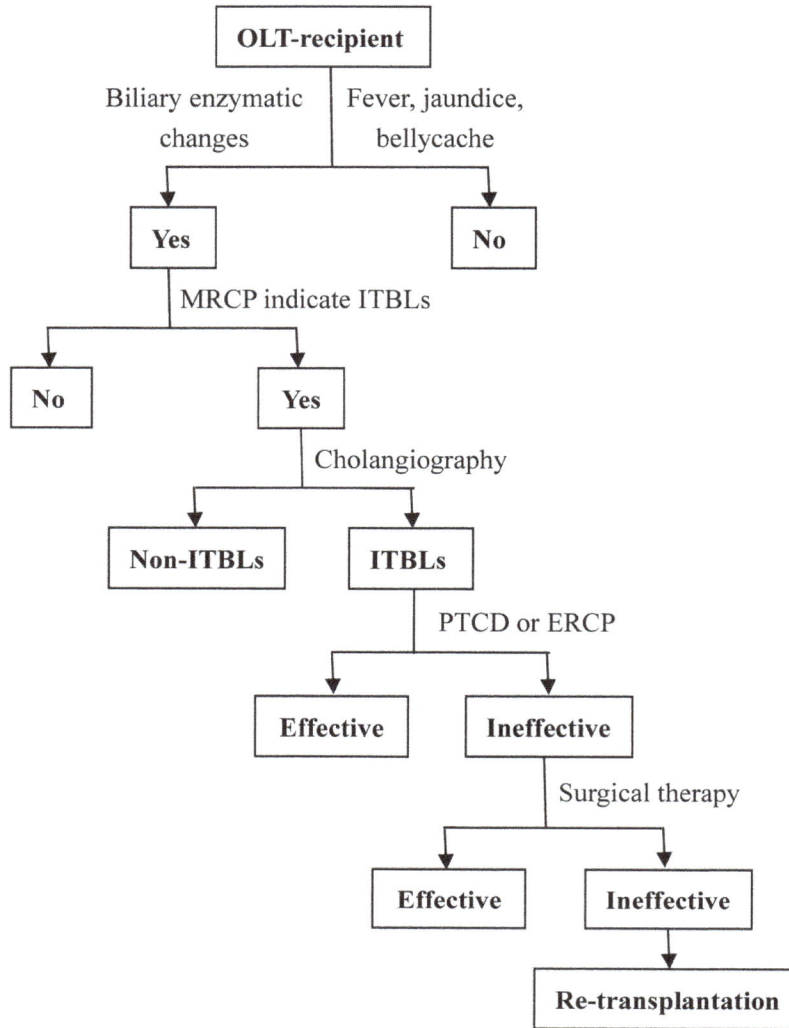

Figure 2. Algorithm for the diagnosis and treatment of ITBLs after OLT in the EDIM group. CEUS, contrast-enhanced ultrasonography; EDIM, early diagnosis and intervention mode; ERCP, endoscopic retrograde cholangio-pancreatography; ITBLs, ischemic-type biliary lesion; MRCP, magnetic resonance cholangiopancreatography; OLT, orthotopic liver transplantation; PTCD, percutaneous transhepatic cholangiodrainage.

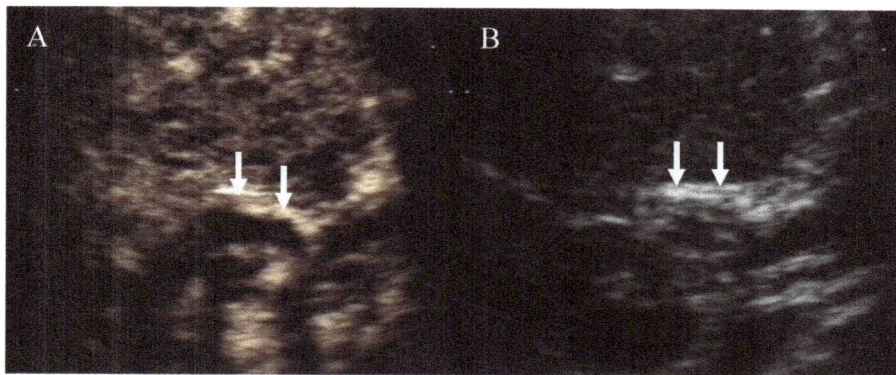

Figure 3. Ultrasound image of the hilar bile duct in a patient without ITBLs. B: Regular ultrasound image showing a thickened hilar bile duct wall with a high echogenicity (arrow) and an obscure lumen. **A:** Arterial stage of CEUS showing high enhancement of the bile duct (arrow) and a clear lumen. CEUS: contrast-enhanced ultrasound; OLT: orthotopic liver transplantation.

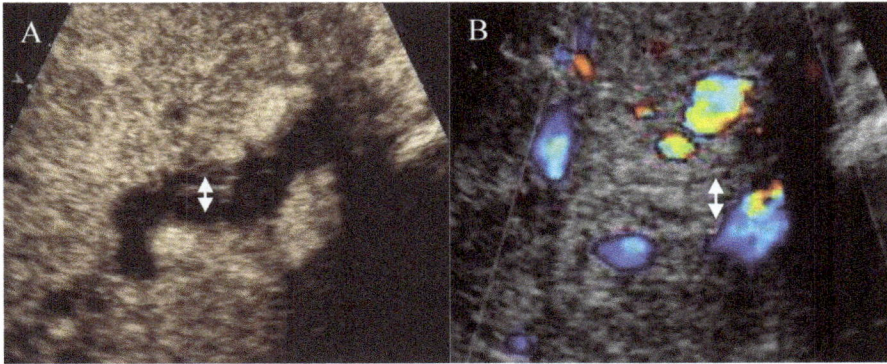

Figure 4. Ultrasound image of the hilar bile duct in a patient with ITBLs. B: Regular ultrasound image showing a thickened hilar bile duct wall with equal echogenicity (arrow) and an obscure lumen. **A:** Arterial stage of CEUS showing low enhancement in the bile duct wall (arrow) and a clear lumen.

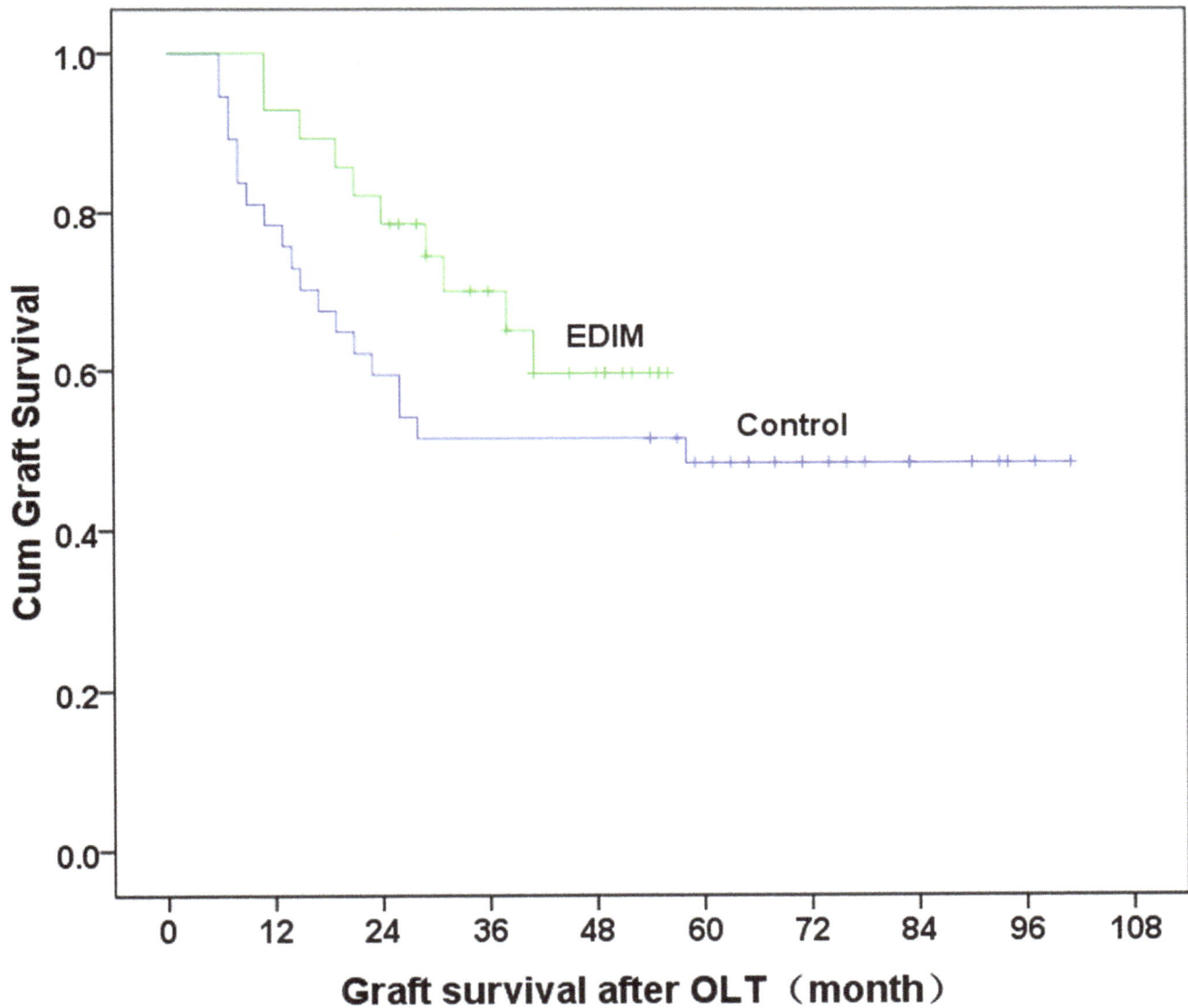

Figure 5. Survival times of liver grafts in the two groups. The 1- and 3-year graft survival rates were 78.4% and 53.2% in the control group and 92.9% and 78.6% in the EDIM group ($P = 0.008$).

important to develop an easy and a non-invasive method for early diagnosis of ITBLs.

CEUS is an ultrasonic examination method that increases the difference in echogenicity, between blood and tissue by injection of ultrasonic contrast agent into the blood. Animal and clinical experiments have shown that the microbubble-to-tissue signal ratio after injection of ultrasonic contrast agent can be used to observe flow that may be difficult to detect on color Doppler ultrasonography, such as in deep vessels or in low-velocity vessels such as the microcirculation [18,19]. CEUS is therefore an important investigation for the diagnosis of hepatic artery and portal vein complications after OLT, and reduces the need for more invasive investigations such as angiography [18,20–23]. However, few studies have focused on using CEUS for the diagnosis of biliary complications such as ITBLs after OLT. The blood supply of the bile ducts depends entirely on the arterial peribiliary plexus, which is perfused by the gastroduodenal and hepatic arteries. Damage to the peribiliary vascular plexus may cause microcirculatory changes, resulting in necrosis, fibrosis, and stenosis of the biliary tract [9,24–26]. SonoVue, the ultrasonic contrast agent used for CEUS, differs from the contrast used for computed tomography and magnetic resonance imaging, Sono-Vue is a blood pool agent that gives a more reliable depiction of tissue microcirculation because the microbubbles are not small enough to pass through the microvascular endothelial gap [27]. Use of CEUS to monitor microcirculatory changes to the peribiliary vascular plexus after OLT may enable early diagnosis of ITBLs.

Our previous study showed a significant difference in the enhancement of the hilar bile duct on CEUS between patients with and without ITBLs. During the arterial phase of CEUS, there was no or low enhancement of the wall of the hilar bile duct in patients with ITBLs. In patients without ITBLs, there was more enhancement of the hilar bile duct walls than of the hepatic parenchyma in the arterial phase, followed by similar or lower enhancement of the hilar bile duct walls compared with the hepatic parenchyma in the portal venous and late phases [28]. The CEUS finding reflects the extent of damage to the peribiliary vascular plexus, and the extent of decreased perfusion to the bile duct. These changes help to diagnose ITBLs before the development of morphological changes to the bile duct. Another study by our group showed that CEUS had a sensitivity of 64.6%, specificity of 88.9%, and accuracy of 75.0% for diagnosing ITBLs [29]. It therefore seems feasible to diagnose ITBLs during the period of functional changes to the bile duct.

This study also evaluated a new model for the treatment of for ITBLs. Previously, medication, interventional and other therapies were administered after ITBLs was diagnosed by ERCP or PTCD. It usually takes 3–5 months to confirm the diagnosis of ITBLs using these methods. Unfortunately, delayed diagnosis is a major risk factor for the irreversible biliary damage. Bile salt retention is a major risk factor for the hepatocellular and biliary injury after OLT [1]. Hertl et al. reported that damage to the intrahepatic biliary duct after OLT was significantly increased when pig livers were flushed with saline containing hydrophobic bile salts compared with being flushed with saline alone [30]. Hoekstra et al. found that intrahepatic bile salt retention was an important mechanism of graft damage after OLT in transgenic mice [31]. In humans, damage to the bile duct is associated with toxic bile, characterized by a high cholate/phospholipid ratio [32]. Salt retention also results in bacterial growth and an increased risk of biliary tract infection. Considering the findings of these previous studies, we believe that it is important to maintain the patency of the biliary tree to prevent salt retention and protect the bile duct epithelium by performing early biliary intervention (PTCD or ERCP). In February 2008, we started to administer oral ursodeoxycholic acid and ademetionine immediately after OLT to prevent bile deposition and gallstone formation, and intravenous prostaglandin-E to improve the microcirculation of the peribiliary vascular plexus and to reduce damage to the biliary epithelial cells. When the CEUS findings indicated ITBLs, PTCD or ERCP were routinely performed to confirm the diagnosis and maintain biliary drainage. The EDIM achieved early diagnosis and treatment of ITBLs, resulting in reduced damage to the bile ducts, a lower incidence of biliary tract infection, longer survival time of liver grafts, and reduced graft loss compared with traditional treatment methods.

In summary, the traditional methods of follow-up and diagnosis result in delayed diagnosis and treatment of ITBLs after OLT compared with regular monitoring with CEUS. Prophylactic medications, earlier detection, and earlier intervention may lead to improved outcomes in patients with ITBLs.

Author Contributions

Conceived and designed the experiments: YZ RZ YY GC. Performed the experiments: YZ EQ. Analyzed the data: JR QZ. Contributed reagents/materials/analysis tools: RZ YY GC. Wrote the paper: YZ EQ JR QZ.

References

1. Buis CI, Hoekstra H, Verdonk RC, Porte RJ (2006) Causes and consequences of ischemic-type biliary lesions after liver transplantation. J Hepatobiliary Pancreat Surg 13: 517–524.

2. Sawyer RG, Punch JD (1998) Incidence and management of biliary complications after 291 liver transplants following the introduction of transcystic stenting. Transplantation 66: 1201–1207.

3. Turrion VS, Alvira LG, Jimenez M, Lucena JL, Nuno J, et al. (1999) Management of the biliary complications associated with liver transplantation: 13 years of experience. Transplant Proc 31: 2392–2393.

4. Rizk RS, McVicar JP, Emond MJ, Rohrmann CA Jr, Kowdley KV, et al. (1998) Endoscopic management of biliary strictures in liver transplant recipients: effect on patient and graft survival. Gastrointest Endosc 47: 128–135.

5. Ward EM, Kiely MJ, Maus TP, Wiesner RH, Krom RA (1990) Hilar biliary strictures after liver transplantation: cholangiography and percutaneous treatment. Radiology 177: 259–263.

6. Campbell WL, Sheng R, Zajko AB, Abu-Elmagd K, Demetris AJ (1994) Intrahepatic biliary strictures after liver transplantation. Radiology 191: 735–740.

7. Feller RB, Waugh RC, Selby WS, Dolan PM, Sheil AG, et al. (1996) Biliary strictures after liver transplantation: clinical picture, correlates and outcomes. J Gastroenterol Hepatol 11: 21–25.

8. Otto G, Roeren T, Golling M, Datsis K, Hofmann WJ, et al. (1995) [Ischemic type biliary lesions after bile ducts after liver transplantation: 2 years results]. Zentralbl Chir 120: 450–454.

9. Sanchez-Urdazpal L, Gores GJ, Ward EM, Maus TP, Wahlstrom HE, et al. (1992) Ischemic-type biliary complications after orthotopic liver transplantation. Hepatology 16: 49–53.

10. Guichelaar MM, Benson JT, Malinchoc M, Krom RA, Wiesner RH, Charlton MR (2003) Risk factors for and clinical course of non-anastomotic biliary strictures after liver transplantation. Am J Transplant 3: 885–890.

11. Sanchez-Urdazpal L, Gores GJ, Ward EM, Maus TP, Buckel EG, et al. (1993) Diagnostic features and clinical outcome of ischemic-type biliary complications after liver transplantation. Hepatology 17: 605–609.

12. Kok T, Van der Sluis A, Klein JP, Van der Jagt EJ, Peeters PM, et al. (1996) Ultrasound and cholangiography for the diagnosis of biliary complications after orthotopic liver transplantation: a comparative study. J Clin Ultrasound 24: 103–115.

13. Boraschi P, Braccini G, Gigoni R, Sartoni G, Neri E, et al. (2001) Detection of biliary complications after orthotopic liver transplantation with MR cholangiography. Magn Reson Imaging 19: 1097–1105.

14. Boraschi P, Donati F, Gigoni R, Urbani L, Femia M, et al. (2004) Ischemic-type biliary lesions in liver transplant recipients: evaluation with magnetic resonance cholangiography. Transplant Proc 36: 2744–2747.

15. Ward J, Sheridan MB, Guthrie JA, Davies MH, Millson CE, et al. (2004) Bile duct strictures after hepatobiliary surgery: assessment with MR cholangiography. Radiology 231: 101–108.

16. Boraschi P, Donati F (2004) Complications of orthotopic liver transplantation: imaging findings. Abdom Imaging 29: 189–202.

17. Sherman S, Lehman GA (1991) ERCP- and endoscopic sphincterotomy-induced pancreatitis. Pancreas 6: 350–367.

18. Leen E, McArdle CS (1996) Ultrasound contrast agents in liver imaging. Clin Radiol 51 Suppl 1: 35–39.

19. Park J, Zhang Y, Vykhodtseva N, Akula JD, McDannold NJ (2012) Targeted and reversible blood-retinal barrier disruption via focused ultrasound and microbubbles. PLOS ONE 7: e42754.

20. Sidhu PS, Shaw AS, Ellis SM, Karani JB, Ryan SM (2004) Microbubble ultrasound contrast in the assessment of hepatic artery patency following liver transplantation: role in reducing frequency of hepatic artery arteriography. Eur Radiol 14: 21–30.

21. Herold C, Reck T, Ott R, Schneider HT, Becker D, et al. (2001) Contrast-enhanced ultrasound improves hepatic vessel visualization after orthotopic liver transplantation. Abdom Imaging 26: 597–600.

22. Worthy SA, Olliff JF, Olliff SP, Buckels JA (1994) Color flow Doppler ultrasound diagnosis of a pseudoaneurysm of the hepatic artery following liver transplantation. J Clin Ultrasound 22: 461–465.

23. Schlosser T, Pohl C, Kuntz-Hehner S, Omran H, Becher H, et al. (2003) Echoscintigraphy: a new imaging modality for the reduction of color blooming and acoustic shadowing in contrast sonography. Ultrasound Med Biol 29: 985–991.

24. Takasaki S, Hano H (2001) Three-dimensional observations of the human hepatic artery (Arterial system in the liver). J Hepatol 34: 455–466.

25. Qian YB, Liu CL, Lo CM, Fan ST (2004) Risk factors for biliary complications after liver transplantation. Arch Surg 139: 1101–1105.

26. Doppman JL, Girton M, Kahn R (1978) Proximal versus peripheral hepatic artery embolization experimental study in monkeys. Radiology 128: 577–588.

27. Isozaki T, Numata K, Kiba T, Hara K, Morimoto M, et al. (2003) Differential diagnosis of hepatic tumors by using contrast enhancement patterns at US. Radiology 229: 798–805.

28. Ren J, Lu MD, Zheng RQ, Lu MQ, Liao M, et al. (2009) Evaluation of the microcirculatory disturbance of biliary ischemia after liver transplantation with contrast-enhanced ultrasound: preliminary experience. Liver Transpl 15: 1703–1708.

29. Ren J, Zheng BW, Wang P, Liao M, Zheng RQ, et al. (2013) Revealing impaired blood supply to the bile ducts on contrast-enhanced ultrasound: a novel diagnosis method to ischemic-type biliary lesions after orthotropic liver transplantation. Ultrasound Med Biol 39: 753–760.

30. Hertl M, Hertl MC, Kluth D, Broelsch CE (2000) Hydrophilic bile salts protect bile duct epithelium during cold preservation: a scanning electron microscopy study. Liver Transpl 6: 207–212.

31. Hoekstra H, Porte RJ, Tian Y, Jochum W, Stieger B, et al. (2006) Bile salt toxicity aggravates cold ischemic injury of bile ducts after liver transplantation in Mdr2+/- mice. Hepatology 43: 1022–1031.

32. Geuken E, Visser D, Kuipers F, Blokzijl H, Leuvenink HG, et al. (2004) Rapid increase of bile salt secretion is associated with bile duct injury after human liver transplantation. J Hepatol 41: 1017–1025.

19

Serum Sphingolipids Reflect the Severity of Chronic HBV Infection and Predict the Mortality of HBV-Acute-on-Chronic Liver Failure

Feng Qu[1][9], Su-Jun Zheng[2][9], Shuang Liu[2], Cai-Sheng Wu[1], Zhong-Ping Duan[2]*, Jin-Lan Zhang[1]*

1 State Key Laboratory of Bioactive Substance and Function of Natural Medicines, Institute of Materia Medica, Chinese Academy of Medical Sciences & Peking Union Medical College, Beijing, China, 2 Artificial Liver Center, Beijing YouAn Hospital, Capital Medical University, Beijing, China

Abstract

Patients with HBV-acute-on-chronic liver failure (HBV-ACLF) have high mortality and frequently require liver transplantation; few reliable prognostic markers are available. As a class of functional lipids, sphingolipids are extensively involved in the process of HBV infection. However, their role in chronic HBV infection remains unknown. The aim of this study was to determine the serum sphingolipid profile in a population of patients with chronic HBV infection, paying special attention to exploring novel prognostic markers in HBV-ACLF. High performance liquid chromatography tandem mass spectrometry was used to examine the levels of 41 sphingolipids in 156 serum samples prospectively collected from two independent cohorts. The training and validation cohorts comprised 20 and 28 healthy controls (CTRL), 29 and 23 patients with chronic hepatitis B (CHB), and 30 and 26 patients with HBV-ACLF, respectively. Biometric analysis was used to evaluate the association between sphingolipid levels and disease stages. Multivariate analysis revealed difference of sphingolipid profiles between CHB and HBV-ACLF was more drastic than that between CTRL and CHB, which indicated that serum sphingolipid levels were more likely to associate with the progression HBV-ACLF rather than CHB. Furthermore, a 3-month mortality evaluation of HBV-ACLF patients showed that dhCer(d18:0/24:0) was significantly higher in survivors than in non-survivors (including deceased patients and those undergoing liver transplantation, $p<0.05$), and showed a prognostic performance similar to that of the MELD score. The serum sphingolipid composition varies between CTRL and chronic HBV infection patients. In addition, dhCer(d18:0/24:0) may be a useful prognostic indicator for the early prediction of HBV-ACLF.

Editor: Ashley Cowart, Medical University of South Carolina, United States of America

Funding: The work was supported by Ministry of Science and Technology of People's Republic of China (2012ZX09301002-006), National Science and Technology Key Project on "Major Infectious Diseases such as HIV/AIDS, Viral Hepatitis Prevention and Treatment" (2012ZX10002004-006, 2012ZX10004904-003-001, 2013ZX10002002-006-001), Beijing Municipal Natural Science Foundation (7102085), Beijing Municipal Science & Technology Commission (No. Z131107002213019); and High Technical Personnel Training Item in Beijing Health System (2011-3-083). The funders had no role in study design, data collection and analysis, decision to publish, or preparation of the manuscript.

Competing Interests: The authors have declared that no competing interests exist.

* Email: zhjl@imm.ac.cn (JLZ); duan2517@163.com (ZPD)

[9] These authors contributed equally to this work.

Introduction

HBV infection is globally endemic. Among the types of chronic HBV infection, HBV-acute-on-chronic liver failure (HBV-ACLF) is one of the most severe end stages [1,2]. Characteristic features of HBV-ACLF include rapid disease progression and a high incidence (50–90%) of short and medium term mortality [3]. However, the pathogenesis of HBV-ACLF remains unclear [4,5].

All animal viruses rely on constituents of the host cell to provide the energy, macromolecules, and structural organization necessary for survival, and they must cross membranes either by transient local disruption of membrane integrity or by cell lysis [6,7]. Sphingolipids are highly bioactive compounds that serve as core components of biological structures, such as membranes and lipoproteins; they also regulate cell proliferation, differentiation, interaction, migration, intracellular and extracellular signaling, membrane trafficking, autophagy, and cell death [8]. A number of

studies show that sphingolipids are involved in the progression of liver disorders, including viral hepatitis, fibrosis, reperfusion following ischemia (in mice), nonalcoholic steatosis hepatitis, and hepatic cell carcinoma [9–15]. Sphingolipid metabolism is highly interconnected, and ceramides and their primary metabolites occupy the central position of the network (**Figure 1**), which is well summarized in recent reviews [16,17]. Inhibition of hepatitis B virus replication by blocking host sphingolipid biosynthesis has recently been suggested as a therapeutic strategy [15]. Although sphingolipids participate in several aspects of the HBV life cycle, the changes that occur in the serum sphingolipid profile during disease progression, and whether/how these changes play a role in chronic HBV infection, have yet to be defined.

ACLF in patients with chronic HBV infection is increasingly recognized and associated with a poor outcome, with an in-hospital mortality rate of more than 70% if liver transplantation is not possible [5,18]. Early prognostic prediction is critical for

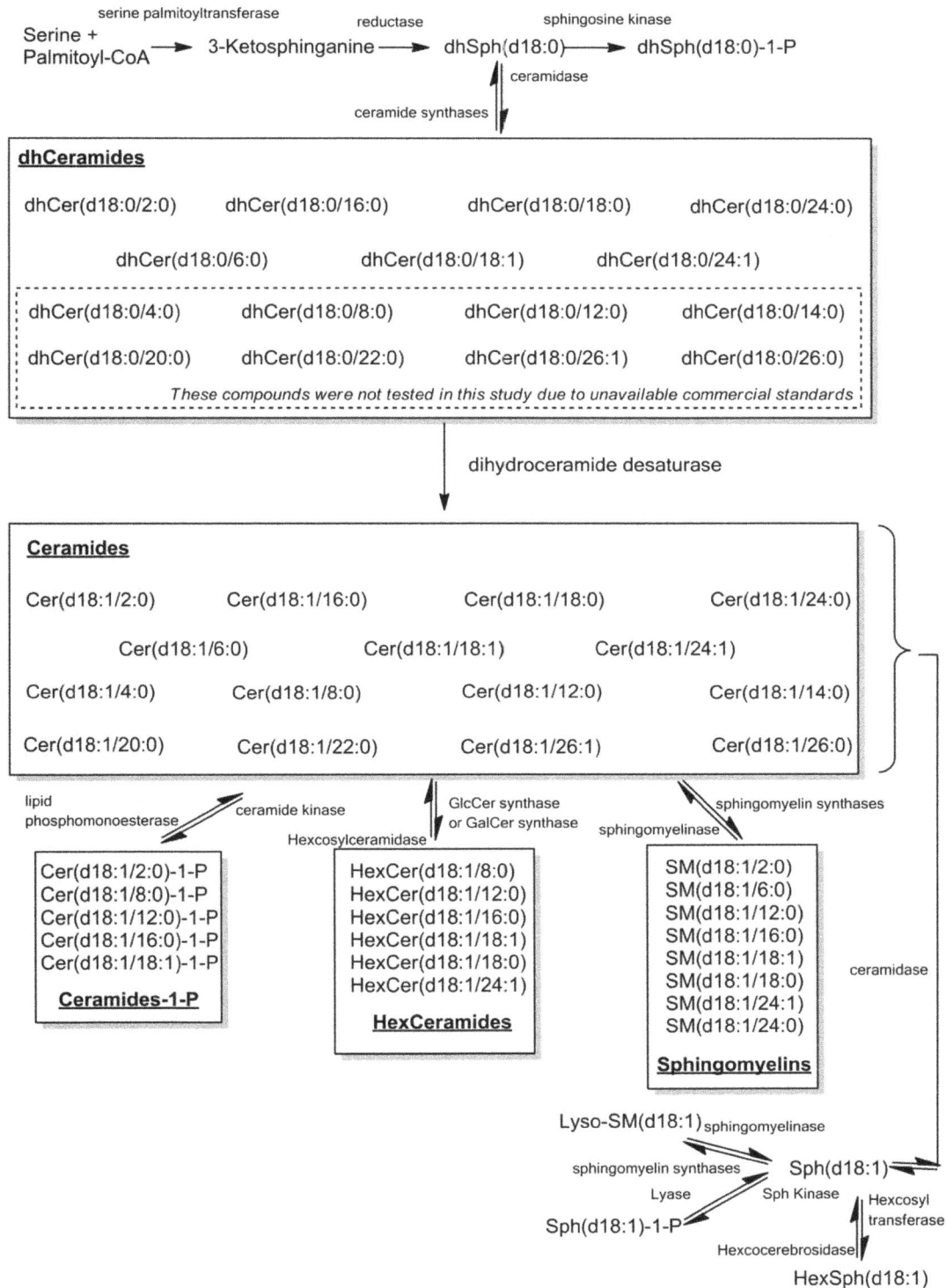

Figure 1. Metabolic pathways of sphingolipids. The sphingolipids examined in this study comprise the core components of sphingolipid metabolism.

distinguishing patients who require transplantation from those who will survive following intensive medical care alone. Presently, the Child-Pugh score and the Model of End-Stage Liver Disease (MELD) are the most commonly used models to assess the severity

of liver disease. However, both of these classification systems were initially designed to evaluate cirrhotic patients. Therefore, the identification of novel prognostic markers remains an important target before a breakthrough appears on HBV-ACLF surveillance and early intervention. Based on the existing results of the study (in the below), we speculated that certain specific sphingolipids are associated with clinical outcomes in ACLF patients.

Because clinical reports on the relationship between sphingolipids and chronic HBV infection are very rare we did not know which one or which subclass of sphingolipids should be our focus. Therefore, with the help of modern metabolomics technologies we first investigated all the sphingolipids of their core network, finding differential metabolites between different stages of chronic HBV infection, and further evaluating their prognostic value in HBV-ACLF. In brief, the aims of the present study were to determine the serum sphingolipid composition in a population of patients with chronic HBV infection, paying special attention to differential sphingolipid metabolites among disease stages, and to further explore novel prognostic markers in HBV-ACLF.

Methods

Patient selection

Between July, 2008, and January, 2013, two independent cohorts comprising a total of 108 patients with chronic HBV infection were recruited from Beijing YouAn Hospital (Capital Medical University, Beijing, China). The training cohort comprised 29 patients with chronic hepatitis B (CHB) and 30 patients with HBV-ACLF, whereas the validation cohort comprised 23 patients with CHB and 26 patients with HBV-ACLF. Age- and sex-matched healthy controls (CTRLs) were also enrolled (n = 20 for the training cohort and n = 28 for the validation cohort). CTRLs were community-dwelling individuals who presented for their yearly physical examinations and had no specific complaints or illnesses requiring treatment. All subjects underwent a physical examination, biochemical screening, blood coagulation testing, lipid testing (not available for CTRLs), and liver function testing. 25 of total 52 CHB patients received hepatic puncture biopsy guided by ultrasound. The diseased liver tissues were collected by hepatectomy from the HBV-ACLF patients who underwent the liver transplantation (n = 8). The result of pathologic analysis is shown in **Figure S1**. The baseline characteristics of the all the subjects are summarized in **Table 1**.

Diagnosis and definitions

All patients included in the study were either positive for HBsAg or HBV DNA (by real-time PCR assay) for more than 6 months before enrollment. Patients with other forms of viral hepatitis, hemochromatosis, Wilson's disease, autoimmune hepatitis, primary biliary cirrhosis, sclerosing cholangitis, biliary obstruction, alpha-1 antitrypsin deficiency, or malignancies were excluded. All CTRLs showed normal liver function and were negative for viral hepatitis; none were alcoholic.

The inclusion criteria for the CHB patients were as follows: all showed a persistent elevation of ALT levels, or repeated elevation of ALT levels and/or evidence of inflammation on histological examination of liver biopsy samples [19].

Patients with HBV-ACLF fulfilled the recommendations for the definition of ACLF established by the Chinese Society of Hepatology [20], in which ACLF is described as the acute decompensation of liver function in patients with chronic pre-existing liver diseases (CHB or cirrhosis in this study). ACLF was defined as the presence of severe jaundice (total bilirubin ≥ 171 µmol/L), coagulopathy (prolonged prothrombin time, prothrombin activity ≤40%). This diagnostic criteria is mostly consistent with that released by Asian Pacific Association for the study of the liver [5], except the total bilirubin ≥85 µmol/L is required by the later one. Precipitating factors of HBV-ACLF

include spontaneous HBV reactivation of CHB, drinking and other unknown reasons. All patients with ACLF received standard ACLF-modifying medical treatment during their hospital stay. This included absolute bed rest, antiviral treatment, intravenous infusion of albumin via a drip, and maintenance of proper hydration and electrolyte and acid-base balance. All patients with HBV-ACLF were followed-up for at least 3 months to record the 3-month mortality rates. The patients who died or underwent liver transplantation during the admission period were recorded directly, and patients who were discharged before the end of the follow-up period were monitored via telephone. Survivors were defined as patients with HBV-ACLF who survived for more than 3 months, whereas non-survivors were defined as patients with HBV-ACLF who died within 3 months or received a liver transplant during this time. The 3 month start point was set as the day on which the serum was collected. The baseline characteristics of the two groups are shown in **Table 2**.

The study protocol was reviewed and approved by the Institutional Review Board of Beijing YouAn Hospital. Written informed consent was obtained from each participant before initiation of the study. The study was carried out according to the Declaration of Helsinki and the guidelines of the International Conference on Harmonization for Good Clinical Practice.

Obtention of serum

Fasted blood samples were prospectively collected in 16×100 mm×10 mL BD Vacutainer glass serum tubes (Becton Dickinson, Franklin Lakes, NJ) in the morning of the second day after the subjects were admitted to the hospital. The tubes were incubated at room temperature for 20 min to allow the blood to clot, and then centrifuged at 750×g for 15 min to obtain the serum. Serum samples were stored at −80°C immediately after collection. Baseline characteristics were acquired on the same day by using the same blood. Sphingolipidomic assays were performed at the Institute of Materia Medica, Peking Union Medical College (Beijing, China).

Determination of sphingolipids

The high performance liquid chromatography coupled to tandem mass spectrometry (HPLC-MS/MS) was performed using an Agilent 6410B Triple Quad mass spectrometer (Agilent Technologies Inc., Santa Clara, CA) comprising a triple quadrupole MS analyzer equipped with an electrospray ionization interface and an Agilent 1200 RRLC system (HPLC-MS/MS). The HPLC-MS/MS methodology used in this study was described in our previous report [21].

MELD-based scoring systems

Disease severity in patients with HBV-ACLF was evaluated using the MELD score, which uses the patient's serum bilirubin and creatinine concentrations and the INR for prothrombin time to predict survival. MELD scores were calculated using the web site calculator (http://www.mayoclinic.org/gi-rst/mayomodel7.html).

Statistical analysis

Sphingolipids were quantified by comparing the peak area ratio (the peak area of the analyte divided by that of its corresponding internal standard) using a standard curve. Analysis was performed on SPSS 18.0 (Chicago, IL, USA) unless otherwise specified. Differences between the groups were analyzed by One-way ANOVA with Tukey post-hoc analyses. For the baseline study, all normally distributed data are expressed as the mean (SEM),

Table 1. Baseline characteristics of the study subjects.

	Training Cohort (n=79)				Validation Cohort (n=77)			
	CTRL	CHB	HBV-ACLF	P value	CTRL	CHB	HBV-ACLF	P value
	(n=20)	(n=29)	(n=30)		(n=28)	(n=23)	(n=26)	
Age: mean (SEM)	37 (3)	37 (2)	39 (2)	0.783	40 (3)	38 (4)	45 (4)	0.435
Gender: M; F (%)	80; 20	69; 31	87; 13	0.200	68; 32	83; 17	85; 15	0.200
ALT (U/L): median (range)	16 (4–31)	75 (13–1988)	83 (37–2400)	0.083	19(3–30)	166(13–782)	683(39–3374)	0.000
AST (U/L): median (range)	20 (13–27)	47 (16–973)	103 (37–1235)	0.023	21(12–27)	108(16–767)	508(57–2599)	0.000
TB (μmol/L): mean (SEM)	13 (0.9)	21 (3)	464 (39)	0.000	11 (1)	24 (5)	390(38)	0.000
AB (g/L): median (range)	45 (41–47)	39 (34–52)	32 (26–41)	0.000	46.2(42–51)	39.7(33–47)	32.0(24–39)	0.000
INR: median (range)	-	0.98(0.88–2.1)	2.1(0.90–5.1)	0.470	-	1.0 (0.93–1.43)	2.2(1.2–3.2)	0.000
HBV DNA (10³ cps/mL): median (range)	-	3E4 (1E2–8E8)	5E3 (2E1–4E9)	0.462	-	3E4(5E1–1E5)	2E4(5E1–3E5)	0.704
Creatinine (μmol/L): median (range)	-	64 (43–93)	68 (47–590)	0.066	-	74(58–100)	76(40–149)	0.119
PT (s): median (range)	-	12 (10–164)	25 (2–75)	0.014	-	12 (11–16)	26 (2–40)	0.000
PTA (%): mean (SEM)	-	94 (5)	31 (3)	0.000	-	98(4)	34(2)	0.000
WBC (/mm³): median (range)	-	5.2 (3–7)	9 (3–113)	0.055	-	5.4(3–9)	8.7 (3–20)	0.002
PLT (/L): median (range)	-	166 (94–297)	91 (35–1107)	0.908	-	154(57–236)	105.4(25–283)	0.000
CHOL (mmol/L): mean (range)	-	4.2 (3–6)	2.3 (0.8–5)	0.000	-	4.2 (3–5)	2.1(1–3)	0.000
TG (mmol/L): mean (range)	-	0.93 (0.33–1.5)	0.69 (0.22–2.9)	0.887	-	0.98 (0.58–1.1)	0.85 (0.3–1.8)	0.715
HDL (mmol/L): mean (range)	-	1.0 (0.88–2.0)	0.30 (0.05–1.2)	0.000	-	1.3 (1.2–2.1)	0.43 (0.06–1.6)	0.000
LDL (mmol/L): mean (range)	-	2.2 (1.1–2.6)	0.95 (0.19–2.7)	0.001	-	2.1 (1.9–2.2)	0.95 (0.32–1.8)	0.000
ApoA1 (g/L): mean (range)	-	96 (89–149)	24 (1.7–71)	0.000	-	109 (76–163)	21 (5.0–46)	0.000
ApoB (g/L): mean (range)	-	65 (50–89)	52 (18–133)	0.351	-	53 (52–56)	53.4 (16.3–84.9)	0.115
A1/B: mean (range)	-	1.7 (1.0–2.3)	0.73 (0.02–1.8)	0.000	-	2 (1.5–3)	0.41 (0.18–2.82)	0.000
Antiviral treatment: (%)		None (76)	None (60)	0.116		None (74)	None (69)	0.151
(before admission)		Enticavir (14)	Enticavir (27)	-		Enticavir (13)	Enticavir (8)	-
		Adefovir dipivoxil (3)	Adefovir dipivoxil (3)	-		Adefovir dipivoxil (9)	Adefovir dipivoxil (8)	-
		Lamivudine (3)	Lamivudine (7)	-		Lamivudine (0)	Lamivudine (4)	-
		Interferon (3)	Interferon (3)	-		Interferon (4)	Interferon (4)	-
		Telbivudine (0)	Telbivudine (0)	-		Telbivudine (0)	Telbivudine (4)	-
MELD: mean (range)			24(8–55)	-			24(15–36)	-
Encephalopathy grade: Grade 0; 1; 2; 3; 4 (%)			53; 30; 10; 7; 0	-			29; 32; 13; 13; 13	-
Spontaneous bacterial peritonitis: (%)			65	-			73	-
Precipitating factors: (%)			HBV reactivation (67)	-			HBV reactivation (70)	-
			Drinking (10)	-			Drinking (5)	-
			Unknown (23)	-			Unknown (25)	-
The basic of ACLF: (%)			Cirrhosis (47)	-			Cirrhosis (65)	-
			CHB (53)	-			CHB (35)	-

Abbreviations: A1/B: apolipoprotein A1 divided by apolipoprotein B; AB, albumin; HBV-ACLF, HBV-acute-on-chronic liver failure; ALT, alanine aminotransferase; AST, aspartate aminotransferase; ApoA1, apolipoprotein A1; ApoB, apolipoprotein B; CHB, chronic hepatitis B; CHOL, cholesterol; HDL, high density lipoprotein; INR, International Normalized Ratio; LC, liver cirrhosis; LDL, low density lipoprotein; MELD, Model for End-Stage Liver Disease; PLT, blood platelet; PT, prothrombin time; PTA, prothrombin activity; TB, total bilirubin; TG, triglyceride; WBC, white blood cell.

Table 2. Baseline characteristics of patients with HBV-ACLF.

	Survivors	Non-survivors	P value
	(n = 25)	(n = 31)	
Age: mean (SEM)	39 (2)	35 (3)	0.394
Gender: M; F (%)	85; 15	88; 12	0.157
ALT (U/L): mean (SEM)	453 (120)	422 (118)	0.857
AST (U/L): median (range)	135 (42–2599)	157 (37–1323)	0.317
TB (μmol/L): mean (SEM)	389 (37)	480 (36)	0.088
AB (g/L): mean (SEM)	33 (1)	31 (1)	0.274
INR: mean (SEM)	2.0 (0.09)	2.4 (0.1)	0.012
HBV DNA (10^3cps/mL): median (range)	1E5 (1E2–3E8)	5E3 (5E2–4E9)	0.452
Creatinine (μmol/L): mean (SEM)	68 (4)	97 (16)	0.124
PT (s): mean (SEM)	24 (1)	28 (2)	0.158
PTA (%): mean (SEM)	38 (3)	28 (2)	0.007
WBC (/mm^3): median (range)	8.2 (3.5–113)	7.2 (3.0–66)	0.608
PLT (/L): median (range)	103 (29–856)	80 (25–1107)	0.903
CHOL (mmol/L): mean (SEM)	2.4 (0.2)	2.1 (0.1)	0.228
TG (mmol/L): mean (SEM)	0.96 (0.1)	0.91 (0.1)	0.707
HDL (mmol/L): mean (SEM)	0.47 (0.06)	0.39 (0.07)	0.425
LDL (mmol/L): mean (SEM)	1.2 (0.1)	0.82 (0.08)	0.006
ApoA1 (g/L): mean (SEM)	25 (2)	20 (3)	0.178
ApoB (g/L): mean (SEM)	57 (4)	53 (5)	0.509
A1/B: mean (SEM)	0.47 (0.05)	0.48 (0.1)	0.896
MELD: mean (SEM)	22 (1)	27 (1)	0.004
Encephalopathy grade: Grade 0; 1; 2; 3; 4 (%)	55; 33; 11; 4; 0	32; 29; 12; 15; 12	0.273
Precipitating factors: (%)	HBV reactivation (59)	HBV reactivation (68)	0.159
	Drinking (7)	Drinking (6)	
	Unknown (33)	Unknown (26)	
The basic of ACLF: (%)	Cirrhosis (48)	Cirrhosis (63)	0.261
	CHB (52)	CHB (37)	
Antiviral treatment: (%)	None (56)	None (71)	0.213
(before admission)	Enticavir (15)	Enticavir (20)	
	Adefovir dipivoxil (7)	Adefovir dipivoxil (3)	
	Lamivudine (11)	Lamivudine (6)	
	Interferon (7)	Interferon (0)	
	Telbivudine (4)	Telbivudine (0)	
Antiviral treatment: (%)	Enticavir (68)	Enticavir (77)	0.238
(after admission)	Lamivudine (24)	Lamivudine (16)	
	Adefovir dipivoxil & lamivudine (8)	Adefovir dipivoxil & lamivudine (3)	
	Refuse antiviral treatment (0)	Refuse antiviral treatment (3)	
Other special treatments: (after admission)			0.303
Steroid pulse therapy [a] (%)	32	45	
Plasmapheresis (%)	80	93	
Immunomodulator therapy [b] (%)	52	48	

[a]Medicine: Methylprednisolone.
[b]Medicine: Thymic peptide α1 or Thymopentin.

and were analyzed by one-way ANOVA (for more than two groups) or an independent sample T-test after Levene's test for equality of variances was performed (for two groups). Non-normally distributed data are expressed as the median (range) and were analyzed by the Kruskal-Wallis test (for more than two groups) or the Mann-Whitney U test (for two groups). Normality was checked by the Shapiro-Wilk test. For categorical variables the chi-square or Fisher's exact test were used. Orthogonal partial least squares discriminant analysis (OPLS-DA), a multivariate analysis method was used to visually discriminate between patients at different HBV disease stages and healthy controls using SIMCA 13.0 software (Umetrics, Umeå, Sweden). Sphingolipidomic data were mean-centered and UV-scaled. The modeling process was run in the auto-fit mode, whereas the components were calculated automatically. Principal component analysis was used to visualize overall clustering or outliers. The quality of each OPLS-DA model was examined using the R2Y(cum) and Q2(cum) values, which are used to assess the stability and predictability of the model, respectively[22]. The criteria for the selection of potential biomarkers were as follows: the value of the variable importance in projection was greater than 1; the jack-knife uncertainty bar excluded zero; and the absolute value of Pcorr in the S-plot was > 0.58 [23]. The cross-validation parameter, Q^2, was calculated as in partial least squares discriminant analysis by permutation testing using 100 random permutations to test the validity of the model against over-fitting. Independent t-test was used to determine whether biomarker candidates obtained from OPLS-DA modeling were significantly different between the groups in the validation cohort. To determine the prognostic value of sphingolipid biomarkers, all patients with ACLF in the two cohorts were combined. Sphingolipids showing marked differences between survivors and non-survivors (identified by independent t-test) were selected as potential predictors. The correlation between the sphingolipid potential predictors and the MELD score was evaluated by Spearman's correlation analysis. The receiver operating characteristic (ROC) curve was obtained and the area under the curve (AUC) was calculated to identify the ability of certain sphingolipid potential predictors and the MELD score to predict 3-month mortality in patients with HBV-ACLF. The Delong method was used to test the significance of the differences between the areas under the ROC curves (MedCalc, Ostend, Belgium) [24]. For all the statistical analyses described above, a two-sided p value of <0.05 signified statistical significance.

Results

Patient Population

Table 1 depicts the baseline characteristics of the study subjects from two cohorts. The groups were selected to ensure approximately equal sample size either for groups (n = 20~30) or for cohorts (n = 70~80). For each cohort, groups were matched in terms of age and gender (**Table 1**). For all the HBV-ACLF patients, the survivor and non-survivor groups were matched in terms of age, gender, ALT, AST, TB and creatinine (**Table 2**). In addition, significant differences of INR, PTA and MELD between these groups are likely to be explained by they are all reported prognosis marker of ACLF [25–27]. The significant decreasing low density lipoprotein (LDL) of non-survivor group can be explained by more cirrhosis based HBV-ACLF patients in this group because it is reported that the decreasing of serum LDL in patients with liver disease was related to the increasing severity of the disease [28]. Antiviral treatment (before admission) may influence the serum sphingolipids, while encephalopathy grade, precipitating factors, the basic of ACLF, antiviral treatment (after admission) and other special treatment (steroid pulse therapy, plasmapheresis and immunomodulator therapy) may influence the outcome of HBV-ACLF. The chi-square or Fisher's exact test shows that there are no significant difference of serum sphingo-lipids between CHB and HBV-ACLF or between survivors and non-survivors. This means the patient groups were matched in term of antiviral treatment (**Table 2**).

HPLC-MS/MS profiling identified significant differences and potential biomarkers in serum sphingolipid profiles among the three groups

We measured the serum sphingolipid profiles in patients with chronic HBV infection by HPLC-MS/MS. In the training cohort, marked differences were observed between groups (**Figure 2**). Detailed data was shown in **Table S1**. In brief, compared with healthy control serum, a total of 10 and 19 sphingolipids were with significant differences in the CHB and HBV-ACLF groups, respectively (p<0.05, **Figure 2**). Compared with the CHB group, totally 17 sphingolipids were with significant differences in HBV-ACLF groups (p<0.05, **Figure 2**).

To maximize the separation between sample groups, we performed a supervised multivariate analysis using OPLS-DA. The results revealed distinct clustering between patients at each disease stage in the training cohort (**Figure 3A,B**). According to the criterias used to select potential biomarkers (described in the Methods section), serum obtained from CHB patients could be discriminated from that from healthy controls according to the levels of dhSphingosine and HexCer(d18:1/18:0), whereas serum from HBV-ACLF patients could be discriminated from that of CHB patients according to the levels of Cer(d18:1/20:0), Cer(d18:1/22:0), Cer(d18:1/24:0), Cer(d18:1/26:0), dhCer(d18:0/24:0), dhSphingosine, dhSphingosine-1-P, HexCer(d18:1/24:1), and SM(d18:1/18:1). After internal cross-validation, all OPLS-DA models showed excellent stability [R2Y(cum)>0.7] and good predictability [Q2(cum)>0.6] (**Figure 3A,B**). Validation using 100 random permutation tests generated intercepts of $R^2 = 0.093$ and $Q^2 = -0.145$ for CTRL versus CHB, and $R^2 = 0.234$ and $Q^2 = -0.356$ for CHB versus HBV-ACLF (**Figure 3D,E**). The potential biomarkers were then selected for verifying in the validation cohort. A bar-plot of the sphingolipid composition in the validation cohort is shown in **Figure 4** (Detailed data was shown in **Table S2**). The results of independent t-tests (p<0.05) between groups excluded all the potential biomarkers identified between the CTRL and CHB groups, whereas all nine potential biomarkers identified between the CHB and HBV-ACLF groups were confirmed; thus, these were regarded as potential, reliable diagnostic biomarkers. Furthermore, sphingolipidomic data obtained from the validation cohort was plotted on the OPLS-DA score plot obtained for the training cohort. As shown in **Figure 3C,D**, the OPLS-DA model correctly predicted 86% of CTRL and 83% of CHB patients within the 95% confidence interval (CI), and correctly predicted 100% of CHB and 100% of CTRL subjects within the 95% CI. This independent external validation confirms the feasibility of LC-MS/MS-based serum sphingolipidomics as a potential diagnostic tool for HBV-ACLF. The results above suggested that sphingolipidome profiles can be used to indicate the progression of liver disease (HBV-ACLF) rather than the development of CHB; this is because nine validated biomarkers could discriminate between CHB and HBV-ACLF patients whereas none could discriminate between CTRL subjects and CHB patients. Thus, we speculated that specific sphingolipids may have some prognostic performance in HBV-ACLF patients, e.g. predicting 3-month mortality, which is a considerable challenge in clinical practice.

dhCer(d18:0/24:0) as a predictor of 3-month mortality in ACLF patients

Indeed, when all HBV-ALCF patients were divided into two groups, survivors and non -survivors, we observed significant differences in the circulating levels of dhCer(d18:0/24:0). The chemical structure of dhCer(d18:0/24:0) was shown in **figure 5**.

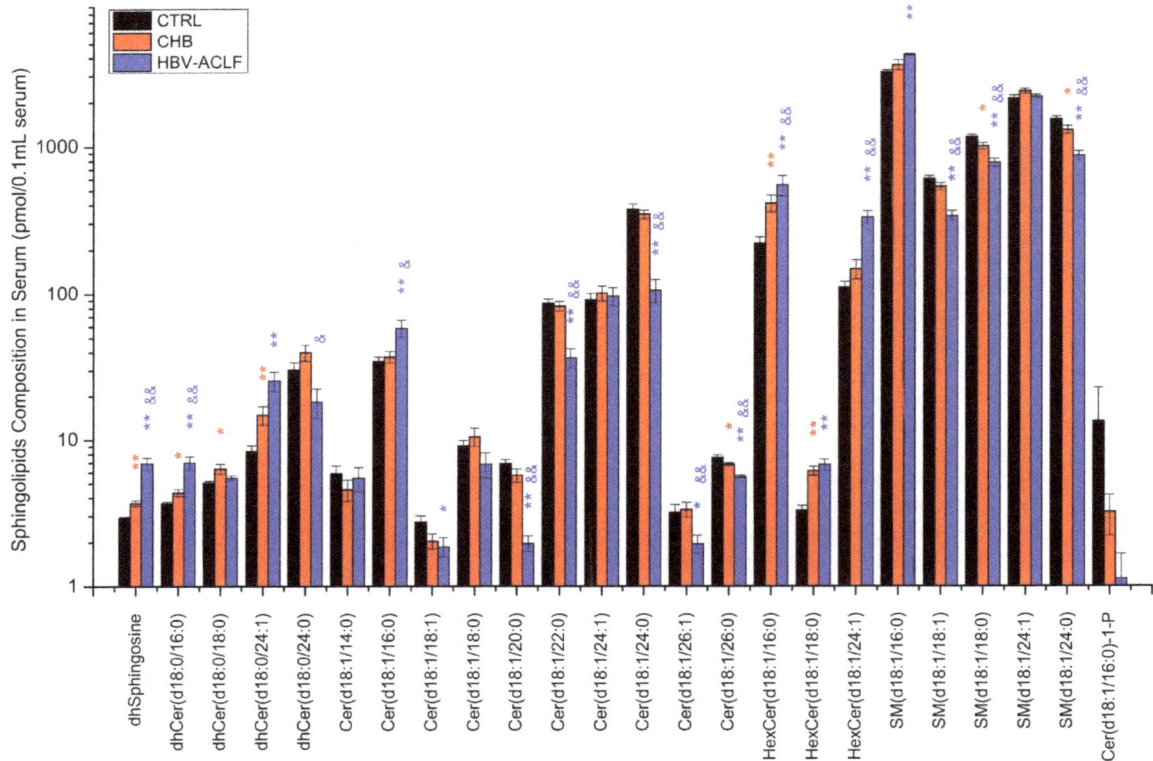

Figure 2. Serum sphingolipid levels in the training cohort (healthy controls, chronic hepatitis patients, and HBV-ACLF patients). Data are expressed as the mean ± SEM. *, significant difference compared with healthy controls (* =p<0.05, ** =p<0.01); &, significant difference compared with CHB (& =p<0.05, && =p<0.01).

An independent t-test showed that dhCer(d18:1/24:0) was the only sphingolipid that showed a significant difference in expression level between survivors and non-survivors (30.2±24.7 pmol/0.1 mL serum in survivors and 14.1±11.4 pmol/0.1 mL serum in non-survivors, $p = 0.005$; **Figure 6A**). This is an excellent indication that decreasing dhCer(d18:0/24:0) concentrations may serve as an independent predictor of 3-month mortality in patients with HBV-ACLF. Over the past decade, the MELD score was the most widely used method for predicting mortality and determining organ allocation in liver transplantation [29]. A previous study reported that the model for the MELD score was related to the prognosis of patients with HBV-related ACLF [30]. In the present study, we compared the performance of dhCer(d18:0/24:0) levels with that of the MELD scores for predicting 3-month mortality. First, the MELD scores for non-survivors were significantly higher than those of survivors (22.1±5.1 in survivors vs. 27.2±7.0 in non-survivors, $p = 0.004$; **Figure 6C**). As shown in **Figure 6B**, ROC analysis revealed that the AUC for dhCer(d18:0/24:0) was 0.759 (95% CI: 0.624-0.893), whereas that for the MELD scores was 0.732 (95% CI: 0.599-0.865). Thus, there was no significant statistical difference between the prognostic performance of dhCer(d18:0/24:0) levels and that of the MELD scores ($p>0.05$, by Delong method) [24]. Furthermore, Spearman's correlation analysis showed that, among 55 HBV-ACLF patients, dhCer(d18:0/24:0) levels significantly correlated with the MELD scores (R = -0.517, $p = 0.00003$; **Figure 6D**). Thus, we conclude that dhCer(d18:0/24:0) levels are associated with the severity of liver disease, and exhibit a prognostic performance similar to that of the MELD score. We further conducted logistic regression and model fitting to investigate whether adding dhCER(d18:0/24:0) to

a prognostic model including MELD improve discrimination. The answer is no. Here is the reason. According to above result, dhCer(d18:0/24:0) correlated significantly with MELD (R = -0.527, p = 0.00003). Therefore, both of them represents the severity of liver failure and would not generated more discrimination power to combine them.

Discussion

Sphingolipids are extensively involved HBV infection pathways and have a significant influence on the life of hepatocytes [15,31]. This study was designed to examine changes in the serum sphingolipidome of patients with chronic HBV infection, and is the first to demonstrate the utility of serum sphingolipidomic profiling to identify novel prognostic biomarkers of 3-month mortality in patients with HBV-ACLF.

Because perturbations in the levels of certain compounds may initiate a cascade of changes in the levels of multiple lipids, which is called the "ripple effect", metabolic homeostasis of sphingolipids is key for maintaining the physical health of an organism [16]. To our knowledge, this is the first study to perform serum sphingolipidomic profiling in patients with chronic HBV infection. In the training cohort, multivariate analysis identified potential biomarkers that could discriminate CHB patients from CTRL subjects and HBV-ACLF patients from CHB patients. In the validation cohort, however, all of the potential biomarkers that discriminated CHB patients from HBV-ACLF patients were confirmed, whereas those that potentially differentiated CTRL subjects from CHB patients were screened out. These results

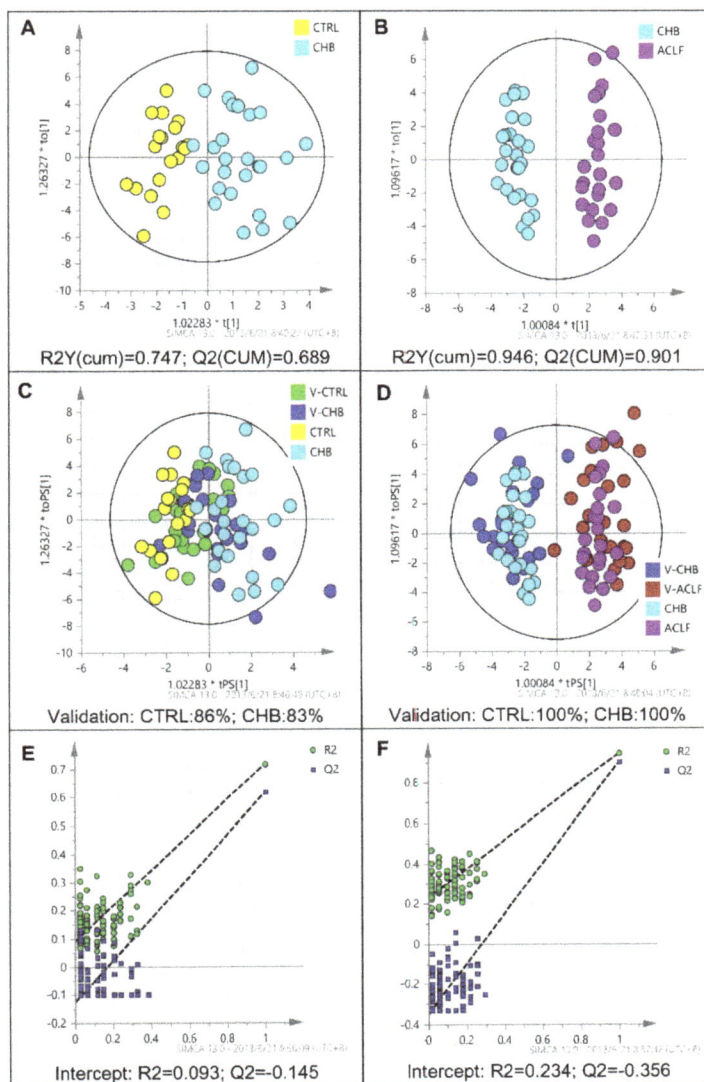

Figure 3. Identification of potential biomarkers through OPLS-DA. (A),(B). Score plots obtained from the training cohort by OPLS-DA. R2Y(cum) and Q2(cum) values are displayed below each panel; these values have a range of 0 to 1 and represent the stability and predictability of the model, respectively. Dots with different colors representing different groups are well separated based on their sphingolipidome data, indicating serum sphingolipidome varied among groups significantly. **(C),(D)**. T-predicted scatter plot of the OPLS-DA model using sphingolipidome data obtained from the validation cohort. The result shows that the OPLS-DA models correctly predicted 86% of V-CTRL and 83% of V-CHB patients within the 95% CI (panel C, CTRL vs. CHB), and correctly predicted 100% of V-CHB and 100% of V-CTRL subjects within the 95% CI (panel D, CHB vs. ACLF). **(E),(F)**. Validation plot of the PLS-DA models obtained using 100 permutation tests to reveal the risk of overfit from the model. The intercept for the blue Q2 line should be below 0.1. Note: V-: corresponding validation group in the validation cohort.

suggested that the ripple effect is more significant in patients showing disease progression.

These results allowed us to speculate on the role played by sphingolipids in disease progression. Because the liver plays an essential role in the metabolism of sphingolipids, it is not surprising that liver diseases are associated with major changes in serum sphingolipid concentrations [32]. Progression of HBV-ACLF ultimately leads to increased hepatocyte apoptosis and/or necrosis, which is a hallmark of liver failure. Cellular debris released by necrotic or apoptotic hepatocytes into the circulation may also cause substantial changes in serum sphingolipid composition [33]. Thus, the use of cell death-related sphingolipids to indicate HBV-ACLF status might represent a novel prognostic marker that can

be used to better identify patients that require a liver transplant. On the other hand, sphingolipids are extensively involved in the function of the immune system [34]. Increasing evidence suggests that non-HBV-specific inflammation of the liver is likely responsible for the hepatic pathology observed in patients with CHB [35].

Perhaps the most interesting finding from the present study is that decreasing dhCer(d18:0/24:0) concentrations can serve as an independent predictor of 3-month mortality in patients with HBV-ACLF. The mechanism underlying the association between serum dhCer(d18:0/24:0) concentrations and death in ACLF patients is unclear. However, inflammation in an HBV-infected liver is mediated by cytokines, which are regulated by sphingolipids

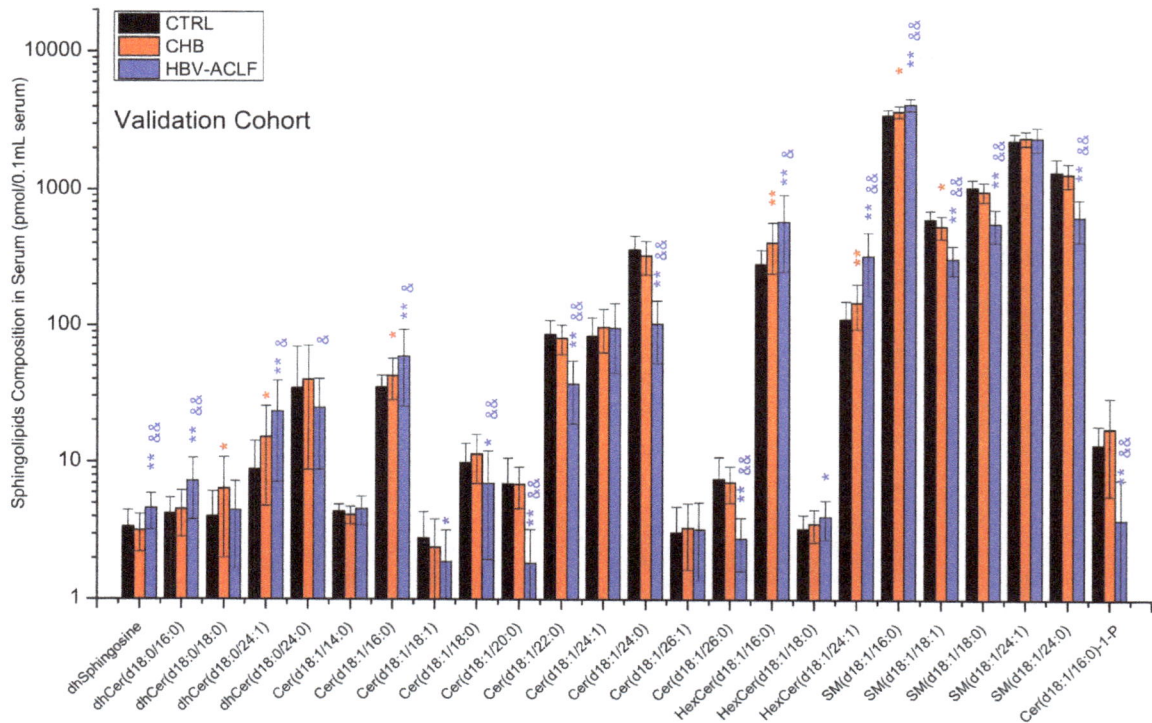

Figure 4. Serum sphingolipid levels in the validation cohort. Data are expressed as the mean ± SEM. *, significant difference compared with healthy control subjects (* =$p<0.05$, ** =$p<0.01$); &, significant difference compared with CHB (& =$p<0.05$, && =$p<0.01$).

[36,37]. The specific cause of this association requires further study. On the other hand, liver failure of other etiologies such as alcohol, acetaminophen, drug-induced hepatitis and autoimmune hepatitis and shock etc. may also have similar associations with serum sphingolipidome. However, it is just a speculation and not our focus. In order to eliminate such uncertainty, we only included HBV induced ACLF patients. Liver failure of other etiologies will be our future focus.

From the perspective of a global metabolomics strategy, metabolites screened with highly differential performance are always identified in a mass to charge ratio form, which could represent whole compounds or fragment ions [38]. Thus, it is necessary to confirm the identity of these metabolites using multi-stage MS or nuclear magnetic resonance. Such confirmation procedures are time-consuming and require significant effort. Here, confirmation was performed in parallel with HPLC-MS/MS quantification, and required no further effort. Sphingolipids were confirmed according to their retention time and fragment pattern that was comparable with that of the reference compounds. Therefore, these results are reliable, and may lead to further metabolic pathway research, or even to the development of simple kits that can be used to evaluate chronic HBV infection.

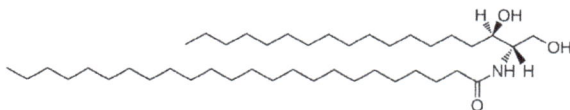

Figure 5. Chemical structure of dhCer(d18:0/24:0).

OPLS-DA is a multivariate classification technique that is used for predicting groupings for observations and for characterizing the groups [39]. The traditional view of disease relationships and subsequent classification is based largely on anatomy and symptoms [40]. OPLS-DA modeling results showed that each stage of chronic HBV infection might have its own sphingolipid profile, or fingerprint. These data-driven efforts to establish disease relationships can offer new opportunities to identify molecular or clinical indices of commonalities or distinctions within each stage of chronic HBV infection. It should be noted that the potential biomarkers identified herein may not be practical for the diagnosis of chronic HBV infection because an easier method already exists (i.e., HBsAg, ALT). Here, we used OPLS-DA to search for potential biomarkers by identifying lipids whose expression levels may correlate with the severity or progression of HBV infection by making full use of the features of OPLS-DA. Nevertheless, it should also be noted that the discovery of a potential biomarker is only the start of the lengthy process of validating them for clinical application or diagnostic purposes.

This study has some limitations. First, it was a single center study and the sample size was relatively small. The findings need to be confirmed in larger multi-center studies before clinical application. Second, due to some economic reasons, details of HBV factors were not tested on all the enrolled patients, for example, genotype, precore mutation and core promoter mutation that were reported as the factors associated with fulminant hepatitis B and may be related to HBV-ACLF [41]. Neither the patients' health insurance nor our grant covered this part. Their relationship with sphingolipids was not revealed in this study. Third, the mechanisms underlying the correlations observed herein remain unclear. Although there were significant differences in the concentrations of many sphingolipids at different stages of

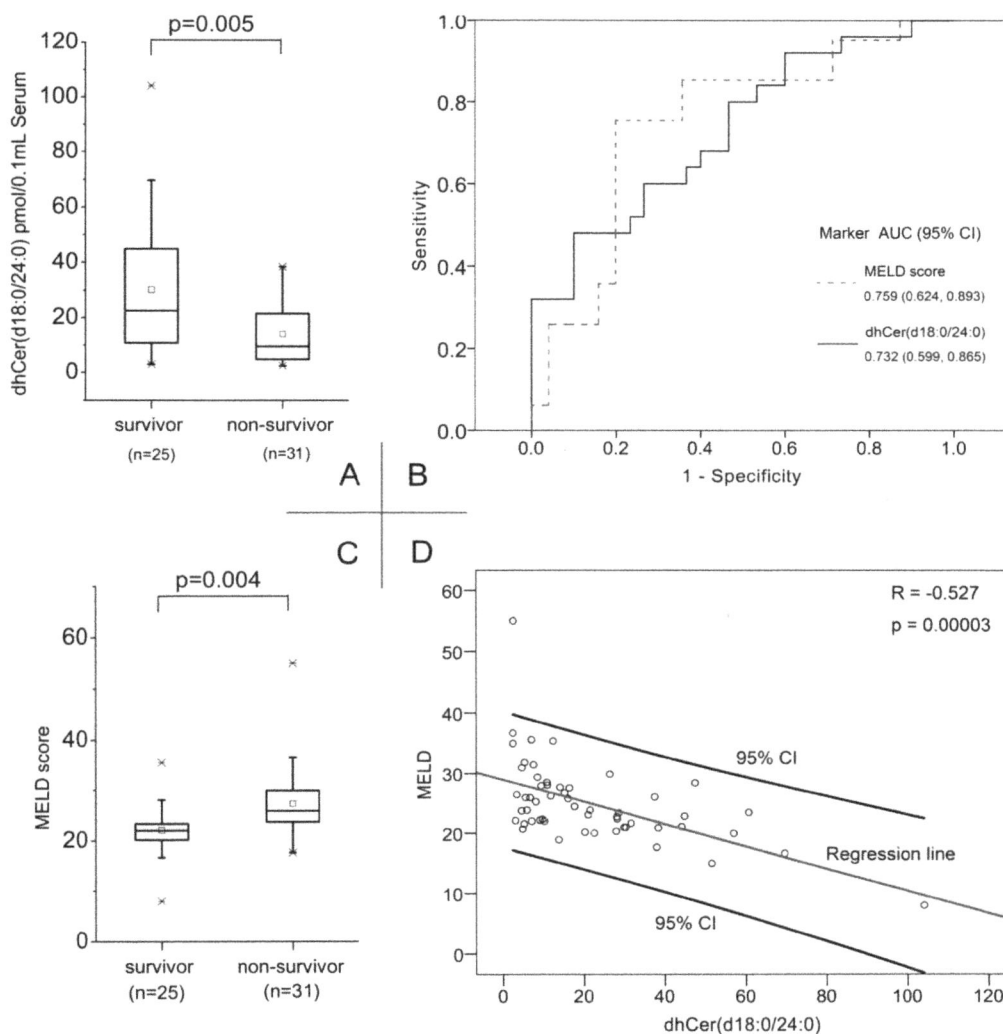

Figure 6. Prognostic performance of dhCer(d18:0/24:0) in HBV-ACLF patients in both cohorts. (A). The serum levels of dhCer(d18:0/24:0) were significantly lower in the non-survivor group compared with those in the survivor group (p = 0.005). Box refers to the 25th and 75th percentile values, with a line indicating median levels, whereas the interquartile range extends outside the box. Points outside the interquartile range are outliers. **(B).** ROC curves of dhCer(d18:0/24:0) and MELD score with the 95% CIs, for survivors versus non-survivors in HBV-ACLF patients. **(C).** The MELD scores of non-survivors with HBV-ACLF were significantly higher than those of survivors. **(D).** Serum levels of dhCer(d18:0/24:0) in all HBV-ACLF patients significantly and negatively correlated with the MELD scores (R = −0.517, p = 0.00003).

chronic HBV infection, the paucity of published clinical reports makes it difficult to connect these results to specific pathological effects and explain their role in HBV development. Given the complexity of sphingolipid metabolism, further *in vitro* and *in vivo* studies are needed.

In conclusion, profiling the sphingolipidome in human serum showed that sphingolipid levels are tightly associated with disease severity in chronic HBV infection. Meanwhile, the data identified reduced serum dhCer(d18:0/24:0) concentration as an indicator of poor prognosis in ACLF patients. Assessment of dhCer(d18:0/24:0) concentration may have prognostic utility as an early predictor of disease progression, and could contribute to the development of better treatment strategies, such as liver transplantation for patients with low dhCer(d18:0/24:0) concentrations in order to reduce their pain and improve the cure rate and intensive medical care alone for patients with high dhCer(d18:0/

24:0) concentrations in order to reduce the waste of the precious donated livers. However, such decision needs comprehensive evaluating the patient's situation. The procedure can be further optimized to measure dhCer(d18:0/24:0) specifically and more rapidly, and can be included in the routine clinical evaluation of patients with HBV-ACLF. This would also allow clinicians to evaluate the prognosis of HBV-ACLF patients in most clinical settings, and potentially improve the reliability of the MELD score rankings.

Supporting Information

Figure S1   Histology of liver tissue samples in representative patients. (A) CHB, mild. Moderate interface hepatitis with enlarged portal tract. Spot necrosis is in the lobule (left, HE×100). Portal tract shows mild fibrosis with short thin septa (right, Masson trichrome ×100). **(B) HBV-ACLF based on**

CHB. Massive necrosis of parenchyma (left, HE×100) without cirrhotic nodule (right, Masson trichrome ×100). (**C**) **HBV-ACLF based on cirrhosis.** Massive necrosis of parenchyma with cirrhotic nodule remaining (left, HE×100). Cirrhotic nodule is surrounded by fibrous tissue (Arrow) (right, Masson trichrome ×100).

References

1. Ganem D, Prince AM (2004) Hepatitis B virus infection—natural history and clinical consequences. N Engl J Med 350: 1118–1129.
2. Organization WH (2012) World Health Organization Fact Sheet 204 dex. (Revised July 2012). http://wwwwhoint/mediacentre/factsheets/fs204/en/indexhtml.
3. Jalan R, Williams R (2002) Acute-on-chronic liver failure: pathophysiological basis of therapeutic options. Blood Purif 20: 252–261.
4. Jalan R, Gines P, Olson JC, Mookerjee RP, Moreau R, et al. (2012) Acute-on chronic liver failure. J Hepatol 57: 1336–1348.
5. Sarin SK, Kumar A, Almeida JA, Chawla YK, Fan ST, et al. (2009) Acute-on-chronic liver failure: consensus recommendations of the Asian Pacific Association for the study of the liver (APASL). Hepatol Int 3: 269–282.
6. Diamond DL, Syder AJ, Jacobs JM, Sorensen CM, Walters KA, et al. (2010) Temporal proteome and lipidome profiles reveal hepatitis C virus-associated reprogramming of hepatocellular metabolism and bioenergetics. PLoS Pathog 6: e1000719.
7. Lorizate M, Krausslich HG (2011) Role of lipids in virus replication. Cold Spring Harb Perspect Biol 3: a004820.
8. Merrill AH, Jr., Stokes TH, Momin A, Park H, Portz BJ, et al. (2009) Sphingolipidomics: a valuable tool for understanding the roles of sphingolipids in biology and disease. J Lipid Res 50 Suppl: S97–102.
9. Moles A, Tarrats N, Morales A, Domínguez M, Bataller R, et al. (2010) Acidic Sphingomyelinase Controls Hepatic Stellate Cell Activation and in Vivo Liver Fibrogenesis. CORD Conference Proceedings 177: 1214–1224.
10. Llacuna L, Mari M, Garcia-Ruiz C, Fernandez-Checa JC, Morales A (2006) Critical role of acidic sphingomyelinase in murine hepatic ischemia-reperfusion injury. Hepatology 44: 561–572.
11. Morales A, Mari M, Garcia-Ruiz C, Colell A, Fernandez-Checa JC (2012) Hepatocarcinogenesis and ceramide/cholesterol metabolism. Anticancer Agents Med Chem 12: 364–375.
12. Tagaram HR, Divittore NA, Barth BM, Kaiser JM, Avella D, et al. (2011) Nanoliposomal ceramide prevents in vivo growth of hepatocellular carcinoma. Gut 60: 695–701.
13. Aizaki H, Morikawa K, Fukasawa M, Hara H, Inoue Y, et al. (2008) Critical role of virion-associated cholesterol and sphingolipid in hepatitis C virus infection. J Virol 82: 5715–5724.
14. Umehara T, Sudoh M, Yasui F, Matsuda C, Hayashi Y, et al. (2006) Serine palmitoyltransferase inhibitor suppresses HCV replication in a mouse model. Biochem Biophys Res Commun 346: 67–73.
15. Tatematsu K, Tanaka Y, Sugiyama M, Sudoh M, Mizokami M (2011) Host sphingolipid biosynthesis is a promising therapeutic target for the inhibition of hepatitis B virus replication. J Med Virol 83: 587–593.
16. Brice SE, Cowart LA (2011) Sphingolipid metabolism and analysis in metabolic disease. Adv Exp Med Biol 721: 1–17.
17. Merrill AH, Jr. (2011) Sphingolipid and glycosphingolipid metabolic pathways in the era of sphingolipidomics. Chem Rev 111: 6387–6422.
18. Marrero J, Martinez FJ, Hyzy R (2003) Advances in critical care hepatology. Am J Respir Crit Care Med 168: 1421–1426.
19. Chinese Society of Hepatology, Chinese Society of Infectious Diseases, Chinese Medical Association (2005) [The guidelines of prevention and treatment for chronic hepatitis B]. Chinese journal of hepatology 13: 881–891.
20. Liver Failure and Artificial Liver Group, Severe Liver Diseases and Artificial Liver Group, Chinese Society of Hepatology, Chinese Medical Association (2006) [Diagnostic and treatment guidelines for liver failure]. Chinese journal of hepatology 14: 643–646.
21. Qu F, Wu C-S, Hou J-F, Jin Y, Zhang J-L (2012) Sphingolipids as New Biomarkers for Assessment of Delayed-Type Hypersensitivity and Response to Triptolide. PLoS ONE 7: e52454.
22. Eriksson L, Byrne T, Johansson E, Trygg J, Vikström C (2013) Multi- and Megavariate Data Analysis Basic Principles and Applications: Umetrics Academy; 3rd Edition edition (October 10, 2013).
23. Jia W (2009) Medical Metabonomics. Shanghai: Shanghai Scientific & Technical Publishers.
24. DeLong ER, DeLong DM, Clarke-Pearson DL (1988) Comparing the areas under two or more correlated receiver operating characteristic curves: a nonparametric approach. Biometrics 44: 837–845.
25. Garg H, Kumar A, Garg V, Sharma P, Sharma BC, et al. (2012) Clinical profile and predictors of mortality in patients of acute-on-chronic liver failure. Dig Liver Dis 44: 166–171.
26. Sun QF, Ding JG, Xu DZ, Chen YP, Hong L, et al. (2009) Prediction of the prognosis of patients with acute-on-chronic hepatitis B liver failure using the model for end-stage liver disease scoring system and a novel logistic regression model. J Viral Hepat 16: 464–470.
27. Zheng YB, Xie DY, Gu YR, Yan Y, Wu YB, et al. (2012) Development of a sensitive prognostic scoring system for the evaluation of severity of acute-on-chronic hepatitis B liver failure: a retrospective cohort study. Clin Invest Med 35: E75–85.
28. Cicognani C, Malavolti M, Morselli-Labate AM, Zamboni L, Sama C, et al. (1997) Serum lipid and lipoprotein patterns in patients with liver cirrhosis and chronic active hepatitis. Arch Intern Med 157: 792–796.
29. Freeman RB, Jr., Wiesner RH, Harper A, McDiarmid SV, Lake J, et al. (2002) The new liver allocation system: moving toward evidence-based transplantation policy. Liver Transpl 8: 851–858.
30. Yu J-W, Sun L-J, Zhao Y-H, Li S-C (2008) Prediction value of model for end-stage liver disease scoring system on prognosis in patients with acute-on-chronic hepatitis B liver failure after plasma exchange and lamivudine treatment. Journal of Gastroenterology and Hepatology 23: 1242–1249.
31. Chatzakos V, Rundlof AK, Ahmed D, de Verdier PJ, Flygare J (2012) Inhibition of sphingosine kinase 1 enhances cytoxicity, ceramide levels and ROS formation in liver cancer cells treated with selenite. Biochem Pharmacol 84: 712–721.
32. Mari M, Fernandez-Checa JC (2007) Sphingolipid signalling and liver diseases. Liver Int 27: 440–450.
33. Malhi H, Gores GJ, Lemasters JJ (2006) Apoptosis and necrosis in the liver: a tale of two deaths? Hepatology 43: S31–44.
34. Sun WY, Bonder CS (2012) Sphingolipids: A Potential Molecular Approach to Treat Allergic Inflammation. Journal of Allergy 2012: 1–14.
35. Wu XX, Sun Y, Guo WJ, Gu YH, Wu XF, et al. (2012) Rebuilding the balance of STAT1 and STAT3 signalings by fusaruside, a cerebroside compound, for the treatment of T-cell-mediated fulminant hepatitis in mice. Biochem Pharmacol 84: 1164–1173.
36. Bertoletti A, D'Elios MM, Boni C, De Carli M, Zignego AL, et al. (1997) Different cytokine profiles of intrahepatic T cells in chronic hepatitis B and hepatitis C virus infections. Gastroenterology 112: 193–199.
37. Malagarie-Cazenave S, Andrieu-Abadie N, Segui B, Gouaze V, Tardy C, et al. (2002) Sphingolipid signalling: molecular basis and role in TNF-alpha-induced cell death. Expert Rev Mol Med 4: 1–15.
38. Seijo S, Lozano JJ, Alonso C, Reverter E, Miquel R, et al. (2013) Metabolomics Discloses Potential Biomarkers for the Noninvasive Diagnosis of Idiopathic Portal Hypertension. Am J Gastroenterol.
39. Trygg J, Wold S (2002) Orthogonal projections to latent structures (O-PLS). Journal of Chemometrics 16: 119–128.
40. Dudley JT, Butte AJ (2010) Biomarker and drug discovery for gastroenterology through translational bioinformatics. Gastroenterology 139: 735–741, 741 e731.
41. Ozasa A, Tanaka Y, Orito E, Sugiyama M, Kang JH, et al. (2006) Influence of genotypes and precore mutations on fulminant or chronic outcome of acute hepatitis B virus infection. Hepatology 44: 326–334.

Acknowledgments

We wish to thank Dr. Jian-Dong Jiang (Institute of Materia Medica, Peking Union Medical College, Beijing 100050,China) for critically evaluating the manuscript and providing useful comments. The authors thank all patients for their participation in the study.

Author Contributions

Conceived and designed the experiments: FQ SJZ JLZ ZPD. Performed the experiments: FQ SJZ SL CSW. Analyzed the data: FQ SJZ. Contributed reagents/materials/analysis tools: FQ SJZ CSW. Contributed to the writing of the manuscript: FQ SJZ JLZ SL.

20

Butyrate Protects Rat Liver against Total Hepatic Ischemia Reperfusion Injury with Bowel Congestion

Bin Liu[1]◕, Jianmin Qian[1]◕, Qingbao Wang[2], Fangrui Wang[1], Zhenyu Ma[1], Yingli Qiao[3,2]*

1 Department of General Surgery, Huashan Hospital, Fudan University, Shanghai, China, **2** Department of General Surgery, Affiliated Hospital of Taishan Medical College, Taian, Shandong, China, **3** Department of General Surgery, Liaocheng People's Hospital, Affiliated Liaocheng Hospital of Taishan Medical College, Liaocheng, Shandong, China

Abstract

Hepatic ischemia/reperfusion (I/R) injury is an unavoidable consequence of major liver surgery, especially in liver transplantation with bowel congestion, during which endotoxemia is often evident. The inflammatory response aggravated by endotoxin after I/R contributes to liver dysfunction and failure. The purpose of the present study was to investigate the protective effect of butyrate, a naturally occurring four-carbon fatty acid in the body and a dietary component of foods such as cheese and butter, on hepatic injury complicated by enterogenous endotoxin, as well as to examine the underlying mechanisms involved. SD rats were subjected to a total hepatic ischemia for 30 min after pretreatment with either vehicle or butyrate, followed by 6 h and 24 h of reperfusion. Butyrate preconditioning markedly improved hepatic function and histology, as indicated by reduced transaminase levels and ameliorated tissue pathological changes. The inflammatory factors levels, macrophages activation, TLR4 expression, and neutrophil infiltration in live were attenuated by butyrate. Butyrate also maintained the intestinal barrier structures, reversed the aberrant expression of ZO-1, and decreased the endotoxin translocation. We conclude that butyrate inhibition of endotoxin translocation, macrophages activation, inflammatory factors production, and neutrophil infiltration is involved in the alleviation of total hepatic I/R liver injury in rats. This suggests that butyrate should potentially be utilized in liver transplantation.

Editor: Helge Bruns, University Hospital Heidelberg, Germany

Funding: This study was supported by the National Natural Science Foundation of China (NO81270530) and Specialized Research Fund for the Health Care (NO201002004). The funders had no role in study design, data collection and analysis, decision to publish, or preparation of the manuscript.

Competing Interests: The authors have declared that no competing interests exist.

* Email: qiao-ying-li@126.com

◕ These authors contributed equally to this work.

Introduction

Hepatic ischemia/reperfusion (I/R) injury remains a major complication of major liver surgery, including liver transplantation and hepatectomy [1]. I/R resulting in Kupffer cell/neutrophil activation and cytokine release often leads to liver dysfunction, and even acute and chronic rejection after transplantation, especially when grafts from non-heart-beating donors are used [2,3]. Moreover, portal triad clamping interrupts the flow of mesenteric blood, resulting in intestinal ischemia, congestion, and damage to the intestinal barriers, thereby accelerating bacterial translocation and intestinal endotoxemia, which complicates I/R-induced injury [4,5,6]. It has been demonstrated that endotoxin can aggravate I/R-induced liver injury by oxidative stress, free radical formation, and the release of inflammatory mediators [7]. Therefore, it is worthwhile to investigate novel agents that can protect against total hepatic I/R injury, especially that aggravated by endotoxemia.

Butyrate, a four-carbon short-chain fatty acid (SCFA) derivative found in foods such as parmesan cheese and butter, which is also normally produced by bacterial fermentation of unabsorbed carbohydrates, has received considerable attention as a potential therapeutic agent for cancers because of its histone deacetylase (HDAC) inhibition activity [8]. In addition to the anticancer activity of SCFAs, recent data have demonstrated that they have potent anti-inflammatory or immunomodulatory and anti-oxidant effects at non-cytotoxic dosing levels [9]. Moreover, SCFAs are the favored energy source for colonic epithelial cells and are important for normal intestinal biology [10]. Furthermore, in physiological concentrations, SCFAs-and especially butyrate-can establish and maintain the intestinal mucosal barrier, as shown in previous in vitro studies [11,12].

We have demonstrated that the dose of 300 mg/kg of butyrate exhibits anti-inflammatory and hepatoprotective effects in a rat model of partial hepatic ischemic reperfusion [13]. However, its effect on total hepatic injury complicated by endotoxin translocation from the intestinal lumen in the setting of liver transplantation has not been previously evaluated. Since impaired intestinal barriers may further promote endotoxin release, thereby aggravating damage to liver tissues induced by I/R, and butyrate can enhance intestinal barrier function, we hypothesize that butyrate may also ameliorate total hepatic injury through the inhibition of endotoxin gut leakage.

Materials and Methods

Animals

Male Sprague-Dawley rats (200–250 g) were housed in the Department of Laboratory Animal Science at Fudan University

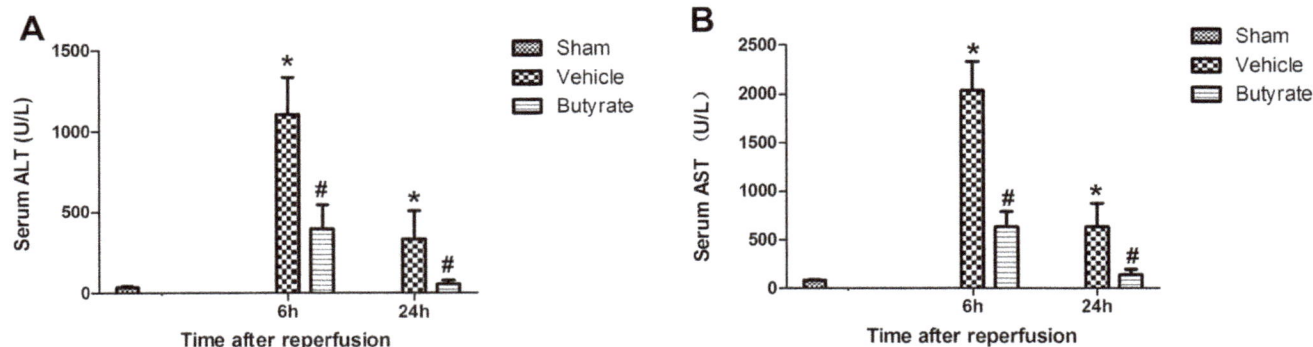

Figure 1. Effect of butyrate on serum ALT and AST levels after reperfusion. Rats were subjected to total warm liver I/R injury or sham operation and pretreated with butyrate or vehicle. Serum ALT (A) and AST (B) levels were analyzed as measures of hepatocellular injury at 6 h and 24 h after reperfusion. Data represent means ± SD, N = 3–5 rats per group. *P<0.05 vs. the sham group, #P<0.05 vs. the vehicle group.

with a laminar flow, specific pathogen-free atmosphere. Animal protocols were approved by the Fudan University Animal Care Committee, and the experiments were performed in adherence to the guidelines provided by the National Institutes of Health for the use of animals in laboratory experiments.

Total hepatic warm I/R

Total hepatic warm ischemia was induced as previously described [14]. All surgical procedures were carried out under sterile conditions. In brief, rats were laparotomized and a sterile pediatric vessel loop was placed around the portal triad for 30 min to induce total hepatic ischemia and mesenteric congestion. Sham controls underwent the same procedure without vascular occlusion. Reperfusion was initiated by removal of the loop. The rectal temperature was maintained at 37°C throughout surgery by a warming pad. For the pretreatment experiments, some rats were injected intravenously with 300 mg/kg of sodium butyrate (Sigma, Saint Louis, USA), as we previously described [13], or vehicle (normal saline solution) at 30 min prior to ischemia.

Serum aminotransferase assessment

To assess hepatic function and cellular injury following total liver ischemia, serum aspartate aminotransferase (AST) and alanine aminotransferase (ALT) activities were measured in blood

samples obtained at predetermined time points (6 and 24 h) after reperfusion with a standard automatic analyzer (type 7150; Hitachi, Tokyo, Japan).

Histological examination

Liver tissues and the last 10 cm of the ileum were harvested, fixed by immersion in 4% buffered paraformaldehyde, and embedded in paraffin. Sections (4 μm) were stained with hematoxylin-eosin (HE) and assessed for inflammation and tissue damage.

Liver myeloperoxidase activity

Tissue-associated myeloperoxidase (MPO) activity, an indicator of neutrophil infiltration, was determined as previously described [15].

Real-time reverse-transcriptase polymerase chain reaction

Total RNA was extracted from the liver using TRIzol reagent (Life Technologies, Carlbad, USA) according to the manufacturer's instructions. The mRNA for tumor necrosis factor-alpha (TNF-a), interleukin-6 (IL-6), and glyceraldehyde 3-phosphate dehydrogenase (GAPDH) was quantified in duplicate by SYBR green two-step, real-time reverse-transcriptase polymerase chain reaction (RT-PCR) with an ABI-Prism 7500 Sequence Detector (Applied Biosystems, Foster City, USA) using the primers previously described [15]. GAPDH mRNA levels were used as the invariant control for each sample.

Enzyme-linked immunosorbent assay

TNF-α, IL-6, and endotoxin levels in serum were measured using enzyme-linked immunosorbent assay (ELISA) kits (R&D Systems, Minneapolis, USA).

Immunohistochemistry

Anti-ZO-1 antibody (Abcam, Cambridge, UK) was used for immunohistochemical staining. Immunohistochemical detection was performed using a two-step visualization system (DAKO, Glostrup, Denmark).

Immunofluorescence

Anti-CD68 antibody (AbD Serotec, Kidlington, UK) was used for immunofluorescent staining. Secondary antibody was FITC-

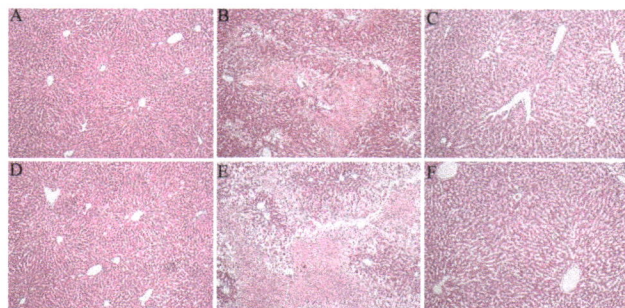

Figure 2. Histopathologic analyses of livers after reperfusion. Rats were subjected to total warm liver I/R injury or sham operation and pretreated with butyrate or vehicle. HE-stained liver sections from the sham (A, D), vehicle (B, E), and butyrate (C, F) groups at 6 h (B, C) and 24 h (E, F) after reperfusion (×200).

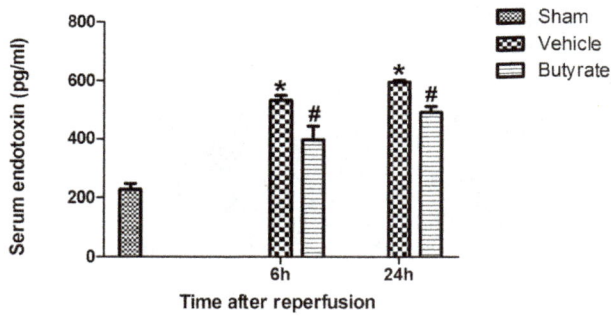

Figure 7. Effect of butyrate on serum endotoxin concentration. Rats were subjected to total liver I/R injury or sham operation and pretreated with butyrate or vehicle. Serum endotoxin concentration was measured by Elisa after reperfusion. Data represent means ± SD, N = 3–5 rats per group. *P<0.05 vs. the sham group, #P<0.05 vs. the vehicle group.

AST levels significantly increased in the vehicle group at 6 and 24 h after reperfusion (Figure 1). In contrast, pretreatment with butyrate significantly decreased the serum levels of AST and ALT at the observation points. The protection was also confirmed by liver pathology after reperfusion (Figure 2). Severe lobular distortion with massive necrosis, increased swelling, cytoplasmic vacuolization, hemorrhage, and neutrophil infiltration were present in the portal area of liver tissue in the vehicle group. In contrast, pretreatment with butyrate markedly reduced the above pathologic changes; mild damage characterized by interstitial edema and less neutrophil infiltration were observed only in a few areas of the liver in the butyrate group.

Butyrate decreases liver I/R-induced inflammatory cytokines production

Inflammatory cytokines such as TNF-α and IL-6 contribute to the pathophysiology of hepatic I/R injury. We analyzed the rats' mRNA expression patterns in the liver following I/R using RT-PCR. As shown in Figure 3A and 3B, butyrate significantly decreased the intrahepatic expression of mRNA coding for TNF-α and IL-6 at 6 and 24 h after reperfusion in comparison with the vehicle group. Furthermore, the serum levels of TNF-α and IL-6 assessed by ELISA were consistent with the mRNA results (Figure 3C, D).

Butyrate inhibits macrophages activation, TLR4 expression in live

Kupffer cells and liver-infiltrating monocyte-derived macrophages play important roles during liver I/R injury [16]. CD68 was detected as the marker of activated macrophages [17]. Immunofluorescent staining showed that only a few CD68-positive cells in the sham group (Figure 4); the CD68-positive cells in the vehicle hepatic tissue increased prominently. However, butyrate treatment significantly inhibited the macrophages activation at 6 and 24 h post-reperfusion (Figure 4). The protein expression assessed by Western blot revealed that the CD68 expression in the liver was upregulated significantly after total hepatic I/R, which was remarkably downregulated compared with the vehicle group by butyrate (Figure 5).

Hepatic I/R injury and LPS signaling are largely TLR4 dependent [16,18]. The expression of TLR4 was determined by Western blot. As shown in Figure 5., there was a marked increase in the expression of TLR4 after total hepatic I/R, but less so in the

butyrate group, indicting the inhibition of inflammation cascade by butyrate.

Butyrate inhibits neutrophil infiltration in live

Based on the pivotal mediators of neutrophils in inflammatory response during I/R injury, we also tested the role of neutrophils infiltration in butyrate live protecting. Neutrophil infiltration after reperfusion in the vehicle group, as analyzed by MPO activity (U/g tissue), increased significantly. Compared to the vehicle group at 6 to 24 h after reperfusion, butyrate pretreatment reduced MPO activity (Figure 6), suggesting that butyrate may inhibit neutrophil infiltration.

Butyrate attenuates serum endotoxin concentration

The link between endotoxin and liver injury has been well demonstrated in other studies. In our study, the endotoxin level in the portal vein was found to be remarkably increased after reperfusion (Figure 7); however, it was decreased in the butyrate group.

Butyrate attenuates intestinal mucosal injury and epithelial apoptosis

Histopathologic analysis of the control rats showed a normal mucosal pattern with packed, tall, and intact villi (Figure 8A, D). Compared with the control animals, total hepatic I/R insult caused significant mucosal damage, that is, epithelial shedding, villi fracturing, mucosal atrophy, and edema (Figure 8B, E). However, butyrate treatment significantly attenuated the mucosal damage at 6 and 24 h post-reperfusion (Figure 8C, F).

To further determine the intestinal epithelial barrier integrity after total hepatic I/R, TUNEL staining was performed. After 6 h of reperfusion, the vehicle group demonstrated the highest number of apoptotic cells when compared with the sham group (Figure 9). In contrast, butyrate significantly inhibited the epithelial apoptosis when compared with the vehicle group (Figure 9).

Butyrate prevents ultrastructure alteration of tight junctions

The intestinal ultrastructure was evaluated to analyze the influence of butyrate on tight junctions (TJs). The 30 min ischemia and sequent 6 h reperfusion resulted in obvious ultrastructural changes in the intestinal mucosa, including epithelial sparsely distributing, disarranging, and distorting cell microvilli; epithelial cell edema or shrinkage; dilation of the rough endoplasmic

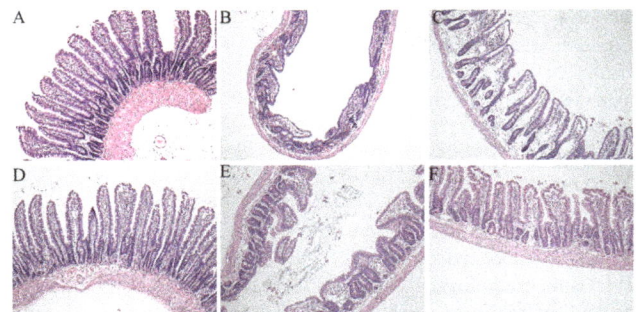

Figure 8. Histopathologic analyses of intestinal mucosa after reperfusion. Rats were subjected to total warm liver I/R injury or sham operation and pretreated with butyrate or vehicle. HE-stained intestinal mucosa from the sham (A, D), vehicle (B, E), and butyrate (C, F) groups at 6 h (B, C) and 24 h (E, F) after reperfusion (×200).

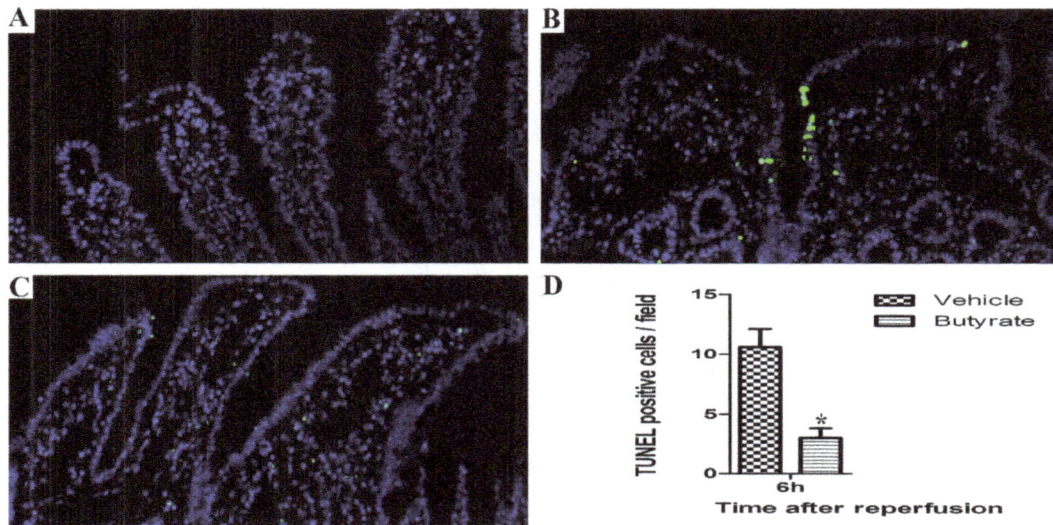

Figure 9. Effects of butyrate on intestinal mucosal epithelial cell apoptosis after I/R. Rats were subjected to total liver I/R injury or sham operation and pretreated with butyrate or vehicle. TUNEL staining was performed to detect intestinal mucosal epithelial cell apoptosis in the sham (A), vehicle (B), and butyrate (C) groups at 6 h after reperfusion (×200). The number of positive cells is presented as means ± SD (D), N = 3–5 rats per group. *P<0.05 vs. the sham group, #P<0.05 vs. the vehicle group.

reticulum, mitochondrial swelling and crista fragmentation; and TJs membrane fusion disruption (Figure 10B, E). In contrast, butyrate supplementation alleviated these ultrastructural pathological changes (Figure 10C, F).

Butyrate protect of the TJs protein ZO-1 after I/R injury

TJs proteins play a critical role in the maintenance of mucosal barrier function, whose deficiency is associated with the altered expression and distribution of TJs proteins. Immunohistochemistry demonstrated the expression of TJs protein ZO-1 in linear fashion at the apical surface of the epithelium with a typical reticular pattern in a normal state (Figure 11A, C). After reperfusion, the expression of ZO-1 showed a significantly disrupted, diffuse staining pattern (Figure 11B, E). Western blot analysis confirmed that ZO-1 expression decreased more significantly after reperfusion, particularly at 6 h (Figure 11G, H). However, butyrate improved the aberrant expression of ZO-1 following I/R, and the reticular structures were subtotally maintained (Figure 11C, F). Consistent with the immunohistochemical results, the expression of ZO-1 was reversed by supplementation with butyrate, as shown by Western blot analysis (Figure 11G, H). These results suggest that butyrate can exert a protective effect on the TJs proteins after reperfusion injury with bowel congestion.

Discussion

The present study demonstrated that I/R resulted in liver injury, as evidenced by the elevated serum levels of AST, ALT, and tissue pathologic changes. Previous research has shown a marked increase in sensitivity to endotoxin after liver injury, leading to further hepatic damage and even systemic endotoxemia or septic shock [19]. Several studies have demonstrated that I/R-induced liver injury was aggravated by exogenous LPS [6,20,21]. Thus, decreasing the levels of endotoxin may protect the liver from injury. The results presented here are promising, as pretreatment with butyrate attenuates liver injury induced by I/R aggravated by

endotoxin translocated from the intestinal lumen due to dysfunction of the gut barrier function, as indicated by the reduced transaminase levels and improved tissue pathology.

What calls for special attention here is that our model of total hepatic I/R with bowel congestion differs from other models involving partial hepatic ischemia with or without LPS administration. In the setting of liver transplantation, portal vein interrupt and bowel congestion are unavoidable. To better reflect the pathophysiology but simplify the procedure of hepatic transplantation, we employed the total hepatic I/R model in our study.

HDAC inhibition is emerging as a novel approach to treat a variety of diseases. Recently, butyrate has been shown to have anti-inflammatory effects both in vitro and in vivo [22,23,24]. HDAC inhibitors have previously shown robust neuroprotective effects in a focal cerebral ischemia model of rats [25], protecting the heart against ischemic injury [26]. Our previous study also supported the pivotal role of butyrate in protection of hepatic injury in the rat partial I/R model [13]. We are also interested in whether butyrate can attenuate total hepatic I/R injury compli-

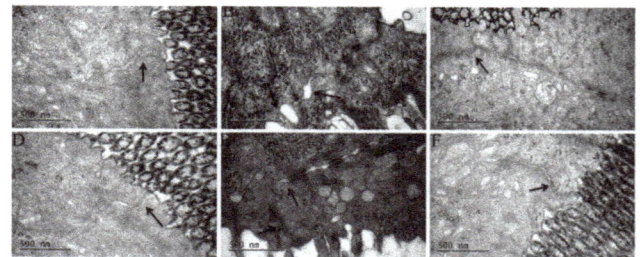

Figure 10. Transmission electron microscopy of intestine. Rats were subjected to total warm liver I/R injury or sham operation and pretreated with butyrate or vehicle. Transmission electron microscopy of rat intestine from the sham (A, D), vehicle (B, E), and butyrate (C, F) groups at 6 h (B, C) and 24 h (E, F) after reperfusion, focusing on tight junctions (↑).

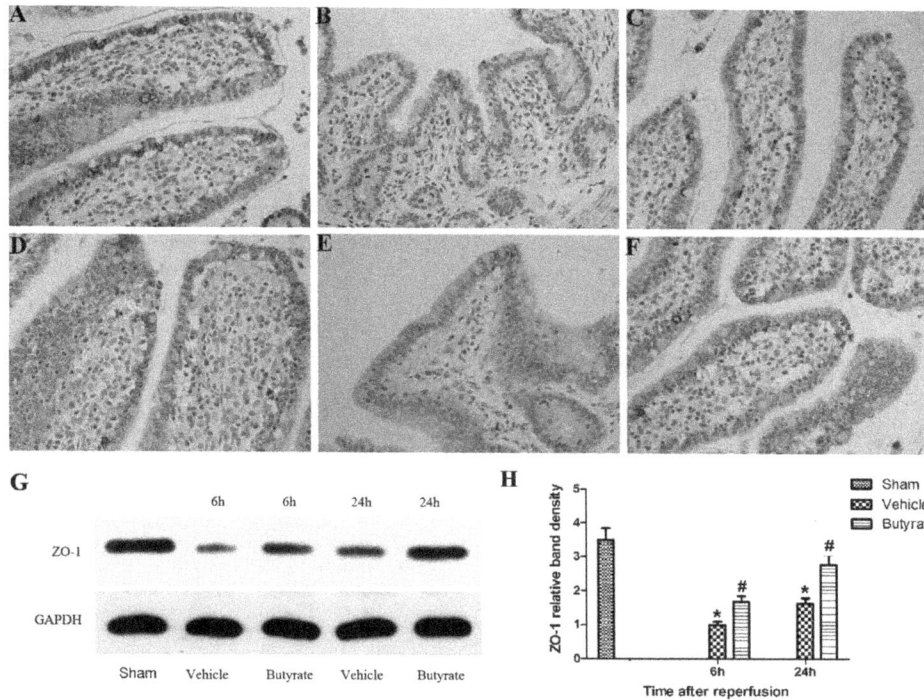

Figure 11. Effects of butyrate on expression of ZO-1. Rats were subjected to total liver I/R injury or sham operation and pretreated with butyrate or vehicle. Immunohistochemical staining of ZO-1 was detected in the sham (A, D), vehicle (B, E), and butyrate (C, F) groups at 6 h (B, C) and 24 h (E, F) after reperfusion (×400). Representative Western blots analysis (G) and quantitative evaluation (H) of the expression of ZO-1 in intestinal mucosa after I/R. GAPDH was run as an internal standard. Data represent means ± SD, N = 3–5 rats per group. *$P < 0.05$ vs. the sham group, #$P < 0.05$ vs. the vehicle group.

cated by endotoxin from the intestinal lumen.

Endotoxin is normally prevented from entering the intestinal lumen because of the intestinal barrier. The intestinal barrier function depends on TJs between intact epithelial cells [27,28]. The disruption of the epithelial barrier because of bowel congestion in total hepatic I/R results in increased intestinal permeability, permitting endotoxin to translocate from the lumen into the portal blood. This, in turn, causes secondary insult to hepatic injury, and even liver failure. Therefore, in the early phase of reperfusion injury, if we can attenuate intestinal barrier injury to inhibit endotoxin translocation, the secondary insult may be reduced.

Few studies have examined intestinal barrier injury and the TJs ultrastructure during total hepatic I/R injury, and butyrate's role and mechanism of action in total hepatic I/R injury remain unclear. In the present study, we observed gross morphological changes and the ultrastructure of microvilli in intestinal tissue. Obvious morphological changes were found, including the shedding and apoptosis of epithelial cells, fracturing and fusion of villi, mucosal atrophy, and edema. This histological damage indicated intestinal barrier function injury, possibly resulting in increased permeability. Moreover, we indeed observed increased endotoxin levels after reperfusion, with simultaneous disruption to TJs integrity. Additionally, these pathological changes were mitigated with butyrate administration, and the endotoxin levels were reduced. Therefore, the increase in intestinal permeability may be attributed to the disruption of TJs between intestinal mucosal epithelial cells, whereas butyrate reversed this pathological change.

To analyze the mechanism of TJs disruption, we assessed the expression of the TJs-related protein ZO-1 by immunohistochemistry and western blot. ZO-1 has been demonstrated to interact between transmembrane protein occlusion and the actin cytoskeleton and play a crucial role in the maintenance of the integrity of the intestinal mucosal barrier and TJs in numerous pathological and physiological processes [29]. In this study, total hepatic I/R injury resulted in the abnormal distribution of ZO-1 and significantly decreased ZO-1 expression in the intestinal mucosa, whereas butyrate pretreatment led to a reversal of aberrant ZO-1 expression, which was probably associated with the mechanisms by which butyrate inhibits gut leakage induced by bowel congestion in total hepatic I/R.

KCs, the resident macrophages in the liver, have been identified as the primary cell type in the initiation and perpetuation of I/R injury [16], which can be further activated by endotoxin through TLR4. Indeed, activated KCs produce reactive oxygen species, proinflammatory cytokines and chemokines. These recruit and activate circulating macrophages, neutrophils, lymphocytes, and sinusoidal endothelial cells, all of which contribute to the inflammation associated with liver damage [1]. We found that CD68, the marker of peripheral or liver-resident macrophages (KCs), is increased in the liver tissue after reperfusion, suggesting that total I/R had induced more macrophages activation, which was confirmed by the remarkable heightened TNF-α and IL-6 levels. Meanwhile, MPO activity, which is a widely used marker of neutrophil infiltration, was rapidly upregulated. However, pre-administration of butyrate downregulated the expression of CD68 protein and MPO activity, decreased inflammatory cytokines, which obviously indicates inhibition of KC activation and neutrophil infiltration, thereby ameliorating the liver injury.

Increasing evidence suggests that TLR4, the detector of bacterial endotoxin and other endogenous ligands including high-mobility group box 1, plays a critical role in LPS signaling and pathogenesis of liver I/R injury [16]. We further detected the increased expression of TLR4 and downregulation by butyrate administration, confirming the hepatoprotection of butyrate.

In conclusion, our study suggests that butyrate hepatoprotection in a rat model of total hepatic I/R injury may be associated with decreased endotoxin translocation via protection of gut barrier function injury and suppressing macrophages activation, inflam-

matory factor production and neutrophil infiltration. Given that butyrate is a naturally occurring product in the body with low toxicity, it may be an effective hepatoprotective agent and a promising candidate in liver transplantation.

Author Contributions

Conceived and designed the experiments: YLQ JMQ. Performed the experiments: FRW ZYM QBW. Analyzed the data: YLQ JMQ BL. Contributed reagents/materials/analysis tools: ZYM QBW. Wrote the paper: YLQ BL.

References

1. Zhai Y, Busuttil RW, Kupiec-Weglinski JW (2011) Liver ischemia and reperfusion injury: new insights into mechanisms of innate-adaptive immune-mediated tissue inflammation. Am J Transplant 11: 1563–1569.
2. Reich DJ, Hong JC (2010) Current status of donation after cardiac death liver transplantation. Curr Opin Organ Transplant 15: 316–321.
3. Foley DP, Fernandez LA, Leverson G, Chin LT, Krieger N, et al. (2005) Donation after cardiac death: the University of Wisconsin experience with liver transplantation. Ann Surg 242: 724–731.
4. Xing HC, Li LJ, Xu KJ, Shen T, Chen YB, et al. (2005) Effects of Salvia miltiorrhiza on intestinal microflora in rats with ischemia/reperfusion liver injury. Hepatobiliary Pancreat Dis Int 4: 274–280.
5. Watanabe M, Chijiiwa K, Kameoka N, Yamaguchi K, Kuroki S, et al. (2000) Gadolinium pretreatment decreases survival and impairs liver regeneration after partial hepatectomy under ischemia/reperfusion in rats. Surgery 127: 456–463.
6. Fernandez ED, Flohe S, Siemers F, Nau M, Ackermann M, et al. (2000) Endotoxin tolerance protects against local hepatic ischemia/reperfusion injury in the rat. J Endotoxin Res 6: 321–328.
7. Zhang F, Mao Y, Qiao H, Jiang H, Zhao H, et al. (2010) Protective effects of taurine against endotoxin-induced acute liver injury after hepatic ischemia reperfusion. Amino Acids 38: 237–245.
8. Hinnebusch BF, Meng S, Wu JT, Archer SY, Hodin RA (2002) The effects of short-chain fatty acids on human colon cancer cell phenotype are associated with histone hyperacetylation. J Nutr 132: 1012–1017.
9. Meijer K, de Vos P, Priebe MG (2010) Butyrate and other short-chain fatty acids as modulators of immunity: what relevance for health? Curr Opin Clin Nutr Metab Care 13: 715–721.
10. Koruda MJ, Rolandelli RH, Bliss DZ, Hastings J, Rombeau JL, et al. (1990) Parenteral nutrition supplemented with short-chain fatty acids: effect on the small-bowel mucosa in normal rats. Am J Clin Nutr 51: 685–689.
11. Peng L, He Z, Chen W, Holzman IR, Lin J (2007) Effects of butyrate on intestinal barrier function in a Caco-2 cell monolayer model of intestinal barrier. Pediatr Res 61: 37–41.
12. Peng L, Li ZR, Green RS, Holzman IR, Lin J (2009) Butyrate enhances the intestinal barrier by facilitating tight junction assembly via activation of AMP-activated protein kinase in Caco-2 cell monolayers. J Nutr 139: 1619–1625.
13. Qiao YL, Qian JM, Wang FR, Ma ZY, Wang QW (2013) Butyrate protects liver against ischemia reperfusion injury by inhibiting nuclear factor kappa B activation in Kupffer cells. J Surg Res.
14. Ellett JD, Atkinson C, Evans ZP, Amani Z, Balish E, et al. (2010) Murine Kupffer cells are protective in total hepatic ischemia/reperfusion injury with bowel congestion through IL-10. J Immunol 184: 5849–5858.
15. Ma ZY, Qian JM, Rui XH, Wang FR, Wang QW, et al. (2010) Inhibition of matrix metalloproteinase-9 attenuates acute small-for-size liver graft injury in rats. Am J Transplant 10: 784–795.
16. Tsung A, Hoffman RA, Izuishi K, Critchlow ND, Nakao A, et al. (2005) Hepatic ischemia/reperfusion injury involves functional TLR4 signaling in nonparenchymal cells. J Immunol 175: 7661–7668.
17. Rabinowitz SS, Gordon S (1991) Macrosialin, a macrophage-restricted membrane sialoprotein differentially glycosylated in response to inflammatory stimuli. J Exp Med 174: 827–836.
18. Zhai Y, Shen XD, O'Connell R, Gao F, Lassman C, et al. (2004) Cutting edge: TLR4 activation mediates liver ischemia/reperfusion inflammatory response via IFN regulatory factor 3-dependent MyD88-independent pathway. J Immunol 173: 7115–7119.
19. Tsuji K, Kwon AH, Yoshida H, Qiu Z, Kaibori M, et al. (2005) Free radical scavenger (edaravone) prevents endotoxin-induced liver injury after partial hepatectomy in rats. J Hepatol 42: 94–101.
20. Kaibori M, Yanagida H, Uchida Y, Yokoigawa N, Kwon AH, et al. (2004) Pirfenidone protects endotoxin-induced liver injury after hepatic ischemia in rats. Transplant Proc 36: 1973–1974.
21. Caraceni P, Pertosa AM, Giannone F, Domenicali M, Grattagliano I, et al. (2009) Antagonism of the cannabinoid CB-1 receptor protects rat liver against ischaemia-reperfusion injury complicated by endotoxaemia. Gut 58: 1135–1143.
22. Liu T, Li J, Liu Y, Xiao N, Suo H, et al. (2012) Short-chain fatty acids suppress lipopolysaccharide-induced production of nitric oxide and proinflammatory cytokines through inhibition of NF-kappaB pathway in RAW 264.7 cells. Inflammation 35: 1676–1684.
23. Park JS, Lee EJ, Lee JC, Kim WK, Kim HS (2007) Anti-inflammatory effects of short chain fatty acids in IFN-gamma-stimulated RAW 264.7 murine macrophage cells: involvement of NF-kappaB and ERK signaling pathways. Int Immunopharmacol 7: 70–77.
24. Zhang LT, Yao YM, Lu JQ, Yan XJ, Yu Y, et al. (2007) Sodium butyrate prevents lethality of severe sepsis in rats. Shock 27: 672–677.
25. Kim HJ, Rowe M, Ren M, Hong JS, Chen PS, et al. (2007) Histone deacetylase inhibitors exhibit anti-inflammatory and neuroprotective effects in a rat permanent ischemic model of stroke: multiple mechanisms of action. J Pharmacol Exp Ther 321: 892–901.
26. Granger A, Abdullah I, Huebner F, Stout A, Wang T, et al. (2008) Histone deacetylase inhibition reduces myocardial ischemia-reperfusion injury in mice. FASEB J 22: 3549–3560.
27. Samak G, Suzuki T, Bhargava A, Rao RK (2010) c-Jun NH2-terminal kinase-2 mediates osmotic stress-induced tight junction disruption in the intestinal epithelium. Am J Physiol Gastrointest Liver Physiol 299: G572–G584.
28. Strauman MC, Harper JM, Harrington SM, Boll EJ, Nataro JP (2010) Enteroaggregative Escherichia coli disrupts epithelial cell tight junctions. Infect Immun 78: 4958–4964.
29. Han X, Fink MP, Yang R, Delude RL (2004) Increased iNOS activity is essential for intestinal epithelial tight junction dysfunction in endotoxemic mice. Shock 21: 261–270.

21

Bone Marrow Transplantation Concurrently Reconstitutes Donor Liver and Immune System across Host Species Barrier in Mice

Ziping Qi[1], Lu Li[1,2], Xuefu Wang[1], Xiang Gao[3], Xin Wang[4], Haiming Wei[1,2], Jian Zhang[5], Rui Sun[1,2], Zhigang Tian[1,2,6]*

1 Department of Immunology, School of Life Sciences, University of Science and Technology of China, Hefei, Anhui, China, 2 Hefei National Laboratory for Physical Sciences at Microscale, Hefei, Anhui, China, 3 Model Animal Research Center, Nanjing University, Nanjing, China, 4 Institute of Biochemistry and Cell Biology, Shanghai Institute for Biological Sciences, Chinese Academy of Sciences, Shanghai, China, 5 School of Pharmaceutical Sciences, Shandong University, Jinan, China, 6 Collaborative Innovation Center for Diagnosis and Treatment of Infectious Diseases, Hangzhou, Zhejiang, China

Abstract

Liver immunopathologic mechanisms during hepatotropic infection, malignant transformation, and autoimmunity are still unclear. Establishing a chimeric mouse with a reconstituted liver and immune system derived from a single donor across species is critical to study regional donor immune responses in recipient liver. Using a strain of mice deficient in tyrosine catabolic enzyme fumarylacetoacetate hydrolase ($fah^{-/-}$) and bone marrow transplantation (BMT), we reconstituted the donor's hepatocytes and immune cells across host species barrier. Syngeneic, allogeneic or even xenogeneic rat BMT rescued most recipient $fah^{-/-}$ mice against liver failure by donor BM-derived FAH[+] hepatocytes. Importantly, immune system developed normally in chimeras, and the immune cells together with organ architecture were intact and functional. Thus, donor BM can across host species barrier and concurrently reconstitutes MHC-identical response between immune cells and hepatocytes, giving rise to a new simple and convenient small animal model to study donor's liver immune response in mice.

Editor: Pranela Rameshwar, Rutgers - New Jersey Medical School, United States of America

Funding: This work was supported by Ministry of Science & Technology of China (Basic Science Project #2013CB531503, #2013CB944902), Natural Science Foundation of China (#31390433), and National Science & Technology Major Projects(#2012ZX10002006). The funders had no role in study design, data collection and analysis, decision to publish, or preparation of the manuscript.

Competing Interests: The authors have declared that no competing interests exist.

* Email: tzg@ustc.edu.cn

Introduction

The liver diseases caused by hepatitis B virus and hepatitis C virus infection are among the most important human health problems [1]. The immunopathogenesis of virus infection and the development of antiviral drugs are hampered by the lack of suitable mouse models for both pathogens, because the mouse cannot be infected by HBV or HCV. Although chimpanzees are susceptible to both infections, their usage is limited by cost, availability, and ethical considerations [2,3]. Other surrogate hepatotrophic viruses that infect ducks [4], woodchucks [5], and ground squirrels [6] have been widely used to study virus biology, however, they suffer from two important limitations: (1) on the microbial side, surrogate viruses are genetically divergent from highly restricted human counterparts; and (2) on the host side, the immunological studies in genetically outbred and immunologically uncharacterized hosts are difficult. HBV-transgenic mice have provided invaluable information on immunopathogenesis of HBV, whereas transgenic mice are immunologically tolerant to transgene products [7]. Hydrodynamic transfection of the mouse liver by the HBV genome has also been reported to study HBV immunobiology [8], but it does not support bona fide viral infection.

Therefore, a robust and reproducible mouse model of HBV or HCV infection is desperately needed, and studies based on chimeric mice appear to be the most promising.

Establishing a chimeric mouse with a reconstituted liver and immune system derived from a single donor is critical to study MHC-restricted immune responses against pathogen-infected, transformed or autoimmune hepatocytes in a physiologic setting. In the separate experiments [9–12], it was reported that donor hematopoietic stem cell (HSC) can differentiate into not only immune cells but also hepatocytes, which greatly helps understanding the maturation of donor immune system, and virus-infected donor hepatocytes, respectively; however, from our knowledge, no experiment was practically economically carried out to exhibit the donor immune response against their own hepatocyte-presented antigens because lacking chimeras mouse with a MHC-matched response between immune cells and hepatocytes which needs a dual reconstitution from a single donor.

A widely accepted method to construct chimeras with a complete donor immune system is hematopoietic stem cell (HSC) transplantation into lethally irradiated or immunodeficient recipients, such as NOD-$scid$-$Il2r\gamma^{-/-}$ (NOG) [13,14] or BALB/c-

$Rag2^{-/-}$—$Il2r\gamma^{-/-}$ mice [10]. These two kinds of mice were highly deficient in immune system, leaving the space for donor's HSC engraftment, especially for the development of human immune system (HIS) in humanized mouse. Chimeras with donor-derived hepatocytes can also be created by transplanting exogenous hepatocytes or embryonic stem cells, like in the uroplasminogen-activator (uPA) transgenic [15] or fumarylacetoacetate hydrolase (FAH)-deficient models [16]. Both uPA transgenic mouse and FAH deficient mouse suffer from progressive liver failure, so that donor's hepatocytes could engraft and repopulate in recipient mouse more easily. However, neither the immune- nor liver-reconstituted chimera alone is sufficient to further evaluate the interaction between the immune system and the pathogen-infected or inflamed liver organs.

There is a significant need for a model system, with MHC-identity between donor immune cells and pathogen-targeting organs, to further investigate the pathology, immune correlates, and mechanisms of highly specialized pathogens like HBV, HCV and malaria (at liver stage). To avoid the potential complication from histocompatibility, hematopoietic and hepatic (or any other organ origin) progenitors had better to be from the same donor. It was recently reported that HSC may also differentiate into hepatocytes in bone marrow transplanted (BMT) mice [9,17–20]. We therefore hypothesized that donor HSCs may concurrently differentiate into immune cells and hepatocytes in recipients that have open tissue space, which will greatly benefit exploiting the donor's MHC-restricted interaction between immune cells and hepatocytes.

Here, using fah-deficient mice and BMT, we reconstituted donor hepatocytes and immune cells across host species barrier. All recipient $fah^{-/-}$ mice survived without NTBC feeding at least 5 months after syn-, allo- and xeno- BMT (rat), and donor BM-derived hepatocytes were detected in liver sections. Importantly, donor immune systems developed normally in MHC-identical chimeras, and the immune cells together with organ architecture were intact and functional. Thus, donor BM can across host species barrier and concurrently reconstitutes MHC-identical response between immune cells and hepatocytes. Thus, this method gives rise to a new simple and convenient small animal model to study donor's liver immune response across host species barrier in mice.

Materials and Methods

Mice

C3H/HeJSlac mice and Sprague-Dawley (S.D.) rats were purchased from the Shanghai Experimental Center, Chinese Science Academy (Shanghai, China). EGFP-transgenic mice were purchased from the Model Animal Research Center (Nanjing, China), who originally obtained them from the Jackson Laboratory (Bar Harbor, ME, USA). $Fah^{-/-}$ mice (a gift from Xin Wang) were normally treated with NTBC in the drinking water at a concentration of 7.5 mg/L.

Ethics Statement

All animals were housed in a specific pathogen-free facility and used according to the animal care regulations of the University of Science and Technology of China. The study was approved by the Local Ethics Committee for Animal Care and Use at University of Science and Technology of China (Permit Number: USTCACUC 1201009). Surgery mice were anesthetized by intraperitoneal injection of 30 μg/g body weight sodium pentobarbital, and the surgeries were performed by skillful experimenter. Sacrificed animals were euthanized by CO_2, and all efforts were made to minimize suffering. For survival study, mice were monitored daily. A humane endpoint was always used, and moribond animals were euthanised by CO_2. The clinical criteria used to determine the endpoint include: a). Rapid or progressive weight loss. b). Rough hair coat/unkempt appearance. c). Hunched posture, dehydration, and hypothermia. d). Lethargy or persistent recumbency, immobility. e). Decreased food or water intake. f). Opacity eyes, lack of responsiveness to manual stimulation.

BMC harvest and transplantation

BMCs were harvested by flushing long bones of mice or rats with 1640 medium (Gibco, New York, USA) and then washed with phosphate-buffered saline and counted. Cell concentrations were adjusted for transplantation by tail vein injection, with 2 million BMCs in 300 μl 1640 medium per mouse. $Fah^{-/-}$ recipient mice were lethally irradiated with a dose of 14 Gy total body irradiation in a split dose with a 4-hour interval (200 cGy/min, 7Gy×2) the day before transplantation. Anti-AsGM1 (Wako Pure Chemicals Industries, Osaka, Japan) was administered (50 μg, i.v.) to deplete NK cells in recipient mice.

Analysis of mice

Mice were monitored and body weight changes were recorded after cell transplantation. To obtain peripheral blood cells and plasma, mice were bled from the tail. When sacrificed, single cell suspensions from organs were prepared, and red blood cells were lysed. Liver mononuclear cells (MNCs) were prepared as described [21].

Assay for metabolic parameters of mice

Serum biochemical markers, including alanine aminotransferase (ALT), aspartate aminotransferase (AST), alkaline phosphatase (ALP), gamma-glutamyl transpeptidase (GGT), total bilirubin (TBILI), creatinine (CRE), and albumin (ALB), were assessed by the standard photometric method using the biochemical detection kits (Rong Sheng, Shanghai, China) following the manufacturer's instructions.

Isolation of mouse hepatocytes

Mouse hepatocytes were isolated as described [22]. Briefly, mice were anesthetized by intraperitoneal injection of 30 μg/g body weight sodium pentobarbital. The portal vein was cannulated, and the liver was subsequently perfused with ethylene glycol tetraacetic acid (EGTA) solution and digested with 0.075% collagenase solution. Viable hepatocytes suspended in Dulbecco's Modified Eagle's Medium (DMEM) (Gibco, NY, USA) solution were separated by a 40% Percoll (Gibco, NY, USA) solution with centrifugation at 400×g for 10 min at 4°C.

Flow cytometry assay

Single-cell suspensions were blocked and incubated with the indicated fluorescent monoclonal antibodies (mAbs). Samples were acquired by a BD FACScalibur cytometer and analyzed by FlowJo software. The anti-mouse mAbs used for flow cytometry included the following: anti-mouse CD16/CD32; FITC-conjugated anti-CD49b (DX5), anti-CD8 (H35-17.2), anti-H-2K^k (AF3-12.1); PE-conjugated anti-CD49b (DX5), anti-CD8 (H35-17.2), anti-H-2D^d (34-2-12), anti-H-2D^b (KH95); PerCP-conjugated anti-CD19 (ID3); PE-Cy^{TM}7-conjugated anti-NK1.1 (PK136), anti-CD45 (30-F11); APC-conjugated anti-CD3 (145-2C11); and APC-Cy^{TM}7-conjugated anti-CD4 (GK1.5). The anti-rat mAbs used for flow cytometry included: FITC-conjugated anti-RT1A (C3); PE-conjugated anti-CD161a (10/78); PerCP-conjugated anti-

CD8α (OX-8); PE-Cy^{TM}7-conjugated anti-CD4 (OX-35); and APC-conjugated anti-CD3 (1F4). Appropriate isotype-matched, irrelevant control mAbs were used to determine the level of background staining. All the antibodies were purchased from BD Biosciences (San Diego, CA, USA).

Histological examination

Liver, spleen, and lymph node samples were fixed in 10% neutral-buffered formalin and embedded in paraffin. Sections of 6- μm thickness were affixed to slides, deparaffinized, dehydrated, and then stained with hematoxylin and eosin (H&E) using routine methods.

Immunohistochemistry

Commercially available monoclonal antibodies to mouse CD3 (Abcam, Cambridge, UK), mouse CD19 (Abcam), EGFP (Clontech, Otsu, Japan), and a polyclonal antibody to FAH (Abnova, CA, USA) were used for immunohistochemistry staining. After heat- or protease-induced antigen retrieval, formalin-fixed and paraffin-embedded liver tissue sections were stained with primary antibodies overnight at 4°C. The slides were subsequently incubated with ImmPRES anti-rabbit Ig or anti-mouse Ig (Vector Laboratories, Burlingame, CA) at room temperature for 30 min, stained with peroxidase substrate 3, 3'-diaminobenzidine chromogen (Vector Laboratories), and finally counterstained with hematoxylin.

Vaccination of transplanted mice

For HBV vaccination, mice were vaccinated intramuscularly with 1 μg recombinant HBsAg protein vaccine (Biokangtai Company, Shenzhen, China) twice at a two-week interval. For OVA immunization, mice received two vaccinations subcutaneously at a two-week interval with 5 μg OVA protein (Sigma, St. Louis, MO, USA) dissolved in complete Freund's adjuvant (Sigma). Blood samples were obtained 1 week after booster vaccination by tail bleeding, and sera were kept at -20°C until used.

RIA and ELISA

Serum anti-HBs levels were assessed using corresponding radioimmunoassay (RIA) kits (Beijing North Institute of Biological Technology, China) according to the manufacturer's instructions. OVA-specific antibodies were detected by ELISA. In brief, stripwell flat bottom polystyrene plates (Corstar, NY, USA) were coated with 1 μg/μl OVA (Sigma) overnight at 4°C, and then the membranes were blocked by a 5% BSA solution in a 200 μl volume. After being washed, plates were filled with 100 μl mice sera at appropriate dilution ratios for 1 hour followed by incubation with an HRP-conjugated goat anti-mouse IgG (Boster, Wuhan, China). Antibody levels were visualized by TMB substrate (eBioscience, San Diego) and collected as OD450 values.

Statistical analysis

The two-tailed unpaired Student's t-test or ANOVA was used for statistical analyses. The experimental data was expressed as mean ± SEM, and the data are representative of at least 3 independent experiments. $p < 0.05$ was considered statistically significant.

Results

Syngeneic BMT rescure fah$^{-/-}$ mice from liver failure by BM-derived FAH$^+$ hepatocytes

The *fah*$^{-/-}$ mouse is a useful animal model for liver regeneration. Without administering a chemical (2-(2-nitro-4-trifluoromethyl-benzoyl) cyclohexane-1, 3-dione, NTBC) to keep hepatocytes alive, *fah*-deficient hepatocytes die of accumulated toxic metabolites [23], and *fah*$^{-/-}$ mice therefore suffer from progressive liver failure and death (Figure S1).

By carefully combining lethal irradiation and NTBC withdrawal in *fah*$^{-/-}$ mice, space is created in both the bone marrow (BM) and in the liver compartments in recipient mice. To determine whether BMCs from a single syngeneic donor can dually reconstitute the immune and hepatic system in recipient *fah*$^{-/-}$ mice after syn-BMT, we transplanted BM from *EGFP-Tg* mice (haplotype H-2^b, *fah*$^{+/+}$) into *fah*$^{-/-}$/129SvJ (H-2^b) recipients. Though transplanted mice initially lost approximately 15% of their body weight, they soon recovered and maintained 100% of their initial weight for 150 days (Fig. 1A). Serum alanine aminotransferase (ALT) levels gradually increased after NTBC withdrawal and finally reduced to 80 IU/L, which differed from *fah*$^{-/-}$ mice without NTBC feeding (Fig. 1B and Figure S1C). All BMT mice survived at least 5 months after NTBC withdrawal beginning at day 28 (Fig. 1C). So syngeneic BMT could reduce liver injury and protect recipient *fah*$^{-/-}$ mice from death.

To evaluate hepatic reconstitution, long-term survivors were sacrificed and analyzed. Hepatocytes from BMT mice partially expressed EGFP, suggesting that they provided the neccessory FAH to restore liver function in recipient *fah*$^{-/-}$ mice (Fig. 1D). EGFP$^+$ hepatocytes, which grow green under fluorescent microscope, were also found in freshly isolated hepatocytes. Liver histology revealed that the EGFP- and FAH-positive cells were organized into a cell cluster, reflecting a gradual reconstitution (Fig. 1E).

Syngeneic BMT reconstitutes a functional immune system in recipient fah$^{-/-}$ mice

Surviving recipients also showed stable multi-lineage hematopoietic reconstitution after syn-BMT. Nearly 100% of the PBMCs from the chimeras expressed EGFP, similar to the PBMCs from *EGFP-Tg* mice (Fig. 2A), and there was little difference in erythroid and lymphoid development between the chimeras and normal mice (Figure S2). PBMC subsets monitored at the indicated time points showed that NK, B, CD4$^+$, and CD8$^+$ T cells reconstituted normally in chimeras (Fig. 2B). Furthermore, we examined lymphocytes in thymus, spleen, and liver at week 9 after BMT and found a similar ratio of T cell subsets between syn-BMT and donor mice in all immune organs (Fig. 2C). Spleen and inguinal lymph node (LN) histology further confirmed successful immune reconstitution in BMT mice. Spleens from chimeras possessed white pulp structures, containing central arterioles surrounded by T and B cells. In some cases, typical germinal center formation was observed in both spleen and LN (Fig. 2D). To directly test the immune response after reconstitution, chimeric mice were immunized twice with an HBV vaccine. All recipient mice produced specific anti-HBsAg antibodies in serum, similar to donor *EGFP-Tg* mice (Fig. 2E), indicating there is a functional immune response. Together, these data suggest that BMCs from syngeneic donors can concurrently reconstitute both the immune and hepatic systems in recipient *fah*$^{-/-}$ mice.

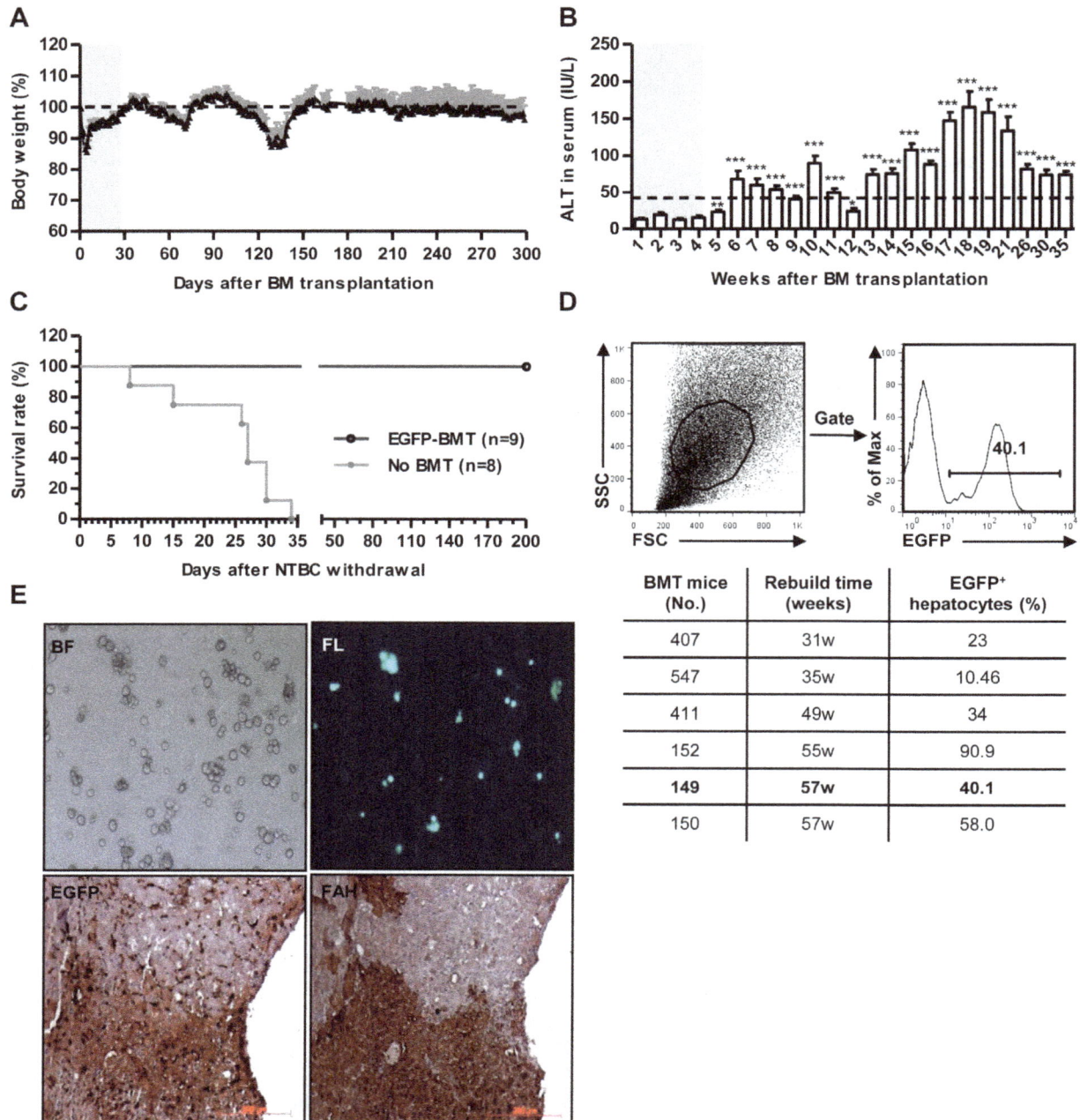

Figure 1. Syngeneic BMT rescue *fah*^{-/-} mice from liver failure by BM-derived hepatocytes. (A-B) Body weight (A) and serum ALT (B) from recipient *fah*^{-/-} mice after syn-BMT. NTBC was withdrawn on day 28 after BMT, and initial body weight was set as 100% (dotted line). Gray areas indicate NTBC administration, white areas indicate NTBC withdrawal. *p<0.05, **p<0.01, ***p<0.001. (mean ± SEM, n=9). (C) Survival rate measurements from recipient *fah*^{-/-} mice after NTBC withdrawal. No BMT *fah*^{-/-} mice without NTBC treatment were set as a control. (D) EGFP+ hepatocytes from a BMT mouse by FACS (rebuild 57w). EGFP+ hepatocytes in other BMT mice are shown in the table below. (E) Donor-derived hepatocytes in BMT mouse 407. Freshly isolated mouse hepatocytes in bright field (left) and under fluorescence (right) are shown above, and EGFP (left) and FAH (right) immunohistochemistry in liver are shown below (brown staining indicates positive cells).

Allogeneic BMC reconstitutes a dual immune and hepatic system in recipient *fah*^{-/-} mice

After successful liver and immune reconstitution in syn-BMT *fah*^{-/-} mice, we next tested whether BMT using allogeneic donors would also concurrently reconstitute in *fah*^{-/-} recipients. We transplanted BM from C3H/HeJSlac mice (H-2^k, *fah*^{+/+}) into *fah*^{-/-}/129SvJ (H-2^b) recipients. Approximately 60% of the allo-

BMT mice survived for at least 5 months after NTBC withdrawal. Although these mice experienced an initial body weight loss of 10%, they soon recovered and maintained normal body weight for at least 150 days, whereas no-BMT mice lost their body weight day by day, and finally died when their body weight was less than 70% of the initial weight (Fig. 3A). Surviving recipients also exhibited stable multi-lineage hematopoietic reconstitution after

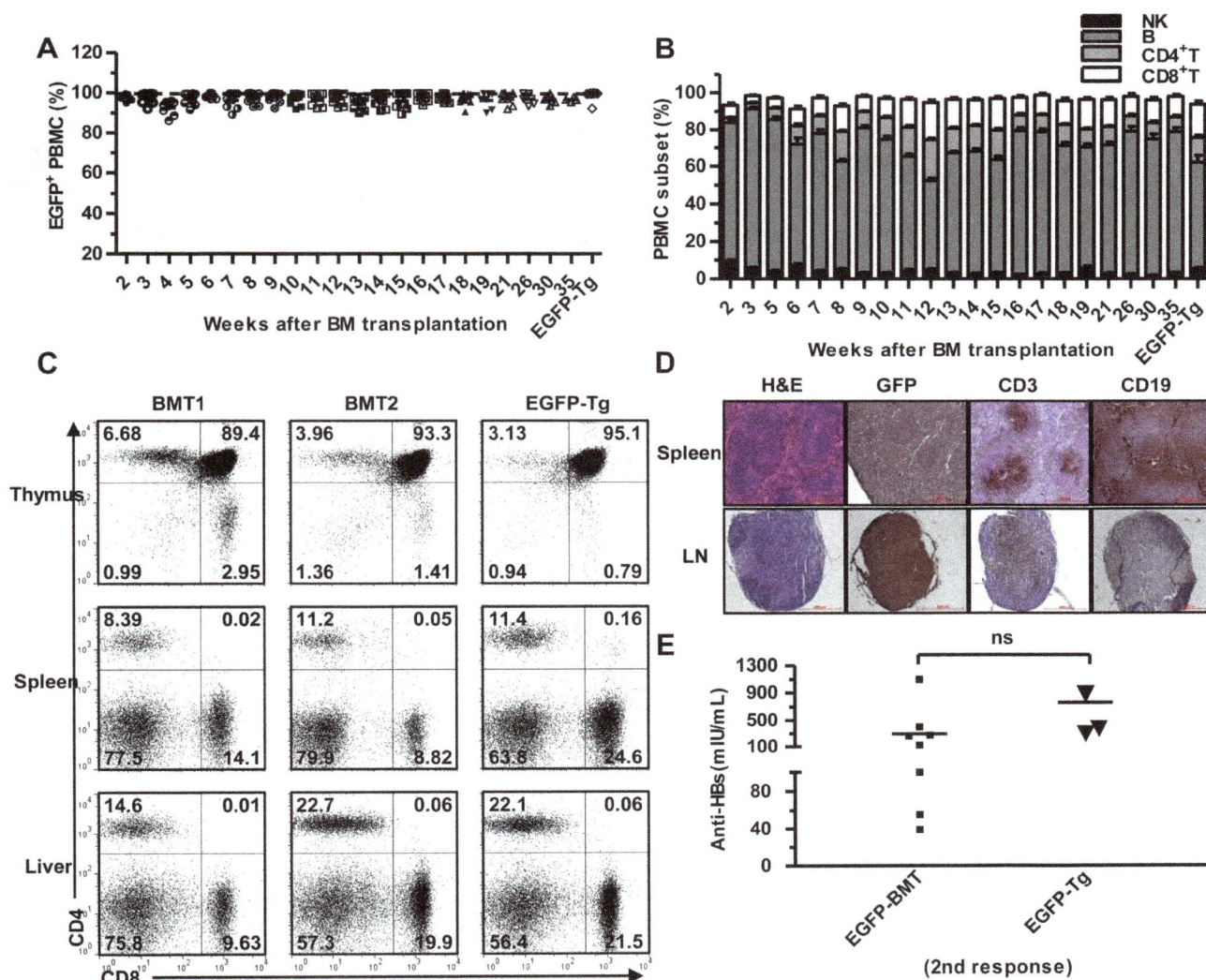

Figure 2. Immune reconstitution in recipient *fah⁻/⁻* mice after syngeneic BMT. (A) Donor-derived EGFP⁺ PBMC measurements from BMT mice at the indicated time points. (B) PBMC subset (NK, B, CD4⁺, and CD8⁺ T) measurements from BMT mice at the indicated times. PBMC from EGFP-Tg mice was set as a positive control. (mean ± SEM, n = 9). (C) Thymus, spleen, and liver CD4⁺ or CD8⁺ T lymphocyte detection in BMT mice (rebuild 9w) or *EGFP-Tg* donor mice by FACS. (D) Spleen and inguinal LN histology of serial sections of BMT mice (rebuild 9w). From L-R, H&E stain, EGFP, CD3, and CD19 immunohistochemistry. Brown staining indicates positive cells. (Original magnification 100×). (E) Serum anti-HBsAg levels in *EGFP-BMT* and *EGFP-Tg* mice after twice HBV vaccine immunizations.

allo-BMT, as nearly 100% of the PBMCs in the chimeras were H-2K^{k+}, similar to C3H donors (Figure S3A), and there was little difference in total erythroid and lymphoid cell counts between chimeras and normal *fah⁻/⁻* mice (Figure S3B–C). Furthermore, the relative percentages of NK, B, CD4⁺, and CD8⁺ T cells subsets in PBMCs became normal over time (Fig. 3B). Spleen and inguinal LN histology further confirmed successful immune reconstitution in allo-BMT mice (Fig. 3C). The reconstituted immune response was functional in allo-BMT mice, as they produced specific anti-OVA antibodies in serum after immunization with OVA protein, similar to donor C3H mice (Fig. 3D).

Hepatocytes from allo-BMT mice also partially expressed donor MHC class I antigen (H-2K^{k+}) (Fig. 3E), suggesting liver allo-repopulation with C3H mice's BM cells. Liver histology further showed that FAH⁺ hepatocytes were detected and organized in a cell cluster (Fig. 3F). From the above, allo-BMT successfully reconstituted both the immune system and hepatocytes in

recipient *fah⁻/⁻* mice, indicating that chimeras with an MHC-matched immune system and liver from a single allogeneic donor can be created.

Xenogeneic rat BMC concurrently reconstitutes their own immune and hepatic system in recipient *fah⁻/⁻* mice

We next attempted to define whether xenogeneic BMC could successfully reconstitute the immune and hepatic system in *fah⁻/⁻* mice. We transplanted Sprague-Dawley rat (RT1A, *fah⁺/⁺*) BM into *fah⁻/⁻* / 129SvJ (H-2^b) recipients. Approximately 50% of xeno-BMT mice survived for at least 5 months after NTBC withdrawal, and serum ALT levels were maintained (Fig. 4). Surviving recipients also showed stable multi-lineage hematopoietic reconstitution. Nearly 100% of the PBMCs were RT1A⁺ in chimeras, and there was little difference in erythroid and lymphoid cell counts between chimeras and recipient mice, NK, CD4⁺, and

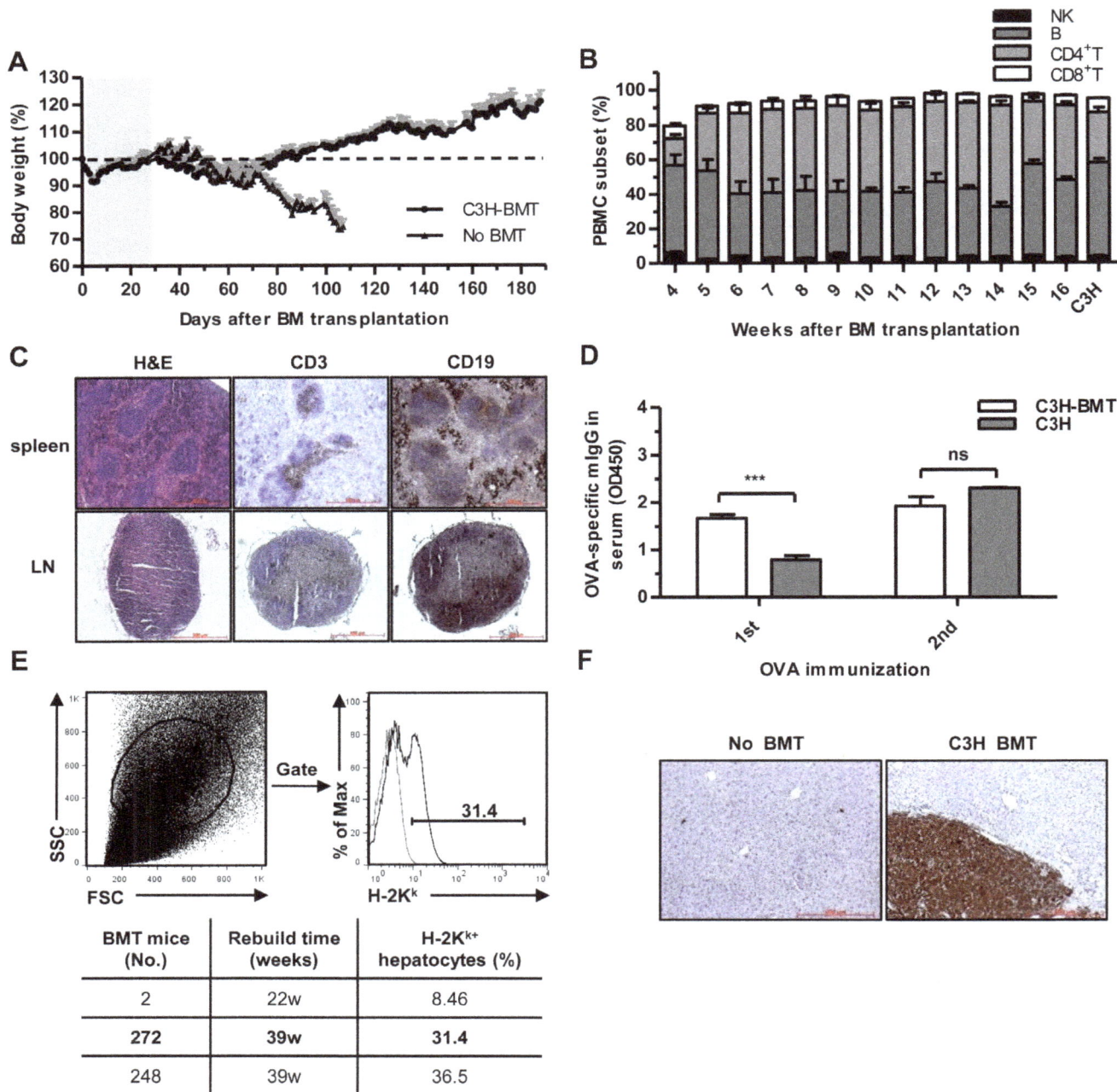

Figure 3. Immune and hepatic reconstitution in recipient *fah^-/-* mice after allogeneic *C3H-BMT*. (A) Body weight in recipient *fah^-/-* mice after allo-BMT. NTBC was withdrawn on day 28 after BMT, and initial body weight was set as 100% (dotted line). No BMT *fah^-/-* mice without NTBC treatment were set as controls. Gray areas indicate NTBC administration, white areas indicate NTBC withdrawal. (mean ± SEM, n=9). (B) PBMC subsets (NK, B, CD4^+, and CD8^+ T) from BMT mice over time. Donor C3H mice's PBMC was set as a positive control. (mean ± SEM, n=5). (C) Spleen and inguinal LN histology of serial sections in BMT mice (rebuild 16w). From L-R: H&E stain, CD3, and CD19 immunohistochemistry. Brown staining indicates positive cells. (Original magnification 100×). (D) Serum anti-OVA levels from *C3H-BMT* and C3H mice after 1 or 2 OVA protein immunizations. (mean ± SEM, n=4, ns: p>0.05, ***p<0.001). (E) Gating and MHC class I expression in hepatocytes from BMT mice (rebuild 39w) by FACS. Gray line indicates isotype control. H-2K^k+ hepatocytes in other BMT mice are shown in the table below. (F) FAH immunohistochemistry in BMT mice (rebuild 16w). Liver section from No BMT *fah^-/-* mice was set as a control. Brown staining indicates FAH^+ cells.

CD8^+ T cells in peripheral blood reconstituted normally over time (Fig. 5A–D). Furthermore, we found a similar ratio of T cell subsets in thymus, spleen, and liver between xeno-BMT mice and donor rat at week 11 after BMT (Fig. 5E). Anti-RT1A antibody staining demonstrated that hepatocytes from rat-BMT mice were partially positive for donor MHC class I antigen (Fig. 5F), suggesting that rat BM-derived hepatocytes were generated. Liver histology also showed that FAH^+ cells were organized in a cell cluster (Fig. 5G). Taken together, BMC from rat could indeed reconstitute both immune and hepatic systems in *fah^-/-* mice.

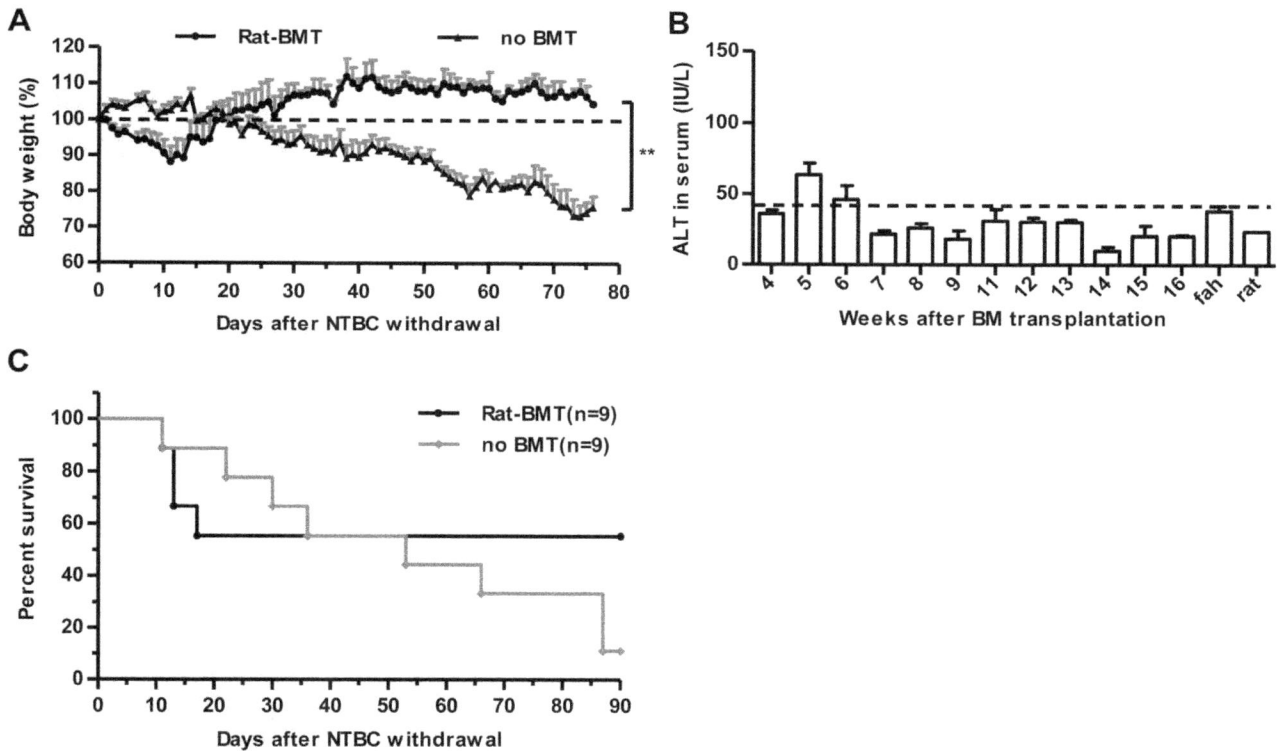

Figure 4. Xenogeneic BMT rescure fah$^{-/-}$ mice from liver failure and death. (A–B) Body weight (A) and serum ALT (B) from recipient fah$^{-/-}$ mice after xeno-BMT. NTBC was withdrawn on day 28 after BMT, and initial body weight was set as 100% (dotted line). **p<0.01. (mean ± SEM, n = 9). (C) Survival rate measurements from recipient fah$^{-/-}$ mice after NTBC withdrawal. No BMT fah$^{-/-}$ mice without NTBC treatment were set as controls.

BM-derived hepatocytes resulted from fusion between donor BM-derived myelomonocytic cells and host hepatocytes

Finally, we investigated whether BM-derived hepatocytes were generated by *in vivo* fusion process between liver infiltrating hematopoietic cells and host hepatocytes. As shown in Fig. 6A, donor MHC class I antigen and recipient MHC class I antigen as well as CD45 antigen were concurrently expressed on BM-derived hepatocytes, suggesting cellular fusion occurred between BM-derived myelomonocytic progenitors and resident hepatocytes, which is known to occur after BMT [19]. Further analysis showed that EGFP$^+$ donor derived hepatocytes were mostly CD45$^+$F4/80$^+$Gr-1$^+$CD11b$^+$CD11c$^-$, while EGFP$^-$ recipient derived hepatocytes were negative for all the above markers (Fig. 6B). Thus, after BM transplantation, BMC might differentiate into CD11b$^+$ myelomonocytic progenitors and entry into the liver, and then fuse with host hepatocytes under the selection pressure.

Metabolic parameters of transplanted animals

Additionally, we assessed serum biochemical markers for *EGFP-BMT (syn-)*, *C3H-BMT (allo-)*, and *rat-BMT (xeno-)* mice 20 weeks after NTBC withdrawal, and compared with levels in *fah$^{-/-}$* mice with NTBC on and off. As shown in Fig. 7, after NTBC withdrawal, no-BMT *fah$^{-/-}$* mice showed a significantly increase in serum ALT, AST, ALP, GGT, TBILI, CRE, with a largely decrease in serum ALB, which indicated the impaired hepatocytes metabolism. However, *syn/allo/xeno-BMT* mice showed a substantial improvement in all tested parameters to levels near that found in NTBC on *fah$^{-/-}$* mice. Thus, metabolic

parameters of BM-derived hepatocytes resembled those of NTBC on *fah$^{-/-}$* mice.

Discussion

In summary (Table 1), our major finding is that BMCs from a single individual can successfully differentiate into both immune cells and hepatocytes, and functionally repopulate the immune system and liver in irradiated *fah$^{-/-}$* mice. From our knowledge, it is the first mouse model with immune and liver reconstitution from a single BMC donor across the host species barrier, which was carried out by using syngeneic, allogeneic, or xenogeneic BMT. These findings also provide a further approach for establishing a dual humanized mouse model with HLA-matched human immune cells and human hepatocytes by using a more immunodeficient *fah$^{-/-}$* mouse, such as *fah$^{-/-}$ NOG*, in the future.

Development of humanized mice provides insights into *in vivo* human biology, which would otherwise be severely limited by ethical and/or technical constraints. Human immune system (HIS) mice are already established, showing a potential as the available model for the study of human immune response and human lymphotropic pathogens in mice [24–26], and human liver chimeric mice were developed for study of human hepatotropic pathogens [27–29] or preclinical evaluation of anti-hepatitis virus drug candidates [30]. However, further investigation of the pathology, immune correlates, and mechanisms of highly specialized pathogens like HBV, HCV and malaria (at liver stage) needs an excellent mouse model engrafted with MHC-restricted human immune system and pathogen-targeting organs. Recently, AFC8-hu HSC/Hep mice model was developed by meeting this

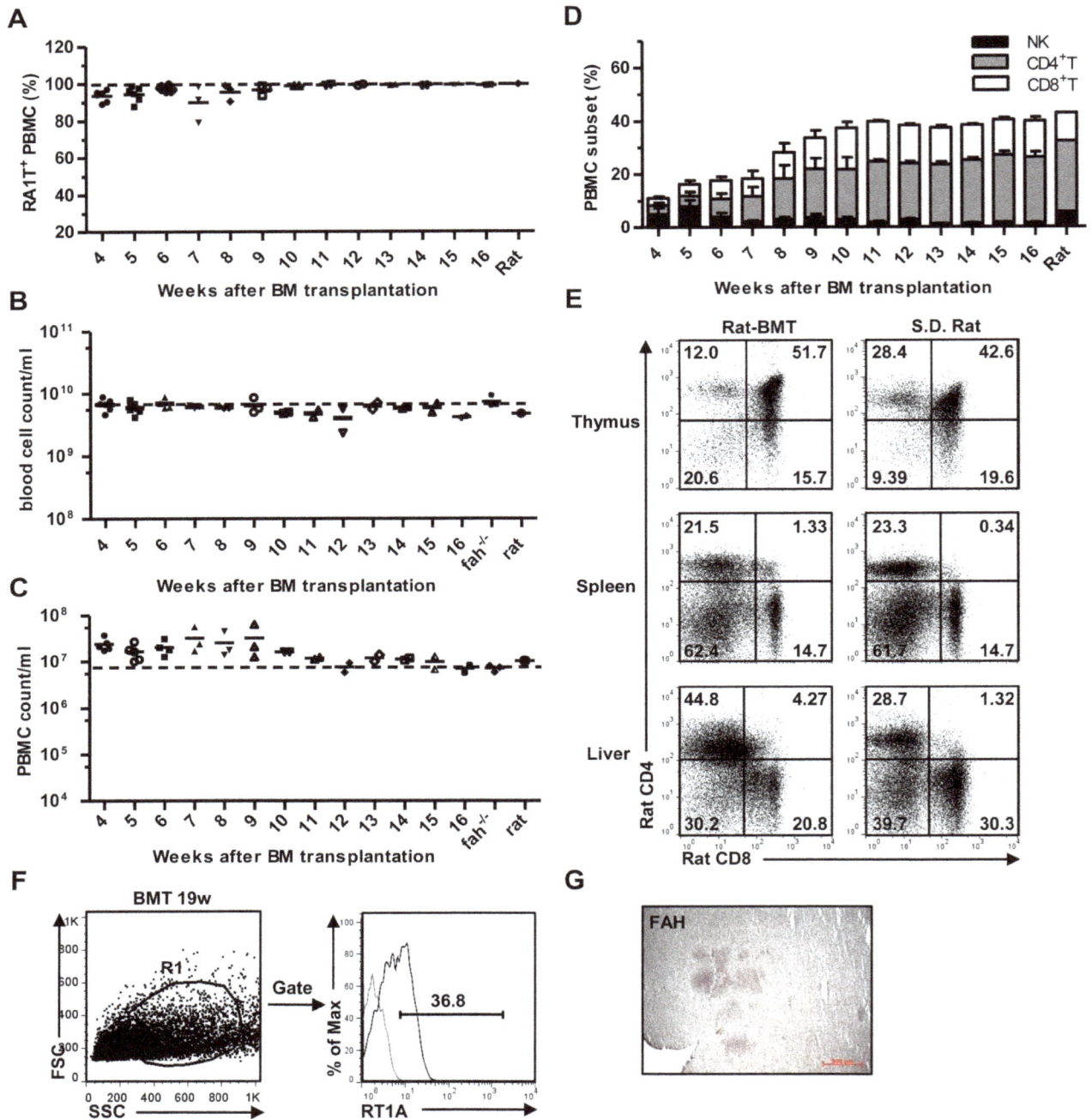

Figure 5. Immune and hepatic reconstitution in recipient fah⁻/⁻ mice after xenogeneic BMT. (A) Donor-derived PBMC (RT1A⁺) measurements from BMT mice at the indicated time points. PBMC from S.D. donor rat was set as a positive control (dotted line). (mean, n = 5). (B–C) Blood cell (B) and PBMC (C) cellularity in peripheral blood from *rat-BMT* mice at the indicated time points. Normal *fah⁻/⁻* mice and S.D. rats were set as positive controls (dotted line). (mean, n = 5). (D) PBMC subset (NK, CD4⁺, and CD8⁺ T) measurements from BMT mice at the indicated time points. PBMC from SD donor rats was set as a positive control. (mean ± SEM, n = 5). (E) Thymus, spleen, and liver CD4⁺ or CD8⁺ T lymphocytes in xeno-BMT mice (rebuild 11w) or donor rats. (F) Gating and MHC class I expression in hepatocytes from BMT mice (rebuild 19w) by FACS. Gray line indicates isotype control. (G) FAH immunohistochemistry in BMT mice (rebuild 19w). Brown staining indicates FAH⁺ cells.

requirement through co-implantation of human CD34⁺ HSCs and hepatocyte progenitor cells from a 15–18 weeks old fetal liver tissue into BALB/c-*Rag2⁻/⁻Il2rγ⁻/⁻* mice [31]. Although this approach successfully provides immune system and liver cells together in recipients, its extensive utilization is limited by obtaining human fetal liver tissues. In our model, syngeneic,

allogeneic and xenogeneic BMT mice may reconstitute the immune system and liver from donor's BMCs, and based on these findings, it is possible that a more practical dual humanized mouse (e.g.HIS/HuHep mice) could be created in near future. Like AFC8-hu HSC/Hep mice model, HBV or HCV could infect

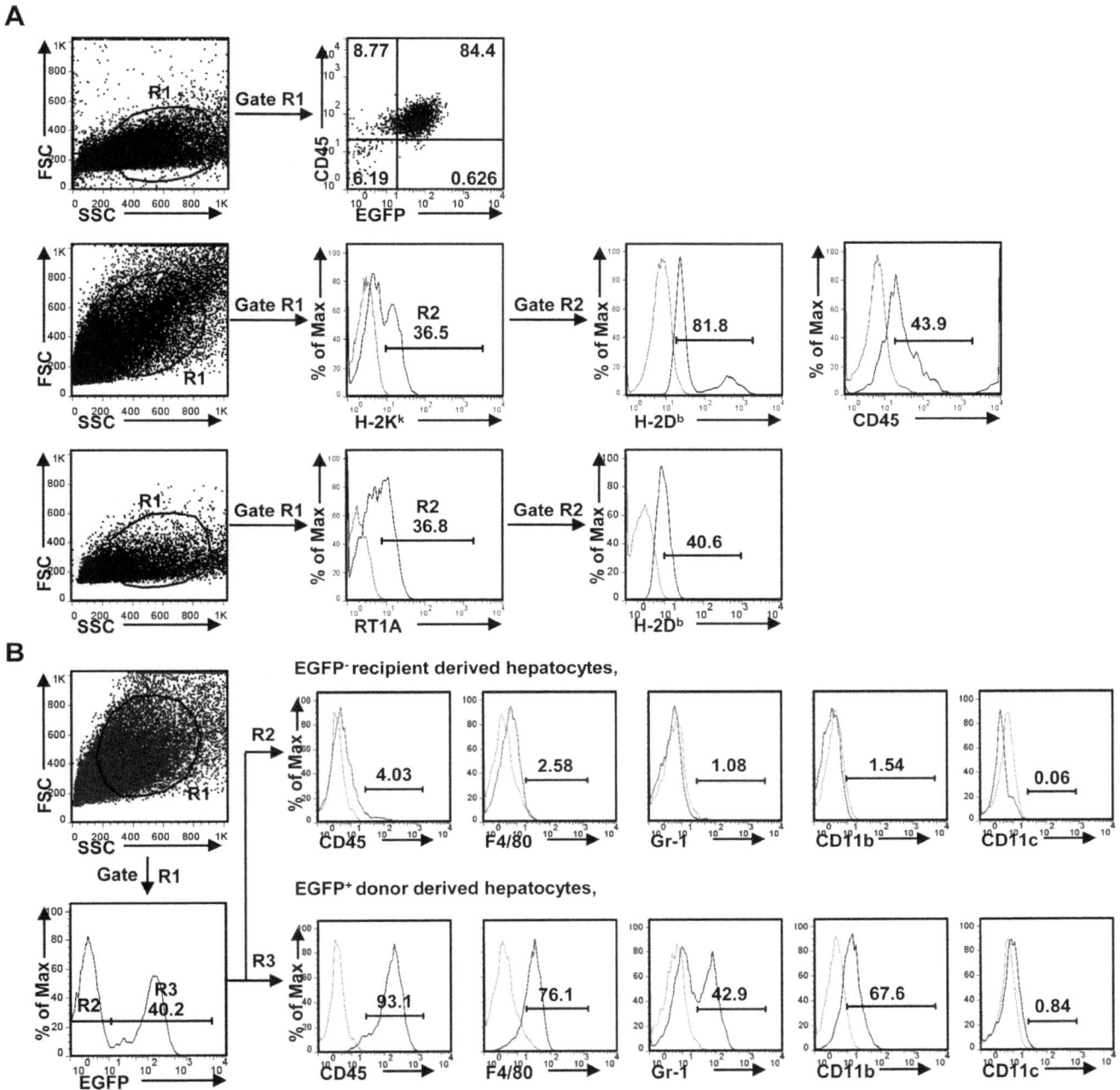

Figure 6. BM-derived hepatocytes emerged from fusion between donor BM-derived myelomonocytic cells and host hepatocytes.
(A) Donor-derived hepatocyte measurements from *EGFP-BMT* (top), *C3H-BMT* (middle), and *rat-BMT* mice (bottom). Gated donor-derived hepatocytes mostly expressed CD45, and the same hepatocytes were partially positive for recipient MHC class I antigen. EGFP+, H-2K^{k+}, or RT1A+ hepatocytes represent donor antigen, while H-2D^{b+} represent recipient MHC antigen. (B) Immunophenotyping of bone marrow-derived hepatocytes in *EGFP-BMT* mice. Recipient derived hepatocytes (R2) were negative for CD45, F4/80, Gr-1, CD11b, CD11c staining, while donor derived hepatocytes (R3) were mostly positive for CD45, F4/80, Gr-1, and CD11b, but negative for CD11c. (Numbers indicate the percentage of each population).

and replicate in HIS/HuHep mice's liver, more similar to that of HBV or HCV clinical infection.

Despite its advantages, further improvements of our model can be envisioned. Firstly, it took a long time to create such a model, typically more than 20 weeks. Perhaps HSC differentiated slowly *in vivo*, *in vitro* cultivation the HSCs into hepatic progenitor cells and hematopoietic progenitor cells before transplantation may partially solve this problem. However, HSCs *ex vivo* cultivation

then became another key challenge for us. Secondly, we observed that hematopoietic stem cells generated hepatocytes by cell fusion at a low frequency, which are in agreement with the former studies [9]. Macrophage depletion using chemicals [32], cytokines [33,34], HLA expression [35] or even immunosuppressive drugs [36] treatments may properly further refine our model. Thirdly, GVHD was major issue in *allo/xeno-BMT* mice. Actually, 17 in 36 rat-BMT mice died in the first 28 days after bone marrow

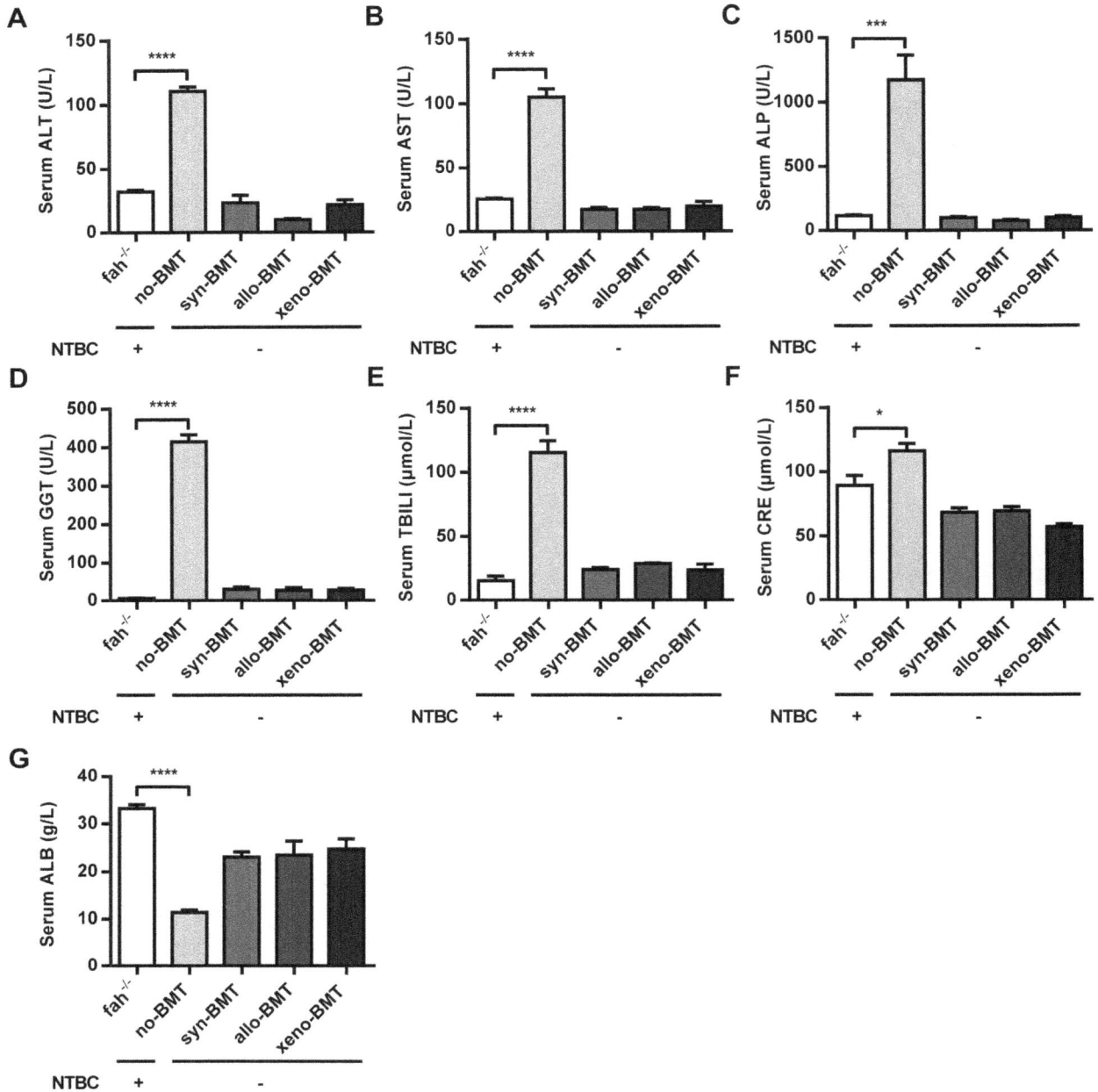

Figure 7. Analysis of metabolic serum parameters. Serum samples, collected from *EGFP-BMT* (syn-), *C3H-BMT* (allo-), and *rat-BMT* (xeno-) mice 20 weeks after NTBC withdrawal, were assessed. *Fah*[-/-] mice with NTBC on and off (4 weeks after NTBC withdrawal) were set as controls. (A) Alanine aminotransferase (ALT, U/L). (B) Aspartate aminotransferase (AST, U/L). (C) Alkaline phosphatase (ALP, U/L). (D) Gamma-Glutamyl Transpeptidase (GGT, U/L). (E) Total bilirubin (TBILI, μmol/L). (F) Creatinine (CRE, μmol/L). (G) Albumin (ALB, g/L). *p<0.05, ***p<0.001, ****p<0.0001. (mean ± SEM, n = 5).

transplantation but before NTBC withdrawal (NTBC was cut off on day 28), which were considered to die from GVHD. Purification HSC from bone marrow before transplantation may reduce the incidence of GVHD [9]. Administration of cyclophosphamide, OKT3, or Il-21 signaling inhibitor was also reported to ameliorate xenogeneic GVHD [37–39]. Finally, the background strain of the mice (129S4.B6) is not optimal for xenorepopulation [40]. Although further improvements of our model are likely, we successfully reconstituted donor hepatocytes and immune cells across host species barrier using *fah*-deficient mice and simple

BMT. We took a key step to construct the ideal model, and provided experimental evidence for the next HIS/HuHep mice model development.

HSCs have been reported to generate hepatocytes [41], cardiac myocytes [42], skeletal muscle [43], gastrointestinal epithelium [44], endothelium [45], and nerve cells [46] *in vivo*. Our new technique would make "multi-tissue" humanized mouse [47] model available, provided that the recipient mouse has open tissue space for donor-cell replacement, similar to the *fah*[-/-] mice used here for hepatocyte. Such a tool will not only be invaluable to

Table 1. Donor MHC-restricted dual reconstitution of immune system and liver across species in mouse.

Transplantation Type	Donor (MHC haplotype)	Recipient (MHC haplotype)	Survival after NTBC withdrawal[1]	Immune reconstitution[2]	Hepatic reconstitution	
No-BMT, *fah*-/- host	No	129s4 (H-2^b)	No	No	No	
Syn-BMT, *fah*-/- host	EGFP-Tg (H-2^b)	129s4 (H-2^b)	ALL (45/45)	Yes	31-35w	10-23%
					49w	~34%
					55-57w	40-90%
Allo-BMT, *fah*-/- host	C3H/HeJSlac (H-2^k)	129s4 (H-2^b)	Partial (16/27) [3]	Yes	22w	~8.5%
					39w	31-36%
Xeno-BMT, *fah*-/- host	Rat (RT-1)	129s4 (H-2^b)	Partial (10/36) [4]	Yes	19w	~36.8%

[1]Survivors in total bone marrow transplanted (BMT) animals for at least 4 months after NTBC withdrawal.
[2]BMT animals exhibited donor-derived immune cells and organ structure, and could respond to antigen immunization.
[3]7 in 27 *allo*-BMT mice died from GVHD in the first 28 days before NTBC withdrawal, only 4 mice died after NTBC cutoff.
[4]17 in 36 rat-BMT mice died in the first 28 days before NTBC withdrawal, and 9 in the rest 19 mice died after NTBC cutoff.

study MHC-restricted interaction between immune cells and their targeted organ/tissue from a single donor, but also critical to developing effective and affordable vaccines and other immunotherapeutic approaches.

Supporting Information

Figure S1 *Fah*-/- mice exhibit progressive liver failure and death unless treated with NTBC. (A) Body weight measurements from mice with or without 2-(2-nitro-4-tifluoro-methylbenzyol)-1, 3-cyclohexanedione (NTBC) treatment for hepatocyte survival. Initial body weight was set as 100% (dotted line). ***p<0.001. (B–C) Survival rate (B) and serum ALT (C) measurements in mice with or without NTBC treatment. ns: p> 0.05, **p<0.01, ***p<0.001. (mean ± SEM, n = 10).

Figure S2 Blood cell and PBMC reconstitution in peripheral blood of recipient *fah*-/- mice after syngeneic EGFP-BMT. (A–B) Blood cell (A) and PBMC (B) cellularity from the peripheral blood of *EGFP-BMT* mice. Normal *fah*-/- mice with NTBC treatment were set as the positive control (dotted line). (mean, n = 5).

Figure S3 Blood cell and PBMC reconstitution in peripheral blood of recipient *fah*-/- mice after allogeneic

C3H-BMT. (A) Donor-derived PBMC (H-2K^{k+}) measurements from BMT mice at the indicated time points. C3H donor mice were set as the positive control (dotted line). (B–C) Blood cell (B) and PBMC (C) cellularity from peripheral blood of *C3H-BMT* mice at the indicated time points. (mean, n = 4). Normal *fah*-/- mice with NTBC treatment were set as the positive control (dotted line).

Acknowledgments

We are grateful to Xin Wang for providing *fah*-/- mice. We thank Xiang Gao for providing the *EGFP-Tg* mice. We also would like to thank Zhiying He (Department of Cell Biology, Second Military Medical University, Shanghai, China) for his useful suggestions of breeding *fah*-/- mice.

Author Contributions

Conceived and designed the experiments: ZPQ ZGT. Performed the experiments: ZPQ LL XFW. Analyzed the data: ZPQ LL ZGT. Contributed reagents/materials/analysis tools: XG XW HMW JZ RS. Wrote the paper: ZPQ ZGT.

References

1. Guidotti LG, Chisari FV (2006) Immunobiology and pathogenesis of viral hepatitis. Annu Rev Pathol 1: 23–61.
2. Abe K, Inchauspe G, Shikata T, Prince AM (1992) Three different patterns of hepatitis C virus infection in chimpanzees. Hepatology 15: 690–695.
3. Guidotti LG, Rochford R, Chung J, Shapiro M, Purcell R, et al. (1999) Viral clearance without destruction of infected cells during acute HBV infection. Science 284: 825–829.
4. Mason WS, Seal G, Summers J (1980) Virus of Pekin ducks with structural and biological relatedness to human hepatitis B virus. J Virol 36: 829–836.
5. Summers J, Smolec JM, Snyder R (1978) A virus similar to human hepatitis B virus associated with hepatitis and hepatoma in woodchucks. Proc Natl Acad Sci U S A 75: 4533–4537.
6. Marion PL, Oshiro LS, Regnery DC, Scullard GH, Robinson WS (1980) A virus in Beechey ground squirrels that is related to hepatitis B virus of humans. Proc Natl Acad Sci U S A 77: 2941–2945.
7. Guidotti LG, Matzke B, Schaller H, Chisari FV (1995) High-level hepatitis B virus replication in transgenic mice. J Virol 69: 6158–6169.
8. Huang LR, Wu HL, Chen PJ, Chen DS (2006) An immunocompetent mouse model for the tolerance of human chronic hepatitis B virus infection. Proc Natl Acad Sci U S A 103: 17862–17867.
9. Lagasse E, Connors H, Al-Dhalimy M, Reitsma M, Dohse M, et al. (2000) Purified hematopoietic stem cells can differentiate into hepatocytes in vivo. Nat Med 6: 1229–1234.
10. Traggiai E, Chicha L, Mazzucchelli L, Bronz L, Piffaretti JC, et al. (2004) Development of a human adaptive immune system in cord blood cell-transplanted mice. Science 304: 104–107.
11. Ishikawa F, Yasukawa M, Lyons B, Yoshida S, Miyamoto T, et al. (2005) Development of functional human blood and immune systems in NOD/SCID/IL2 receptor {gamma} chain(null) mice. Blood 106: 1565–1573.
12. Ito R, Takahashi T, Katano I, Ito M (2012) Current advances in humanized mouse models. Cell Mol Immunol 9: 208–214.
13. Ito M, Hiramatsu H, Kobayashi K, Suzue K, Kawahata M, et al. (2002) NOD/SCID/gamma(c)(null) mouse: an excellent recipient mouse model for engraftment of human cells. Blood 100: 3175–3182.
14. Shultz LD, Lyons BL, Burzenski LM, Gott B, Chen X, et al. (2005) Human lymphoid and myeloid cell development in NOD/LtSz-scid IL2 gamma null mice engrafted with mobilized human hemopoietic stem cells. J Immunol 174: 6477–6489.
15. Mercer DF, Schiller DE, Elliott JF, Douglas DN, Hao C, et al. (2001) Hepatitis C virus replication in mice with chimeric human livers. Nat Med 7: 927–933.

16. Azuma H, Paulk N, Ranade A, Dorrell C, Al-Dhalimy M, et al. (2007) Robust expansion of human hepatocytes in Fah-/-/Rag2-/-/Il2rg-/- mice. Nat Biotechnol 25: 903–910.

17. Vassilopoulos G, Wang PR, Russell DW (2003) Transplanted bone marrow regenerates liver by cell fusion. Nature 422: 901–904.

18. Wang X, Willenbring H, Akkari Y, Torimaru Y, Foster M, et al. (2003) Cell fusion is the principal source of bone-marrow-derived hepatocytes. Nature 422: 897–901.

19. Camargo FD, Finegold M, Goodell MA (2004) Hematopoietic myelomonocytic cells are the major source of hepatocyte fusion partners. J Clin Invest 113: 1266–1270.

20. Willenbring H, Bailey AS, Foster M, Akkari Y, Dorrell C, et al. (2004) Myelomonocytic cells are sufficient for therapeutic cell fusion in liver. Nat Med 10: 744–748.

21. Chen Y, Wei H, Sun R, Dong Z, Zhang J, et al. (2007) Increased susceptibility to liver injury in hepatitis B virus transgenic mice involves NKG2D-ligand interaction and natural killer cells. Hepatology 46: 706–715.

22. Jaruga B, Hong F, Sun R, Radaeva S, Gao B (2003) Crucial role of IL-4/STAT6 in T cell-mediated hepatitis: up-regulating eotaxins and IL-5 and recruiting leukocytes. J Immunol 171: 3233–3244.

23. Grompe M, Lindstedt S, al-Dhalimy M, Kennaway NG, Papaconstantinou J, et al. (1995) Pharmacological correction of neonatal lethal hepatic dysfunction in a murine model of hereditary tyrosinaemia type I. Nat Genet 10: 453–460.

24. Sun Z, Denton PW, Estes JD, Othieno FA, Wei BL, et al. (2007) Intrarectal transmission, systemic infection, and CD4+ T cell depletion in humanized mice infected with HIV-1. J Exp Med 204: 705–714.

25. Kumar P, Ban HS, Kim SS, Wu H, Pearson T, et al. (2008) T cell-specific siRNA delivery suppresses HIV-1 infection in humanized mice. Cell 134: 577–586.

26. Zhang L, Su L (2012) HIV-1 immunopathogenesis in humanized mouse models. Cell Mol Immunol 9: 237–244.

27. Sugiyama M, Tanaka Y, Sakamoto T, Maruyama I, Shimada T, et al. (2007) Early dynamics of hepatitis B virus in chimeric mice carrying human hepatocytes monoinfected or coinfected with genotype G. Hepatology 45: 929–937.

28. Bissig KD, Wieland SF, Tran P, Isogawa M, Le TT, et al. (2010) Human liver chimeric mice provide a model for hepatitis B and C virus infection and treatment. J Clin Invest 120: 924–930.

29. Lutgehetmann M, Mancke LV, Volz T, Helbig M, Allweiss L, et al. (2012) Humanized chimeric uPA mouse model for the study of hepatitis B and D virus interactions and preclinical drug evaluation. Hepatology 55: 685–694.

30. Tateno C, Yoshizane Y, Saito N, Kataoka M, Utoh R, et al. (2004) Near completely humanized liver in mice shows human-type metabolic responses to drugs. Am J Pathol 165: 901–912.

31. Washburn ML, Bility MT, Zhang L, Kovalev GI, Buntzman A, et al. (2011) A humanized mouse model to study hepatitis C virus infection, immune response, and liver disease. Gastroenterology 140: 1334–1344.

32. Schiedner G, Hertel S, Johnston M, Dries V, van Rooijen N, et al. (2003) Selective depletion or blockade of Kupffer cells leads to enhanced and prolonged hepatic transgene expression using high-capacity adenoviral vectors. Mol Ther 7: 35–43.

33. Chen Q, Khoury M, Chen J (2009) Expression of human cytokines dramatically improves reconstitution of specific human-blood lineage cells in humanized mice. Proc Natl Acad Sci U S A 106: 21783–21788.

34. Quintana-Bustamante O, Alvarez-Barrientos A, Kofman AV, Fabregat I, Bueren JA, et al. (2006) Hematopoietic mobilization in mice increases the presence of bone marrow-derived hepatocytes via in vivo cell fusion. Hepatology 43: 108–116.

35. Shultz LD, Saito Y, Najima Y, Tanaka S, Ochi T, et al. (2010) Generation of functional human T-cell subsets with HLA-restricted immune responses in HLA class I expressing NOD/SCID/IL2r gamma(null) humanized mice. Proc Natl Acad Sci U S A 107: 13022–13027.

36. He Z, Zhang H, Zhang X, Xie D, Chen Y, et al. (2010) Liver xeno-repopulation with human hepatocytes in Fah-/-Rag2-/- mice after pharmacological immunosuppression. Am J Pathol 177: 1311–1319.

37. Hippen KL, Bucher C, Schirm DK, Bearl AM, Brender T, et al. (2012) Blocking IL-21 signaling ameliorates xenogeneic GVHD induced by human lymphocytes. Blood 119: 619–628.

38. Luznik L, Bolanos-Meade J, Zahurak M, Chen AR, Smith BD, et al. (2010) High-dose cyclophosphamide as single-agent, short-course prophylaxis of graft-versus-host disease. Blood 115: 3224–3230.

39. Wunderlich M, Brooks RA, Panchal R, Rhyasen GW, Danet-Desnoyers G, et al. (2014) OKT3 prevents xenogeneic GVHD and allows reliable xenograft initiation from unfractionated human hematopoietic tissues. Blood 123: e134–144.

40. Legrand N, Weijer K, Spits H (2006) Experimental models to study development and function of the human immune system in vivo. J Immunol 176: 2053–2058.

41. Kakinuma S, Tanaka Y, Chinzei R, Watanabe M, Shimizu-Saito K, et al. (2003) Human umbilical cord blood as a source of transplantable hepatic progenitor cells. Stem Cells 21: 217–227.

42. Ishikawa F, Shimazu H, Shultz LD, Fukata M, Nakamura R, et al. (2006) Purified human hematopoietic stem cells contribute to the generation of cardiomyocytes through cell fusion. FASEB J 20: 950–952.

43. Torrente Y, Belicchi M, Sampaolesi M, Pisati F, Meregalli M, et al. (2004) Human circulating AC133(+) stem cells restore dystrophin expression and ameliorate function in dystrophic skeletal muscle. J Clin Invest 114: 182–195.

44. Ishikawa F, Yasukawa M, Yoshida S, Nakamura K, Nagatoshi Y, et al. (2004) Human cord blood- and bone marrow-derived CD34+ cells regenerate gastrointestinal epithelial cells. FASEB J 18: 1958–1960.

45. Droetto S, Viale A, Primo L, Jordaney N, Bruno S, et al. (2004) Vasculogenic potential of long term repopulating cord blood progenitors. FASEB J 18: 1273–1275.

46. Taguchi A, Soma T, Tanaka H, Kanda T, Nishimura H, et al. (2004) Administration of CD34+ cells after stroke enhances neurogenesis via angiogenesis in a mouse model. J Clin Invest 114: 330–338.

47. Legrand N, Ploss A, Balling R, Becker PD, Borsotti C, et al. (2009) Humanized mice for modeling human infectious disease: challenges, progress, and outlook. Cell Host Microbe 6: 5–9.

22

The Role of miR-34a in the Hepatoprotective Effect of Hydrogen Sulfide on Ischemia/Reperfusion Injury in Young and Old Rats

Xinli Huang, Yun Gao, Jianjie Qin, Sen Lu*

Center of Liver Transplantation, The First Affiliated Hospital of Nanjing Medical University, The Key Laboratory of Living Donor Liver Transplantation, Ministry of Health, Nanjing, China

Abstract

Hydrogen sulfide (H_2S) can protect the liver against ischemia-reperfusion (I/R) injury. However, it is unknown whether H_2S plays a role in the protection of hepatic I/R injury in both young and old patients. This study compared the protective effects of H_2S in a rat model (young and old animals) of I/R injury and the mechanism underlying its effects. Young and old rats were assessed following an injection of NaHS. NaHS alone reduced hepatic I/R injury in the young rats by activating the nuclear erythroid-related factor 2 (Nrf2) signaling pathway, but it had little effect on the old rats. NaHS pretreatment decreased miR-34a expression in the hepatocytes of the young rats with hepatic I/R. Overexpresion of miR-34a decreased Nrf-2 and its downstream target expression, impairing the hepatoprotective effect of H_2S on the young rats. More importantly, downregulation of miR-34a expression increased Nrf-2 and the expression of its downstream targets, enhancing the effect of H_2S on hepatic I/R injury in the old rats. This study reveals the different effects of H_2S on hepatic I/R injury in young and old rats and sheds light on the involvement of H_2S in miR-34a modulation of the Nrf-2 pathway.

Editor: Edward J. Lesnefsky, Virginia Commonwealth University, United States of America

Funding: This work was supported by grant from the Priority Academic Program of Jiangsu Higher Education Institutions. The funders had no role in study design, data collection and analysis, decision to publish, or preparation of the manuscript.

Competing Interests: The authors have declared that no competing interests exist.

* Email: senlusen@163.com

Introduction

Hepatic warm ischemia-reperfusion (I/R) injury is a dynamic process that frequently occurs during a variety of clinical situations, including liver transplantation and liver surgery [1]. A series of events, such as the formation of reactive oxygen species (ROS), depletion of ATP, production of inflammatory mediators, and apoptosis of hepatocytes are involved in the pathophysiology of hepatic I/R [2]. Several risk factors (aging and liver steatosis) can exacerbate liver failure during I/R [3]. Therefore, effective treatment of hepatic I/R injury is difficult.

The gasotransmitter hydrogen sulfide (H_2S), similar to nitric oxide and carbon monoxide, is implicated in a wide range of physiological activities [4]. Endogenous H_2S can be produced from L-cysteine in several organs, such as the brain, heart, kidney, and liver [5]. H_2S has been reported to protect these tissues against I/R injury by maintaining mitochondrial function, inhibiting proinflammatory factors, neutralizing ROS and reducing apoptosis [6]. Treatment with H_2S can be via inhalation of H_2S or administration of NaHS by intravenous injection. However, it is difficult to control the concentration of inhaled H_2S, resulting in potential toxicity to animals [7]. The administration of NaHS by intravenous injection has become the common treatment method in I/R injury because the concentration can be controlled [8].

MicroRNAs (miRNAs) are 20–25 nucleotides long non-coding RNAs that modulate a variety of biological processes, such as development, apoptosis, metabolism, and proliferation [9]. Aberrant miRNA expression is associated with a large number of pathophysiological conditions, including liver diseases [10]. In recent years, the role of miR-34a in the regulation of liver function and survival has received a great deal of attention [11–12]. An increase in the expression of miR-34a was reported to be involved in age-dependent loss of oxidative defense in the liver [13]. In addition, miR-34a expression was regulated in a partial hepatectomy model, which resulted in the inhibition of hepatocyte proliferation [14]. However, the role of miR-34a in hepatic I/R damage remains largely unknown.

As a target gene of miR-34a, nuclear erythroid-related factor 2 (Nrf-2) is involved in the detoxification process. Studies have shown that this transcription factor exerts an antioxidant effect by regulating the expression of antioxidant enzymes genes, such as glutathione S-transferase (GST), superoxide dismutases (SODs) and heme oxygenase-1 (HO-1), and NAD(P)H: quinine oxidoreductase-1 (NQO1) [15–17]. Nrf-2 provides cytoprotection by inducing an anti-inflammatory response [18]. It is activated by a variety of factors, including oxidative stress. The activation of Nrf-2 predominantly occurs via the release of the Nrf-2/Keap1 (Kelch-like ECH associating protein 1) complex in the cytosol of cells [19]. It has been reported that the administration of H_2S can have beneficial effects on cardiac I/R injury by activating Nrf-2 [20]. In the liver, activation of Nrf-2 was reported to prevent or ameliorate toxin-induced injury and fibrosis [21].

Due to decreased endogenous antioxidants production and an increased inflammatory response, the ability of the liver cells of aged animals to combat I/R injury is significantly weakened [22]. Increasing evidence has shown that hepatic I/R injury is enhanced in aged animals and patients [23]. Although the effect of age on I/R-induced hepatic damage is well known, it is unknown whether the effect of therapy differs in aged and young patients with I/R injury. Here, we investigated if H_2S protected the liver against I/R damage both in aged and young rats and whether miR-34a was involved in this effect.

Materials and Methods

Ethics statement

All the animals were treated humanely, using approved procedures in accordance with the guidelines of the Institutional Animal Care and Use Committee at Nanjing Medical University. The study was approved by the Experimental Animal Ethics Committee of Nanjing Medical University and the animal protocol was approved by the Ethics Review of Lab Animal Use Application of Nanjing Medical University (Permit Number: NJMU-ERLAUA-20120107).

Chemicals and reagents

RPMI 1640 and DMEM were obtained from GIBCO (Invitrogen Company). Fetal bovine serum (FBS) was obtained from Hyclone (Logan, UT, USA). Lipofectamine 2000 transfection reagent was obtained from Invitrogen Life Technologies (Grand Island, NY, USA). NaHS was purchased from Sigma Aldrich (St. Louis, MO, USA). Antibodies against Nrf-2, GST, SOD, HO-1, and β-Actin were purchased from Santa Cruz Biotechnology (Santa Cruz, CA, USA). The Detergent Compatible (DC) Protein Assay kit was purchased from Bio-Rad Laboratories (Hercules, CA, USA).

Animals and surgery

Young and old male Sprague-Dawley (SD) rats aged 3 months and 20 months, respectively, were obtained from Vital River Laboratories (VRL) in China. The young rats (3 months) were randomly and equally divided into six groups: sham, hepatic I/R, hepatic I/R +20 μmol/kg of NaHS, hepatic I/R+ a negative control oligonucleotide (NC), hepatic I/R+ an miR-34a mimic, hepatic I/R+NaHS+NC, and hepatic I/R+NaHS+an miR-34a mimic. The old rats (20 months) were also randomly and equally divided into six groups: sham, hepatic I/R, hepatic I/R + 20 μmol/kg of NaHS, hepatic I/R+ anti-NC, hepatic I/R+ an miR-34a inhibitor, hepatic I/R+NaHS+anti-NC, and hepatic I/R+NaHS+an miR-34a inhibitor. The rats in the sham group underwent laparotomy, and the abdominal cavity was closed without hepatic I/R. Hepatic warm I/R was induced according to the previous reports [24]. Briefly, the rats were subjected to overnight fasting (with free access to water) before the surgery, and they were anaesthetized with 7% chloral hydrate (1 ml per 100 g of 7% chloral hydrate, intraperitoneal injection). After the midline laparotomy and anatomy of the hepatic portal, the left and median hepatic artery and the portal vein branches were blocked by no-damage artery clips to create a model of partial ischemia (70%). The right hepatic artery was opened to prevent the mesenteric venous congestion by permitting portal decompression through the right and caudate lobes. Under such circumstances of occluding, liver lobes were subjected to warm ischemia for 90 min. Reperfusion for 120 min was initiated by the removal of the clamp. The rats in the hepatic I/R+NaHS group received an intraperitoneal injection of 1 ml of NaHS solution 30 min before

hepatic I/R. An miR-34a mimic (5′-UGGCAGUGUCUUAG-CUGGUUGU-3′, 10 nmol) or miR-34a inhibitor (5′-ACAAC-CAGCUAAGACACUGCCA-3′, 10 nmol) in 0.1 ml of saline buffer was injected into the tail vein of the rats for 48 h before the administration of NaHS and subsequent liver I/R. A cholesterol-conjugated miR-34a mimic or an miR-34a inhibitor (both from RiboBio, Guangzhou, China) was used for in vivo RNA delivery. At each of the indicated time points (1, 3, 6 and 24 hours after I/R), six rats (per group) were randomly sacrificed, and blood and liver samples were collected.

Measurement of serum H_2S concentrations

Serum H_2S concentrations were measured according to a previously reported method [24]. Briefly, 75 μl of sera were mixed with 300 μl of 10% trichloroacetic acid, 100 μL of distilled water and 150 μl of 1% zinc acetate. Then, 133 μl of N-dimethyl-p-phenylenediamine sulfate (20 μmol/L) and 133 μl of $FeCl_3$ (30 μmol/L) were added to the mixture. After incubation at room temperature (25°C) for 15 min, the absorbance of the resulting solution was read at 670 nm. All the samples were assayed in duplicate, and serum H_2S concentrations were calculated based on the calibration curve of NaHS.

Measurement of serum ALT and AST

The serum samples were separated from rat blood by centrifugation at 1500 g for 15 min, and aspartate aminotransferase (AST) and alanine aminotransferase (ALT) were measured using an automated biochemistry analyzer (HITACHI 7600-020, Tokyo, Japan) to assess the hepatic function.

Histopathological evaluation

Liver samples were frozen first and fixed in 10% neutral buffered formalin, embedded in paraffin, sliced into 5 μm thickness, and stained with hematoxylin-eosin. The histopathological scoring analysis was performed blindly according to previously described methods [25].

Isolation of rat hepatocytes

Hepatocytes were isolated from the young and old rats according to a previous report [26]. Briefly, the liver was perfused retrogradely with 250 ml of 135 mmol/l NaCl, 7 mmol/l KCl, 12 mmol/l glucose, and 10 mmol/l HEPES, pH 7.4, followed by 250 ml of the same medium supplemented with collagenase (150 U/ml) and 1 mmol/l $CaCl_2$. The Hepatocytes were diluted into William's E medium supplemented with 10% fetal calf serum, 50 mg/ml penicillin-streptomycin, 5 mg/ml insulin and 4 ng/ml dexamethasone, 10 mmol/l HEPES and 1 mmol/l $CaCl_2$.

Western blot analysis

The rat hepatocytes and liver tissue samples were lysed with ice-cold lysis buffer containing the following: 50 mmol/l Tris-HCl, pH 7.4; 1% NP-40; 150 mmol/l NaCl; 1 mmol/l EDTA; 1 mmol/l phenylmethylsulfonyl fluoride; and complete proteinase inhibitor mixture (one tablet per 10 ml; Roche Molecular Biochemicals, Indianapolis, IN, USA). The lysates were sonicated using the Sonicator VCX130 (Sonics & Materials) on ice, followed by centrifuging at 12000 g for 10 minutes at 4°C and the supernatants were retained. The protein concentration in the cell lysate was quantified using the DC protein assay kit (Bio-Rad). After determination of the protein content with the DC Protein Assay kit. Western blot analysis was performed.

Real-time PCR Assay

Mature miRNAs were isolated and purified using Trizol reagent (Invitrogen, USA), according to the manufacturer's protocol. The levels of miRNAs (miR-34a, miR-28, miR-155, miR-27a, miR-144 and miR-153) were quantified with a TaqMan PCR kit. Real-time PCR was performed with LightCycler 480, using U6 small nuclear RNA as an internal normalized reference. The mature miRNAs were amplified using specific miR primers and an miScript universal primer (Qiagen, Hilden, Germany). The average expression levels of the miRNAs were normalized against U6 using the $2^{-\Delta\Delta Ct}$ method. Differences between the groups were presented as ΔCt, indicating the difference between the Ct value of the miRNAs and the Ct value of U6. To ensure consistent measurements throughout all the assays, for each PCR amplification reaction, three independent RNA samples were loaded as internal controls to account for any plate-to-plate variation, and the results from each plate were normalized against internal normalization controls.

The mRNA expression of Nrf-2, HO-1, NQO1, SOD2 and GST was assessed using SYBR GREEN PCR Master Mix (Applied Biosystems). The specific primers were as follows: Nrf-2 5'-GCTATTTTCCATTCCCGAGTTAC-3' (forward), 5'-ATTG CTGTCCATCTCTGTCAG-3' (reverse); HO-1 5'-CTTTCAGAAGGGTCAGGTG TC-3' (forward), 5'-TGCTTGTTTCGCTCTATCTCC-3' (reverse); NQO1 5'-CATCATTTGGGCAAGTCC-3' (forward), 5'-ACAGCCGTGGCAGAACTA-3' (reverse); SOD2 5'-GAGAAGTACCAGGAGGCGTTG-3' (forward), 5'-GAGCCTTGGACACCAACAGAT-3' (reverse); GST,5'-GCTCTATGGGAAG GACCAG-3' (forward), 5'-CTCAAAAGGCTTCAGTTGC-3' (reverse); GAPDH 5'-TATCGGACGCCTGGTTAC-3' (forward), 5'-CTGTGCCGTTGAACTTGC-3' (reverse). All the data were analyzed using GAPDH gene expression as an internal standard.

Statistical analysis

The statistical analysis was performed with the statistical analysis software SPSS 13.0. Statistical analyses were performed using either an analysis of variance (ANOVA) or a Student's t-test. Data were expressed as the mean $\pm$ standard deviation. $P<0.05$ was considered significant.

Results

H$_2$S reduced hepatic I/R injury in young rats but has no effect in old rats

To identify the effect of H$_2$S on hepatic injury according to the age of the rats, the animals were treated with 20 µmol/kg NaHS. The serum levels of H$_2$S, ALT and AST were measured 1, 3, and 6 hours after I/R. Treatment with NaHS 30 minutes prior to the ischemia markedly increased the serum concentration of H$_2$S both in young and in old rats (Figure 1A and B, $P<0.01$). NaHS significantly reduced the serum levels of ALT and AST in young rats after 6 h reperfusion (Figure 1C, $P<0.01$). However, NaHS only slightly decreased the serum levels of ALT and AST in old rats (Figure 1D, $P>0.05$). These results imply that the protective effect of H$_2$S on the hepatic I/R-induced damage differs in young and old rats. The level of ALT or AST in old rats was significantly higher than that of young rats without NaHS treatment, suggesting that old rats were prone to damage after hepatic I/R.

Hematoxylin and Eosin (HE) staining was performed on the liver tissues after 24 h of reperfusion. As shown in figure 1E and F, NaHS could improve liver damage in young rats ($P<0.01$) but had little effect in old rats ($P>0.05$).

H$_2$S stimulated Nrf-2-mediated signaling pathway in the hepatocytes of the young rats but has no effect in old rats

The antioxidant effects of the transcription factor Nrf-2 play a crucial role in the protection of hepatic I/R damage [27]. To measure whether Nrf-2 was involved in the effect of H$_2$S on hepatic I/R, we measured the expression of Nrf-2 in the hepatocytes of young and old rats. The results showed that the mRNA level of Nrf-2 was significantly decreased in the hepatocytes of the young rats after 6 h I/R, and this decrease was reversed by NaHS treatment ($P<0.01$). The mRNA level of Nrf-2 was slightly changed in the hepatocytes of the old rats following I/R and the NaHS treatment compared to that of the untreated animals (Figure 2A, $P>0.05$). Consistent with the observed alteration in mRNA levels, NaHS treatment increased Nrf-2 protein levels in the hepatocytes of the young rats after I/R (Figure 2B). More importantly, the protein level of Nrf-2 in the hepatocytes of the young rats was significantly higher than that from old rats at baseline (Figure 2B).

It has been well documented that the transcription factor Nrf-2 up-regulates the expression of NQO1, GST and HO-1 [17]. Thus, we measured mRNA and protein levels of NQO1, GST and HO-1. After I/R, the expression of NQO1, GST and HO-1 was significantly reduced in the livers of the young rats, and the reduction was reversed by NaHS treatment (Figure 2C and 2D, $P<0.01$). However, no differences were observed in mRNA and protein levels of NQO1, GST and HO-1 in the old rats (Figure 2E and 2F, $P>0.05$). These results indicate that H$_2$S can stimulate Nrf-2-mediated signaling pathway to protect the liver against I/R injury in young rats.

H$_2$S reduced miR-34a expression in hepatocytes of the young rats but has no effect in old rats

To further study the mechanism of H$_2$S on Nrf-2 expression in the liver after I/R, we detected the expression of many miRNAs including miR-34a, miR-28, miR-155, miR-27a, miR-144 and miR-153, which may be involved in regulating the expression of this transcription factor [28]. Real-time PCR assays showed that, among these miRNAs, miR-34a was significantly up-regulated in the hepatocytes of the young and old rats after I/R (Figure 3A and B). Interestingly, the level of miR-34a was remarkably increased in the old rats compared to that in the young rats in the sham group and the I/R group (Figure 3C and D, $P<0.01$).

We also measured the expression of miR-34a in the liver following I/R and treatment with NaHS. As shown in Figure 3E and 3F, NaHS significantly decrease miR-34a expression in hepatocytes from young rats after I/R, but it had no effect on miR-34a expression in the hepatocytes of the old rats.

Overexpression of miR-34a could inhibit hepatoprotective effect of H$_2$S on young rats

Next, the role of miR-34a in the hepatoprotective effect of H$_2$S on young rats was further explored. After a tail vein injection of the cholesterol-conjugated miR-34a mimic, a slight increase in the serum levels of ALT and AST was observed in hepatic I/R young rats. However, the miR-34a mimic significantly reversed the effect of H$_2$S on hepatic I/R injury (Figure 4A, $P<0.01$). In addition, the expression of miR-34a was significantly increased in the hepatocytes of the young rats administered NaHS and the miR-34a mimic (Figure 4B, $P<0.01$). These results indicate that miR-34a was involved in the hepatoprotective effect of H$_2$S on hepatic I/R in the young rats.

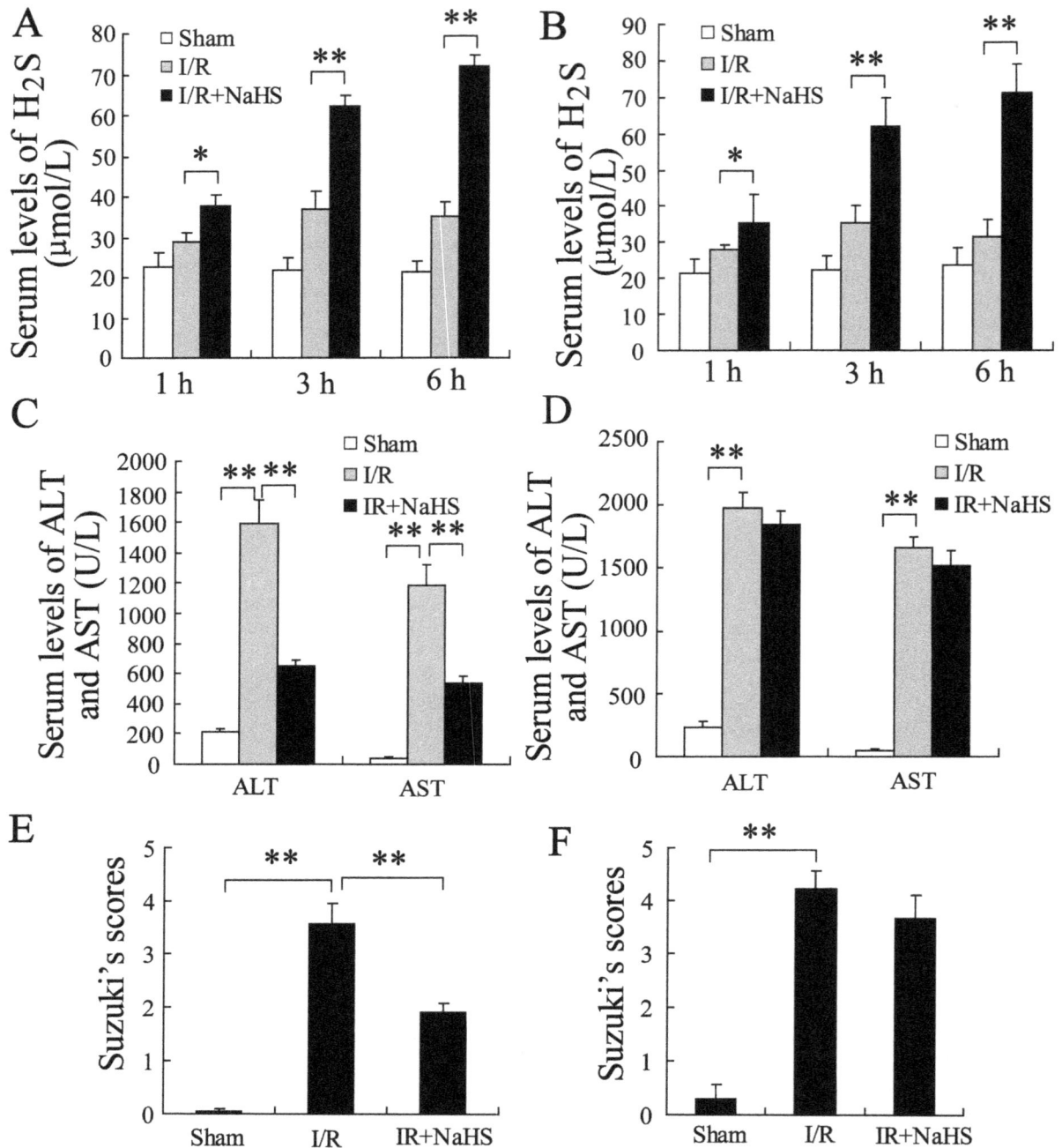

Figure 1. The effect of H₂S on hepatic I/R injury in young and old rats. (A) The serum levels of H2S were significantly increased in the young rats that received a preconditioning dose of 20 μmol/kg NaHS compared to rats in the I/R group. (B) The serum levels of H2S were significantly increased in the old rats that received a preconditioning dose of 20 μmol/kg NaHS compared to the rats in the I/R group. (C) The serum levels for alanine aminotransferase (ALT) and aspartate aminotransferase (AST) were determined in the young rats after 6 h of reperfusion. (D) The serum levels for ALT and AST were determined in the old rats after 6 h of reperfusion. (E) Suzuki's scores for the livers of the young rats after 24 h of reperfusion. (F) Suzuki's scores for the livers of the old rats after 24 h of reperfusion. **P<0.01, indicates significant differences from the respective control groups.

Knockout of miR-34a expression enhanced the hepatoprotective effect of H₂S on old rats

As the expression of miR-34a is abundant in hepatocytes of the old rats, we wondered whether the hepatoprotective effect of H₂S would be enhanced if its expression was down-regulated by an miR-34a inhibitor. As expected, the administration of the miR-34a inhibitor administration decreased serum levels of ALT and

AST in the old rats with hepatic I/R. Hepatoprotective effect were improved in the I/R group treated with NaHS and the miR-34a inhibitor compared to those in the miR-34a inhibitor-only group (Figure 5A, P<0.01), with the inhibitor further attenuating the pathological changes in the livers of the NaHS-treated old rats (Figure 5B, P<0.01).

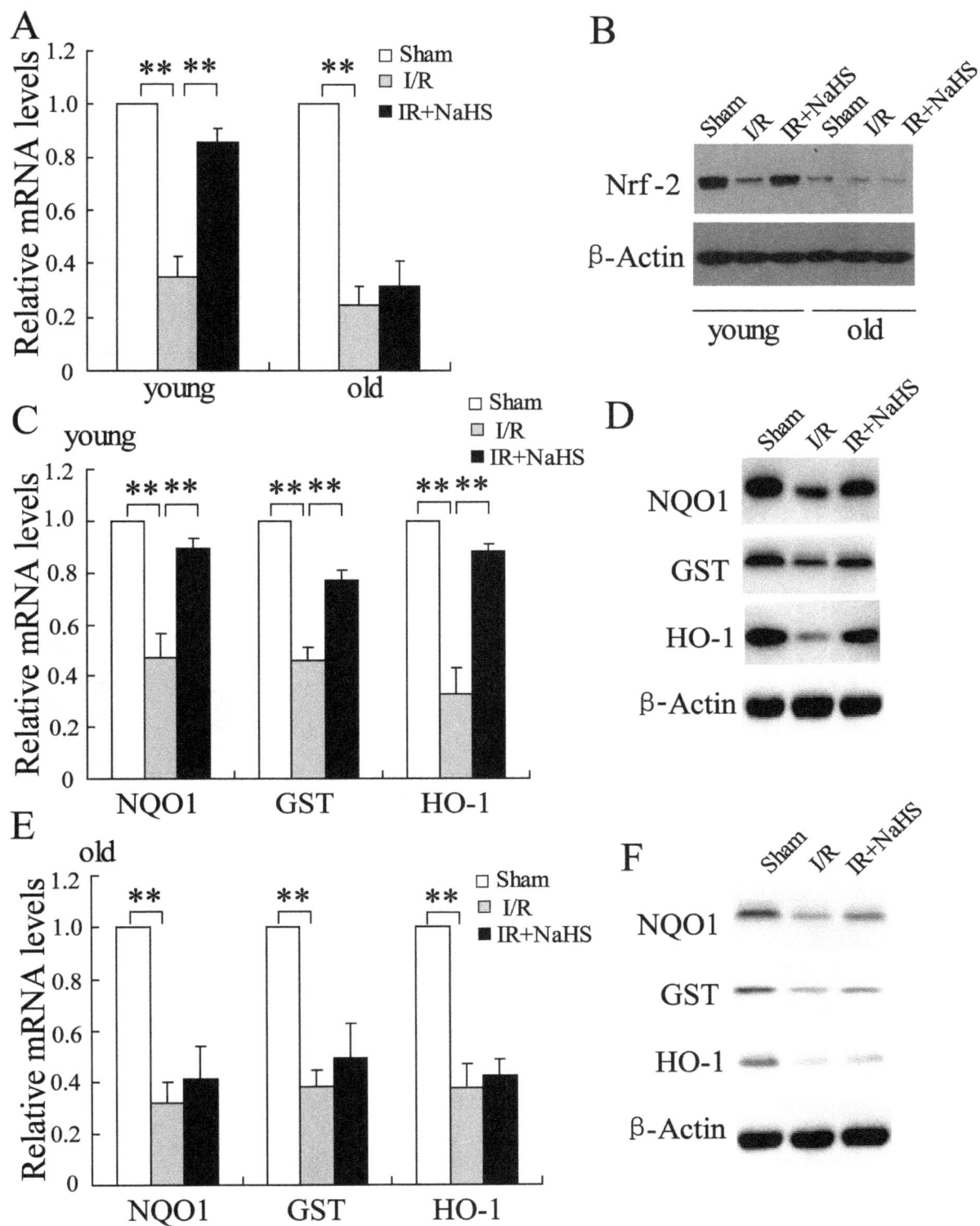

Figure 2. The effect of H₂S on Nrf-2-mediated signaling pathway. Relative mRNA levels of Nrf-2 were assayed in the young and old rats. Pretreatment with NaHS (20 μmol/kg) significantly increased Nrf-2 mRNA (A) and protein (B) levels in the young rats treated with I/R, but it had little effect on those in the old rats. Pretreatment with 20 μmol/kg NaHS significantly increased mRNA (C) and protein (D) levels of NQO1, GST, and HO-1 in the young rats treated with I/R. Pretreatment of 20 μmol/kg NaHS slightly increased mRNA (E) and protein (F) levels of NQO1, GST and HO-1 in the old rats treated with I/R. **P<0.01, indicate significant differences from the respective control groups.

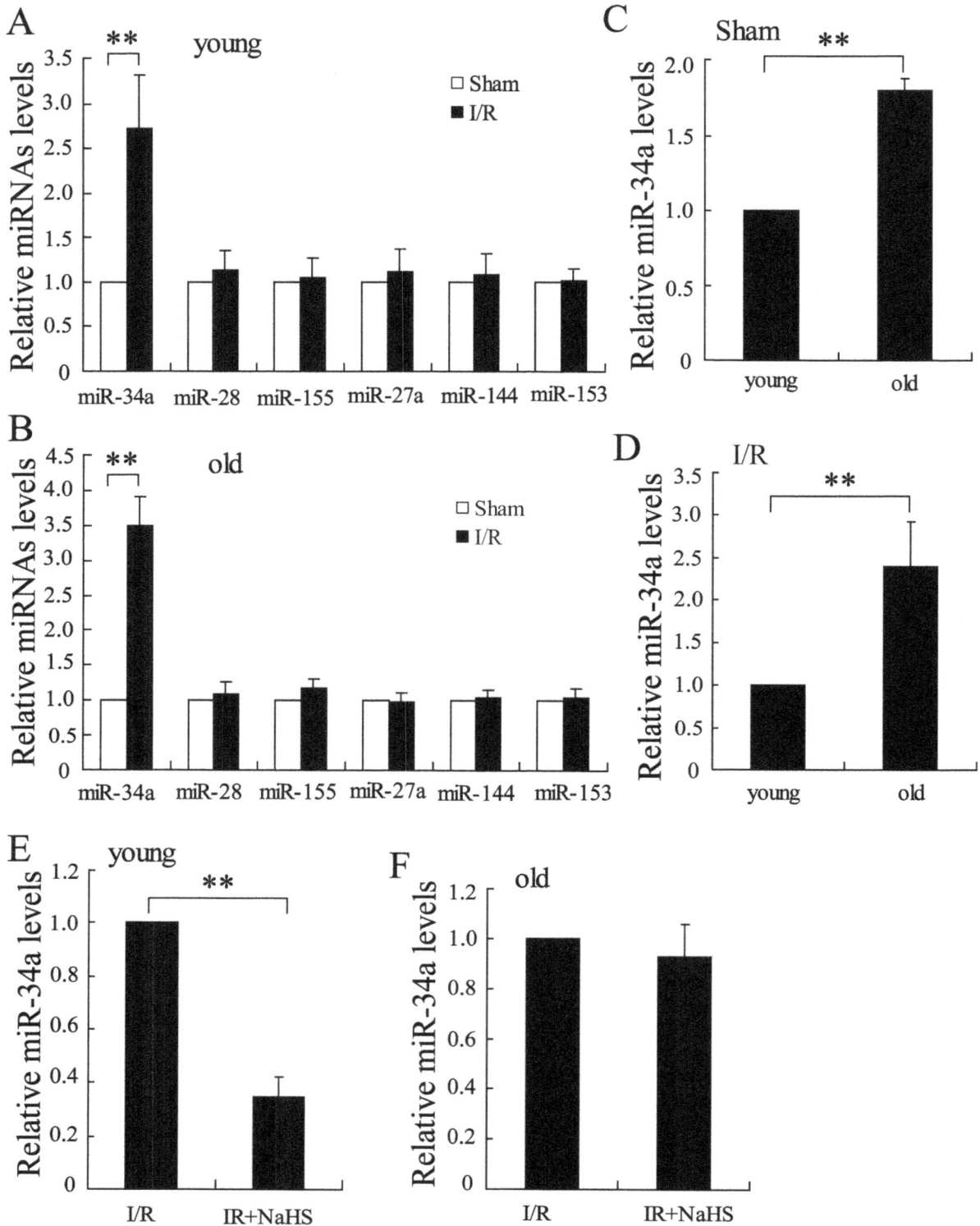

Figure 3. The effect of H₂S on miR-34a expression in the I/R liver. Relative levels of miR-34a, miR-28, miR-155, miR-27a, miR-144, and miR-153 were assayed in young rats (A) and old rats (B) after I/R. Levels of miR-34a were lower in the young rats in the sham group (C) and the in I/R group (D) than in the old rats. (E and F) Pretreatment with 20 μmol/kg NaHS significantly decreased miR-34a levels in the young rats (E), but it had little effect on those in the old rats. **P<0.01, indicates significant differences from the respective control groups.

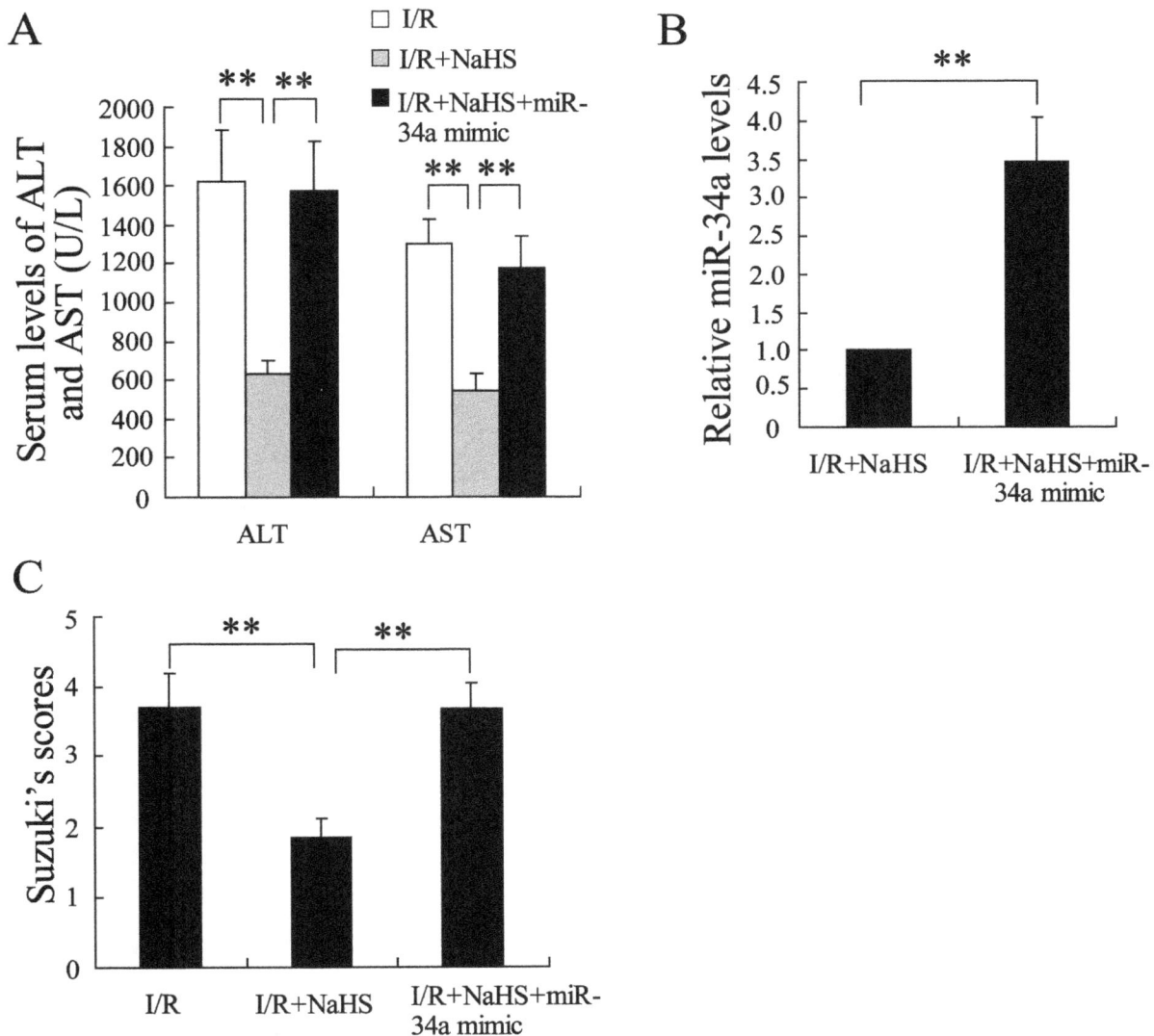

Figure 4. Overexpression of miR-34a inhibited the hepatoprotective effect of H₂S on young rats. (A) The serum levels of ALT and AST were assayed in the young rats. The serum levels of ALT and AST were significantly decreased in the young rats following the pretreatment with NaHS, and this decrease was reversed by miR-34a mimic. (B) The injection of miR-34a mimic clearly increased miR-34a levels. (C) Suzuki's scores for the livers of the young rats. **P<0.01, indicates significant differences from the respective control groups.

miR-34a mediation of Nrf-2 signaling pathway was implicated in the hepatoprotective effects of H₂S

To explore the mechanism of miR-34a in the hepatoprotective effects of H₂S, the expression of Nrf-2, NQO1, GST and HO-1 was measured in the young and old rats after injection of miR-34a mimic or inhibitor. As shown in Figure 6A and 6B, miR-34a mimic could reduce the expressions of Nrf-2, NQO1, GST and HO-1 in the young rats after hepatic I/R pretreated with NaHS, suggesting that the promotion of Nrf-2-mediated signaling pathway by NaHS might act through down-regulation of the miR-34a level. On the other hand, miR-34a inhibitor significantly increased the expressions of Nrf-2, NQO1, GST and HO-1 in the old rats after hepatic I/R injury with NaHS treatment (Figure 6C and 6D), suggesting that miR-34a-mediated Nrf-2 signaling pathway is involved in hepatoprotective effects of H₂S.

Discussion

The gasotransmitter H₂S can protect several tissues including the liver against I/R injury [29]. Previous study focused on the protective effect of H₂S on the tissues of young animals. The present study explored the hepatoprotective effect of H₂S on young (3 months) and old rats (20 months). We found that NaHS alone could reduce hepatic I/R injury in young rats, but it had little effect on hepatic I/R injury in old rats. In addition, NaHS pretreatment decreased miR-34a expression in the hepatocytes of the young rats treated with hepatic I/R. Our data also showed that miR-34a was implicated in H₂S-induced prevention of liver damage in the young rats. More importantly, the inhibition of miR-34a expression enhanced the effect of H₂S on hepatic I/R injury in the old rats. H₂S might promote Nrf-2-mediated signaling pathway through the down-regulation of the expression of miR-34a. The levels of miR-34a were higher in the hepatocytes of the old rats than in those of the young rats.

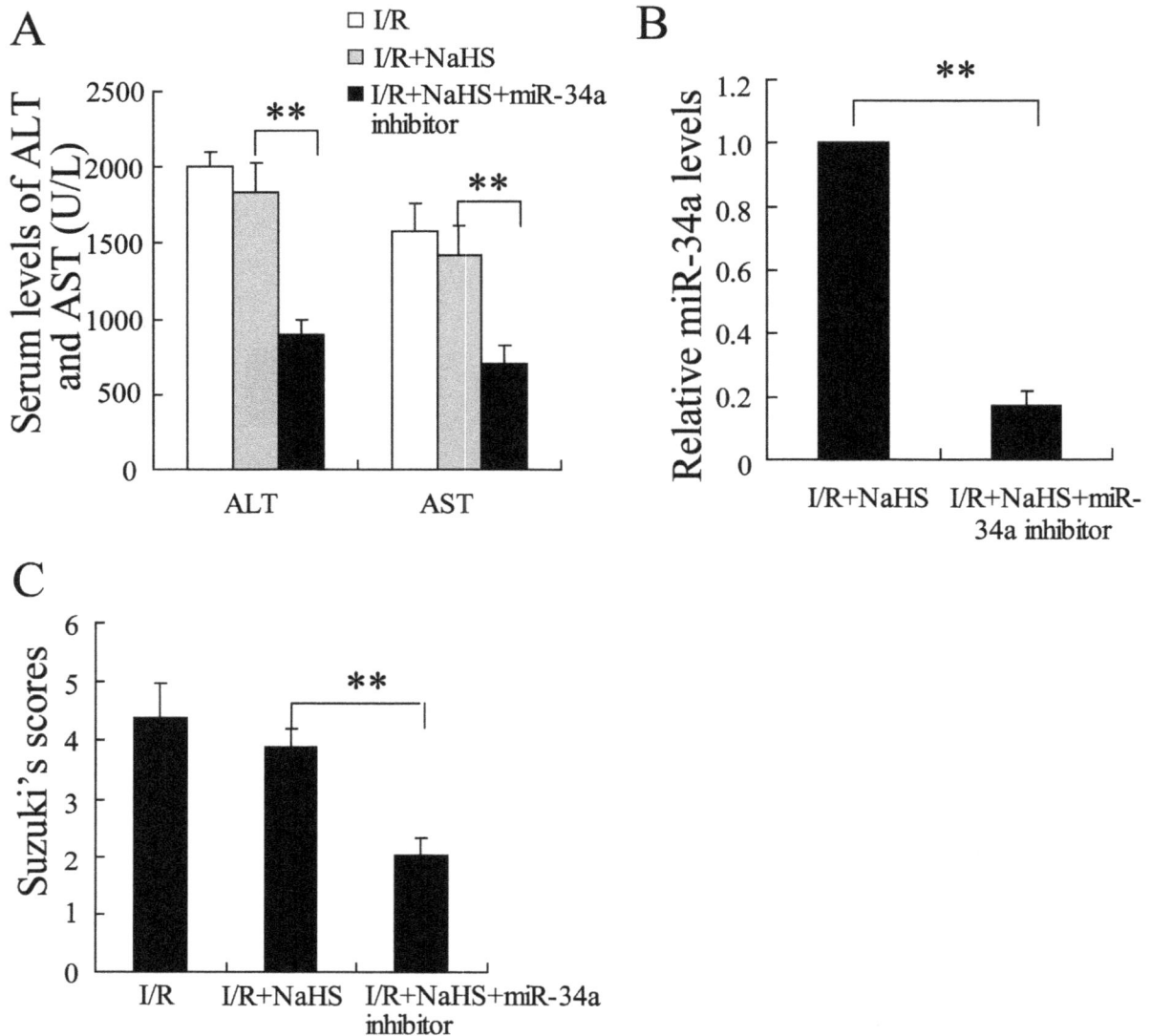

Figure 5. Knockout of miR-34a expression enhanced the hepatoprotective effect of H₂S on the old rats. (A) The serum levels of ALT and AST were assayed in the old rats. Pretreatment with NaHS had little effect on the serum levels of ALT and AST, which were significantly decreased by miR-34a inhibitor in the old rats with I/R. (B) The injection of miR-34a inhibitor clearly decreased miR-34a levels. (C) Suzuki's scores for the livers of the old rats. **P<0.01, indicates significant differences from the respective control groups.

Due to its anti-inflammatory, antioxidative, and cytoprotective activity, H_2S is capable of protecting tissues from I/R-induced injury [30]. The present study has for the first time explored the effect of H_2S on hepatic I/R injury in young and old rats. Our data showed that the administration of NaHS, a donor of H_2S, significantly decreased serum levels of AST and ALT, as well as histopathological alterations after hepatic I/R in young rats. However, NaHS had little effect on I/R-induced liver injury in the old rats. The different effect of NaHS on I/R injury was due to decreased production of endogenous antioxidants with increasing age. Our data demonstrated that NaHS stimulated the expression of Nrf-2 and its downstream target gene in young rats but that it had little effect on the expression of these molecules in old rats.

MiR-34a was previously reported to be involved in the regulation of liver function and survival [11]. In this study, we found that the level of miR-34a was remarkably higher in the hepatocytes of the old rats compared to that of the young rats,

which was consistent with previous findings [12]. NaHS significantly decreased miR-34a expression in the hepatocytes of the young rats but had little effect on miR-34a expression in the old rats due to the hepatoprotective effect of H_2S. To investigate the relationship between miR-34a and the effect of NaHS on hepatic I/R, we used miR-34a mimic and miR-34a inhibitor. Injection with miR-34a mimic diminished the protective effect of NaHS on hepatic I/R injury in the young rats. In the old rats, the combination of NaHS and the miR-34a inhibitor prevented the damage caused by hepatic I/R. MiR-34a has been implicated in liver oxidative stress during aging [12]. Based on that, we believe that the oxidative stress defense function of NaHS might rely on the regulation of miR-34a expression.

Our data also indicated that miR-34a mediation of the Nrf-2 signaling pathway was implicated in the hepatoprotective effect of H_2S. There are several lines of evidence to support this. First, in the young rats, miR-34a mimic reduced the expression of Nrf-2

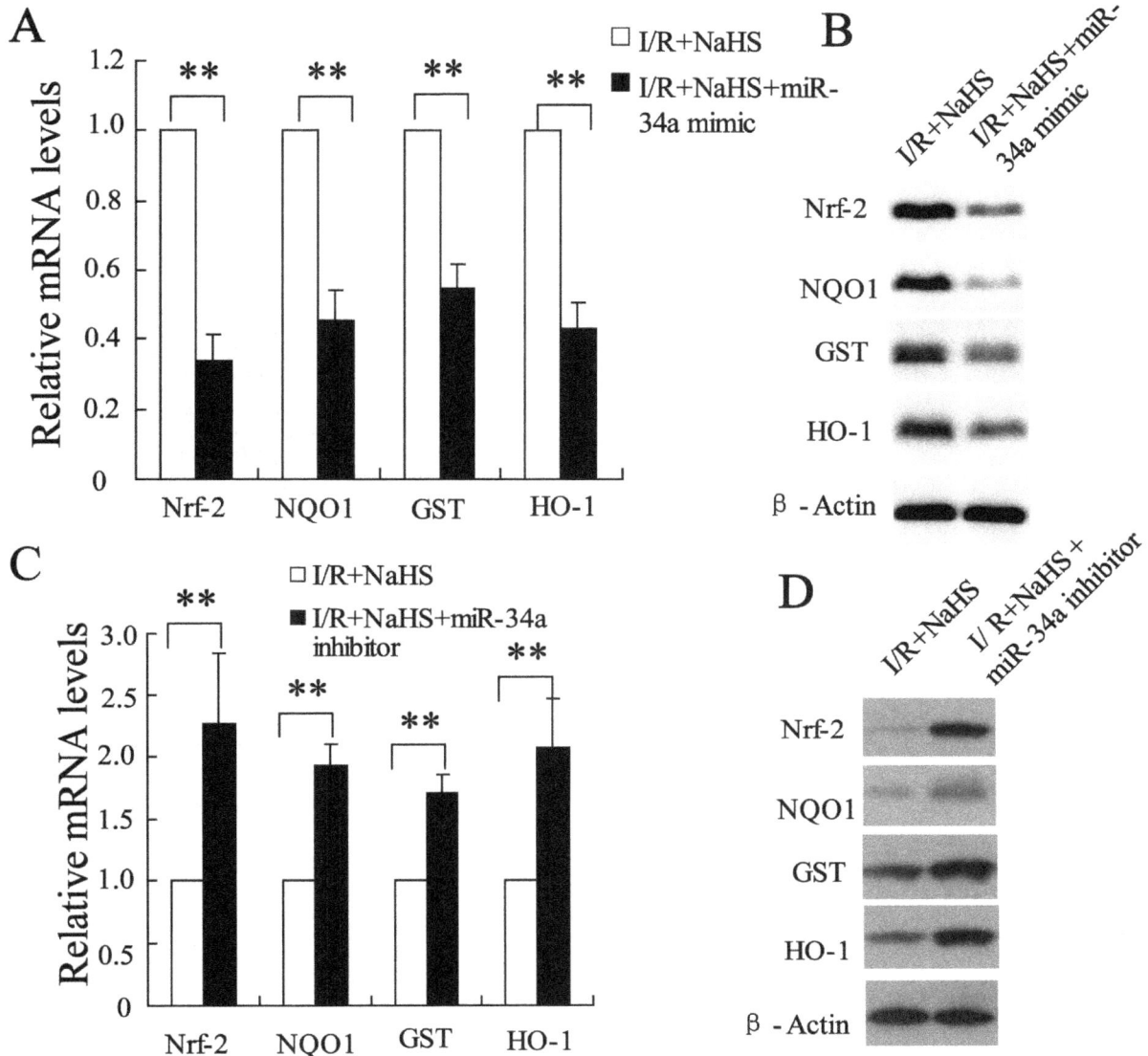

Figure 6. miR-34a mediated Nrf-2 signaling pathway was implicated in the hepatoprotective effects of H₂S. The injection of miR-34a mimic decreased the mRNA (A) and protein (B) levels of Nrf-2, NQO1, GST and HO-1 in the young rats in the I/R+pretreatment with NaHS group. The injection of miR-34a inhibitor increased the mRNA (C) and protein (D) levels of Nrf-2, NQO1, GST and HO-1 in the old rats in the with I/R+pretreatment with NaHS group. **P<0.01, indicates significant differences from the respective control groups.

and its downstream target gene in hepatic I/R pretreated with NaHS. Second, miR-34a inhibitor significantly increased the expression of Nrf-2 and its downstream target gene in the old rats with or without NaHS pretreatment. Third, miR-34a level was negatively correlated with Nrf-2 expression, which is consistent with the finding of a previous report [13].

Our data demonstrated that I/R stress decreased HO-1 mRNA and protein expressions in rat liver (Figure 2), which is inconsistent with the previous report [31]. It is possible that chloral hydrate treatment instead of pentobarbital treatment might affect the expression of some antioxidant gene in the liver. However, more clarification of the specific molecular mechanism involved is needed.

In summary, we demonstrated that NaHS had a different effect on hepatic I/R damage in young and old rats. Our results also

suggested that the hepatoprotective effect of NaHS in the young rats was due to decreased miR-34a expression, which resulted in the promotion of Nrf-2 signaling pathway. The protective effect of NaHS when it was combined with miR-34a inhibitor in the old rats provided further evidence for the role of miR-34a in hepatic I/R. These results may lead to the development of therapeutic strategies to minimize injury after I/R during liver transplantation and liver surgery both in young and aged patients.

Author Contributions

Conceived and designed the experiments: SL. Performed the experiments: XH. Analyzed the data: YG. Contributed reagents/materials/analysis tools: JQ. Contributed to the writing of the manuscript: SL.

References

1. Berrevoet F, Schäfer T, Vollmar B, Menger MD (2003) Ischemic preconditioning: enough evidence to support clinical application in liver surgery and transplantation? Acta Chir Belg 103: 485–489.

2. Papadopoulos D, Siempis T, Theodorakou E, Tsoulfas G (2013) Hepatic ischemia and reperfusion injury and trauma: current concepts. Arch Trauma Res 2: 63–70.

3. Jaeschke H, Woolbright BL (2012) Current strategies to minimize hepatic ischemia-reperfusion injury by targeting reactive oxygen species. Transplant Rev 26: 103–114.

4. Lisjak M, Teklic T, Wilson ID, Whiteman M, Hancock JT (2013) Hydrogen sulfide: environmental factor or signalling molecule? Plant Cell Environ 36: 1607–1616.

5. Kimura H (2013) Physiological role of hydrogen sulfide and polysulfide in the central nervous system. Neurochem Int 63: 492–497.

6. Guo W, Kan JT, Cheng ZY, Chen JF, Shen YQ, et al. (2012) Hydrogen sulfide as an endogenous modulator in mitochondria and mitochondria dysfunction. Oxid Med Cell Longev 2012: 878052.

7. Wagner F, Asfar P, Calzia E, Radermacher P, Szabó C (2009) Bench-to-bedside review: Hydrogen sulfide-the third gaseous transmitter: applications for critical care. Crit Care 13: 213.

8. Henderson PW, Weinstein AL, Sohn AM, Jimenez N, Krijgh DD, et al. (2010) Hydrogen sulfide attenuates intestinal ischemia-reperfusion injury when delivered in the post-ischemic period. J Gastroenterol Hepatol 25: 1642–1647.

9. Inui M, Martello G, Piccolo S (2010) MicroRNA control of signal transduction. Nat Rev Mol Cell Biol 11: 252–263.

10. Miska EA (2005) How microRNAs control cell division, differentiation and death. Curr Opin Genet Dev 15: 563–568.

11. McDaniel K, Herrera L, Zhou T, Francis H, Han Y, et al. (2014) The functional role of microRNAs in alcoholic liver injury. J Cell Mol Med 18: 197–207.

12. Fu T, Choi SE, Kim DH, Seok S, Suino-Powell KM, et al. (2012) Aberrantly elevated microRNA-34a in obesity attenuates hepatic responses to FGF19 by targeting a membrane coreceptor β-Klotho. Proc Natl Acad Sci U S A 109: 16137–16142.

13. Li N, Muthusamy S, Liang R, Sarojini H, Wang E (2011) Increased expression of miR-34a and miR-93 in rat liver during aging, and their impact on the expression of Mgst1 and Sirt1. Mech Ageing Dev 132: 75–85.

14. Chen H, Sun Y, Dong R, Yang S, Pan C, et al. (2011) Mir-34a is upregulated during liver regeneration in rats and is associated with the suppression of hepatocyte proliferation. PLoS One 6: e20238.

15. Suzuki T, Takagi Y, Osanai H, Li L, Takeuchi M, et al. (2005) Pi class glutathione S-transferase genes are regulated by Nrf 2 through an evolutionarily conserved regulatory element in zebrafish. Biochem J 388: 65–73.

16. Sahin K, Orhan C, Tuzcu M, Sahin N, Ali S, et al. (2014) Orally Administered Lycopene Attenuates Diethylnitrosamine-Induced Hepatocarcinogenesis in Rats by Modulating Nrf-2/HO-1 and Akt/mTOR Pathways. Nutr Cancer [Epub ahead of print].

17. Zeng T, Zhang CL, Song FY, Zhao XL, Yu LH (2013) The activation of HO-1/Nrf-2 contributes to the protective effects of diallyl disulfide (DADS) against ethanol-induced oxidative stress. Biochim Biophys Acta 1830: 4848–4859.

18. Park SY, Kim JH, Lee SJ, Kim Y (2013) Involvement of PKA and HO-1 signaling in anti-inflammatory effects of surfactin in BV-2 microglial cells. Toxicol Appl Pharmacol 268: 68–78.

19. MacLeod AK, McMahon M, Plummer SM, Higgins LG, Penning TM, et al. (2009) Characterization of the cancer chemopreventive NRF2-dependent gene battery in human keratinocytes: demonstration that the KEAP1-NRF2 pathway, and not the BACH1-NRF2 pathway, controls cytoprotection against electrophiles as well as redox-cycling compounds. Carcinogenesis 30: 1571–1580.

20. Peake BF, Nicholson CK, Lambert JP, Hood RL, Amin H, et al. (2013) Hydrogen sulfide preconditions the db/db diabetic mouse heart against ischemia-reperfusion injury by activating Nrf2 signaling in an Erk-dependent manner. Am J Physiol Heart Circ Physiol 304: H1215–H1224.

21. Lu YF, Liu J, Wu KC, Qu Q, Fan F, et al. (2014) Overexpression of Nrf2 Protects against Microcystin-Induced Hepatotoxicity in Mice. PLoS One 9: e93013.

22. Schiesser M, Wittert A, Nieuwenhuijs VB, Morphett A, Padbury RT, et al. (2009) Intermittent ischemia but not ischemic preconditioning is effective in restoring bile flow after ischemia reperfusion injury in the livers of aged rats. J Surg Res 152: 61–68.

23. van der Bilt JD, Kranenburg O, Borren A, van Hillegersberg R, Borel Rinkes IH (2008) Ageing and hepatic steatosis exacerbate ischemia/reperfusion-accelerated outgrowth of colorectal micrometastases. Ann Surg Oncol 15: 1392–1398.

24. Zhang Q, Fu H, Zhang H, Xu F, Zou Z, et al. (2013) Hydrogen sulfide preconditioning protects rat liver against ischemia/reperfusion injury by activating Akt-GSK-3β signaling and inhibiting mitochondrial permeability transition. PLoS One 8: e74422.

25. Suzuki S, Toledo-Pereyra LH, Rodriguez FJ, Cejalvo D (1993) Neutrophil infiltration as an important factor in liver ischemia and reperfusion injury. Modulating effects of FK506 and cyclosporine. Transplantation 55: 1265–1272.

26. Tulsawani R, Gupta R, Misra K (2013) Efficacy of aqueous extract of Hippophae rhamnoides and its bio-active flavonoids against hypoxia-induced cell death. Indian J Pharmacol 45: 258–263.

27. Ke B, Shen XD, Zhang Y, Ji H, Gao F, et al. (2013) KEAP1-NRF2 complex in ischemia-induced hepatocellular damage of mouse liver transplants. J Hepatol. 2013; 59(6): 1200–1207.

28. Cheng X, Ku CH, Siow RC (2013) Regulation of the Nrf2 antioxidant pathway by microRNAs: New players in micromanaging redox homeostasis. Free Radic Biol Med 64: 4–11.

29. Kimura H, Shibuya N, Kimura Y (2012) Hydrogen sulfide is a signaling molecule and a cytoprotectant. Antioxid Redox Signal 17: 45–57.

30. Nicholson CK, Calvert JW (2010) Hydrogen sulfide and ischemia-reperfusion injury. Pharmacol Res 62: 289–297.

31. Tanaka Y, Maher JM, Chen C, Klaassen CD (2007) Hepatic ischemia-reperfusion induces renal heme oxygenase-1 via NF-E2-related factor 2 in rats and mice. Mol Pharmacol 71: 817–825.

23

Criteria for Viability Assessment of Discarded Human Donor Livers during *Ex Vivo* Normothermic Machine Perfusion

Michael E. Sutton[1,2,◊], Sanna op den Dries[1,2,◊], Negin Karimian[1,2], Pepijn D. Weeder[1,2], Marieke T. de Boer[1], Janneke Wiersema-Buist[2], Annette S. H. Gouw[3], Henri G. D. Leuvenink[2], Ton Lisman[1,2], Robert J. Porte[1]*

1 Section of Hepatobiliary Surgery and Liver Transplantation, Department of Surgery, University of Groningen, University Medical Center Groningen, Groningen, The Netherlands, 2 Surgical Research Laboratory, University of Groningen, University Medical Center Groningen, Groningen, The Netherlands, 3 Department of Pathology, University of Groningen, University Medical Center Groningen, Groningen, The Netherlands

Abstract

Although normothermic machine perfusion of donor livers may allow assessment of graft viability prior to transplantation, there are currently no data on what would be a good parameter of graft viability. To determine whether bile production is a suitable biomarker that can be used to discriminate viable from non-viable livers we have studied functional performance as well as biochemical and histological evidence of hepatobiliary injury during *ex vivo* normothermic machine perfusion of human donor livers. After a median duration of cold storage of 6.5 h, twelve extended criteria human donor livers that were declined for transplantation were *ex vivo* perfused for 6 h at 37°C with an oxygenated solution based on red blood cells and plasma, using pressure controlled pulsatile perfusion of the hepatic artery and continuous portal perfusion. During perfusion, two patterns of bile flow were identified: (1) steadily increasing bile production, resulting in a cumulative output of $\geq$30 g after 6 h (high bile output group), and (2) a cumulative bile production <20 g in 6 h (low bile output group). Concentrations of transaminases and potassium in the perfusion fluid were significantly higher in the low bile output group, compared to the high bile output group. Biliary concentrations of bilirubin and bicarbonate were respectively 4 times and 2 times higher in the high bile output group. Livers in the low bile output group displayed more signs of hepatic necrosis and venous congestion, compared to the high bile output group. In conclusion, bile production could be an easily assessable biomarker of hepatic viability during *ex vivo* machine perfusion of human donor livers. It could potentially be used to identify extended criteria livers that are suitable for transplantation. These *ex vivo* findings need to be confirmed in a transplant experiment or a clinical trial.

Editor: Déla Golshayan, Centre Hospitalier Universitaire Vaudois (CHUV), Université de Lausanne, Switzerland

Funding: This work was supported by: 1. Innovatief Actieprogramma Groningen (author SODD), http://www.provinciegroningen.nl/servicelinks-provincie-groningen/english/; 2. Jan Kornelis de Cock Stichting, http://www.decockstichting.nl/subsidies.html (authors: SODD MES); 3. Tekke Huizingafonds, http://tekkehuizingafonds.nl/ (author SODD). The funders had no role in study design, data collection and analysis, decision to publish, or preparation of the manuscript.

Competing Interests: The authors have declared that no competing interests exist.

* Email: r.j.porte@umcg.nl

◊ These authors contributed equally to this work.

Introduction

Donor liver shortage remains a limiting factor in liver transplant programs in most parts of the world. In an attempt to reduce the discrepancy between donor liver availability and demand, criteria for organ acceptance have gradually widened with increasing acceptance of livers that carry a higher risk of early graft failure or transmission of an infectious or malignant disease (so called extended criteria donor (ECD) livers). The types of ECD livers most frequently considered for transplantation are livers with mild-moderate steatosis, livers from older donors or donors with a high body mass index, and livers donated after cardiac death (DCD) [1], [2], [3]. Although livers from ECD donors are increasingly considered for transplantation, many of them are still declined. A recent study in the US has shown that the proportion of donor livers not used for transplantation is increasing since 2004 [4]. The proportion of nonuse attributable to DCD increased from 9% in 2004 to 28% in 2010, probably because in many cases the risk of early graft failure after transplantation is considered to be too high [4].

The decisions to either accept or decline a potential donor liver for transplantation is currently based on the interpretation of donor data, obtained before or during procurement, by the physician. Parameters such as donor past medical history, last known laboratory values, findings during liver procurement, and other procurement variables such as expected ischemia times primarily determine acceptability of the graft. Once a donor liver is retrieved and stored in an organ box for transportation functional assessment is no longer possible until after transplantation. The uncertainty about how much additional damage a liver will sustain during the hours of cold storage poses an important hurdle for accepting many ECD livers.

During the past decade, machine perfusion of donor livers has received increasing attention as a tool to improve organ preservation and improve outcome after transplantation [5], [6], [7], [8], [9]. Several experimental studies have shown superiority of machine perfusion compared to static cold storage with respect to reduction of ischemia/reperfusion (IR) injury [10], [11], [12]. Apart from providing better graft protection against IR injury, machine perfusion provides the possibility of functional assessment of a liver graft short before implantation in a recipient. Although machine perfusion can be performed at various temperatures, only normothermic oxygenated machine perfusion (NMP) may allow a full functional assessment of an organ prior to transplantation. During NMP the liver is offered physiological amounts of oxygen and nutrients supporting a full functional metabolic activity [13]. The possibility of functional assessment of an ECD liver after static cold storage and transportation would be of great importance in the judgment of livers that would otherwise be declined for transplantation based on the current criteria.

Despite the growing amount of literature on the role of machine perfusion as an alternative and better preservation method compared to static cold storage, there are no data on what would be reliable parameters for functional assessment of human donor livers during NMP. Based on a porcine model of normothermic liver perfusion, Imber et al. have suggested that bile production is directly attributed to liver viability and could therefore be used as a predictive marker of liver function [11]. In addition, bile production has long been recognized as an important clinical parameter to predict early graft dysfunction (including primary non-function and delayed graft function) after liver transplantation [14]. We, therefore, hypothesized that bile production during NMP of human donor livers is a suitable and easy to assess biomarker of hepatic viability that can be used to discriminate a potentially transplantable from a non-transplantable graft. To test this hypothesis we have studied functional performance as well as biochemical and histological signs of hepatobiliary injury during ex vivo NMP of human donor livers that were declined for transplantation. Secondary aim of this study was to determine the minimal duration of NMP needed to discriminate viable and potentially transplantable livers from non-viable livers.

Materials and Methods

Liver Donors

Between May 2012 and May 2013 twelve human livers that were declined for transplantation by all three liver transplant centers in The Netherlands, as well as other centers within the Eurotransplant region, were included in this study. Of these, ten were obtained from a DCD donor and two were obtained from donors after brain death (DBD). The donor risk index (DRI) was used to assess the chance of graft failure within three months after transplantation [15]. Livers were retrieved using a standard surgical technique of in situ cooling and flush-out with ice cold preservation fluid (University of Wisconsin [UW] or histidine–tryptophan–ketoglutarate [HTK] solution). The surgical procedure was not started until after a five minute 'no touch' period following declaration of cardiac arrest and circulatory death in case of a DCD donor. In case of DBD liver procurement the administration of 25.000 units of heparin was given intravenously before cross clamping. The same dose of heparin was added to the preservation solution in case of DCD liver procurement. Livers were subsequently packed and stored on ice and transported to our center. In all cases, informed consent to use a donor liver for this

study for this study was provided from the relatives. The study protocol was approved by the medical ethical committee of the University Medical Center Groningen and the *Nederlandse Transplantatie Stichting*, the competent authority for organ donation in the Netherlands.

Normothermic Oxygenated Machine Perfusion

Upon arrival at our center, cold preserved livers were prepared on the back table for normothermic oxygenated machine perfusion as described previously [13]. NMP was initiated using a CE marked (European Union certification of safety, health and environmental requirements) device that enables dual perfusion via both the hepatic artery and the portal vein in a closed circuit (Liver Assist Organ Assist, Groningen, Netherlands). Livers were perfused for 6 h with a perfusion solution based on heparinized human plasma and red blood cells fortified with nutrients, trace elements and antibiotics as described previously [13]. Two rotary pumps provided pulsatile flow to the hepatic artery and a continuous flow to the portal vein. Two hollow fiber membrane oxygenators provided oxygenation of the perfusion solution, as well as removal of CO_2. The system was temperature and pressure controlled, allowing auto-regulation of the blood flow through the liver. Pressure was limited to a mean of 60 mmHg in the hepatic artery and 11 mmHg in the portal vein. The temperature was set to 37°C and a new sterile disposable set of tubing, reservoir and oxygenators was used for each liver. Before connecting the liver to the device, the perfusion fluid was primed with the addition of an 8.4% sodium bicarbonate solution to obtain a stable physiological pH. A summary of the composition of perfusion fluid prior to initiation of NMP is provided in Table 1.

Assessment of Hepatobiliary Function and Injury

Bile samples were collected from a catheter in the donor common bile duct and bile production was measured gravimetrically at 30 min intervals. Bile production was expressed as g/30 min. Concentration of bilirubin in bile was determined as a marker of hepatic secretory function, using standard biochemical methods. Biliary concentration of bicarbonate and glucose were determined as markers of biliary epithelial cell (cholangiocyte) function. For this purpose, bile samples were collected under mineral oil and analyzed immediately using an ABL800 FLEX analyzer (Radiometer, Brønhøj, Denmark).

During NMP, samples were taken from the perfusion fluid at 30 min intervals and analyzed immediately for blood gas parameters (pO_2, pCO_2, sO_2, HCO^{3-} and pH) and for biochemical parameters (glucose, calcium, lactate, potassium, sodium, and hemoglobin) by an ABL800 FLEX analyzer (Radiometer, Brønhøj, Denmark). Oxygen consumption was calculated based on the difference between the venous oxygen content and the arterial oxygen content of the perfusion fluid. The oxygen content of the perfusion fluid was calculated by adding the free dissolved oxygen fraction to the Hb-bound oxygen fraction using the following formula: O_2 cont = $(pO_2 \times K) + (sO_2 \times Hb \times c)$, where pO_2 is partial oxygen pressure in kPa, K equals 0,027 for O_2 in water at 37°C, sO_2 is the saturation expressed as a fraction, Hb is the concentration in mmol/L and c equals 91,12 mlO_2/mmol for the oxygen binding capacity of hemoglobin. Oxygen consumption was expressed in mlO_2/min/kilogram liver tissue. Next to this, hepatic concentration of adenosine-5′-triphosphate (ATP) was used as an indicator of the energy status of the liver grafts. Liver samples were immediately frozen in liquid nitrogen. Frozen tissue was cut into 20 μm slices and a total amount of ±50 mg was homogenized in 1 mL of SONOP (0.372 g EDTA in 130 mL H_2O and NaOH (ph 10.9)+370 mL 96% ethanol) and

Table 1. Biochemical Composition of Perfusion Fluid Used For Normothermic Machine Perfusion of Donor Livers.

Variable	Median	IQR	Reference values in blood
pH	7.40	7.34–7.45	7.35–7.45
pCO$_2$ (kPa)	4.1	3.5–4.6	4.6–6.0
pO$_2$ (kPa)	71	65–75	9.5–13.5
sO$_2$ (%)	100	99–100	96–99
HCO3- (mmol/L)	19	17–21	21–25
Base Excess (mmol/L)	−4.6	−6.7–−3.5	−3 to 3.0
Na$^+$ (mmol/L)	150	145–154	135–145
K$^+$ (mmol/L)	4.4	3.8–5.6	3.5–5.0
Free Ca^{2+} (mmol/L)	0.67	0.61–0.72	1.15–1.29
Glucose (mmol/L)*	14	13–15	4–9
Lactate (mmol/L)*	6	6–7	0.5–2.2
Hemoglobin (mmol/L)*	4.7	4.6–4.9	8.7–10.6
Albumin (mmol/L)	31	29–33	35–50
Chloride (mmol/L)	97	91–98	97–107
Urea (mmol/L)	3.5	2.9–3.6	2.5–7.5
Phosphate (mmol/L)	1.8	1.5–2.2	0.7–1.5
Magnesium (mmol/L)	0.55	0.51–0.63	0.70–1.00
Alanine-aminotransferase (U/L)	9	8–11	0–45
Aspartate-aminotransferase (U/L)	13	13–17	0–40
Alkaline phosphatase (U/L)	24	23–28	0–120
Gamma-glutamyltransferase (U/L)	9	7–16	0–40
Lactate dehydrogenase (U/L)	101	93–114	0–250
Total bilirubin (µmol/L)*	2	2–3	0–17

* To convert values for glucose to mg/dL, multiply by 18.02. To convert values for lactate to mg/dL, multiply by 9.01. To convert values for hemoglobin to g/dL, multiply by 1.650. To convert the value for bilirubin to mg/dL, divide by 17.1.

sonoficated. Precipitate was removed by centrifugation (13,000 rcf for 10 min). Supernatant was diluted with SONOP to attain a protein concentration of 200–300 µg/mL (Pierce BCA Protein Assay Kit, Thermo Scientific, Rockford, IL) and mixed with 450 µL of 100 mM phosphate buffer (Merck; ph 7.6–8.0). Fifty microliters of phosphate buffered supernatant was used for ATP measurement using ATP Bioluminescence assay kit CLS II (Boehringer, Mannheim, Germany) and a luminometer (Victor[3] 1420 multilabel counter, PerkinElmer). ATP concentrations were calculated from a calibration curve constructed on the same plate, corrected for amount of protein, and values were expressed as µmol/g protein.

In addition, plasma from the perfusion fluid was collected (after 5 min centrifugation at 2700 rpm at 4°C), frozen and stored at −80°C for determination of alkaline phosphatase (ALP), gamma-glutamyl transferase (gamma-GT), alanine aminotransferase (ALT), lactate dehydrogenase (LDH), total bilirubin, and albumin, using standard biochemical methods.

Histological Evaluation

Biopsies were obtained from the liver grafts before and after 6 h of machine perfusion and stored in formalin for histological evaluation. Paraffin-embedded slides of liver biopsies were prepared for hematoxylin and eosin (H&E) staining, and assessed in a semi-quantitative fashion for the presence or absence of venous congestion or >30% hepatocellular necrosis. All liver and slides were examined in a blinded fashion by an experienced liver pathologist (ASHG) using light microscopy.

Statistical Analysis

Continuous variables are presented as medians and interquartile range (IQR). Categorical variables are presented as number and percentage. Continuous variables were compared between groups using the Mann-Whitney U test. Categorical variables were compared with the Pearson chi-square. Total course of ATP concentration starting at baseline (before NMP) through 6 h of NMP was analyzed between the groups by comparing the area under the curve (AUC, using the trapezium rule). A p-value <0.05 was considered to indicate statistical significance. All statistical analyses were performed using SPSS software version 16.0 for Windows (SPSS, Inc., Chicago, IL).

Results

Bile Production as Discriminating Variable during Machine Perfusion

First aim of this study was to determine whether bile production is a suitable marker of hepatic viability that can be used during NMP to discriminate a potentially transplantable from a non-transplantable graft. Therefore, we determined the evolution of bile production during 6 h of NMP for all twelve livers. Two distinct patterns of bile flow could be identified: 1) a steadily increasing bile production, resulting in a cumulative bile output of

≥30 g during the 6 h of perfusion, and 2) an initially increasing bile production during the first 2–3 hours, followed by a diminishing production, resulting in a cumulative bile production in 6 h <20 g (Figure 1). Based on this finding of two distinct profiles of bile production a cutoff value of 20 g cumulative bile production during 6 h of NMP was chosen to separate high from low bile output. There were six livers in each group and these two groups were used for further analyses.

A comparison of donor characteristics between livers with a high bile output versus livers with a low bile output during *ex vivo* machine perfusion is provided in Table 2. There were no statistically significant differences for any of these variables. Most livers were declined for transplantation because of a combination of DCD and age (>60 years) or DCD and high BMI. Two livers were declined because of macrovesicular steatosis >30% and both livers were in the low bile output group. It was obvious from this comparison that one would not have been able to identify livers with a high versus low bile output before organ procurement based on conventional donor characteristics alone.

Comparison of Hepatic Function and Injury

We next examined whether the differences in bile production correlated with other markers of hepatobiliary function and injury during NMP. First, we compared perfusion characteristics between the two groups. During NMP the flow in the portal vein and hepatic artery increased rapidly during the first 30 min and flows remained stable thereafter for the entire 6 h perfusion period (Figure 2). There were no significant differences in portal flow and although median arterial flow was constantly lower in livers with a low bile output, compared to the high bile output group, this did not reach statistical significance.

Biochemical markers of hepatobiliary function and injury after 6 h of *ex vivo* perfusion are presented in Table 3. Most striking differences were significantly higher concentrations of transaminases and a higher potassium level in the perfusion fluid of the low bile output group, compared to the high bile output group. These findings are compatible with a higher degree of IR injury and

hepatocellular lysis in the former group. Bicarbonate concentration in perfusion fluid of livers with high bile output was 26 mmol/L (22–28 mmol/L), compared to 18 mmol/L (13–29 mmol/L) in the group of low bile output livers. Although this difference was not statistically different, it should be noted that about 4-times more sodium bicarbonate solution (8.4%) had been added during perfusion in the low bile output group to maintain a physiological pH. After initiation of machine perfusion, glucose and lactate concentrations in the perfusion fluid initially increased in all cases. In the group of livers with high bile output glucose and lactate levels subsequently decreased rapidly and levels were normal at 6 h of NMP. In contrast, glucose and lactate levels in the low bile output group did not normalize during machine perfusion. Albumin levels decreased during all liver perfusions. After 6 h of NMP, albumin levels in the high bile output group were 23 g/L (22–24 g/L), compared to 26 (25–29 g/L) in the low bile output group (Table 3).

At the start of NMP, median pO_2 in the perfusate was 71 kPa (or 533 mmHg) with an interquartile range of 65–75 kPa (or 488–563 mmHg). After the start of NMP, the pO_2 dropped in 4 out of the 6 livers with low bile output and median pO_2 in this group after 6 hours of NMP was 35 kPa (or 263 mmHg). This was not significantly different from pO_2 values in the high bile output group (Table 3) and this value is still far above the upper limit of normal arterial pO_2 *in vivo* (13.5 kPa or 101 mmHg). After 6 hr of NMP, there was a small, but significant difference in sO_2 between the two groups (100% versus 98%), yet median values never fell below the normal range *in vivo* (normal values arterial sO_2: 96–99%). In parallel with these changes, total hepatic ATP content was significantly higher during the course of NMP in the livers with high bile output, compared to those with low bile output. At baseline, all livers were ATP depleted with a median in the high bile output group 7 μmol/g protein compared to 8 μmol/g in the low bile output group. After 2 h of NMP the ATP had increased to 50 μmol/g in the high bile output group and to 15 μmol/g in the low bile output group. This difference in ATP content persisted during the course of NMP and the AUC analysis

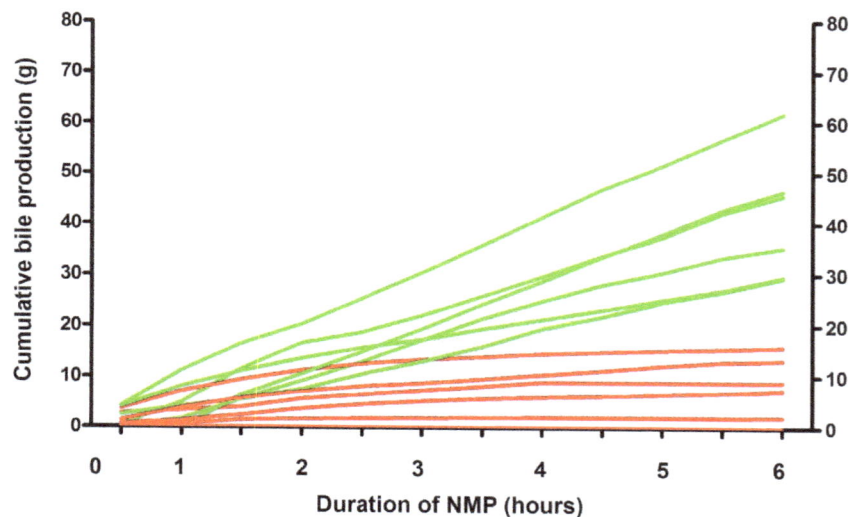

Figure 1. Cumulative bile production during *ex vivo* **normothermic machine perfusion of human donor livers.** Presented are individual values for 12 livers that were declined for transplantation. *Ex vivo* machine perfusion and viability testing was started after a median cold storage of 6.5 hours. Two distinct patterns of bile flow could be identified: 1) a steadily increasing bile production, resulting in a cumulative bile output of ≥ 30 g during the 6 h of perfusion (green lines), and 2) an initially increasing bile production during the first 2–3 hours, followed by a diminishing production, resulting in a cumulative bile production in 6 h <20 g (red lines).

Table 2. Donor Characteristics.

	Total group	Low Bile Output	High Bile Output	P-value
	(n = 12)	(n = 6)	(n = 6)	
Type of donor				0.12
DCD	10 (83%)	4 (67%)	6 (100%)	
DBD	2 (17%)	2 (33%)	0 (0%)	
Age (years)	61 (50–64)	55 (48–65)	63 (51–65)	0.47
Gender				0.22
Male	8 (67%)	3 (50%)	1 (17%)	
Female	4 (33%)	3 (50%)	5 (83%)	
Height (m)	1.77 (1.67–1.80)	1.77 (1.64–1.81)	1.78 (1.71–1.81)	0.69
Weight (kg)	88 (76–98)	90 (85–100)	78 (75–95)	0.20
Reason for rejection				0.25
DCD + age>60 years	5 (41%)	1 (17%)	4 (67%)	
DCD + high BMI	3 (25%)	2 (33%)	1 (17%)	
DCD + other reason*	2 (17%)	1 (17%)	1 (17%)	
Severe steatosis**	2 (17%)	2 (33%)	0 (0%)	
Donor Risk Index	2.35 (2.01–2.54)	2.48 (2.23–2.61)	2.20 (1.83–2.42)	0.35
ALT (U/L) *	38 (24–59)	59 (34–104)	25 (14–49)	0.05
GGT (U/L) *	90 (39–130)	111 (62–144)	65 (30–130)	0.27
Prothrombin time (sec)	14.0 (12.3–16.3)	15.0 (14.0–16.8)	12.9 (9.1–39.7)	0.20
Preservation Solution				1.00
UW solution	6 (50%)	3 (50%)	3 (50%)	
HTK solution	6 (50%)	3 (50%)	3 (50%)	
Time between switch-off and cardiac death (min)	24 (15–52)	30 (2–53)	24 (17–53)	0.27
Donor warm ischemia time (min)†	17 (16–20)	19 (9–26)	17 (15–18)	0.31
Total donor warm ischemia (min) †	43 (33–71)	51 (27–72)	43 (34–68)	0.35
Cold ischemia time (min)	389 (458–585)	530 (431–750)	409 (363–473)	0.11
Liver weight (kg)	2.09 (1.60–2.24)	2.17 (1.60–2.31)	2.03 (1.71–2.18)	0.63

* One DCD donor with history of iv drug abuse (low bile output group) and one donor with prolonged s0$_2$<30% after withdrawal of life support (high bile output group).
** defined as macrovesicular steatosis with more than 60% of hepatocytes involved.
*** last known value before procurement.
†Donor warm ischemia times was defined as the time interval between cardiac arrest and start of *in situ* cold perfusion. Total donor warm ischemia time was defined as the time interval between switch -off and start of *in situ* cold perfusion.
Continuous variables are presented as median and interquartile range, categorical variables are presented as numbers and percentage.
Abbreviations used: DCD, donation after cardiac death; DBD, donation after brain death; ALT, alanine aminotransferase; GGT, gamma glutamate transferase; UW, university of Wisconsin; HTK, Histidine- tryptophan-ketoglutarate.

revealed statistical significant difference (p = 0.04; Figure 3). In addition, pO$_2$ and sO$_2$, oxygen consumption was higher in the group of livers with low bile output, compared to those with high bile output, but this did not reach statistical significance.

Biochemical analysis of bile samples during 6 h of NMP revealed a 4-times higher concentration of bilirubin and a 2-times higher biliary concentration of bicarbonate in the high bile output group, compared to the low bile output group (Table 3). These findings indicate that a better secretory function of hepatocytes (bilirubin) coincides with that of cholangiocytes (bicarbonate).

Histological Comparison

Finally, we compared histology of liver grafts after 6 h of NMP between the two groups. In accordance with the observed differences in biochemical markers of hepatic injury, livers in the low bile output group displayed more signs of hepatic necrosis and venous congestion, compared to the high bile output group (Figure 4 A-D). Venous congestion was present in 5 out of 6 livers (83%) in the low bile output group and in 2 out of 6 livers (33%) in the high bile output group (p = 0.08). Necrosis >30% was observed in 4/6 (66%) of the livers in the low bile output group and in 2/6 (33%) livers in the high bile output group (p = 0.25). Despite these differences in hepatic parenchymal damage between the two groups, there were no major differences in the degree of biliary damage (Figure 4 E-F).

Minimal Duration of NMP Needed for Viability Assessment

Secondary aim of this study was to determine the minimal duration of NMP needed to discriminate viable and potentially transplantable livers from non-viable livers. For this, we used the individual data on cumulative bile production as depicted in Figure 1. It can be deduced from this figure that livers in the low and high bile output groups can be discriminated from each other

A

B

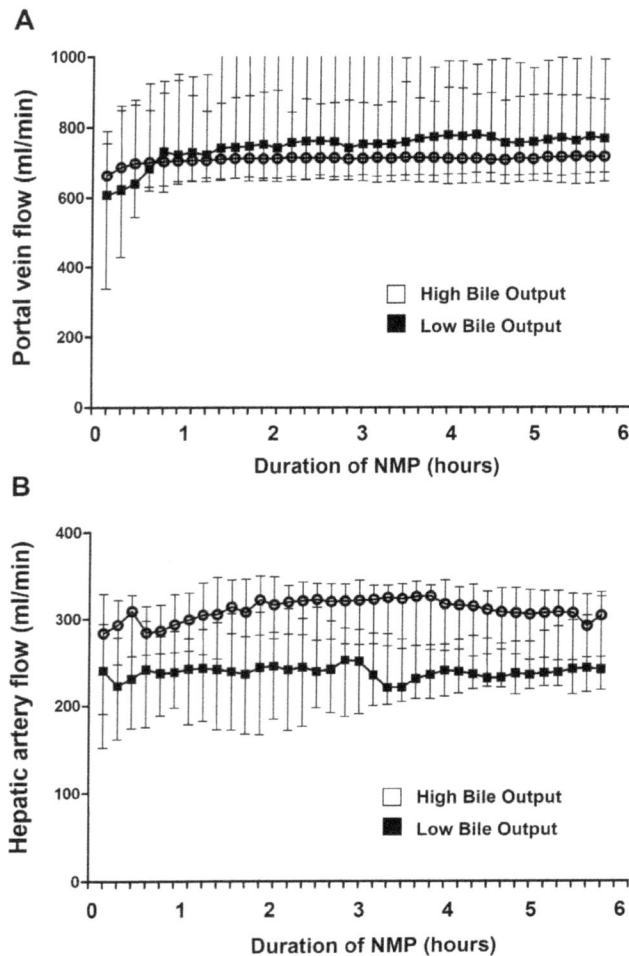

Figure 2. Changes in portal flow (panel A) and arterial flow (panel B) during *ex vivo* normothermic machine perfusion of human donor livers, using a pressure controlled device. Flow in the portal vein and hepatic artery increased rapidly during the first 30 min and flows remained stable thereafter for the entire 6 h perfusion period. There were no significant differences in portal flow and although median arterial flow was constantly lower in livers with a low bile output, compared to the high bile output group, this did not reach statistical significance.

as early as 150 min after *ex vivo* machine perfusion. The combination of a cumulative bile production of ≥10 grams at 150 min and a bile production of ≥4 grams in the preceding hour identified 100% of the livers that would be considered as a high bile output liver after 6 h (Table 4). This finding indicates that after cold storage of a donor liver, a short period of 2.5 hours of *ex vivo* assessment during NMP is sufficient to identify a liver that may been preserved well enough to be transplanted successfully.

Discussion

Machine perfusion of donor livers is receiving increasing attention as experimental studies have suggested that this method can provide better protection during storage and transportation, compared to static cold storage [10], [11], [12]. Especially ECD livers have been shown to be more susceptible to IR injury, requiring the introduction of novel and more complex preservation techniques [7], [16]. Besides the potential benefits of machine

perfusion in providing better protection against preservation injury, this technique also provides the possibility of viability testing of a donor organ prior to transplantation. Pretransplant viability testing may become an important new tool to compensate for the increasing proportion of ECD livers (i.e. livers from donors with advanced age, elevated body mass index, diabetes, or livers from DCD donors), which has resulted in an increasing proportion of non-use of donor livers during the last decade [4].

The main finding in this study is that bile production can be used as an easy assessable marker of liver graft viability during *ex vivo* NMP. Cumulative bile production of ≥30 g during 6 h of NMP was associated with significantly lower release of transaminases and potassium into the perfusion fluid and better hepatobiliary function as reflected by a normalization of glucose and lactate levels and higher biliary secretion of bilirubin. In addition, histology of grafts with a high bile output showed less signs of venous congestion and hepatocellular necrosis, compared to livers with a low cumulative bile output. The second novel finding of this study is that the minimal duration of NMP needed to discriminate viable and potentially transplantable livers from non-viable livers is 2.5 hours. This relatively short time period facilitates a timely selection and preparation of a potential recipient, making this new selection method clinically applicable.

The results of this study open interesting new avenues for the clinical application of *ex vivo* viability testing of ECD livers that, based on conventional criteria, are declined for transplantation. This method has the potential to have a significant impact on the number of donor liver available for transplantation. Of the twelve discarded livers included in this study, 6 (50%) displayed improving function and normalization of hepatobiliary metabolism. Although all livers were declined for transplantation because they were considered ECD livers with a too high risk of primary non-function after transplantation (as indicated by a high DRI), 50% of these may have functioned well after transplantation. All livers were retrieved from a donor outside our hospital and the median duration of cold storage prior to initiation of *ex vivo* viability testing was 6.5 hours. This time sequence can also be expected when this technique is introduced in clinical practice.

In an experimental study using pig livers, Imber *et al* have previously suggested that bile production is probably the most important parameter of liver function [11]. The amount of bile production correlated strongly with the degree of hepatic IR injury. Our experience with discarded human donor livers is in line with this experimental study.

The significant higher release of potassium and ALT in low-bile output livers reflects a higher degree of hepatocellular injury. The absolute concentrations of ALT measured in the perfusion fluid may seem relatively high; however, these results cannot be compared directly with values usually obtained after clinical liver transplantation. First of all, livers were perfused *ex vivo* in a closed circuit and values represent the cumulative release of ALT without any clearance from the system. Secondly, the perfusion circuit contained only 2 liters compared to an average of 5 liters of blood *in vivo*.

In addition to bile production alone, good liver function was reflected by a normalization of glucose and lactate levels in the perfusion fluid, as well as an increasing production of bicarbonate in the livers with high bile output. The latter was reflected by an increasing median concentration of bicarbonate in perfusion fluid from 19 mmol/L at baseline to 26 mmol./L after 6 h of NMP in the high bile output group. In the low bile output group median bicarbonate concentration in the perfusion fluid at 6 h was only 18 mmol/L, despite the addition of a 4-times higher amount of sodium bicarbonate 8.4% during perfusion to maintain a

Table 3. Biochemical Composition of Perfusion Fluid and Bile after 6 hour of *Ex Vivo* Normothermic Machine Perfusion.

	High Bile Output (n = 6)	Low Bile Output (n = 6)	P- value
Blood gas variables			
pH	7.36 (7.25–7.40)	7.34 (7.29–7.40)	1.00
pCO$_2$ (kPa)*	6.7 (5.9–7.8)	5.0 (3.4–6.3)	0.08
pO$_2$(kPa)*	64 (54–65)	35 (10–67)	0.42
sO$_2$ (%)	100 (99–100)	98 (94–99)	**0.04**
HCO$_3^-$ (mmol/L)	26 (22–28)	18 (13–29)	0.20
Added HCO$_3^-$ 8.4% (mL)	8 (0–20)	25 (4–86)	0.24
Base excess (mmol/L)	+0.1 (−3.6–+3.6)	−6.8 (−12.0−−4.0)	0.34
Hemoglobin (mmol/L)*	4.2 (3.7–4.3)	4.3 (4.1-4.6)	0.26
Oxygen consumption** (mlO$_2$/min/kilogram liver)	21 (16–22)	60 (27–119)	0.30
Electrolytes and Metabolites			
Na$^+$ (mmol/L)	154 (143–155)	142 (139–151)	0.26
K$^+$ (mmol/L)	4 (2–8)	13 (8–18)	**0.01**
Urea (mmol/L)	14 (11–16)	15 (12–22)	0.63
Albumin (g/L)	23 (22–24)	26 (25–29)	**0.01**
Glucose (mmol/L)*	10 (8–19)	23 (16–32)	0.07
Lactate (mmol/L)*	2 (1–4)	6 (3–11)	**0.03**
Injury markers			
ALT (U/L)	2795 (1761–3972)	11074 (6144–16050)	**0.04**
ALP (U/L)	36 (25–44)	154 (82–258)	**0.01**
GGT (U/L)	35 (20–55)	124 (107–187)	0.06
LDH (U/L)	6227 (5151–6703)	22119 (9584–34558)	0.06
Total bilirubin (μmol/L)	3 (3–3)	5 (3–7)	0.20
*Variables measured in bile***			
Biliary pH	7.58 (7.56–7.70)	7.37 (7.05–7.71)	0.10
Biliary HCO$_3^-$ (mmol/L)	44 (35–50)	20 (7–41)	0.09
Bilirubin in bile (μmol/L)*	1100 (968–1398)	270 (215–525)	**0.02**

* To convert values for glucose to mg/dL, multiply by 18.02. To convert values for lactate to mg/dL, multiply by 9.01. To convert values for hemoglobin to g/dL, multiply by 1.650. To convert the value for bilirubin to mg/dL, divide by 17.1. To convert kPa to mmHg, multiply by 7.5.
** Peak values during 6 h of machine perfusion.
Abbreviations used: ALT, alanine aminotransferase; ALP, alkaline phosphatase; GGT, gamma-glutamate transferase; LDH, lactate dehydrogenase.

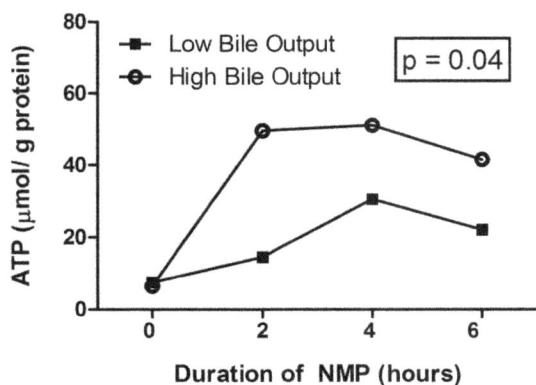

Figure 3. Changes in hepatic energy content as reflected by hepatic ATP content. In contrast to livers with low bile output, livers in the high bile output group showed a significantly higher hepatic ATP content during the course of NMP. (AUC p = 0.04).

physiologic pH. These finding are in accordance with a previous animal study that has indicated that autoregulation of the acid-base balance is a reflection of a well-functioning liver [17].

During 6 h of NMP albumin levels decreased in all perfusions. Although levels after 6 h of NMP were slightly (but significantly) lower in the high bile output group compared to the low bile output group, this cannot be used as a marker of hepatic synthetic function because of the overall decline in albumin during all perfusions.

Interestingly, oxygen consumption appeared to be higher in livers with low bile production, compared with those with high bile production. This finding is in agreement with observations made by Imber *et al.* during NMP of porcine livers [11]. These investigators found significantly higher oxygen consumption during NMP of livers that were severely injured after prolonged cold preservation, compared to well preserved donor livers. Imber *et al.* explained this difference in oxygen consumption by the respiratory burst and subsequent oxygen debt that occurs in severely injured post-ischemic livers [11]. In addition, ATP concentration appeared to be significantly higher in livers with

Low Bile Output Liver   High Bile Output Liver

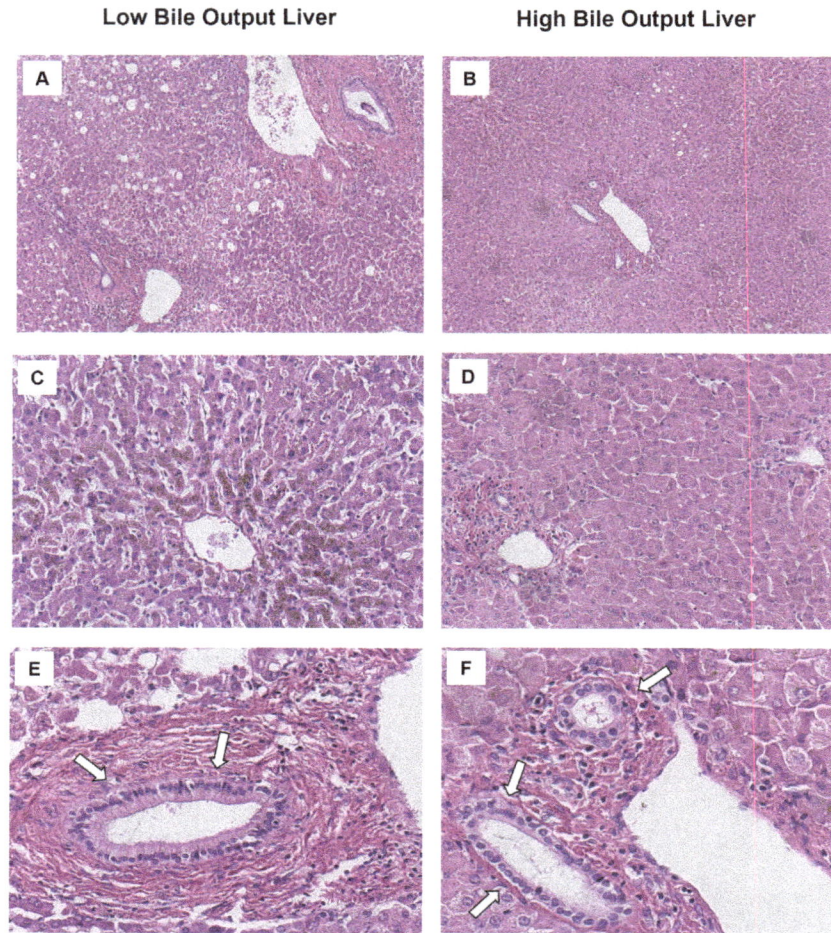

Figure 4. Histology of livers after 6 hours of normothermic machine perfusion. In comparison to livers with high bile output, livers in the low bile output group displayed more signs of hepatic necrosis (panels A and B) and venous congestion (panels C en D). Despite these differences in hepatic parenchymal damage between the two groups, there were no major differences in the degree of biliary damage (panels E and F).

Table 4. Criteria to Assess Bile Production after 2.5 hours of Normothermic Machine Perfusion.

Liver (Number)	Cumulative Bile Output After 2.5 h (g)	Bile Output Between 1.5 h and 2.5 h (g)	Meets Both Criteria
Low-bile output			
1	6.54	2.52	No
2	12.53	3.14	No
3	1.86	0.37	No
4	4.66	2.19	No
5	0.00	0.00	No
6	8.14	2.36	No
High-bile output			
7	18.77	7.22	Yes
8	12.93	7.33	Yes
9	14.92	8.50	Yes
10	10.55	5.00	Yes
11	15.72	4.66	Yes
12	25.35	8.85	Yes

Criteria are: 1) Cumulative bile production of ≥ 10 grams after 2.5 h and 2) a bile production of ≥ 4 grams in the preceding hour (1.5–2.5 h of perfusion).

high bile production reflecting a higher energy status upon reperfusion compared to livers with low bile output.

In the current study, we did not add bile salts to the perfusion fluid. Hepatocellular secretion of bile salts into bile canaliculi is an important driving force of bile flow [18], [19]. *In vivo*, bile salts are reabsorbed from the gut and transported back to the liver through the enterohepatic circulation. Bile salts are subsequently secreted again into the bile, causing a choleretic increase in total bile flow. Obviously, this enterohepatic circulation is interrupted during *ex vivo* NMP and this could theoretically lead to bile salt depletion and a subsequent decline in bile production. However, experimental studies using pig livers have shown that bile salt depletion does not occur until after 10 hours of NMP [19]. In the current study, livers were perfused for 6 hours and we did not observe a decline in bile output. Therefore, we do not believe the addition of bile salts is necessary when livers are perfused for less than 10 hours. In fact, hydrophobic bile salts have been demonstrated to play a role in bile duct epithelial injury after liver transplantation and this could be considered an additional argument not to add bile salts to the perfusion fluid [19], [20], [21], [22]. On the other hand, due to the strong choleric effect of bile salts, bile production during *ex vivo* NMP will be higher when bile salts are added to the perfusion fluid. This should be kept in mind when comparing bile output values obtained in different studies.

Bile production is an energy consuming, multi-step process that requires an intact network of sinusoidal cells, hepatocytes and cholangiocytes. Therefore, intuitively, bile production is a strong and reliable indicator of overall liver quality and viability. In clinical liver transplantation, poor initial bile production has been associated with poor outcomes. In one study, graft survival at one year was only 45% for livers that failed to produce bile in the operating room [14]. In addition to bile volume, we have shown a higher biliary secretion of bilirubin in grafts with high bile output, reflecting a better quality of bile produced by these livers.

Although some studies on kidney and liver machine perfusion have suggested that a decline in arterial flow in a pressure controlled system of machine perfusion can be used as a marker of decreasing graft viability [23], [24], [25], we found stable flows in both high and low bile output livers. Apparently, change in perfusion flow is not a reliable parameter of graft viability in human liver machine perfusion. However, in livers with a low bile production we did observe a lower arterial flow during the entire 6 h of NMP, compared to the low bile output group, but this did not reach statistical significance. In general, we do not advise to use flow values as an indicator of liver damage and viability during human liver machine perfusion.

A limitation of *ex vivo* NMP is the inability to assess bile duct viability. Although the main aim of the current study was to assess hepatocyte viability, ischemic cholangiopathy, resulting in non-anastomotic biliary strictures, remains a major complication after liver transplantation [3]. Unfortunately, reliable markers or other tools that help predict ischemic cholangiopathy before transplantation are still lacking. Therefore, we cannot rule out that some of the livers that we considered viable based on *ex vivo* bile production may still have developed non-anastomotic biliary strictures if they had been transplanted. Clearly, there is a need to develop non-invasive methods that enable assessment of the biliary epithelium during organ preservation and before implantation. An attractive option could be the development of molecular imaging techniques using near-infrared fluorescence that allow a non-invasive assessment of the biliary epithelium. If such molecular imaging techniques are combined with visible light cholangioscopy this could provide a tool for assessment of the biliary tree during NMP [26], [27].

A second limitation of the study is the relative small number of liver grafts. Unfortunately human livers do not come available for research in high numbers. This may have caused a statistical type II error, explaining the trend towards significance for some variables as presented in Table 3.

In conclusion, this study suggests that the assessment of bile production is a discriminative indicator of hepatic function and injury during *ex vivo* NMP of human donor livers. It could potentially be used to identify ECD livers that are declined for transplantation based on donor risk factors, but that may still be suitable for transplantation. These findings need to be confirmed in a clinical trial in which the proposed selection criteria are used to accept ECD livers that would otherwise have been declined for transplantation based on an anticipated poor postoperative function. We are currently preparing such a trial.

Acknowledgments

We are grateful to Arjan van der Plaats, Martin Kuizenga and Ron Leuvenink (Organ Assist, Groningen, Netherlands) for their technical support and assistance during the perfusion experiments. Furthermore, we are appreciative to the Dutch transplantation coordinators for identifying the potential discarded livers and obtaining informed consent.

Author Contributions

Conceived and designed the experiments: MES SODD NK HGDL TL RJP. Performed the experiments: MES SODD NK MTDB HGDL TL RJP. Analyzed the data: MES SODD NK PDW JWB ASHG TL RJP. Wrote the paper: MES SODD PDW TL RJP.

References

1. Merion RM, Goodrich NP, Feng S (2006) How can we define expanded criteria for liver donors? J Hepatol 45: 484–488.
2. McCormack L, Dutkowski P, El-Badry AM, Clavien PA (2011) Liver transplantation using fatty livers: always feasible? J Hepatol 54: 1055–1062.
3. Op den Dries S, Sutton ME, Lisman T, Porte RJ (2011) Protection of bile ducts in liver transplantation: looking beyond ischemia. Transplantation 92: 373–379.
4. Orman ES, Barritt AS,4th, Wheeler SB, Hayashi PH (2013) Declining liver utilization for transplantation in the United States and the impact of donation after cardiac death. Liver Transpl 19: 59–68.
5. Bae C, Henry SD, Guarrera JV (2012) Is extracorporeal hypothermic machine perfusion of the liver better than the 'good old icebox'? Curr Opin Organ Transplant 17: 137–142.
6. Brockmann J, Reddy S, Coussios C, Pigott D, Guirriero D, et al. (2009) Normothermic perfusion: a new paradigm for organ preservation. Ann Surg 250: 1–6.
7. Dutkowski P, de Rougemont O, Clavien PA (2008) Machine perfusion for 'marginal' liver grafts. Am J Transplant 8: 917–924.
8. Hessheimer AJ, Fondevila C, Garcia-Valdecasas JC (2012) Extracorporeal machine liver perfusion: are we warming up? Curr Opin Organ Transplant 17: 143–147.
9. Monbaliu D, Brassil J (2010) Machine perfusion of the liver: past, present and future. Curr Opin Organ Transplant 15: 160–166.
10. Fondevila C, Hessheimer AJ, Maathuis MH, Munoz J, Taura P, et al. (2012) Hypothermic oxygenated machine perfusion in porcine donation after circulatory determination of death liver transplant. Transplantation 94: 22–29.
11. Imber CJ, St Peter SD, Lopez de Cenarruzabeitia I, Pigott D, James T, et al. (2002) Advantages of normothermic perfusion over cold storage in liver preservation. Transplantation 73: 701–709.
12. Schlegel A, Rougemont O, Graf R, Clavien PA, Dutkowski P (2013) Protective mechanisms of end-ischemic cold machine perfusion in DCD liver grafts. J Hepatol 58: 278–286.
13. op den Dries S, Karimian N, Sutton ME, Westerkamp AC, Nijsten MW, et al. (2013) Ex vivo normothermic machine perfusion and viability testing of discarded human donor livers. Am J Transplant 13: 1327–1335.

14. Markmann JF, Markmann JW, Desai NM, Baquerizo A, Singer J, et al. (2003) Operative parameters that predict the outcomes of hepatic transplantation. J Am Coll Surg 196: 566–572.

15. Feng S, Goodrich NP, Bragg-Gresham JL, Dykstra DM, Punch JD, et al. (2006) Characteristics associated with liver graft failure: the concept of a donor risk index. Am J Transplant 6: 783–790.

16. Pomfret EA, Sung RS, Allan J, Kinkhabwala M, Melancon JK, et al. (2008) Solving the organ shortage crisis: the 7th annual American Society of Transplant Surgeons' State-of-the-Art Winter Symposium. Am J Transplant 8: 745–752.

17. Reddy SP, Bhattacharjya S, Maniakin N, Greenwood J, Guerreiro D, et al. (2004) Preservation of porcine non-heart-beating donor livers by sequential cold storage and warm perfusion. Transplantation 77: 1328–1332.

18. Portincasa P, Calamita G (2012) Water channel proteins in bile formation and flow in health and disease: when immiscible becomes miscible. Mol Aspects Med 33: 651–664.

19. Imber CJ, St Peter SD, de Cenarruzabeitia IL, Lemonde H, Rees M, et al. (2002) Optimisation of bile production during normothermic preservation of porcine livers. Am J Transplant 2: 593–599.

20. Buis CI, Geuken E, Visser DS, Kuipers F, Haagsma EB, et al. (2009) Altered bile composition after liver transplantation is associated with the development of nonanastomotic biliary strictures. J Hepatol 50: 69–79.

21. Yska MJ, Buis CI, Monbaliu D, Schuurs TA, Gouw AS, et al. (2008) The role of bile salt toxicity in the pathogenesis of bile duct injury after non-heart-beating porcine liver transplantation. Transplantation 85: 1625–1631.

22. Hoekstra H, Porte RJ, Tian Y, Jochum W, Stieger B, et al. (2006) Bile salt toxicity aggravates cold ischemic injury of bile ducts after liver transplantation in Mdr2+/− mice. Hepatology 43: 1022–1031.

23. Obara H, Matsuno N, Enosawa S, Shigeta T, Huai-Che H, et al. (2012) Pretransplant screening and evaluation of liver graft viability using machine perfusion preservation in porcine transplantation. Transplant Proc 44: 959–961.

24. Nyberg SL, Baskin-Bey ES, Kremers W, Prieto M, Henry ML, et al. (2005) Improving the prediction of donor kidney quality: deceased donor score and resistive indices. Transplantation 80: 925–929.

25. Impedovo SV, Martino P, Palazzo S, Ditonno P, Tedeschi M, et al. (2012) Value of the resistive index in patient and graft survival after kidney transplant. Arch Ital Urol Androl 84: 279–282.

26. Moon JH, Terheggen G, Choi HJ, Neuhaus H (2013) Peroral cholangioscopy: diagnostic and therapeutic applications. Gastroenterology 144: 276–282.

27. Karimian N, op den Dries S, Porte RJ (2013) The origin of biliary strictures after liver transplantation: Is it the amount of epithelial injury or insufficient regeneration that counts? J Hepatol 58: 1065–1067.

24

Netrin-1 and Semaphorin 3A Predict the Development of Acute Kidney Injury in Liver Transplant Patients

Lidia Lewandowska[2], Joanna Matuszkiewicz-Rowińska[2], Calpurnia Jayakumar[1], Urszula Oldakowska-Jedynak[3], Stephen Looney[4], Michalina Galas[3], Małgorzata Dutkiewicz[5], Marek Krawczyk[3], Ganesan Ramesh[1]*

1 Vascular Biology Center, Georgia Regents University, Augusta, GA, United States of America, **2** Department of Nephrology, Dialysis & Internal Diseases, Medical University of Warsaw, Warsaw, Poland, **3** Department of General, Transplant and Liver Surgery, Medical University of Warsaw, Warsaw, Poland, **4** Department of Biostatistics and Epidemiology, Georgia Regents University, Augusta, GA, United States of America, **5** Department of General and Nutritional Biochemistry, Medical University of Warsaw, Warsaw, Poland

Abstract

Acute kidney injury (AKI) is a serious complication after liver transplantation. Currently there are no validated biomarkers available for early diagnosis of AKI. The current study was carried out to determine the usefulness of the recently identified biomarkers netrin-1 and semaphorin 3A in predicting AKI in liver transplant patients. A total of 63 patients' samples were collected and analyzed. AKI was detected at 48 hours after liver transplantation using serum creatinine as a marker. In contrast, urine netrin-1 (897.8±112.4 pg/mg creatinine), semaphorin 3A (847.9±93.3 pg/mg creatinine) and NGAL (2172.2±378.1 ng/mg creatinine) levels were increased significantly and peaked at 2 hours after liver transplantation but were no longer significantly elevated at 6 hours after transplantation. The predictive power of netrin-1, as demonstrated by the area under the receiver-operating characteristic curve for diagnosis of AKI at 2, 6, and 24 hours after liver transplantation was 0.66, 0.57 and 0.59, respectively. The area under the curve for diagnosis of AKI was 0.63 and 0.65 for semaphorin 3A and NGAL at 2 hr respectively. Combined analysis of two or more biomarkers for simultaneous occurrence in urine did not improve the AUC for the prediction of AKI whereas the AUC was improved significantly (0.732) only when at least 1 of the 3 biomarkers in urine was positive for predicting AKI. Adjusting for BMI, all three biomarkers at 2 hours remained independent predictors of AKI with an odds ratio of 1.003 (95% confidence interval: 1.000 to 1.006; $P = 0.0364$). These studies demonstrate that semaphorin 3A and netrin-1 can be useful early diagnostic biomarkers of AKI after liver transplantation.

Editor: Giovanni Camussi, University of Torino, Italy

Funding: This work was supported by an R01 grant (1R01DK083379 - 01A3) to Ganesan Ramesh from NIH-NIDDK. The funders had no role in study design, data collection and analysis, decision to publish, or preparation of the manuscript.

* Email: gramesh@gru.edu

Introduction

Acute kidney injury (AKI) is a serious complication after liver transplantation. Several studies have demonstrated that development of AKI has been associated with increased length of hospital stay, morbidity, and mortality [1–3]. The incidence of post liver transplantation AKI has been reported in the range of 50–94% [2–5]. The mechanisms of renal dysfunction in liver transplant recipients are not clearly understood. Calcineurin inhibitors are generally perceived as the most prominent cause; however, the liver transplant procedure itself represents a significant surgical/hemodynamic/inflammatory trauma that, on its own can cause renal dysfunction [1]. Development of therapies has been hindered by lack of early diagnostic biomarkers. Creatinine and creatinine clearance are late markers of AKI, and changes in these parameters occur only after substantial injury has already

occurred. Even a stable creatinine level does not exclude structural kidney damage. Moreover, in the settings of end stage liver disease, creatinine was found to be an unreliable marker of renal function [6]. Several studies have examined urinary neutrophil gelatinase-associated lipocalin (NGAL), IL-8, IL-18 and liver fatty acid binding protein (L-FABP) as biomarkers of AKI in orthotopic liver transplantation (OLT) patients [7,8]. However, their usefulness has not been translated to theclinic. The recent identification of new biomarkers e.g., netrin-1 and semaphorin 3A (sema3A) for the diagnosis of AKI have shown significant promise in a variety of clinical settings [9–12]. However, the use of these biomarkers for the detection of AKI in patients undergoing OLT has not been explored. Netrin-1 and sema3A are neuronal guidance cues known to regulate axons to find their target during development [13–16]. However, these molecules are also expressed in adult tissues, including kidney. Recent studies show that netrin-1 plays a protective role in kidney injury, whereas sema3A may have a pathogenic role [17–19]. Therefore, in this study, we examined these newly identified biomarkers, netrin-1 and sema3A, in OLT patient urine to determine whether they can predict the early development of AKI, much before serum creatinine levels are increased.

Materials and Methods

Patients

All patients over 18 years old who underwent an OLT at the University of Warsaw Medical Center, Poland were eligible for the study. The age of the patient population ranged from 19 to 64 years. The inclusion criteria included liver insufficiency, acute or chronic, such that liver transplantation was required. Patients were excluded from the study if they were unable to provide consent and if they had had a previous transplant procedure. A total of 68 patients were recruited, out of which 4 patients were excluded due to a second transplant procedure and 1 patient was excluded due to incomplete collection of urine samples. I All donors over age 60 years and donors aged 50–59 years with at least two of the three following criteria (1) cause of death was cerebrovascular accident; 2) preexisting history of systemic hypertension; and 3) terminal serum creatinine >1.5 mg/d were identified as extended donor criteria (EDC)). Whether or not the organ donor was an EDC did not appear to affect whether the receipient did or did not develop AKI. Ten patients had preexisting renal dysfunction (mean basal serum creatinine concentration 2.14±1.19 mg/dl; range 1.26–5.31 mg/dl). All transplanted patients received either tacrolimus, cyclosporine, or mycophenolate mofetil as immunosuppressive therapy. All eligible patients were consented according to proper procedures over an 18-month period (2010–2011) were enrolled at the hospital. All study enrollment procedures and subsequent data collection and acquisition were approved by the Institutional Review Board at the Medical University of Warsaw. Written informed consent was obtained from the patients or their legal guardian if they were not capable of consenting before enrollment. The sample processing and data analysis were carried out at Georgia Regents University and were approved by Institutional Review Board.

Sample collection and processing

Pre-operative blood and urine samples (ten milliliters) were collected from each patient within 24 hours of OLT. Additional urine samples (10 milliliter) were collected at 2, 6 and 24 hr after OLT (measured from the time the operation ended). Blood samples were collected at 2, 6 and 24 hr, then every 24 hr thereafter until day 7 after surgery. Collected urine samples were centrifuged at 10000 G for 10 minutes, and the supernatant liquid was aliquoted and stored at −80°C. Blood samples were centrifuged at 10000 RPM for ten minutes, and serum was stored at −80°C.

Biomarker Measurement

Biomarkers were measured on individual, not pooled, samples. Urine netrin-1 levels were measured with a specific enzyme-linked immunosorbent assay (ELISA) kit (Cat #MBS725887, MyBiosource, Inc., San Diego, CA) that specifically detects human netrin-1. Urine sema3A levels were measured with a specific ELISA kit (Cat #MBS732622, MyBiosource, Inc., San Diego, CA). All measurements were made in a blinded fashion. The inter- and intra-assay coefficient variations were 5–10%, corresponding to that reported by the kit manufacturer. Urine NGAL levels were measured using a commercially available ELISA kit (Human Lipocalin-2/NGAL, R&D Systems, Minneapolis, MN, cat no. DLCN20).

Serum creatinine levels were measured daily by the hospital's central laboratory as part of routine peri-operative care, but we performed additional measurements corresponding to same time-points used here for the biomarker measurements, and then additionally for 7 days of follow-up observation. A combination of retrospective and prospective chart reviews was performed to collect demographic and pertinent clinical data. AKI was defined as an increase in serum creatinine level by 50% or greater compared to pre-operative values that occurred within 72 hours of the OLT. Results were also analysed according to the definition of AKI, which was based on the Risk, Injury, Failure, Loss, End-Stage Renal Disease (RIFLE) classification [20,21].

Statistical Analyses

SAS version 9.3 was used for all analyses (SAS Institute, Cary, NC, 2010), and a significance level of 0.05 was used throughout, controlling for multiple comparisons whereever necessary. Demographics and clinical outcomes were compared between patients who developed AKI and patients who did not. Continuous variables were compared using the two-sample t test, and categorical variables were compared using Fisher's exact test. Estimates of mean values of serum creatinine and urinary netrin levels by a group at various time points were calculated using repeated-measures ANOVA, which accounts for correlations of measurements from the same individuals across time. Least square (LS) means and their standard errors (SEMs) are reported. Spearman correlation coefficients were used to examine the correlation between urinary netrin concentrations at various time points (baseline and at 2, 6, and 24 hours after surgery) and the following clinical outcomes: percent change in serum creatinine level, liver transplantation surgery time, length of hospital stay after surgery and days of AKI.

To measure the sensitivity and specificity for urinary netrin-1, a conventional receiver-operating characteristic (ROC) curve was generated for urinary netrin at 2, 6, and 24 hours after liver transplantation. We calculated the area under the curve (AUC) to ascertain the utility of netrin-1 as a biomarker. An area of 0.5 is expected by chance, whereas a value of 1.0 signifies a perfect biomarker. The optimal urinary netrin time point was selected to maximize prediction at the earliest time possible, thus weighing the AUC, timing of measurement, and P value from the predictive logistic model. We then identified the values of urinary netrin level that provided 95% sensitivity, 95% specificity, and optimal sensitivity and specificity using the ROC curve at the best time point.

Univariable and multivariable logistic regression analyses were then performed to assess predictors of AKI. Potential independent predictor variables included urinary netrin concentration at the best time point, age, sex, BMI, surgery time, hospital length of stay and urine output on day 1. Variables were retained in the final model if $P \le 0.05$.

Results

Patient Characteristics and Renal Function Changes

During the enrollment period, 83 subjects underwent a liver transplant at our institution. Of these, 63 subjects met the inclusion criteria for this study. AKI occurred in 35 patients (56%) within a 3-day period. No significant differences were noted between the two groups with respect to gender, BMI, surgery time, or hospital stay (Table 1). Patients who developed AKI were significantly older at baseline compared with those who did not

($P = 0.0475$) and had significantly greater percent change in serum creatinine post surgery ($P<0.0001$), lower urine output on Day 1 ($P = 0.0286$), and greater need for dialysis ($P = 0.0419$). Figure 1 shows the changes of serum creatinine concentrations after liver transplantation for patients who developed AKI and those who did not. During the first 6 hours after transplantation, serum creatinine did not differ significantly between the two groups. Significant differences between groups were seen by 24 hours after surgery and were maintained until 7 days after surgery.

Associations of Biomarkers with Patient Characteristics

Netrin-1 level, but not sema 3A and NGAL levels, was positively associated with patient age at 2 and 6 hours post-surgery (Table 2). Netrin, sema3A and NGAL levels were not significantly associated with any post-surgery outcome at baseline or at 2, 6, or 24 h following liver transplant (Table 2).

Urinary Netrin-1 and Sema3A Levels Predict AKI after Liver Transplantation

The currently used, but late, diagnostic biomarker for AKI, serum creatinine, begins to rise significantly at 24 hr after liver transplant surgery and remains elevated for the remaining study period in patients categorized as AKI (Figure 1). In contrast, urinary netrin-1 and sema3A levels increased significantly ($P = 0.0106$ and $P = 0.0012$, respectively) and peaked at 2 hours following liver transplant surgery in patients who developed AKI and were no longer significantly elevated at 6 hours after surgery (Figure 2 A and B). Patients who did not develop AKI experienced a much smaller increase in concentration of these biomarker after surgery, which did not differ significantly from baseline. However, the netrin-1 level was relatively higher in the AKI group as compared to the non-AKI group at baseline but this did not reach statistical significance.

Conventional ROC curves for AKI *versus* no AKI were generated for urinary netrin-1, sema3A and NGAL at 2, 6, and 24 hours after surgery. The AUCs of the three ROC curves for netrin-1 were 0.658 ($P = 0.0123$), 0.570 ($P = 0.3342$), and 0.594 ($P = 0.1919$), respectively. The AUCs of the three ROC curves for sema3A were 0.631 ($P = 0.0680$), 0.560 ($P = 0.4057$), and 0.523 ($P = 0.7528$) respectively. The AUCs of the three ROC curves were 0.651 ($P = 0.0306$), 0.605 ($P = 0.1369$), and 0.603

($P = 0.1563$), respectively. Thus, the time point for optimal urinary concentration for all three biomarkers was at 2 hours after surgery. Figure 3 displays the unadjusted ROC curve for the three biomarkers at 2 hours after liver transplantation. The sensitivities and specificities for the three biomarkers at optimal concentrations obtained at the 2-hour time point with different combination analyses are listed in Table 3, corresponding to 95% sensitivity, optimal sensitivity and specificity and 95% specificity. All three biomarkers performed equally well when analysed individually. The simultaneous occurrence of levels of 2 urine biomarkers above a designated threshold did not improve the AUC for the prediction of AKI (e.g., when biomarkers were taken in pairs, i.e., 2 by 2), while the AUC improved significantly only when at least 1 of the 3 biomarker urine levels was above threshold.

Among the 35 subjects who developed AKI, 17 (27%) were classified as being in the risk (R) category, 9 (14%) in the injury (I) category, and 9 (14%) in the failure (F) category, on the basis of RIFLE criteria. Analysis of netrin-1 concentrations by RIFLE classification revealed that the injury group differed from no AKI at 2 hours and 6 hours after OLT (all $P<0.0070$; Figure 3). No other significant differences were found among the RIFLE groups. However, analysis of sema3A concentrations by RIFLE classification revealed that the risk group differed significantly from no AKI at 2 hours ($P = 0.0026$; Figure 4).

Univariable logistic regression identified that age ($P = 0.0471$), urine output on Day 1 ($P = 0.0265$), and higher netrin-1 concentrations at 2 hours ($P = 0.0369$) are significantly associated with higher odds of AKI. A stepwise logistic regression analysis was used to determine the most parsimonious model, given a set of potential variables for predicting AKI. Potential variables for this model included age, sex, BMI, urine output on Day 1, surgery time, hospital length of stay and netrin-1 level at the selected optimal time point (i.e., 2 hours after liver transplant surgery). The final model revealed that BMI and biomarker concentrations at 2 hours after surgery were the only significant independent predictors of AKI in our cohort. The estimated odds ratio for every 1- pg/mg of urinary creatinine increase of netrin-1 at 2 hours after surgery was 1.003 (95% confidence interval: 1.000 to 1.006; $P = 0.0364$). The estimated odds ratio for every 1 unit increase in BMI was 1.198 (95% CI: 1.030 to 1.394; $P = 0.0194$). The estimated odds ratio for every 1- pg/mg of urinary creatinine

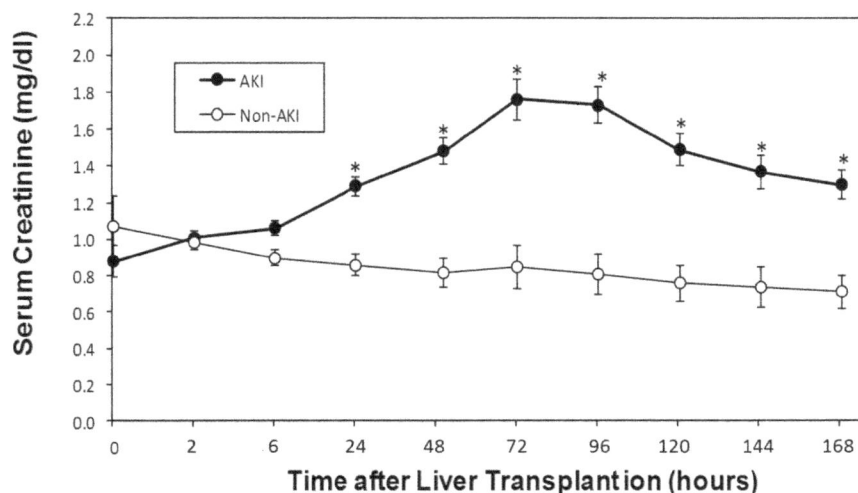

Figure 1. Changes in serum creatinine (LS mean ± SE) at various time points after liver transplantation in the non-AKI and AKI group. *$p \leq 0.0001$ for differences between groups by repeated measures ANOVA.

Table 1. Descriptive statistics of patient characteristics.

Parameter	AKI	No AKI	P
N	35	28	–
Age, yr	49.0±11.2	42.4±13.5	0.0475[a]
Male, %	66	70	0.6870[b]
BMI	26.8±6.3	24.0±4.2	0.0735[a]
Surgery time, h	7.1±1.4	6.9±1.3	0.6339[a]
Creatinine change, %	245.7±98.7	13.9±13.6	<0.0001[a]
Urine output (day 1), ml/24 h	1699.8±1178.2	2687.6±1735.6	0.0286[a]
Duration of AKI, d	3.3±2.0	–	–
Hospital stay, d	19.3±18.5	14.0±5.6	0.1359[a]
Dialysis, %	20	4	0.0419[b]

Means ± standard deviation (SD) are reported for continuous measures, percentages are reported for categorical variables.
[a]Welch modified two-sample t test.
[b]Fisher exact test.

increase of sema3A at 2 hours after surgery was 1.004 (95% confidence interval: 1.001 to 1.007; $P = 0.0166$). The estimated odds ratio for every 1 unit increase in BMI was 1.238 (95% CI: 1.049 to 1.460; $P = 0.0113$). The estimated odds ratio for every 1 ng/mg of urinary creatinine increase of NGAL at 2 hours after surgery was 1.001 (95% confidence interval: 1.000 to 1.002; $P = 0.0069$). The estimated odds ratio for every 1 unit increase in BMI was 1.225 (95% CI: 1.043 to 1.439; $P = 0.0135$).

Discussion

In this study, we validated two new biomarkers that have never been studied in liver transplant patients for the diagnosis of AKI. Based on our earlier studies, we chose to examine biomarkers at very early time points i.e., 2, 6 and 24 hr, after transplantation. Our results show that both netrin-1 and sema3A were able to predict the development of AKI similar to known established biomarkers such as NGAL. Our analysis, based on RIFLE classification, shows that the netrin-1 level is much higher in the injury group whereas the sema3A levels is elevated in the risk, injury and failure groups. Interestingly, different combinations of biomarkers did not improve the sensitivity and specificity, as compared to the individual biomarkers, except when at least one marker was considered positive for the prediction of AKI.

Post-operative serum creatinine level begins to rise by 24 hr and remain significantly elevated until day 7 in the AKI group as compared to the non-AKI group. Interestingly, however, we found that the pre-operative serum creatinine level tends to be lower in the AKI group than in the non-AKI group although the difference

did not reach statistical significance. The baseline creatinine difference before surgery suggests that AKI patients did not harbor any renal dysfunction prior to transplantation, which was further supported by the similar low basal levels of NGAL and sema3A in both groups. It is interesting to note that pre-operative urine netrin-1 levels tended to be higher in the AKI group as compared to the non-AKI group. However, the reason behind this elevation is unknown. Using serum creatinine elevation to define AKI, we found statistically significant elevation in post-operative urine netrin-1, sema3A and NGAL levels at 2 hr, which then decreases in the subsequent time points. These results are remarkably similar to earlier studies in cardiac bypass surgery patients for netrin-1 and sema3A [9,12] and in liver transplant patients for NGAL [22]. ROC curve analysis showed that urine netrin-1 levels had a slightly better diagnostic performance as compared to sema3A and NGAL levels, however, it did not reach statistical significance. A number of studies recently evaluated NGAL, but not netrin-1 and sema3A, as a biomarker of AKI in the OLT population. In 2009, Niemann et al. evaluated plasma NGAL levels in 59 patients undergoing OLT and found that elevation in NGAL levels measured at two hours after reperfusion was predictive of AKI [22]. Among those patients with pre-operative serum creatinine levels of <1.5 mg/dL, the plasma NGAL level at two hours post-perfusion was associated with the subsequent development of AKI. The following year, Portal et al. evaluated both urinary and serum NGAL levels in 95 patients undergoing OLT and found that post-operative serum NGAL (but not urinary NGAL) was a predictor of severe AKI using multiple logistic regression analysis [23]. In 2011, Wagener et al. examined urinary NGAL/creatinine ratios in

Table 2. Spearman correlation coefficients of netrin with clinical characteristics.

	Age	Percent Change in Serum Creatinine	Surgery Time	Hospital Length of Stay	Days AKI
Baseline	0.20	0.10	0.01	−0.08	0.19
2 h	0.30[a]	0.15	−0.04	0.04	0.21
6 h	0.32[a]	0.08	0.11	0.02	0.09
24 h	0.08	0.03	0.03	−0.15	0.12

[a]$P \leq 0.05$.

A

B

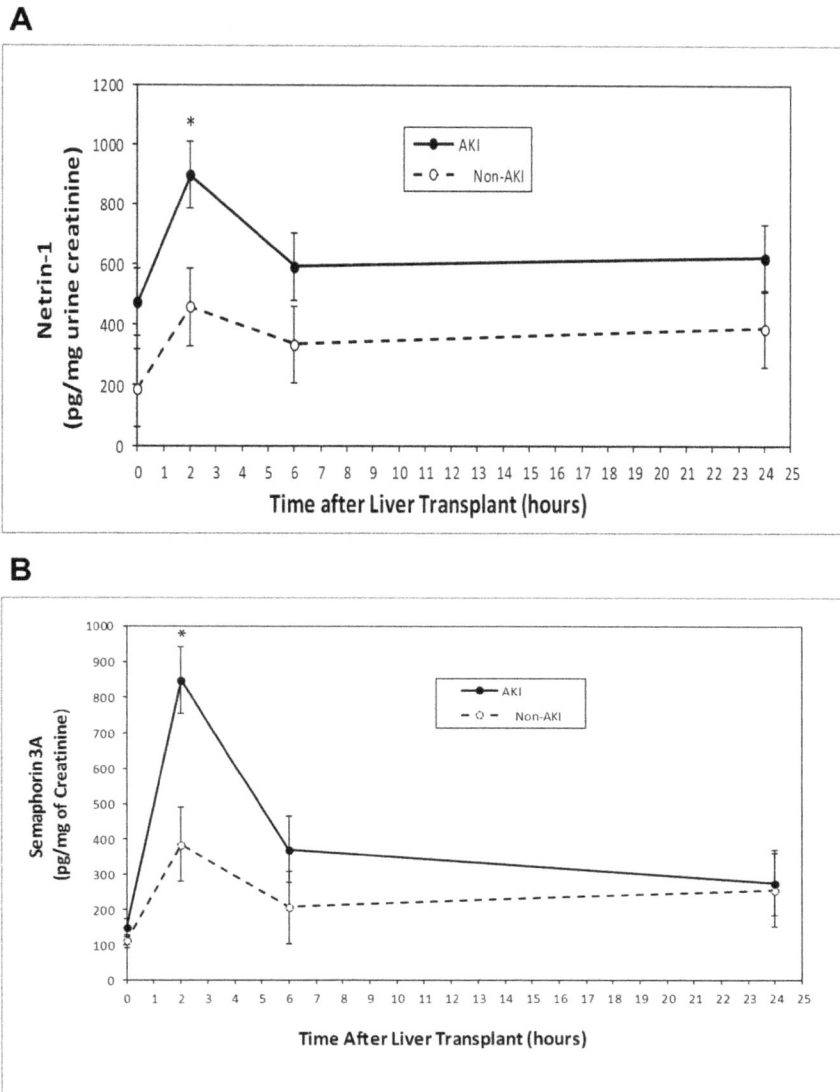

Figure 2. Changes in urinary netrin-1 (A) and sema3A (B) concentrations at various time points after liver transplant surgery in non-AKI and AKI patients. Error bars are LS mean ± SEM. *P = <0.001 for differences between groups (non-AKI and AKI) by repeated-measures ANOVA.

Table 3. Test characteristics for various combinations of biomarkers at 2 hr post-surgery.

Biomarker or Combination	AUC	Sensitivity	Specificity	Positive Predictive Value	Negative Predictive Value
SEMA at 464.5	0.631	0.57	0.79	0.77	0.59
NETRIN at 621.9	0.658	0.47	0.82	0.76	0.56
NGAL at 1225.3	0.651	0.51	0.89	0.86	0.60
SEMA + NETRIN	0.582	0.34	0.82	0.71	0.50
SEMA + NGAL	0.707	0.49	0.93	0.89	0.59
NETRIN + NGAL	0.625	0.29	0.96	0.91	0.52
At Least 1 Positive	**0.732**	**0.71**	**0.75**	**0.78**	**0.68**
At Least 2 Positive	0.664	0.54	0.79	0.76	0.58
All 3 Positive	0.625	0.29	0.96	0.91	0.52

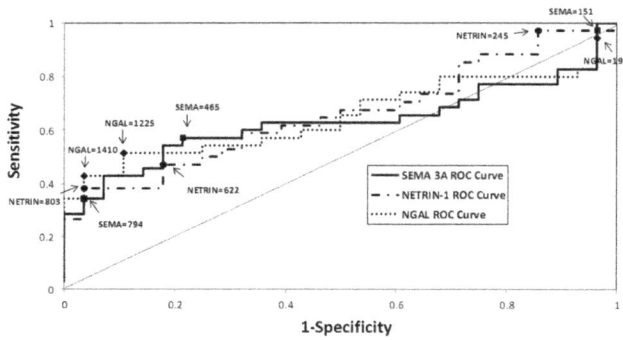

Figure 3. ROC curve analysis for urinary semaphorin 3A, Netrin-1, and NGAL at 2 hours after liver transplantation. The values are urinary concentrations at 2 hours after liver transplant, which correspond to 95% sensitivity, optimal sensitivity and specificity, and 95% specificity, respectively, for each biomarker.

92 patients undergoing OLT [24]. Elevations in urinary NGAL/creatinine ratios were detected three hours after reperfusion and were more pronounced in patients who developed AKI. Urinary NGAL/creatinine ratios were evaluated again in a recent study by Jeong et al. [25]. Elevated urinary NGAL/creatinine ratios were seen two hours after reperfusion in 11 patients who developed AKI after liver transplantation from a living, related donors and peak elevation was preceded by a rise in serum creatinine in these patients by 19 hours. However, NGAL itself has a varying degree of performance in different settings. Therefore, there is a need to study other biomarkers to determine their relative performance and to see whether a combination of biomarkers can be used for the diagnosis of AKI.

It is interesting to note that the baseline level of netrin-1 in the AKI group was relatively higher than the non-AKI group. The reason for this difference is not clear. However it could be due to the presence of higher levels of renal stressors including circulating factors, hemodymic changes or other unknown factors that may have influence netrin-1 expression in this group. Further studies are required to determine the significance of this observation.

A

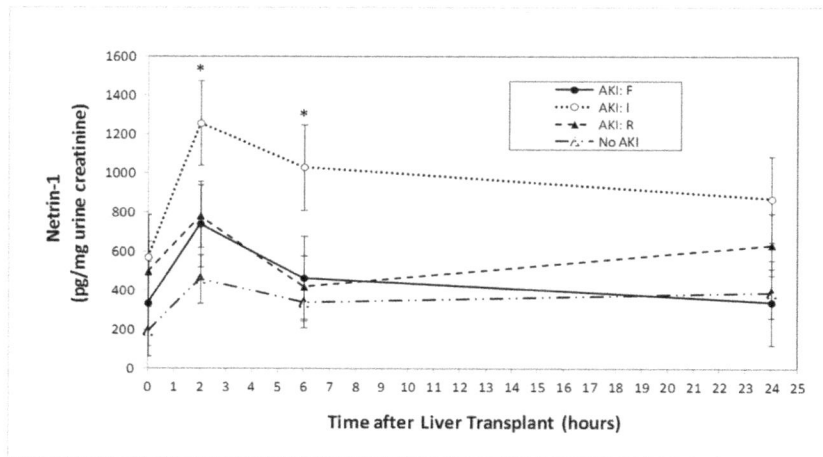

B

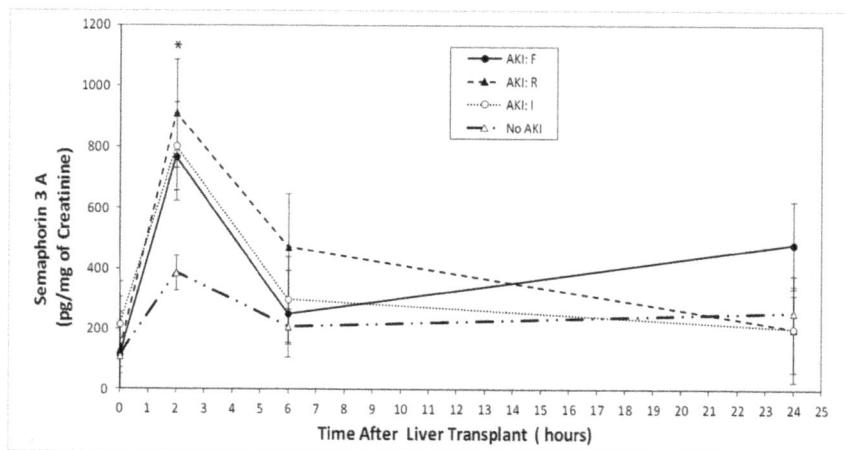

Figure 4. Changes in urinary netrin-1 (A) and sema3A (B) concentrations at various time points after liver transplant surgery in non-AKI and AKI patients, stratified by RIFLE categories. *$p \leq 0.0070$ for differences between groups (non-AKI and each of the RIFLE categories) by repeated-measures ANOVA.

Previous studies suggest that netrin-1 is also induced and excreted after kidney transplantation [10] as well other forms of AKI. The induction of netrin-1 was localized in the proximal tubular epithelial cells in response to injury [26], whereas sema3A expression is localized in distal and collecting tubules [12], which is similar to NGAL expression. Based on previous studies, urine netrin-1 most likely comes from proximal tubular epithelium of the kidney. The contribution of serum netrin-1 to urine netrin-1 is unlikely due to its large size (72 KDa). Similarly, the mature form of sema3A has a molecular weight of 95 KDa, which may not be filtered under normal conditions. However, it is also possible that due to a change in hemodynamics, netrin-1 and sema3A may be filtered from the blood and may contribute to urine netrin-1 and sema3A levels in the disease state. This needs to be clarified by future studies. Animal studies show that netrin-1 plays a protective role in epithelial cells [18,19] whereas sema3A may have a pathogenic role [17] in kidney disease. The molecular mechanism of sema3A induction is less clear. However, netrin-1 expression was shown to be regulated at the translational level [27]. Recently, two biomarkers, insulin like growth factor binding protein-1 (IGFBP-1) and tissue inhibitor of metalloprotease-2 (TIMP-2), were shown to have high specificity and sensitivity for detecting AKI in two different studies, as compared to other previously described biomarkers such as NGAL, KIM-1, IL-18, NAG and liver fatty acid binding protein-1 [28,29]. However, the performance of IGFBP-1 and TIMP-2 was not validated in OLT patients. Moreover, no studies have compared these biomarkers with netrin-1 and sema3A. Further studies are needed to determine whether netrin-1 and sema3A, either alone or in combination with IGFBP-1 and TIMP-2, can perform better for early diagnosis of AKI in different settings.

Our study has several noteworthy strengths. First, the incidence of AKI in our OLT patient population is 56%, which is similar to what was reported in the literature [5,22,25,30]. Second, netrin-1 and sema3A were examined in an OLT patient population for the first time. Third, netrin-1 performed better than NGAL and sema3A performed similarly to NGAL. Fourth, by examining earlier time points, we found peaks levels of biomarkers that would have been overlooked in previous studies [8]. Our study also has limitations. It is a single-center study. Second, the AUC achieved with all three biomarkers is moderate. Third, the absence of an evaluation of renal function (e.g., serum creatinine, eGFR) months after OLT makes it difficult to know the real clinical impact of the early netrin-1 and sema3a urine levels on the long-term outcome of renal function in OLT recipients.

Conclusion

The present study establishes the utility of measuring the newly discovered biomarkers netrin-1 and sema3A as biomarkers of AKI in liver transplantation patients. This work should prompt further research into the use of these biomarkers along with urine NGAL to detect AKI prior to the randomization of therapeutic strategies in clinical studies. Given the prevalence of AKI associated with OLT and its associated morbidity and mortality, therapeutic studies based on the diagnosis of AKI using a panel of biomarkers including netrin-1, sema3A, IGFBP-1 and TIMP-2 [28] may be possible in the future.

Author Contributions

Conceived and designed the experiments: LL JM GR. Performed the experiments: LL CJ UO MG. Analyzed the data: LL SL JM GR. Contributed reagents/materials/analysis tools: UO MG MD MK GR. Wrote the paper: LL JM CJ GR.

References

1. Lima EQ, Zanetta DM, Castro I, Massarollo PC, Mies S, et al. (2003) Risk factors for development of acute renal failure after liver transplantation. Ren Fail 25: 553–560.
2. Bilbao I, Charco R, Balsells J, Lazaro JL, Hidalgo E, et al. (1998) Risk factors for acute renal failure requiring dialysis after liver transplantation. Clin Transplant 12: 123–129.
3. Cabezuelo JB, Ramirez P, Rios A, Acosta F, Torres D, et al. (2006) Risk factors of acute renal failure after liver transplantation. Kidney Int 69: 1073–1080.
4. Utsumi M, Umeda Y, Sadamori H, Nagasaka T, Takaki A, et al. (2013) Risk factors for acute renal injury in living donor liver transplantation: evaluation of the RIFLE criteria. Transpl Int 26: 842–852.
5. Barri YM, Sanchez EQ, Jennings LW, Melton LB, Hays S, et al. (2009) Acute kidney injury following liver transplantation: definition and outcome. Liver Transpl 15: 475–483.
6. Caregaro L, Menon F, Angeli P, Amodio P, Merkel C (1994) Limitations of serum creatinine level and creatinine clearance as filtration markers in cirrhosis. Arch Intern Med 154: 201–205.
7. Li Y, Zhu M, Xia Q, Wang S, Qian J, et al. (2012) Urinary neutrophil gelatinase-associated lipocalin and L-type fatty acid binding protein as diagnostic markers of early acute kidney injury after liver transplantation. Biomarkers 17: 336–342.
8. Sirota J, Walcher A, Faubel S, Jani A, McFann K, et al. (2013) Urine IL-18, NGAL, IL-8 and serum IL-8 are biomarkers of acute kidney injury following liver transplantation. BMC Nephrology 14: 17.
9. Ramesh G, Krawczeski CD, Woo JG, Wang Y, Devarajan P (2010) Urinary netrin-1 is an early predictive biomarker of acute kidney injury after cardiac surgery. Clin J Am Soc Nephrol 5: 395–401.
10. Ramesh G, Kwon O, Ahn K (2010) Netrin-1: a novel universal biomarker of human kidney injury. Transplant Proc 42: 1519–1522.
11. Mishra J, Dent C, Tarabishi R, Mitsnefes MM, Ma Q, et al. (2005) Neutrophil gelatinase-associated lipocalin (NGAL) as a biomarker for acute renal injury after cardiac surgery. Lancet 365: 1231–1238.
12. Jayakumar C, Ranganathan P, Devarajan P, Krawczeski CD, Looney S, et al. (2013) Semaphorin 3A Is a New Early Diagnostic Biomarker of Experimental and Pediatric Acute Kidney Injury. PLoS ONE 8: e58446.
13. Huber AB, Kolodkin AL, Ginty DD, Cloutier JF (2003) Signaling at the growth cone: ligand-receptor complexes and the control of axon growth and guidance. Annu Rev Neurosci 26: 509–563.
14. Barallobre MJ, Pascual M, Del Rio JA, Soriano E (2005) The Netrin family of guidance factors: emphasis on Netrin-1 signalling. Brain Res Brain Res Rev 49: 22–47.
15. Furne C, Rama N, Corset V, Chedotal A, Mehlen P (2008) Netrin-1 is a survival factor during commissural neuron navigation. Proc Natl Acad Sci U S A 105: 14465–14470.
16. de Wit J, Verhaagen J (2003) Role of semaphorins in the adult nervous system. Prog Neurobiol 71: 249–267.
17. Tapia R, Guan F, Gershin I, Teichman J, Villegas G, et al. (2007) Semaphorin3a disrupts podocyte foot processes causing acute proteinuria. Kidney Int 73: 733–740.
18. Wang W, Reeves WB, Ramesh G (2008) Netrin-1 and kidney injury. I. Netrin-1 protects against ischemia-reperfusion injury of the kidney. Am J Physiol Renal Physiol 294: F739–F747.
19. Wang W, Reeves WB, Pays L, Mehlen P, Ramesh G (2009) Netrin-1 overexpression protects kidney from ischemia reperfusion injury by suppressing apoptosis. Am J Pathol 175: 1010–1018.
20. Ricci Z, Cruz DN, Ronco C (2011) Classification and staging of acute kidney injury: beyond the RIFLE and AKIN criteria. Nat Rev Nephrol 7: 201–208.
21. Bellomo R, Ronco C, Kellum JA, Mehta RL, Palevsky P (2004) Acute renal failure - definition, outcome measures, animal models, fluid therapy and information technology needs: the Second International Consensus Conference of the Acute Dialysis Quality Initiative (ADQI) Group. Crit Care 8: R204–R212.
22. Niemann CU, Walia A, Waldman J, Davio M, Roberts JP, et al. (2009) Acute kidney injury during liver transplantation as determined by neutrophil gelatinase-associated lipocalin. Liver Transpl 15: 1852–1860.
23. Portal AJ, McPhail MJ, Bruce M, Coltart I, Slack A, et al (2010) Neutrophil gelatinase-associated lipocalin predicts acute kidney injury in patients undergoing liver transplantation. Liver Transpl 16: 1257–1266.
24. Wagener G, Minhaz M, Mattis FA, Kim M, Emond JC, et al. (2011) Urinary neutrophil gelatinase-associated lipocalin as a marker of acute kidney injury after orthotopic liver transplantation. Nephrol Dial Transplant 26: 1717–1723.

25. Jeong TD, Kim S, Lee W, Song GW, Kim YK, et al. (2012) Neutrophil gelatinase-associated lipocalin as an early biomarker of acute kidney injury in liver transplantation. Clin Transplant 26: 775–781.
26. Reeves WB, Kwon O, Ramesh G (2008) Netrin-1 and kidney injury. II. Netrin-1 is an early biomarker of acute kidney injury. Am J Physiol Renal Physiol 294: F731–F738.
27. Jayakumar C, Mohamed R, Ranganathan PV, Ramesh G (2011) Intracellular Kinases Mediate Increased Translation and Secretion of Netrin-1 from Renal Tubular Epithelial Cells. PLoS ONE 6: e26776.
28. Kashani K, Al Khafaji A, Ardiles T, Artigas A, Bagshaw S, et al. (2013) Discovery and validation of cell cycle arrest biomarkers in human acute kidney injury. Critical Care 17: R25.
29. Bihorac A, Chawla LS, Shaw AD, Al Khafaji A, Davison DL, et al. (2014) Validation of Cell-Cycle Arrest Biomarkers for Acute Kidney Injury Using Clinical Adjudication. Am J Respir Crit Care Med 189: 932–939.
30. Rimola A, Gavaler JS, Schade RR, el Lankany S, Starzl TE, et al. (1987) Effects of renal impairment on liver transplantation. Gastroenterology 93: 148–156.

25

Scoring Systems for Predicting Mortality after Liver Transplantation

Heng-Chih Pan[1], Chang-Chyi Jenq[1,4], Wei-Chen Lee[3,4]*, Ming-Hung Tsai[2,4], Pei-Chun Fan[1], Chih-Hsiang Chang[1], Ming-Yang Chang[1,4], Ya-Chung Tian[1,4], Cheng-Chieh Hung[1,4], Ji-Tseng Fang[1,4], Chih-Wei Yang[1,4], Yung-Chang Chen[1,4]*

1 Kidney Research Center, Department of Nephrology, Chang Gung Memorial Hospital, Taipei, Taiwan, 2 Division of Gastroenterology, Chang Gung Memorial Hospital, Taipei, Taiwan, 3 Laboratory of Immunology, Department of General Surgery, Chang Gung Memorial Hospital, Taipei, Taiwan, 4 Chang Gung University College of Medicine, Taoyuan, Taiwan

Abstract

Background: Liver transplantation can prolong survival in patients with end-stage liver disease. We have proposed that the Sequential Organ Failure Assessment (SOFA) score calculated on post-transplant day 7 has a great discriminative power for predicting 1-year mortality after liver transplantation. The Chronic Liver Failure - Sequential Organ Failure Assessment (CLIF-SOFA) score, a modified SOFA score, is a newly developed scoring system exclusively for patients with end-stage liver disease. This study was designed to compare the CLIF-SOFA score with other main scoring systems in outcome prediction for liver transplant patients.

Methods: We retrospectively reviewed medical records of 323 patients who had received liver transplants in a tertiary care university hospital from October 2002 to December 2010. Demographic parameters and clinical characteristic variables were recorded on the first day of admission before transplantation and on post-transplantation days 1, 3, 7, and 14.

Results: The overall 1-year survival rate was 78.3% (253/323). Liver diseases were mostly attributed to hepatitis B virus infection (34%). The CLIF-SOFA score had better discriminatory power than the Child-Pugh points, Model for End-Stage Liver Disease (MELD) score, RIFLE (risk of renal dysfunction, injury to the kidney, failure of the kidney, loss of kidney function, and end-stage kidney disease) criteria, and SOFA score. The AUROC curves were highest for CLIF-SOFA score on post-liver transplant day 7 for predicting 1-year mortality. The cumulative survival rates differed significantly for patients with a CLIF-SOFA score ≤8 and those with a CLIF-SOFA score >8 on post-liver transplant day 7.

Conclusion: The CLIF-SOFA score can increase the prediction accuracy of prognosis after transplantation. Moreover, the CLIF-SOFA score on post-transplantation day 7 had the best discriminative power for predicting 1-year mortality after liver transplantation.

Editor: Stanislaw Stepkowski, University of Toledo, United States of America

Funding: The authors have no support or funding to report.

Competing Interests: The authors have declared that no competing interests exist.

* Email: cyc2356@gmail.com (Y-CC); weichen@cgmh.org.tw (W-CL)

Introduction

Liver transplantation is a viable treatment option for patients with end-stage liver disease, hepatocellular carcinoma, and fulminant hepatitis. [1–7] Over the past several decades, the immunosuppression, surgical techniques, and experience in managing liver allograft recipients has gradually matured and the outcome of liver transplantation has greatly improved. [8] However, organ shortage has been a new challenge because of a greater treatment demand. The selection of an adequate transplant candidate is important and the decision-making process for allocation of restricted medical resources is complex and difficult. Clinicians and investigators have, therefore, been persistently looking for objective scoring systems capable of providing accurate information on disease severity and predicting

post-transplant prognosis. Main scoring systems such as the Child-Pugh score, the model for end-stage liver disease (MELD) score, the RIFLE (risk of renal dysfunction, injury to the kidney, failure of the kidney, loss of kidney function, and end-stage kidney disease) criteria, and the sequential organ failure assessment (SOFA) score, have been applied to predict the outcome after liver transplant.

In our previous report, we had compared the above main scoring systems and documented that the SOFA score calculated on post-transplant day 7 had a greater discriminative power for predicting 3-month and 1-year mortality after liver transplantation. [9] However, the SOFA score was developed from a general ICU population rather than patients with end-stage liver disease. In 2009, a group of European investigators decided to create the Chronic Liver Failure (CLIF) consortium, which was dedicated to

Table 1. The sequential organ failure assessment (SOFA) and chronic liver failure (CLIF)-SOFA scores.

SOFA Score	0	1	2	3	4
Respiration					
PaO2/FiO2	>400	>300–≤400	>200–≤300	>100–≤200 with ventilator	≤100 with ventilator
Coagulation					
Platelets, ×10³/mm³	>150	>100–≤150	>50–≤100	>20–≤50	≤20
Liver					
Bilirubin, mg/dL (µmol/L)	<1.2 (<20)	≥1.2–<2.0 (20–32)	≥2.0–<6.0 (33–101)	≥6.0–<12.0 (102–204)	≥12.0 (>204)
Cardiovascular					
Hypotension	MAP≥70 mm Hg	MAP<70 mm Hg	Dopamine ≤5 or dobutamine (any dose)*	Dopamine >5 or epi ≤0.1 or norepi ≤0.1*	Dopamine >15 or epi >0.1 or norepi >0.1*
CNS					
Glasgow Coma Score	15	13–14	10–12	6–9	<6
Renal					
Creatinine, mg/dL (µmol/L) or urine output	<1.2 (<110)	≥1.2–<2.0 (110–170)	≥2.0–<3.5 (171–299)	≥3.5–<5.0 (300–440) or <500 mL/day	≥5.0 (>440) or <200 mL/day

CLIF-SOFA Score	0	1	2	3	4
Respiration					
PaO2/FiO2 or Sp O2/FiO2	>400>512	>300–≤400>357–≤512	>200–≤300>214–≤357	>100–≤200>89–≤214	≤100≤89
Coagulation					
INR	<1.1	≥1.1–<1.25	≥1.25–<1.5	≥1.5–<2.5	≥2.5 or platelet ≤20
Liver	Same as SOFA				
Cardiovascular					
Hypotension	MAP≥70 mm Hg	MAP<70 mm Hg	Dopamine ≤5 or dobutamine (any dose)* or terlipressin	Dopamine >5 or epi ≤0.1 or norepi ≤0.1*	Dopamine >15 or epi >0.1 or norepi >0.1*
CNS					
HE grade	No HE	I	II	III	IV
Renal					
Creatinine, mg/dL	<1.2	≥1.2–<2.0	≥2.0–<3.5	≥3.5–<5.0 or use of RRT	≥5.0

CLIF-C OF Score	1	2	3
Respiration			
PaO2/FiO2 or SpO2/FiO2	>300>357	>200–≤300>214–≤357	≤200**≤214**
Coagulation			
INR	<2.0	≥2.0–<2.5	≥2.5
Liver			
Bilirubin, mg/dL	<6.0	≥6.0–<12.0	≥12.0

Table 1. Cont.

SOFA Score	0	1	2	3	4
Cardiovascular					
Hypotension		MAP≥70 mm Hg	MAP<70 mm Hg	Use of vasopressors	
CNS					
HE grade		No HE	I–II	III–IV	
Renal					
Creatinine, mg/dL		<2.0	≥2.0–<3.5	≥3.5 or use of RRT	

*Abbreviations: CNS, central nervous system; CLIF-C OF: chronic liver failure-consortium organ failure; CLIF-SOFA: chronic liver failure - sequential organ failure assessment; epi, epinephrine; FiO2, fractional inspired oxygen; HE, hepatic encephalopathy; INR, international normalized ratio; MAP, mean arterial pressure; norepi, norepinephrine; PaO2, arterial oxygen tension; RRT, renal replacement therapy; SOFA: sequential organ failure assessment; SpO2, pulse oximetric saturation.

the study of the complication of cirrhosis. The investigators used a modified SOFA score for diagnosis of organ failure, the so-called CLIF-SOFA score. Like the original SOFA score, the CLIF-SOFA score assessed the six organ systems, but it also took into account some specificities of end-stage liver disease (Table 1). [10] The purpose of this investigation was to compare the efficacy of the newly developed CLIF-SOFA score with that of commonly used scoring systems in predicting prognosis after liver transplantation.

Materials and Methods

Ethics statement

The protocol for this clinical study was designed in full compliance with the ethical principles of the Declaration of Helsinki and was consistent with Good Clinical Practice guidelines and with applicable local regulatory requirements. Because this study examined only preexisting data, written informed consent was not obtained from each patient. In its place, we informed patients of their right to refuse enrolment via telephone interview. These procedures for informed consent and enrolment are in accordance with the detailed regulations regarding informed consent described in the guidelines. This study, including the procedure for enrolment, was approved by the Institutional Review Board of Chang Gung Memorial Hospital.

Patient information and data collection

This study was conducted between October 2002 and December 2010 in a 2000-bed tertiary care referral hospital in Taiwan. In this study, we included 323 consecutive patients with end-stage liver disease patients who had undergone liver transplantation. We excluded pediatric patients and patients who had previously undergone liver transplantation.

The following data were collected retrospectively: demographic data, etiologies of liver disease, clinical variables, donor type, intraoperative blood loss, anesthesia time, length of ICU stay and hospitalization, and outcome. The Child-Pugh points, MELD score, SOFA score, and RIFLE criteria were used to assess illness severity on the first day of admission before transplantation and on post-transplantation days 1, 3, 7 and 14. The primary study outcomes were 1-year mortality rates after liver transplantation. Follow-up at 1 year after transplantation was performed via telephone interview or by analyzing the chart records.

Definitions

The severity of the liver disease on admission to the ICU was determined by using the Child–Pugh points and the MELD scoring systems. The MELD score was calculated with the following formula: [11].

MELD score = (0.957 ln[creatinine]+0.378 ln[bilirubin]+1.120 ln[international normalized ratio of prothrombin]+0.643)×10.

Severity of the illness can also be assessed by using the SOFA score, the CLIF-SOFA score, and the CLIF-C OF score (the CLIF-Consortium Organ Failure score, a simplified version of the CLIF-SOFA Score) based on 6 organ systems [12] (Table 1). The worst physiological and biochemical values determined on the first day of ICU admission were recorded. The RIFLE criteria were also used to group patients according to risk, injury, and failure. [13] No patient met the criteria for loss or end-stage renal disease. The following simple model for mortality was constructed: non–acute renal failure (0 points), RIFLE-R (1 point), RIFLE-I (2 points), and RIFLE-F (3 points) [14].

Table 2. Patient demographic data and clinical Characteristics according to In-hospital mortality.

	All patients (n = 323)	Survivors (n = 281)	Non-survivors (n = 42)	P-value
Age (years)	51±10	51±10	50±14	NS (0.187)
Gender (M/F) (%)	231(72)/92(28)	199(71)/82(29)	32(76)/10(24)	NS (0.583)
BMI (kg/m^2)	24.3±4.0	24.7±4.0	21.1±2.4	<0.001
Diabetes mellitus (yes/no) (%)	55(17)/268(83)	46(16)/235(84)	9(21)/33(79)	NS (0.387)
Chronic kidney disease (yes/no) (%)	31(10)/292(90)	22(8)/259(92)	9(21)/33(79)	0.005
Proteinuira on admission (yes/no (%))	45(14)/278(86)	31(11)/250(89)	14(33)/28(67)	<0.001
Variceal bleeding on admission (yes/no) (%)	62(19)/261(81)	50(18)/231(82)	12(29)/30(71)	NS (0.613)
Hemoglobin on admission (g/dL)	10.6±2	10.7±2	9.8±2	0.008
Leukocytes on admission (×10^9/L)	2.9±3.7	2.8±3.5	3.3±4.9	NS (0.569)
Platelets on admission (×10^9/L)	73±46	73±46	71±45	NS (0.809)
Prothrombin time INR on admission	1.8±0.7	1.8±0.7	1.9±0.7	NS (0.050)
Serum sodium on admission (mmol/L)	142±69	142±74	137±8	NS (0.650)
AST on admission (U/L)	89±94	87±79	98±168	NS (0.498)
ALT on admission (U/L)	67±120	67±121	66±118	NS (0.938)
Total bilirubin on admission (mg/dL)	8.5±11.9	7.6±10.8	14.3±16.5	0.003
Lactate on admission (mmol/L)	2.1±0.8	1.5±0.8	2.9±0.9	NS (0.064)
A-a gradient on admission	251±413	233±407	316±430	0.039
Urea on admission (mmol/L)	8.3±10.3	7.8±10.7	10.1±8.82	0.007
Serum creatinine on admission (mg/dL)	1.1±1.0	1.1±1.0	1.3±1.1	NS (0.064)
MAP on admission (mmHg)	86±12	86±13	85±10	NS (0.427)
Child-Pugh points on admission	10±3	10±3	11±2	0.010
MELD score on admission	17±10	17±10	21±10	0.025
RIFLE on admission (No AKI/Risk/Injury/Failure)	286/16/9/12	250/13/9/9	36/3/0/3	NS (0.449)
SOFA on admission	5±3	5±2	7±3	0.001
CLIF-SOFA on admission	6±3	5±3	8±4	0.001
Anesthesia time (hours)	12±2	12±2	12±2	NS (0.362)
Donor type (deceased/splint/living)	51/40/232	42/32/207	9/8/25	NS (0.091)
Length of ICU stay (days)	21±23	19±22	34±27	0.002
Length of hospital stay (days)	48±32	47±30	55±39	NS (0.215)
Graft-to-recipient weight ratio (%)	1.04±0.30	1.03±0.26	1.10±0.44	NS (0.125)
Blood loss volume (ml)	3034±3731	2672±3057	4430±5431	0.014
Reimplantation time	42±11	42±11	43±11	NS (0.801)

*Abbreviations: INR, international normalized ratio; AST: aspartate aminotransferase; ALT: alanine aminotransferase; MAP, mean arterial pressure; MELD: model for end-stage liver disease; SOFA: sequential organ failure assessment; CLIF-SOFA: chronic liver failure - sequential organ failure assessment; RIFLE: the risk of renal failure, injury to the kidney, Failure of kidney function, loss of kidney function, and end-stage renal failure; ICU: intensive care unit.

Statistical analysis

Continuous variables were summarized with means and standard derivations unless otherwise stated. All variables were tested for normal distribution with the Kolmogorov–Smirnov test. Student's t-test was employed to compare the means of continuous variables and normally distributed data; otherwise, the Mann–Whitney U test was employed. Categorical data were tested using the chi-square test. Cumulative survival curves as a function of time were constructed with the Kaplan-Meier approach and compared with the log rank test.

Calibration was assessed by the Hosmer–Lemeshow goodness-of-fit test (C statistic) to compare the number of observed and predicted deaths in risk groups for the entire range of death probabilities. Discrimination was examined using the area under

the receiver operating characteristic curve (AUROC). An AUROC close to 0.5 indicates that the model performance approximates that of flipping a coin. However, the model nears 100% sensitivity and specificity despite any cutoff point as the area nears 1.0. To compare the areas under the two resulting AUROC curves we used a nonparametric approach. AUROC analysis was also performed to calculate the sensitivity, specificity, and overall correctness of the Child–Pugh points, the MELD score, the RIFLE classification, the SOFA score, and the CLIF-SOFA score. Finally, cutoff points were calculated by obtaining the best Youden index (sensitivity + specificity − 1). [15] The scores calculated at pre-OP, post-OP Day1, Day3, and Day7 were compared between 1-year survival and mortality groups by repeated-measurement analysis of variance (ANOVA) using the general linear model

Table 3. Primary liver disease.

Primary liver disease	All patients (n = 323)
Alcoholic, n (%)	47 (14)
Hepatitis B, n (%)	200 (62)
Hepatitis C, n (%)	84 (26)
Hepatoma, n (%)	88 (27)
Single etiology	
Alcoholic, n (%)	16 (5)
Hepatitis B, n (%)	111 (34)
Hepatitis C, n (%)	31 (10)
Hepatoma, n (%)	3 (1)
Multiple etiologies	
Alcoholic + hepatitis B, n (%)	21 (6)
Alcoholic + hepatitis C, n (%)	5 (2)
Alcoholic + hepatoma, n (%)	3 (1)
Hepatitis B + hepatitis C, n (%)	17 (5)
Hepatitis B + hepatoma, n (%)	49 (15)
Hepatitis C + hepatoma, n (%)	31 (10)
Alcoholic + hepatitis B + hepatoma	2 (1)
Other causes, n (%)*	34 (10)
Total (Single etiology + Multiple etiologies)	323(100)

*Biliary cirrhosis, biliary sclerosis, autoimmune hepatitis, Wilson's disease, polycystic liver disease, drugs, and unknown causes.

procedure. All statistical tests were two-tailed and a value of $P < 0.05$ was considered statistically significant. Data were analyzed with the statistical package SPSS 12.0 for Windows 95 (SPSS, Inc., Chicago, IL, USA).

Results

Patient characteristics

We enrolled 323 patients who underwent liver transplantation between October 2002 and December 2010. The overall 3-month and 1-year survival rates were 86.4% (279/323) and 78.3% (253/323), respectively. Patient data and clinical characteristics of survivors and non-survivors according to in-hospital mortality are listed in Table 2. The median age of the patients was 51 years; 231 patients were men (71%) and 92 were women (29%). The median length of ICU stay was 21 days.

The pre-transplant Child-Pugh points, MELD, SOFA, and CLIF-SOFA scores were statistically significant predictors of in-hospital mortality; the pre-transplant.

RIFLE criteria was not. Fifty-one patients (15.8%) received deceased-donor grafts; there was no significant difference in the age or gender between the survivors and non-survivors. The primary liver diseases are listed in Table 3. In this study, hepatitis B virus infection was observed to be the cause of liver diseases in most of the patients

Calibration, Discrimination, and Severity of the Illness Scoring Systems

We have listed the results of goodness-of-fit as measured by the Hosmer-Lemeshow chi-square statistic denoting the predicted mortality risk, the predictive accuracy of the Child-Pugh points, MELD score, RIFLE criteria, SOFA score, and CLIF-SOFA

score in predicting 1-year mortality in Table 4. The comparison between discriminatory values of the 5 scoring systems has also been included in Table 4. Based on the analysis of the AUROC curves, the discriminatory power of the CLIF-SOFA score was excellent. The AUROC curves of the CLIF-SOFA score calculated on post-transplant day 1, 3, 7, and 14 were significantly superior to those of the Child-Pugh points and RIFLE criteria. Moreover, the AUROC curves of the CLIF-SOFA score calculated on post-transplant day 1 and 7 were significantly superior to those of the MELD and SOFA score. The AUROC curves were highest for the CLIF-SOFA score on post-liver transplant day 7 for predicting 1-year mortality (0.877 ± 0.033).

Indices for predicting short-term prognosis

To assess the validity of the scoring methods, we tested the sensitivity, specificity, and overall correctness of prediction at cut-off points that provided the best Youden index (Table 5). On post-liver transplant day 7, the Youden index and overall correctness for predicting 1-year mortality were higher for the CLIF-SOFA score than those for the Child-Pugh points, MELD score, RIFLE criteria, and SOFA score. Figure 1 illustrates that the cumulative survival rates differed significantly for patients with a CLIF-SOFA score ≤ 8 and for those with a CLIF-SOFA score > 8 on post-liver transplant day 7. Figure 2 shows significant increases in the CLIF-SOFA scores between the periods for the 1-year mortality group but not for the 1-year survival group by repeated-measures analysis of variance.

Data not shown

Only the pre-transplant SOFA score and CLIF-SOFA score were statistically significant predictors of 1-year post-transplant

Table 4. Calibration and discrimination for the scoring methods used in predicting 1-year mortality.

	Calibration			Discrimination		
	Goodness-of-fit (x^2)	df	p	AUROC±SE	95% CI	P
On admission						
Child-Pugh points	13.626	7	0.058	0.576±0.046	0.506–0.687	0.060
MELD score	5.519	8	0.701	0.580±0.050	0.482–0.678	0.119
RIFLE				0.566±0.054	0.460–0.671	0.202
SOFA	3.586	5	0.610	0.618±0.054	0.512–0.724	0.022
CLIF-SOFA	2.542	6	0.864	0.635±0.053	0.531–0.739	0.009
CLIF-C OF	23.315	3	<0.001	0.669±0.039	0.592–0.745	<0.001
Postoperative day 1						
Child-Pugh points	4.400	5	0.493	0.629±0.045	0.541–0.718	0.012
MELD score	5.960	8	0.652	0.637±0.049	0.541–0.734	0.008
RIFLE	1.341	2	0.511	0.591±0.054	0.485–0.696	0.078
SOFA	5.359	7	0.616	0.706±0.050	0.608–0.804	<0.001
CLIF-SOFA	9.516	7	0.218	0.788±0.047	0.695–0.880	<0.001
CLIF-C OF	2.316	4	0.678	0.712±0.039	0.635–0.789	<0.001
Postoperative day 3						
Child-Pugh points	1.271	5	0.938	0.714±0.044	0.627–0.801	<0.001
MELD score	9.404	8	0.309	0.733±0.048	0.639–0.827	<0.001
RIFLE	1.297	1	0.255	0.638±0.054	0.531–0.745	0.007
SOFA	9.968	6	0.126	0.769±0.048	0.625–0.813	<0.001
CLIF-SOFA	10.692	7	0.153	0.808±0.041	0.729–0.888	<0.001
CLIF-C OF	4.217	4	0.377	0.820±0.035	0.752–0.888	<0.001
Postoperative day 7						
Child-Pugh points	6.751	4	0.150	0.726±0.051	0.585–0.786	<0.001
MELD score	10.011	8	0.264	0.758±0.046	0.667–0.849	<0.001
RIFLE	11.967	2	0.003	0.656±0.054	0.550–0.761	0.002
SOFA	1.001	6	0.986	0.813±0.040	0.734–0.892	<0.001
CLIF-SOFA	7.395	7	0.389	0.877±0.033	0.813–0.941	<0.001
CLIF-C OF	6.378	3	0.095	0.850±0.033	0.785–0.915	<0.001
Postoperative day 14						
Child-Pugh points	5.710	3	0.127	0.763±0.040	0.685–0.840	<0.001
MELD score	23.453	8	0.003	0.792±0.047	0.700–0.884	<0.001
RIFLE	5.957	2	0.051	0.625±0.053	0.521–0.730	0.015
SOFA	10.075	7	0.184	0.807±0.042	0.724–0.889	<0.001
CLIF-SOFA	15.193	7	0.034	0.853±0.033	0.788–0.918	<0.001
CLIF-C OF	1.266	3	0.737	0.815±0.038	0.740–0.889	<0.001

*Abbreviations: CLIF-C OF: chronic liver failure-consortium organ failure; CLIF-SOFA: chronic liver failure - sequential organ failure assessment; MELD: model for end-stage liver disease; RIFLE: the risk of renal failure, injury to the kidney, Failure of kidney function, loss of kidney function, and end-stage renal failure; SOFA: sequential organ failure assessment.

mortality; the pre-transplant Child-Pugh points, MELD score, and RIFLE criteria were not.

In the study population, 64 patients with CLIF-SOFA score >8 while 254 patients with CLIF-SOFA score ≤8 on day 7 post-transplantation. The patients with CLIF-SOFA score >8 on day 7 post-transplantation had higher rates of acute rejection (29.7% vs. 12.6%, $p = 0.002$), hospital death (51.6% vs. 15.0%, $p<0.001$) and 1-year mortality (75.0% vs. 7.5%, $p<0.001$) than those with CLIF-SOFA score ≤8 on day 7 post-transplantation.

Discussion

In this study, the overall 3-month and 1-year survival rates were 86.4% (279/323) and 78.3% (253/323), which is consistent with that reported previously. [9,16,17] We found that the SOFA score and CLIF-SOFA score on admission day were independent predictors of in-hospital mortality and 1-year mortality after liver transplantation (Table 2). Our results also show that the CLIF-SOFA score is a good scoring system for predicting patient outcome and that it has better discriminatory power than the Child-Pugh points, MELD score, RIFLE criteria, and SOFA

Table 5. Prediction of subsequent 1-year mortality.

Predictive factors	Cutoff point	Youden index	Sensitivity (%)	Specificity (%)	Overall correctness (%)
Child-Pugh points					
On admission	10	0.15	69	46	58
Postoperative day 1	10	0.25	92	34	63
Postoperative day 3	8	0.37	59	77	67
Postoperative day 7	8	0.37	51	85	68
Postoperative day 14	8	0.33	38	94	66
MELD score					
On admission	10	0.18	85	34	60
Postoperative day 1	22	0.25	85	40	63
Postoperative day 3	20	0.41	62	80	71
Postoperative day 7	20	0.43	59	84	72
Postoperative day 14	20	0.50	64	85	75
SOFA					
On admission	5	0.21	46	75	61
Postoperative day 1	9	0.37	69	68	69
Postoperative day 3	7	0.41	74	74	74
Postoperative day 7	7	0.53	67	82	75
Postoperative day 14	7	0.53	56	93	75
CLIF-SOFA					
On admission	5	0.23	59	64	62
Postoperative day 1	8	0.51	72	79	76
Postoperative day 3	8	0.54	67	87	77
Postoperative day 7	8	0.59	64	95	80
Postoperative day 14	8	0.58	67	88	78
CLIF-C OF					
On admission	6	0.35	76	59	68
Postoperative day 1	8	0.34	43	77	60
Postoperative day 3	8	0.56	78	82	80
Postoperative day 7	8	0.59	69	91	80
Postoperative day 14	8	0.53	76	78	77
RIFLE					
On admission	R category	0.13	23	90	57
Postoperative day 1	R category	0.16	36	80	58
Postoperative day 3	R category	0.24	31	94	63
Postoperative day 7	R category	0.28	46	82	64
Postoperative day 14	R category	0.22	46	76	61

*Abbreviations: CLIF-C OF: chronic liver failure-consortium organ failure; CLIF-SOFA: chronic liver failure - sequential organ failure assessment; MELD: model for end-stage liver disease; RIFLE: the risk of renal failure, injury to the kidney, Failure of kidney function, loss of kidney function, and end-stage renal failure; SOFA: sequential organ failure assessment.

scores (Table 4). Moreover, the CLIF-SOFA score had the best Youden index and the highest overall correctness of prediction (Table 5).

Several studies had tried to find the optimal prognostic scores for critically ill cirrhotic patients. Freire P *et al* showed that SOFA and MELD scores had better overall correctness than Child-Pugh score, APACHE II, and SAPS II scores in predicting ICU mortality [18]. Levesque E *et al* reported that SOFA and SAPS II scores predicted ICU mortality better than Child-Pugh score or MELD scores with or without the incorporation of serum sodium levels [19]. Our previous studies also showed the good discrim-

inative power and independent predictive value of the SOFA score in accurately predicting in-hospital mortality [6,20,21]. Since no extrahepatic parameters are included in the determination of the Child-Pugh points, and no liver-specific prognostic factors are included in the determination of the APACHE II score, their discriminative powers are significantly inferior to that of the SOFA score in predicting prognosis for critically ill cirrhotic patients. The prognosis of cirrhotic patients is grave and liver transplantation is the treatment of choice. Liver transplantation improves survival rate of patients with end-stage liver disease dramatically therefore

Post-OP Day 7 Survival Functions

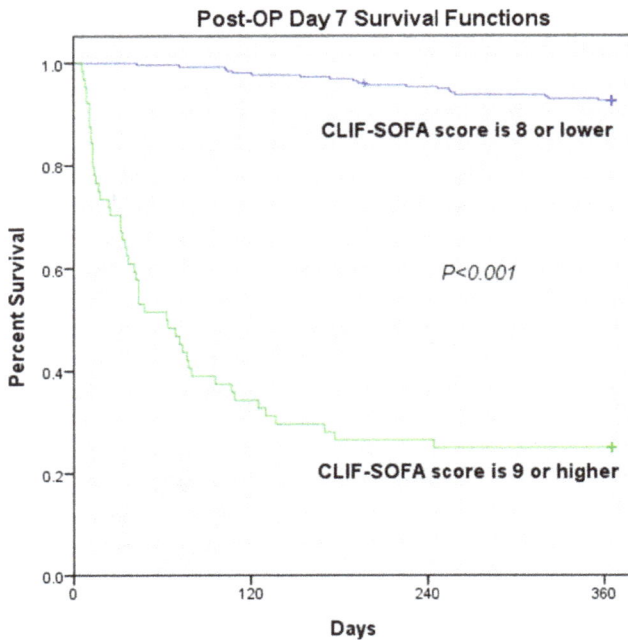

Figure 1. Cumulative survival rate for 323 liver transplant patients according to the CLIF-SOFA scores on day 7 after liver transplantation. *Abbreviations: CLIF-SOFA: chronic liver failure - sequential organ failure assessment.

impacts the capability of pre-transplant scoring systems in predicting short-term prognosis of post-transplant patients.

Theocharidou E et al had proposed the Royal Free Hospital (RFH) Score from a cohort of 635 critically ill cirrhotic patients, which included variceal bleeding, bilirubin, INR, lactate, A-a gradient and urea. The AUROC of the pre-transplant RFH score is 0.600 in predicting 1-year survival for liver transplantation

patients in this study, it is even inferior to that of the pre-transplant SOFA (AUROC = 0.618) and CLIF-SOFA (AUROC = 0.635) scores. Based on our clinical experience, we think the 6 parameters of the RFH score are good predictors in predicting short-term prognosis for patients with portal hypertension. However, liver transplantation dramatically turns the course of disease in decompensated cirrhotic patients and post-OP critical care is the key for post- transplant patient survival. Other mortality risk factors are technical problems (especially vascular and biliary anastomoses), rejection, primary graft failure, opportunistic infection, and drug reaction. CLIF-SOFA and SOFA scores could evaluate parameters related to 6 different important organ systems and provide a global assessment of the patient's clinical condition. It might explain the good prediction value of the CLIF-SOFA and SOFA scores. For lacking of CNS and CV parameters, the performance of RFH score is slightly inferior to that of the SOFA and CLIF-SOFA scores in predicting short-term prognosis for patients undergoing liver transplantation.

Similar to other general ICU scores, the SOFA score was developed for the general ICU population. Many studies have reported that the SOFA score could provide a complete representation of illness dynamics, and patients with a higher SOFA score are associated with a lower probability of receiving liver transplantation. [22,23] However, it is possible that some components of the SOFA score could be influenced by the nature of liver disease. For example, platelet counts are always reduced in cirrhotic patients due to hypersplenism, reduced production of thrombopoeitin, alcohol consumption, or antiviral treatment. [24,25] Relatedly, no association has been reported between low platelet level and outcome of cirrhotic patients. [24–26] The CLIF-SOFA score is a newly developed scoring system that is a modified version of the SOFA score (Table 1), and that is exclusively for patients with end-stage liver disease. It replaces platelet count with an international ratio of prothrombin time as the coagulation parameter, and replaces the Glasgow coma scale with hepatoencephalopathy as the CNS parameter. It also takes into account the usage of terlipressin and renal replacement

CLIF-SOFA

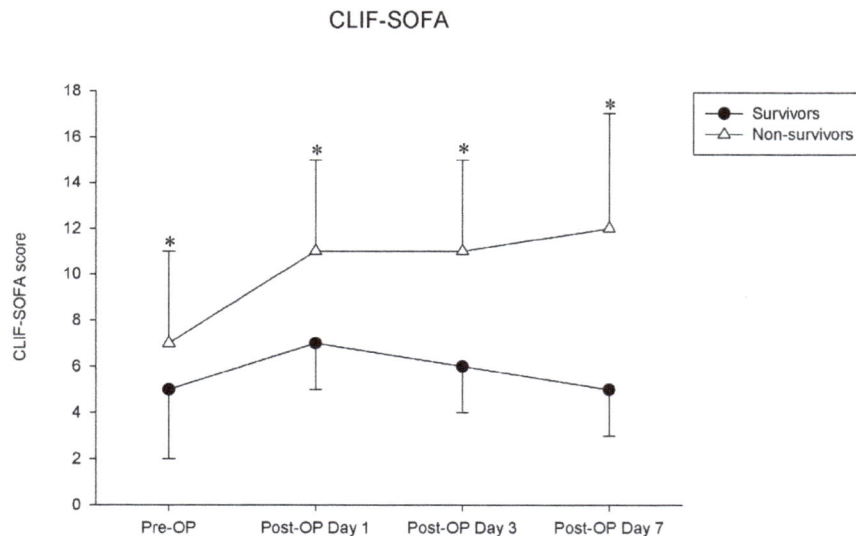

Figure 2. Estimated CLIF-SOFA scores (mean ± standard deviation) for the 1-year survivor group (alive, n = 253) and the 1-year non-survivor group (death, n = 70) during the preoperative period and on postoperative days 1, 3, and 7 (*P<0.05 for survivor group and non-survivor group). By repeated-measures analysis of variance, the CLIF-SOFA scores significantly increased between the period (before transplantation and on postoperative days 1, 3, and 7) in the 1-year non-survivor group but not in the 1-year survivor group. *Abbreviations: CLIF-SOFA: chronic liver failure - sequential organ failure assessment.

therapy in the grading of cardiovascular and renal parameters, respectively. Furthermore, the CLIF-SOFA score added SpO2/FiO2 as an alternative respiration parameter for patients without an A-line. All these modifications were set up especially targeting the disease nature and general treatment protocol of end-stage liver disease [10]. In this study, although both pre-transplant SOFA score and CLIF-SOFA score were statistically significant predictors of 1-year post-transplant mortality, the discriminatory power of CLIF-SOFA score was even superior to that of the SOFA score on post-transplant day 1, 3, 7, and 14 ($p<0.05$ on post-transplant day 1 and day 7). Both SOFA score and CLIF-SOFA score provided a complete representation of illness dynamics in serial assessment before and after transplantation, but the CLIF-SOFA score showed greater numerical differences between the 1-year survivor group and non-survivor group, especially during the post-transplantation period (Figure 2). Moreover, trends in the CLIF-SOFA score reflect a patient's response to therapeutic strategies, [9,23,27] with a CLIF-SOFA score >8 on post-transplant day 7 indicating a delayed recovery of multiple organ dysfunction from operation that is associated with a higher rate of acute rejection and poor 1-year survival rate (Figures 1–2). Because of implications for graft survival, the diagnosis of acute rejection and its prompt treatment is very important for these patients.

Recently, Jalan et al from the CLIF Consortium have generated a simplified version of the CLIF-SOFA Score (the CLIF-Consortium Organ Failure score, CLIF-C OFs, which has only 3-point range per organ system) [12] (Table 1). The performance of the CLIF-C OF score is similar to that of the CLIF-SOFA score and superior to that of the SOFA score significantly (Table 4–5). It is also an excellent scoring system in predicting short-term prognosis for liver transplantation patients. In the same study, Jalan et al also elaborated a specific score for patients with acute-on-chronic liver failure (CLIF-Consortium score for ACLF, CLIF-C ACLFs) that includes the CLIF-C OFs plus age and white-cell count. The accuracy of the CLIF-ACLF score is even superior to that of the CLIF-SOFA and CLIF-C OF scores in the study of Jalan et al. However, the performance of the CLIF-ACLIF is inferior to that of the CLIF-SOFA score in this study (data not shown). There are some explanations for the discrepancy of the study results. First, in this study, age is not significantly associated with in-hospital mortality rate (table 2) and this finding is consistent with our previous reports [6,20,21]. Hepatitis B virus-related liver cirrhosis is the major population in our country, while alcoholic cirrhosis is the major population in Europe. The difference of prediction value of age might be attributed to the different population between our studies and European ones. Second, the usage of prednisolone and other immunosuppressant might impact the application of white blood cell count in predicting outcome for liver transplantation patients. Above 2 reasons might, at least partially, explain why the CLIF-C ACLF score is not an optimal score in predicting prognosis for patients undergoing liver transplantation in our study. Another well-powered trial is required to examine this issue.

In spite of the encouraging results observed in our study, several potential limitations should be recognized. First, the fact that our study was conducted at a single tertiary medical center limits the generalization of the findings to other hospitals with different patient populations. Second, because of the retrospective nature of this investigation, some clinical variables were unavailable. Third, in our study, given that hepatitis B viral infection was the leading cause of liver cirrhosis, the use of our classification system may not be appropriate for patients in North America and in Europe where liver diseases are mostly attributed to hepatitis C viral infection and alcoholism. The patient population contained a high proportion of hepatitis B (62%) patients and hepatoma (27%) patients (Table 3), and may present as a special subgroup in the cirrhotic patient. Finally, the predictive accuracy of logistic regression models had its own limitations.

Conclusion

In conclusion, the short-term prognosis after liver transplantation is best predicted by the CLIF-SOFA score. Our data suggest that the SOFA and CLIF-SOFA scoring systems were independent predictors of 1-year mortality after liver transplantation. The analytical data also showed the CLIF-SOFA score is superior to the Child-Pugh points, MELD score, RIFLE criteria, and SOFA score in predicting short-term prognosis. We confirmed that the pre-transplant and post-transplant CLIF-SOFA scores are accurate and capable of providing an improved prediction of prognosis along with objective information for clinical decision making for treating this subset of patients. On the basis of the observed results, we recommend that a CLIF-SOFA score >8 on post-transplantation day 7 be considered as high risk of acute rejection and negative short-term outcome. Graft biopsy is suggested for these patients to diagnosis and to guide antirejection therapy.

Author Contributions

Conceived and designed the experiments: YCC HCP WCL MYC JTF CWY. Performed the experiments: WCL HCP YCC MHT CCJ PCF. Analyzed the data: YCC HCP CCJ CHC. Contributed to the writing of the manuscript: HCP. Provided intellectual content of the work: CCJ MHT PCF CHC MYC YCT CCH JTF CWY. Edited and revised the manuscript: CCJ MHT PCF CHC MYC YCT CCH JTF CWY.

References

1. Schrier RW (2010) Primary systemic arterial vasodilation in cirrhotic patients. Kidney Int 78: 619; author reply 619–620.

2. Gines P, Guevara M, Arroyo V, Rodes J (2003) Hepatorenal syndrome. Lancet 362: 1819–1827.

3. Iwakiri Y, Groszmann RJ (2006) The hyperdynamic circulation of chronic liver diseases: from the patient to the molecule. Hepatology 43: S121–S131.

4. Martin PY, Ginès P, Schrier RW (1998) Nitric oxide as a mediator of hemodynamic abnormalities and sodium and water retention in cirrhosis. N Engl J Med 339: 533–541.

5. Xu L, Carter EP, Ohara M, Martin PY, Rogachev B, et al. (2000) Neuronal nitric oxide synthase and systemic vasodilation in rats with cirrhosis. Am J Physiol Renal Physiol 279: F1110–1115.

6. Pan HC, Jenq CC, Tsai MH, Fan PC, Chang CH, et al. (2012) Risk models and scoring systems for predicting the prognosis in critically ill cirrhotic patients with acute kidney injury: a prospective validation study. PLoS One 7: e51094.

7. Chen YC, Gines P, Yang J, Summer SN, Falk S, et al. (2004) Increased vascular heme oxygenase-1 expression contributes to arterial vasodilation in experimental cirrhosis in rats. Hepatology 39: 1075–1087.

8. Shellman RG, Fulkerson WJ, DeLong E, Piantadosi CA (1988) Prognosis of patients with cirrhosis and chronic liver disease admitted to the medical intensive care unit. Crit Care Med 16: 671–678.

9. Wong CS, Lee WC, Jenq CC, Tian YC, Chang MY, et al. (2010) Scoring short-term mortality after liver transplantation. Liver Transpl 16: 138–146.

10. Moreau R, Jalan R, Gines P, Pavesi M, Angeli P, et al. (2013) Acute-on-chronic liver failure is a distinct syndrome that develops in patients with acute decompensation of cirrhosis. Gastroenterology 144: 1426–1437, 1437. e1421–1429.

11. Wiesner R, Edwards E, Freeman R, Harper A, Kim R, et al. (2003) Model for end-stage liver disease (MELD) and allocation of donor livers. Gastroenterology 124: 91–96.

12. Jalan R, Saliba F, Pavesi M, Amoros A, Moreau R, et al. (2014) Development and Validation of a Prognostic Score to Predict Mortality in Patients with Acute on Chronic Liver Failure. J Hepatol 17: 00408–00405.

13. Bellomo R, Ronco C, Kellum JA, Mehta RL, Palevsky P, et al. (2004) Acute renal failure - definition, outcome measures, animal models, fluid therapy and information technology needs: the Second International Consensus Conference

of the Acute Dialysis Quality Initiative (ADQI) Group. Critical care 8: R204–R212.

14. Lin CY, Chen YC, Tsai FC, Tian YC, Jenq CC, et al. (2006) RIFLE classification is predictive of short-term prognosis in critically ill patients with acute renal failure supported by extracorporeal membrane oxygenation. Nephrology Dialysis Transplantation 21: 2867–2873.

15. Youden W (1950) Index for rating diagnostic tests. Cancer 3: 32–35.

16. Akyildiz M, Karasu Z, Arikan C, Kilic M, Zeytunlu M, et al. (2004) Impact of pretransplant MELD score on posttransplant outcome in living donor liver transplantation. Transplant Proc 36: 1442–1444.

17. Leppke S, Leighton T, Zaun D, Chen SC, Skeans M, et al. (2013) Scientific Registry of Transplant Recipients: collecting, analyzing, and reporting data on transplantation in the United States. Transplant Rev (Orlando) 27: 50–56.

18. Freire P, Romãozinho JM, Amaro P, Ferreira M, Sofia C (2011) Prognostic scores in cirrhotic patients admitted to a gastroenterology intensive care unit. Revista espanola de enfermedades digestivas: organo oficial de la Sociedad Espanola de Patologia Digestiva 103: 177.

19. Levesque E, Hoti E, Azoulay D, Ichai P, Habouchi H, et al. (2012) Prospective evaluation of the prognostic scores for cirrhotic patients admitted to an intensive care unit. J Hepatol 56: 95–102.

20. Chen Y, Tian Y, Liu N, Ho Y, Yang C, et al. (2006) Prospective cohort study comparing sequential organ failure assessment and acute physiology, age, chronic health evaluation III scoring systems for hospital mortality prediction in critically ill cirrhotic patients. International journal of clinical practice 60: 160–166.

21. Jenq CC, Tsai MH, Tian YC, Lin CY, Yang C, et al. (2007) RIFLE classification can predict short-term prognosis in critically ill cirrhotic patients. Intensive Care Med 33: 1921–1930.

22. Karvellas CJ, Lescot T, Goldberg P, Sharpe MD, Ronco JJ, et al. (2013) Liver transplantation in the critically ill: a multicenter Canadian retrospective cohort study. Crit Care 17: R28.

23. Jalan R, Gines P, Olson JC, Mookerjee RP, Moreau R, et al. (2012) Acute-on chronic liver failure. J Hepatol 57: 1336–1348.

24. Bleibel W, Caldwell SH, Curry MP, Northup PG (2013) Peripheral platelet count correlates with liver atrophy and predicts long-term mortality on the liver transplant waiting list. Transpl Int 26: 435–442.

25. Galbois A, Das V, Carbonell N, Guidet B (2013) Prognostic scores for cirrhotic patients admitted to an intensive care unit: which consequences for liver transplantation? Clin Res Hepatol Gastroenterol 37: 455–466.

26. Das V, Boelle PY, Galbois A, Guidet B, Maury E, et al. (2010) Cirrhotic patients in the medical intensive care unit: early prognosis and long-term survival. Crit Care Med 38: 2108–2116.

27. Goldhill DR, Sumner A (1998) Outcome of intensive care patients in a group of British intensive care units. Crit Care Med 26: 1337–1345.

Permissions

All chapters in this book were first published in PLOS ONE, by The Public Library of Science; hereby published with permission under the Creative Commons Attribution License or equivalent. Every chapter published in this book has been scrutinized by our experts. Their significance has been extensively debated. The topics covered herein carry significant findings which will fuel the growth of the discipline. They may even be implemented as practical applications or may be referred to as a beginning point for another development.

The contributors of this book come from diverse backgrounds, making this book a truly international effort. This book will bring forth new frontiers with its revolutionizing research information and detailed analysis of the nascent developments around the world.

We would like to thank all the contributing authors for lending their expertise to make the book truly unique. They have played a crucial role in the development of this book. Without their invaluable contributions this book wouldn't have been possible. They have made vital efforts to compile up to date information on the varied aspects of this subject to make this book a valuable addition to the collection of many professionals and students.

This book was conceptualized with the vision of imparting up-to-date information and advanced data in this field. To ensure the same, a matchless editorial board was set up. Every individual on the board went through rigorous rounds of assessment to prove their worth. After which they invested a large part of their time researching and compiling the most relevant data for our readers.

The editorial board has been involved in producing this book since its inception. They have spent rigorous hours researching and exploring the diverse topics which have resulted in the successful publishing of this book. They have passed on their knowledge of decades through this book. To expedite this challenging task, the publisher supported the team at every step. A small team of assistant editors was also appointed to further simplify the editing procedure and attain best results for the readers.

Apart from the editorial board, the designing team has also invested a significant amount of their time in understanding the subject and creating the most relevant covers. They scrutinized every image to scout for the most suitable representation of the subject and create an appropriate cover for the book.

The publishing team has been an ardent support to the editorial, designing and production team. Their endless efforts to recruit the best for this project, has resulted in the accomplishment of this book. They are a veteran in the field of academics and their pool of knowledge is as vast as their experience in printing. Their expertise and guidance has proved useful at every step. Their uncompromising quality standards have made this book an exceptional effort. Their encouragement from time to time has been an inspiration for everyone.

The publisher and the editorial board hope that this book will prove to be a valuable piece of knowledge for researchers, students, practitioners and scholars across the globe.

List of Contributors

Chengfen Wang., Kan Chen., Yujing Xia, Weiqi Dai, Fan Wang, Miao Shen, Ping Cheng, Junshan Wang, Jie Lu, Yan Zhang, Jing Yang, Rong Zhu, Huawei Zhang, Jingjing Li, Yuanyuan Zheng, Yingqun Zhou and Chuanyong Guo
Department of Gastroenterology, Shanghai Tenth People's Hospital, Tongji University School of Medicine, Shanghai, China

Shenglin Chen
Department of Hepatobiliary Surgery Ward of General Surgery, The Affiliated Wuhu No. 2 People's Hospital of Wannan Medical College, Wuhu, Anhui Province, China,

Cunhua Shao
Department of Hepatobiliary Surgery, Dongying People's Hospital, Dongying, Shandong Province, China

Tianfu Dong, Hao Chai, Xinkui Xiong, Daoyi Sun, Long Zhang, Yue Yu, Ping Wang and Feng Cheng
Liver Transplantation Center, First Affiliated Hospital of Nanjing Medical University, Nanjing, Jiangsu Province, China
Key Laboratory of Living Donor Liver Transplantation, Ministry of Public Health, Nanjing, Jiangsu Province, China

Theresa Mokry, Nadine Bellemann, Miriam Klauß, Ulrike Stampfl, Boris Radeleff, Hans-Ulrich Kauczor and Christof-Matthias Sommer
Department of Diagnostic and Interventional Radiology, University Hospital Heidelberg, Heidelberg, Germany

Dirk Müller
Philips Healthcare Germany, Hamburg, Germany

Justo Lorenzo Bermejo
Department of Medical Biometry and Informatics, University Hospital Heidelberg, Heidelberg, Germany

Peter Schemmer
Department of General and Transplant Surgery, University Hospital Heidelberg, Heidelberg, Germany

Mattias Mandorfer, Simona Bota, Philipp Schwabl, Theresa Bucsics, Nikolaus Pfisterer, Christian Summereder, Arnulf Ferlitsch, Wolfgang Sieghart, Michael Trauner, Markus Peck-Radosavljevic, Thomas Reiberger
Division of Gastroenterology and Hepatology, Department of Internal Medicine III, Medical University of Vienna, Vienna, Austria
Vienna Hepatic Hemodynamic Lab, Division of Gastroenterology and Hepatology, Department of Internal Medicine III, Medical University of Vienna, Vienna, Austria

Michael Hagmann
Section for Medical Statistics, Center for Medical Statistics, Informatics, and Intelligent Systems, Medical University of Vienna, Vienna, Austria

Alexander Blacky
Clinical Institute of Hospital Hygiene, Vienna General Hospital, Vienna, Austria

Justin C. Wheat
Department of Pediatrics, Divisions of Pediatric Hematology/Oncology and Medical Genetics, Massachusetts General Hospital, Boston, Massachusetts, United States of America
Department of Cell Biology, Albert Einstein College of Medicine, Bronx, New York, United States of America

Daniela S. Krause
Center for Regenerative Medicine and Cancer Center, Massachusetts General Hospital, Boston, Massachusetts, United States of America
Department of Pathology, Massachusetts General Hospital, Boston, Massachusetts, United States of America

Thomas H. Shin
Department of Pediatrics, Divisions of Pediatric Hematology/Oncology and Medical Genetics, Massachusetts General Hospital, Boston, Massachusetts, United States of America
Department of Molecular and Translational Medicine, Boston University School of Medicine, Boston, Massachusetts, United States of America

Xi Chen, Jianfeng Wang, Dacheng Ding, Rae'e Yamin and David A. Sweetser
Department of Pediatrics, Divisions of Pediatric Hematology/Oncology and Medical Genetics, Massachusetts General Hospital, Boston, Massachusetts, United States of America

Yi-kuan Chen., Long-zhi Han., Feng Xue, Cong-huan Shen, Jun Lu, Tai-hua Yang, Jian-jun Zhang and Qiang Xia
Department of Liver Surgery and Liver Transplantation, Ren Ji Hospital, School of Medicine, Shanghai Jiao Tong University, Shanghai, P.R. China

Mei Zhang, Liang Yu and Shengli Wu
Department of Hepatobiliary Surgery, the First Affiliated Hospital of Xi'an Jiaotong University, Xi'an, P.R. China

Wujun Li
Department of General Surgery, the First Affiliatedm Hospital of Xi'an Medical University, Xi'an, P.R. China

Zhenmin Liu, Yi Chen, Renchuan Tao and Xiangzhi Yong
Department of Periodontology and Oral Medicine, College of Stomatology, Guangxi Medical University, Nanning, Guangxi, China

Jing Xv and Jianyuan Meng
Department of Hepato-biliary Surgery, First Affiliated Hospital of Guangxi Medical University, Nanning, Guangxi, China

Jie Lian, Yang Lu, Peng Xu, Ai Ai, Guangdong Zhou, Wei Liu, Yilin Cao and Wen Jie Zhang
Department of Plastic and Reconstructive Surgery, Shanghai 9th People's Hospital, Shanghai Jiao Tong University School of Medicine, Shanghai Key Laboratory of Tissue Engineering, National Tissue Engineering Center of China, Shanghai, China

Yoshinari Asaoka, Ryosuke Tateishi, Ryo Nakagomi, Mayuko Kondo, Naoto Fujiwara, Tatsuya Minami, Masaya Sato, Koji Uchino, Kenichiro Enooku, Hayato Nakagawa, Yuji Kondo, Haruhiko Yoshida and Kazuhiko Koike
Department of Gastroenterology, Graduate School of Medicine, The University of Tokyo, Tokyo, Japan

Shuichiro Shiina
Department of Gastroenterology, Graduate School of Medicine, Juntendo University, Tokyo, Japan

Yoshikuni Kawaguchi, Yasuhiko Sugawara, Nobuhisa Akamatsu, Junichi Kaneko, Takeaki Ishizawa, Sumihito Tamura, Taku Aoki, Yoshihiro Sakamoto, Kiyoshi Hasegawa and Norihiro Kokudo
Artificial Organ and Transplantation Surgery Division, Department of Surgery, Graduate School of Medicine, University of Tokyo, Tokyo, Japan

Tsuyoshi Hamada
Department of Gastroenterology, Graduate School of Medicine, University of Tokyo, Tokyo, Japan

Tomohiro Tanaka
Organ Transplantation Service, University of Tokyo, Tokyo, Japan

Salam Salloum-Asfar, Raú l Teruel-Montoya, Ana B. Arroyo, Nuria García-Barberá, Giné s Luengo-Gil, Vicente Vicente, Rocío González-Conejero and Constantino Martínez
Centro Regional de Hemodonación, University of Murcia, Instituto Murciano de Investigación Biosanitaria Virgen de la Arrixaca, Murcia, Spain

Amarjit Chaudhry and Erin Schuetz
Department of Pharmacology, St. Jude Children's Research Hospital, Memphis, Tennessee, United States of America

Shuaidan Zeng, Peng Sun and Lei Liu
Zhuhai Campus of Zunyi Medical College, Zhuhai, Guangdong, China
Department of General Surgery, Shenzhen Children's Hospital, Shenzhen, Guangdong, China

Zimin Chen, Jianxiong Mao, Jianyao Wang and Bin Wang
Department of General Surgery, Shenzhen Children's Hospital, Shenzhen, Guangdong, China

Ayami Tsuchimoto, Haruka Shinke, Miwa Uesugi, Emina Hashimoto, Tomoko Sato, Kazuo Matsubara and Satohiro Masuda
Department of Clinical Pharmacology and Therapeutics, Kyoto University Hospital, Kyoto, Japan

Mio Kikuchi
Department of Clinical Pharmacology and Therapeutics, Kyoto University Hospital, Kyoto, Japan
Department of Pharmacy, Kagawa University Hospital, Kagawa, Japan

Yasuhiro Ogura, Koichiro Hata, Yasuhiro Fujimoto, Toshimi Kaido and Shinji Uemoto
Division of Hepatobiliary-Pancreatic Surgery and Transplantation, Department of Surgery, Graduate School of Medicine, Kyoto University, Kyoto, Japan

Junji Kishimoto
Department of Research and Development of Next Generation Medicine, Faculty of Medical Sciences, Kyushu University, Fukuoka, Japan

Motoko Yanagita
Department of Nephrology, Graduate School of Medicine, Kyoto University, Kyoto, Japan

Yan Wang, Yang Tian, Jingcheng Wang, Lin Zhou, Haiyang Xie, Hui Chen, Hui Li, Jinhua Zhang and Jiacong Zhao
Key Laboratory of Combined Multi-organ Transplantation, Ministry of Public Health, First Affiliated Hospital, Zhejiang University School of Medicine, Hangzhou, China

Yuan Ding, Sheng Yan and Shusen Zheng
Division of Hepatobiliary and Pancreatic Surgery, First Affiliated Hospital, Zhejiang University School of Medicine, Hangzhou, China

Yingqiang Wang
The Chinese Evidence-based Medicine center/The Chinese Cochrane Centre, West China Hospital, Sichuan University, Chengdu, China
Department of Medical Administration, 363 Hospital, Chengdu, China

Qianqian Luo
National Chengdu Center for Safety Evaluation of Drugs, West China Hospital, Sichuan University, Chengdu, China

Youping Li and Xianglian Li
The Chinese Evidence-based Medicine center/The Chinese Cochrane Centre, West China Hospital, Sichuan University, Chengdu, China

Haiqing Wang
Institute of Preventive Medicine, Yichun University, Yichun, China

Shaolin Deng and Shiyou Wei
West China Medical School, West China Hospital, Sichuan University, Chengdu, China

Wei-Che Lin and Yu-Fan Cheng
Department of Diagnostic Radiology, Kaohsiung Chang Gung Memorial Hospital and Chang Gung University College of Medicine, Kaohsiung, Taiwan

Kun-Hsien Chou
Brain Research Center, National Yang-Ming University, Taipei, Taiwan

Chao-Long Chen
Department of Surgery, Kaohsiung Chang Gung Memorial Hospital and Chang Gung University College of Medicine, Kaohsiung, Taiwan

Hsiu-Ling Chen
Department of Diagnostic Radiology, Kaohsiung Chang Gung Memorial Hospital and Chang Gung University College of Medicine, Kaohsiung, Taiwan
Department of Biomedical Imaging and Radiological Sciences, National Yang-Ming University, Taipei, Taiwan

Cheng-Hsien Lu
Department of Neurology, Kaohsiung Chang Gung Memorial Hospital and Chang Gung University College of Medicine, Kaohsiung, Taiwan

Shau-Hsuan Li
Department of Internal Medicine, Kaohsiung Chang Gung Memorial Hospital and Chang Gung University College of Medicine, Kaohsiung, Taiwan

Chu-Chung Huang
Department of Biomedical Imaging and Radiological Sciences, National Yang-Ming University, Taipei, Taiwan

Ching-Po Lin
Brain Research Center, National Yang-Ming University, Taipei, Taiwan
Department of Biomedical Imaging and Radiological Sciences, National Yang-Ming University, Taipei, Taiwan

Ying-cai Zhang, Yang Yang and Gui-hua Chen
Department of Liver Transplantation, Third Affiliated Hospital of Sun Yat-Sen University, Guangzhou, China

En-ze Qu, Jie Ren and Rong-qin Zheng
Department of Medical Ultrasonics, Third Affiliated Hospital of Sun Yat-Sen University, Guangzhou, China

Qi Zhang
Guangdong Provincial Key Laboratory of Liver Disease, Guangzhou, China

Feng Qu, Cai-Sheng Wu and Jin-Lan Zhang
State Key Laboratory of Bioactive Substance and Function of Natural Medicines, Institute of Materia Medica, Chinese Academy of Medical Sciences & Peking Union Medical College, Beijing, China

Su-Jun Zheng, Shuang Liu and Zhong-Ping Duan
Artificial Liver Center, Beijing YouAn Hospital, Capital Medical University, Beijing, China

Bin Liu, Jianmin Qian, Fangrui Wang and Zhenyu Ma
Department of General Surgery, Huashan Hospital, Fudan University, Shanghai, China

Qingbao Wang
Department of General Surgery, Affiliated Hospital of Taishan Medical College, Taian, Shandong, China

Yingli Qiao
Department of General Surgery, Affiliated Hospital of Taishan Medical College, Taian, Shandong, China
Department of General Surgery, Liaocheng People's Hospital, Affiliated Liaocheng Hospital of Taishan Medical College, Liaocheng, Shandong, China

Ziping Qi and Xuefu Wang
Department of Immunology, School of Life Sciences, University of Science and Technology of China, Hefei, Anhui, China

Lu Li, Rui Sun and Haiming Wei
Department of Immunology, School of Life Sciences, University of Science and Technology of China, Hefei, Anhui, China
Hefei National Laboratory for Physical Sciences at Microscale, Hefei, Anhui, China

Xiang Gao
Model Animal Research Center, Nanjing University, Nanjing, China

Xin Wang
Institute of Biochemistry and Cell Biology, Shanghai Institute for Biological Sciences, Chinese Academy of Sciences, Shanghai, China

Jian Zhang
School of Pharmaceutical Sciences, Shandong University, Jinan, China

Zhigang Tian
Department of Immunology, School of Life Sciences, University of Science and Technology of China, Hefei, Anhui, China
Hefei National Laboratory for Physical Sciences at Microscale, Hefei, Anhui, China
Collaborative Innovation Center for Diagnosis and Treatment of Infectious Diseases, Hangzhou, Zhejiang, China

Xinli Huang, Yun Gao, Jianjie Qin and Sen Lu
Center of Liver Transplantation, The First Affiliated Hospital of Nanjing Medical University, The Key Laboratory of Living Donor Liver Transplantation, Ministry of Health, Nanjing, China

Michael E. Sutton, Sanna op den Dries, Negin Karimian, Pepijn D. Weeder and Ton Lisman
Section of Hepatobiliary Surgery and Liver Transplantation, Department of Surgery, University of Groningen, University Medical Center Groningen, Groningen, The Netherlands
Surgical Research Laboratory, University of Groningen, University Medical Center Groningen, Groningen, The Netherlands

Marieke T. de Boer and Robert J. Porte
Section of Hepatobiliary Surgery and Liver Transplantation, Department of Surgery, University of Groningen, University Medical Center Groningen, Groningen, The Netherlands

Janneke Wiersema-Buist and Henri G. D. Leuvenink
Surgical Research Laboratory, University of Groningen, University Medical Center Groningen, Groningen, The Netherlands

Annette S. H., Gouw
Department of Pathology, University of Groningen, University Medical Center Groningen, Groningen, The Netherlands

Lidia Lewandowska and Joanna Matuszkiewicz-Rowińska
Department of Nephrology, Dialysis & Internal Diseases, Medical University of Warsaw, Warsaw, Poland

Calpurnia Jayakumar and Ganesan Ramesh
Vascular Biology Center, Georgia Regents University, Augusta, GA, United States of America

Urszula Oldakowska-Jedynak, Michalina Galas and Marek Krawczyk
Department of General, Transplant and Liver Surgery, Medical University of Warsaw, Warsaw, Poland

Stephen Looney
Department of Biostatistics and Epidemiology, Georgia Regents University, Augusta, GA, United States of America

Małgorzata Dutkiewicz
Department of General and Nutritional Biochemistry, Medical University of Warsaw, Warsaw, Poland

Heng-Chih Pan, Pei-Chun Fan and Chih-Hsiang Chang
Kidney Research Center, Department of Nephrology, Chang Gung Memorial Hospital, Taipei, Taiwan

Chang-Chyi Jenq, Ming-Yang Chang, Ya-Chung Tian, Cheng-Chieh Hung, Ji-Tseng Fang, Chih-Wei Yang and Yung-Chang Chen
Kidney Research Center, Department of Nephrology, Chang Gung Memorial Hospital, Taipei, Taiwan
Chang Gung University College of Medicine, Taoyuan, Taiwan

Wei-Chen Lee
Laboratory of Immunology, Department of General Surgery, Chang Gung Memorial Hospital, Taipei, Taiwan
Chang Gung University College of Medicine, Taoyuan, Taiwan

Ming-Hung Tsai
Division of Gastroenterology, Chang Gung Memorial Hospital, Taipei, Taiwan
Chang Gung University College of Medicine, Taoyuan, Taiwan

Index